Instructor's Resource Manual

Varcarolis/Carson/Shoemaker

Foundations of Psychiatric Mental Health Nursing: A Clinical Approach

Fifth Edition

Helene S. (Kay) Charron, MS, RN
Professor Emeritus
Monroe Community College
Rochester, New York;
Partner, Initiatives in Nursing Education
West Bloomfield, New York

Lee Murray, RN, MS, CS, CADAC
Associate Professor
Holyoke Community College
Holyoke, Massachusetts

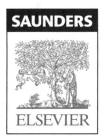

SAUNDERS

ELSEVIER

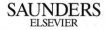
SAUNDERS
ELSEVIER

11830 Westline Industrial Drive
St. Louis, Missouri 63146

INSTRUCTOR'S RESOURCE MANUAL FOR
FOUNDATIONS OF PSYCHIATRIC MENTAL HEALTH NURSING: ISBN-13   978-1-4160-3111-6
A CLINICAL APPROACH, FIFTH EDITION   ISBN-10   1-4160-3111-1
Copyright © 2006, 2002, 1998, 1994 by Elsevier Inc.

ISBN-13   978-1-4160-3111-6
ISBN-10   1-4160-3111-1

Executive Editor: Tom Wilhelm
Developmental Editors: Jill Ferguson, Allison Brock
Publishing Services Manager: Deborah L. Vogel
Senior Project Manager: Deon Lee
Design Manager: Teresa McBryan

Printed in the United States of America

Last digit is the print number: 9   8   7   6   5   4   3   2   1

Contents

Instructor's Manual

Contents, continued

Test Bank

Introduction

This instructor's manual contains resources for instructors using the fifth edition of *Foundations of Psychiatric Mental Health Nursing*. Each chapter provides an annotated outline that can be used as a guide for lecture preparation and suggested teaching strategies.

Seasoned faculty teaching the course may have little need to read about course organization, syllabus preparation, use of a clinical journal, or evaluation of students. However, it is often interesting to learn how other faculties address these issues. The section on Selection of Teaching Strategies will be of interest to instructors who are new to planning courses and those who wish to enhance a course by using strategies that promote active learning.

Test items are available in a Test Bank in the second half of this manual. A computerized Test Bank is available on the *Instructor's Electronic Resource* (CD-ROM) and as part of the Instructor Learning Resources of the Evolve website (http://evolve.elsevier.com/Varcarolis). The computerized Test Bank in ExamView can generate tests and also allows instructors to customize tests to fit local practice or personal preference and perform on-line testing. Items in the Test Bank are categorized by chapter and include correct answer, rationale, phase of the nursing process, cognitive level according to Bloom's taxonomy of learning (most questions are at the application level or higher), and NCLEX category of client need.

ORGANIZING THE COURSE

Impact of Course Length on Choice of Topics

What any instructor or teaching team includes in a course will be as much a function of available time as philosophy. Obviously, a 5-week course and an 8-week course must be organized differently, and a curriculum in which psychiatric mental health material is integrated will be different from a curriculum that teaches psychiatric mental health concepts as a discrete course. Topics often included in an Associate Degree in Nursing (ADN) course in psychiatric nursing include the following:

Basic Psychiatric Mental Health Concepts
    Mental Health and Mental Illness
        Health and Mental Illness on a Continuum
        Epidemiology of Mental Disorders
        DSM-IV-TR
        Nursing Diagnoses

    Major Theories of Personality including: Psychodynamic, Humanistic, Behavioral, Biological, and Nursing Theories. (Some programs assume students have acquired this information in required psychology courses and do not reteach it.)
    Traditional Therapeutic Approaches
    Some of the Traditional Therapeutic approaches include Classical Psychoanalysis, Psychodynamic/Psychoanalytic Psychotherapy, Short-Term Dynamic Psychotherapy, Interpersonal Psychotherapy, Milieu Therapy, and Cognitive Therapy and Behavioral Therapy
    Contemporary Issues and Trends in Psychiatry Affecting Psychiatric Mental Health Nursing (e.g., managed care)

Psychotropic drugs and the physiological affect they have on the individual can be incorporated as the instructor teaches each mental health topic or disorder if it is not taught as a separate Pharmacology course.

Basic Psychiatric Mental Health Nursing Concepts
    Overview of Nursing in Acute Care Settings
        and in the Community
    Developing Communication Skills
    The Clinical Interview
    Phases of the Nurse-Client Relationship
    Stress, Anxiety, and Defenses Against Anxiety
    Culturally Relevant Nursing
    Legal and Ethical Guidelines for Safe Practice
    Suicide
    Anger and Aggression

Nursing of Clients with Clinical Psychiatric Disorders
    and Syndromes
    Mood Disorders: Depression and Mania
    Schizophrenic Disorders
    Severe and Persistent Mental Illness
    Cognitive Impairment Disorders: Dementia
        and Delirium
    The Anxiety Disorders, Somatoform
        and Dissociative Disorders
    Care of the Chemically Impaired
    Personality Disorders

Other Topics Covered to Varying Degrees
(These topics are sometimes considered part of medical surgical or pediatric content in ADN programs.)

    Family Violence
    Rape
    Psychophysiological Disorders
    Eating Disorders
    Care of the Dying and Those Who Grieve
    Psychosocial Needs of the Medically Ill
    Disorders of Children and Adolescents
    Adults Requiring Special Interventions
    Psychosocial Needs of the Older Adult
    Care of the Incarcerated Client
    Alternative and Complementary Therapies
      and Practices

Suggestions for use of *Foundations of Psychiatric Mental Health Nursing* for 5- or 6- and 8-week courses follow. For the purposes of these examples, each class is assumed to be 2 hours in length.

Although the number of the chapter in which each topic is explained is given, realistic reading assignments are important. Assign too much and the students will be defeated before they begin. The students who read at a slower pace will be grateful for instructor selectivity and realistic assignment, and the rapid readers will probably read suggested as well as required readings.

Suggestions for Using *Foundations* in a 5-Week or 6-Week Course

One must assume the learner has taken a basic psychology course, as well as anatomy and physiology, and brings knowledge to this course. Nothing is retaught in so short a course, so there would be no coverage of mental health versus mental illness, theories of growth and development, explanations of common types of psychotherapy, the biological basis of mental illness, or legal issues in general, such as torts. Legal focus would be on new content such as types of admissions, duty to warn, and so on. Cognitive disorders would probably be included in medical-surgical content, rather than this course. Culturally relevant care is incorporated with assessment strategies and the nursing process to help the student learn to include culture in each client's nursing plan of care.

The focus in a short course is on psychiatric mental health, rather than to nursing in general. Information about psychopharmacologic agents and other treatments, such as electroconvulsive therapy (ECT), would be integrated, as shown in the outline.

Evaluation could be handled by carving out time for several 15-minute quizzes at the conclusion of class time and giving a 2-hour comprehensive examination at the end of the course. Most students can easily answer 10 to 12 questions in 15 minutes, but schedule the quizzes at the end of class, so there is less of a tendency to give extra time and lose class time.

The 6-week course would not include additional topics, but would allow the instructor to include more detail in areas of his or her preference. It would also be possible to give two 30-minute quizzes or a 1-hour examination in addition to the comprehensive final.

It is this writer's bias that the learners should be given material about psychotic disorders early in the course, if that is the type of disorder they will be working with in the clinical setting. Thus these courses are arranged to accomplish this. Obviously, other arrangements are possible.

Placement	Topics	Chapter Number
Week 1		
Class 1	Basic Psychiatric Concepts	1
	Psychiatric Nurses: Who We Are and What We Do	4
	Where We Provide Care	
	Mental Health Nursing in Acute Care Settings	5
	Mental Health Nursing in Community Settings	6
Class 2	Assessment Strategies and the Nursing Process	9
	Developing Therapeutic Relationships	10
	The Clinical Interview and Communication Skills	11
	Legal and Ethical Guidelines for Safe Practice	8
	Culturally Relevant Mental Health Nursing	7
Week 2		
Class 3	Caring for Clients with Common Problems	
	Understanding Anxiety and Anxiety Defenses	13
	Anxiety Disorders	14
	The Schizophrenias	20
	Antipsychotic Medications	
Class 4	Mood Disorders: Depression	18
	Antidepressants	
	Mood Disorders: Bipolar	19
	Mood Stabilizers	
Week 3		
Class 5	Care of the Chemically Impaired	27
	Somatoform and Dissociative Disorders	15
	Personality Disorders	16

2

Introduction

Class 6	Suicide	23
	Anger and Aggression	24
Week 4		
Class 7	Crisis	22
	Severe Mental Illness: Crisis Stabilization and Rehabilitation	28
Class 8	Sexual Assault	26
	Family Violence	25
Week 5		
Class 9	Eating Disorders	17
	Therapeutic Groups, Family Therapy	35, 36
Class 10	Comprehensive Examination	

Suggestions for Using *Foundations* in an 8-Week Course

For a course of 8 weeks, the progression is slightly more leisurely and a greater variety of topics can be included.

Placement	Topics	Chapter Number
Week 1		
Class 1	Basic Psychiatric Concepts	
	Mental Health and Mental Illness	1
	Relevant Theories and Therapies for Nursing Practice	2
	Biological Basis for Understanding Psychotropic Drugs	3
Class 2	Psychiatric Mental Health Nursing and Managed Care Issues	4
	Where We Provide Care	
	Mental Health Nursing in Acute Care Settings	5
	Mental Health Nursing in Community Settings	6
Week 2		
Class 3	Developing Therapeutic Relationships	10
	Assessment Strategies and the Nursing Process	9
	The Clinical Interview and Communication Skills	11
Class 4	Legal and Ethical Guidelines for Safe Practice	8
	Culturally Relevant Mental Health Nursing	7
Week 3	Providing Client Care	12
Class 5	Understanding Stress and Holistic Approaches to Stress Management	12
	Understanding Anxiety and Anxiety Defenses	23
Class 6	Suicide	24
	Anger and Aggression	
Week 4		
Class 7	Midterm Examination	18
Class 8	Mood Disorders: Depression	19
	Mood Disorders: Bipolar	
Week 5		
Class 9	The Schizophrenias	20
	Severe Mental Illness: Stabilization and Rehabilitation	28
Class 10	Cognitive Disorders	21
	Care of the Chemically Impaired	27
Week 6		
Class 11	Crisis	22
	Sexual Assault	26
	Family Violence	25
Class 12	Anxiety Disorders	14
	Somatoform and Dissociative Disorders	15
	Personality Disorders	16
Week 7		
Class 13	Eating Disorders	17
	Disorders of Children and Adolescents	32
	Psychological Needs of the Medically Ill	29
	Care for the Dying and for Those Who Grieve	30
Class 14	Adult Issues	33
	Psychosocial Needs of the Older Adult	34
	Psychiatric Forensic Nursing	31
Week 8		
Class 15	Therapeutic Groups	35
	Family Therapy	36
	Integrative Care	37
Class 16	Final Examination	

Writing Theory Objectives

When topics to be taught in the theoretical portion of the course have been determined, course and unit and chapter objectives are written. The objectives should be consistent with the organizing framework of the program as a whole. A program using basic needs and nursing

3

process as major curriculum themes devised the following course objectives:

- Describe alterations in ability to meet their own basic needs demonstrated by selected psychiatric clients demonstrating anxiety, rituals, dissociative patterns, somatization, withdrawal from reality, depression or mania, aggression, pathological suspicion, and abuse of food, chemical substances, and people, characteristic behaviors of borderline or antisocial personality disorders.
- Identify physiological, psychological, and sociological responses that commonly occur when clients exhibit the behaviors stated above.
- Apply the nursing process and theoretical concepts related to psychiatric nursing
    - to assess selected clients;
    - develop nursing diagnoses in order of priority;
    - plan and evaluate client outcomes;
    - plan, prioritize, implement, and evaluate nursing interventions;
    - identify the rationale for therapeutic nursing interventions based on scientific knowledge;
    - collaborate with client and health care team members to individualize client care that includes health counseling, discharge, and self-care information.
- Assume the roles of caregiver (including teacher and communicator), manager of care, and member of the profession within the purview of the psychiatric nursing course and previously taught nursing program content.
- Apply concepts related to levels of prevention by identifying
    - health promotion behaviors and activities;
    - risk behaviors and activities;
    - strategies to reduce risk behaviors and activities.

Unit objectives must be developed with an eye to being consistent with, and meeting, course objectives. For example, the following objectives were written for the unit on Assisting the Anxious Client to Meet Basic Needs:

- Analyze the relationship between anxiety and the use of ego defense mechanisms.
- Define and give examples of the following ego defense mechanisms: repression, suppression, rationalization, denial, projection, identification, introjection, conversion, regression, compensation, reaction formation, displacement, sublimation, and undoing.
- Identify manifestations of mild, moderate, severe, and panic levels of anxiety.
- Examine theories as they relate to the etiology and treatment of an increased anxiety level in clients.
- Identify relevant nurse self-assessment factors when working with clients with an increased anxiety level.

- Specify assessment data for the client with an increased anxiety level.
- Formulate nursing diagnoses, outcome criteria, goals, and nursing interventions (including rationales) for the client with an increased anxiety level.
- Evaluate goal attainment for the client utilizing an actual or simulated client situation.
- Identify the information to be included in a teaching plan for a client receiving anxiolytic medication.

Selecting Written Assignments

One teaching team chose these course assignments for fulfillment of selected course objectives:

- a written assessment of a psychiatric client using form and guidelines included in the syllabus;
- a nursing process paper (nursing care plan);
- progress notes for selected clients based on the day's observations;
- a process recording;
- attendance at a self-help group meeting and submission of a written commentary;
- submission of a weekly written journal of clinical observations.

Selecting Clinical Objectives and Activities

Students can be expected to prepare for clinical experience according to course requirements, including those set forth in the orientation to the clinical agency; to work within the framework of the treatment team; and to accept guidance and supervision from the college faculty member and the agency staff.

In general, clinical objectives and activities are chosen to complement theory. For example, early in a course, topics such as these are common:

Concepts Basic to Psychiatric Nursing
    Therapeutic Use of Self: Knowing Yourself
    Therapeutic Relationships
    Therapeutic Communication
    Common Problems in the One-on-One Relationship
The Therapeutic Milieu

Clinical objectives for the initial clinical day might focus on analyzing one's reactions and beginning interactions with clients, for example:

- Analyze your reactions to beginning psychiatric nursing.
- Participate in a tour of the unit.
- Observe and assess the unit milieu.
- Begin assessment of clients by observing and interacting with at least two clients.
- Begin a therapeutic relationship during interaction with one client.

Selecting Clinical Sites

Sites must provide an opportunity for learners to meet the clinical objectives you have set forth, apply theoretical nursing knowledge, and develop interpersonal and nursing process skills while working with clients with common psychiatric problems. Most schools have placed increasing emphasis on using community-based learning sites. Possible clinical sites include mental health center inpatient units, state hospital units, psychiatric outpatient departments and clinics, emergency departments, special screening clinics (e.g., anxiety screening, dementia screening), psychiatric rehabilitation centers, day care programs, halfway houses, psychosocial clubs, Veterans Administration hospitals and clinics, homeless shelters, special units and clinics for children with psychiatric disorders, self-help group meetings, alcohol and drug detoxification programs, rehabilitation and residential programs, dementia units in long-term care facilities, and brain injury rehabilitation units.

It is the responsibility of the school to provide a contract with the agency stating the responsibilities of both parties. The school is protected by having a contract, since clinical experience cannot be capriciously terminated. It is, however, incumbent upon the instructor to know the contract and to abide by its provisions.

In the past, all students went to psychiatric clinical sites under the direct supervision of the instructor. Now, when students are placed in community agencies, the instructor must find nurses in the agency willing to fulfill the role of preceptor. This task can be simplified by writing the desired qualifications and duties expected of the preceptor and circulating it to agency nurses. After choosing from among the applicants, create a contract stipulating the responsibilities of the student, the preceptor, the agency, and the school. It is rare that a program can pay for the services of the preceptor, so creating good will is important. Regular contacts between the instructor and the preceptor are helpful to give and obtain feedback. Written notes of thanks at the end of the semester help the preceptor feel appreciated, as do luncheons or teas once a year.

Using Preconferences and Postconferences

The model espoused at the inception of ADN programs called for the preconference to be instructor-directed with student participation expected. During the 45 to 60 minutes of preconference, objectives are reviewed, assignments clarified, and plans for the day established. Preconference gives the instructor an opportunity to assess student preparation for the day's activities, discuss client needs and nursing interventions necessary to meet these needs, and explore priorities of care. It is not a time to present new material about a topic in lieu of using class time.

Postconferences give an opportunity for students to share in a discussion of their experiences and the knowledge gained. Other activities include evaluating care given in terms of objectives established in preconference, group problem solving related to problems encountered

during the clinical experience, clarification of relationships between theory and practice, developing generalizations and guidelines for providing nursing care, discussion of the milieu, focusing on clients as individuals, exploring the role of the psychiatric nurse in the roles of manager of care and member of the profession, in addition to the role of caregiver. Sharing learning can be a powerful and effective teaching-learning strategy. Students should be the dominant figures in postconference. This supports the lifelong learning concept with students' taking responsibility for their own learning. The instructor role is that of facilitator: to make comparisons, identify similarities and differences, link accounts to objectives, and to summarize at the end of the conference. Postconference should not be weekly miniclasses given over to the leadership of a person from the clinical agency, as is sometimes seen.

Nursing Care Plans Versus Clinical Pathways

One dilemma to be resolved early in planning is whether to teach learners to develop nursing care plans based on the nursing process or teach the exclusive use of clinical pathways. When one examines the purposes of each of these tools, it seems clear that there is value in learners understanding both.

Care plans are excellent educational tools and are client-centered guides for clinical practice. Use of the nursing process in psychiatric nursing helps novices begin to think as nurses think. Creating nursing care plans fosters the evolution of this "nurse-thinking." Creating care plans helps learners see relationships between and among assessment data and nursing diagnoses, assessment data and desired outcomes, assessment data and planned interventions, and the implementation of interventions and outcomes and their evaluation.

Clinical pathways are excellent practice tools that can enhance student learning. Clinical pathways are "maps" that have been created by expert multidisciplinary practitioners (after assessment data are obtained and analyzed) to identify predetermined times that specific medical, nursing, and other professional interventions will be implemented and the dates by which certain outcomes can be expected. By their specificity they allow us to efficiently allocate scarce resources, and to quickly determine whether or not a client is progressing according to plan.

Care plans and clinical pathways are not mutually exclusive; rather they can be interdependent resources for learning. The learner must understand the logical scientific thinking of the nursing process in order to make use of the pathways. The clinical pathways, in turn, enhance the student's understanding of the importance of efficient, effective treatment that proceeds according to plan. It seems reasonable to point out that nurses must understand their own discipline to be able to collaborate in the writing of clinical pathways.

5

Use of a Clinical Journal

Since faculty cannot be present as each student interacts with clients (and because the instructor's presence would alter the interaction), having students write about the interactions gives a picture of student activity. Some faculty believe students modify "what really happened" to relate an interaction with a favorable outcome. Whenever that is the case, little has been lost, for this action calls for the student to review the interaction and consider ways to arrive at a more favorable outcome. Most students "tell it as it happened" when a climate of trust is present between faculty and student. A positive expectation that the journal will provide helpful feedback serves as the basis for student openness.

The journal should be written in a separate notebook or in a private e-mail so it can be shared with the instructor weekly for the purpose of receiving feedback. The journal describes the learner's interactions during the clinical laboratory. Typical instructions might be the following: Summarize your interactions and activities during the clinical laboratory. Describe your observations of, and impressions about, significant events occurring on the unit or during special assignments (activities therapy, groups, etc.). Remember to include your feelings about the clients or situations you describe. Refer to clients by initials, rather than by name.

Many faculty believe learning is maximized when the learner is given specific topics to address each week in addition to the general directions. Directions for the student's focused writing for the first clinical week might be similar to these:

Describe your reactions to the stress of beginning psychiatric nursing. Note both physiological and behavioral responses.

Describe your reactions to the unit milieu: the physical environment, staff behaviors and attitudes, interactions among clients, and factors that impacted positively or negatively on stress.

Describe the appearance, behavior, and conversation of at least one client with whom you interacted.

Describe client and nurse behaviors that you observed or experienced that are characteristic of the introductory stage of a relationship.

Describe other behaviors you used while on the psychiatric unit and while interacting with clients. Analyze the significance of these behaviors.

Faculty will have much feedback to give, so having students write on the left-hand page, leaving the opposite page for the instructor's comments, works well. Feedback encompasses giving helpful suggestions, asking what the learner thinks might have happened if he or she had said or done . . ., pointing out that something in the journal is an example of theory, as well as pointing out areas of concern to the instructor. Never underestimate the value of positive reinforcement. Give praise to help shape behavior and to build self-esteem. Students depend upon the instructor's feedback to determine what, if any, modifications should be made, so it is important to read and return the journal in the shortest possible time. A 1- to 2-day "turnaround" time is reasonable.

Creating a Course Syllabus

The syllabus is created after course planning is completed. A learner can be likened to a traveler, and a syllabus (course outline) can be likened to a travel itinerary. A travel itinerary tells learners how they're going to go from New York to Los Angeles and what points of interest they'll visit along the way. Just as a travel itinerary tells a traveler where the traveler should be on a given day, a course syllabus informs learners what material is to be learned by a given point in time. A well-organized syllabus assists students to master content.

While most faculty see a syllabus as serving the educational function of providing a learning guide for students, it also has a legal function. It is the legal contract between the college or university and the student. When a syllabus is complete and detailed, students have fewer opportunities to suggest that faculty are being arbitrary or capricious. Grievance committees and courts of law, alike, are reluctant to find in favor of the student if the faculty administered the course in adherence to the syllabus. In addition, the detail of the syllabus produces consistency among faculty. This is particularly helpful when many sections are taught by adjunct faculty who have little contact with full time faculty. A new faculty member once suggested that a detailed syllabus was as helpful as a cookbook; the ingredients were listed and hints were given as to how and when to mix and stir.

What are the elements of the syllabus?

Course identification: Name of the college or university, department, course number and title, semester and year, placement (e.g., third semester), prerequisites and corequisites, credit allotment (list required class hours, conference hours, clinical laboratory hours).

Course description: Taken from the catalog.

Course overview: Elaborates on the course description, if you wish.

Faculty teaching the course: Give names, titles, office numbers, and telephone extensions.

List of clinical laboratory facilities and phone numbers of each: Specific instructions about how to contact the instructor enables students to notify the instructor if he or she is unable to attend the clinical laboratory.

Course outcomes: Usually begin with "At the completion of this course, it is expected that the learner will be able to . . ." Outcomes are written in measurable, behavioral terms. Usually, terminal objectives for a course number between 5 and 10.

Instructional strategies: List methods of instruction such as small-group discussion, lecture, reading assignments, computer assisted instruction, interactive video programs, films and videotapes, simulations, supervised clinical experience, and so on. List required textbooks and optional or recommended texts as well.

Course requirements and final grade determination: Explain the requirements each learner must accomplish for satisfactory course completion. This should include a list of assignments or projects that are to count as part of the grade, criteria for grading each, and a detailed explanation as to how the course grade will be computed. State your policy on class participation, attendance, receipt and grading of late assignments, penalties for late papers, missed examinations, and make-up examinations. Describe the type of examinations that will be given and dates for the examinations.

Explain how the clinical laboratory grade is achieved, e.g., "The clinical laboratory grade will be recorded as satisfactory or unsatisfactory. A satisfactory grade is achieved when the learner prepares for each session by . . .; meets the standard for performance of skills according to criteria established by the department." This is a good place to explain expectations for the student during pre- and postconferences.

If clinical appraisal tools have been developed, include the forms in the syllabus. If formative and summative evaluations are to be conducted, explain the use of the tool and the roles of the student and instructor. The overriding criterion for student competence is client safety. Explain the results of course failure, and where the procedure for grade appeal can be found.

Guidelines for professional behavior: May be included in the syllabus if not included in a student handbook. The teaching team may wish to speak to concepts such as integrity, accountability, responsibility, dependability, courtesy, dress code and personal hygiene, and rules of conduct such as substance use and abuse.

Course progression and assignments: A schedule of lecture topics and conference topics should be given. Learning objectives, written in measurable terms, should be listed for each topic. This helps the student know where to focus, as well as what to study for examinations. List the learning resources for each topic: for example, required reading assignments, films and videos, computer programs, and optional resources that may be used for remediation or enrichment. You may also specify the amount of independent preparation required or suggested to the learner prior to class or clinical experi-

ence. Dates assignments are due should be reiterated in this section also.

Clinical activities and objectives should also be listed to assist the student to see the relationship between theory and clinical practice.

SELECTING TEACHING STRATEGIES FOR THE COURSE

Educational literature pertaining to primary and secondary education consistently speaks to the importance of actively involving learners. Yet, at the collegiate level, many faculty plan courses in which learners are passive recipients of knowledge via the exclusive use of the lecture method. With appropriate thought, lectures can, in fact, be structured to avoid making the student a passive recipient.

Lecture

When instructors choose to teach a particular segment of material via lecture, they will first develop objectives for the lecture and outline the content to be presented. The next step is developing explanations, descriptions, and examples designed to meet the objectives. The lecture outlines prepared for this manual respond to the objectives for each chapter. Each lecture should have an introduction, a body, and a summary. The introduction should explain briefly what is to be addressed and should create a "bridge" between what the learner already knows and the new information that will be presented. The body of the lecture presents the new material. The summary briefly highlights what has been presented and may go on to set the stage for the next facet of learning.

Pointers for spicing up a lecture:
- Think of a lecture as a performance.
- Pace the delivery of your material. Think about what to present. Your students deserve the opportunity to think about it, too, rather than having to write frantically.
- Pause to punctuate. Pause slightly at significant points, after each item in a list, after a key word or phrase.
- Allow students to ask questions
- Many lectures have too much tell and too little show. Plan audiovisuals.
- Pose questions to students. Questions can be used to enter into elaborations, encourage critical analysis, to change direction, and to check understanding. Questions require the student to be an active participant.

Passive Versus Active Learning Strategies

Use of lecture as the exclusive teaching strategy often produces unenthusiastic, even bored, learners. In addition,

7

actively involving learners in the learning process is of great importance both for understanding and retention. For this reason, varying teaching strategies is advisable. Using classroom games, puzzles, structured learning projects, discussions, case studies, experiential learning, role playing, group projects, computer- assisted instruction, and interactive video technology provides learners with options to become actively involved in the teaching-learning process.

Accommodating Preferred Learning Styles

Because the preferred learning styles of students vary, using multiple teaching-learning strategies allows the instructor to address a variety of learning styles. To accommodate various learning styles, provide a variety of learning resources from which the learner can choose. For example, allow learners to address a unit's objectives via textbook readings, completing a computer-assisted instructional program, or by viewing a video or film.

Alternative strategies provide opportunities for learners to interact with theory in different ways. For example, analysis of case studies during class time calls for students to integrate facts and theory with clinical practice.

Examples of various teaching-learning strategies are included in this manual. Take a risk! Try a different technique as part of, or in lieu of, a lecture presentation. Let students tell you what they thought about the strategy. Most students tell faculty they enjoyed the activity.

Meeting Adult Learner Needs

Adult learners are motivated to focus on practical applications of what is learned. The instructor can facilitate integration of content by illustrating or fostering discussion of the relevance of the learned material to nursing practice. Adult learners also welcome opportunities for independent learning. Being able to learn at one's own pace and at the time most conducive to learning is appealing to adult learners.

Bridging

The use of bridging techniques is essential (i.e., linking new topics to familiar material). Possible examples of bridging: relating already learned therapeutic communication techniques to new techniques to be learned in the course, relating pre- and post-ECT care to pre- and post-operative care

Textbook and Other Readings

Most faculty assign textbook readings, then repeat important points in lecture. Students soon learn this and skip the readings. It's permissible to remind students that information relative to objectives x, y, and z can be found in the reading and to concentrate on elaborating on other topics. What are some other ways to motivate students to read?

- Give the students a reason to read. When alternative teaching strategies are used, students become responsible for doing the readings. They cannot assume the instructor will "hit the highlights" during lecture.
- Be optimistic. Assume learners are reading. If one assumes learners are not reading or asks who has read the assignment, the faculty member will teach in ways that reveal the content of the reading by explaining, summarizing, and so on. Again, learners have little reason to read.
- Ask questions, but do not always call on those who volunteer to give the answer. Nonreaders often rely on the readers to supply all the answers. Don't assume that either you or a reader must give the answer to the question. Both you and the readers know the answer. The nonreader does not. Feeling left out can motivate a student to read. Be careful, however, not to be punitive and do not make the nonreaders feel defensive.
- Read aloud a short quotation or give an example and ask learners to explain how it relates to the material in the reading.
- Ask learners to identify the most important idea given in a particular section of the reading.

Critical Thinking

Nursing requires practitioners who are able to think critically and make decisions. Faculty can foster the development of these skills by carefully engineering classroom activities and interactions that go beyond simply learning facts. A number of critical thinking exercises are included in the text and still more can be found on this textbook's companion website at http://evolve.elsevier.com/Varcarolis.

Always be prepared to help learners stretch their minds, rather than stuff their minds.

Ask students for evaluations, for value judgments for cause-and-effect relationships, for comparisons, and for ideas for solutions.

Games

Games, like lectures, highlight important facts and concepts. Students soon learn that they must be prepared or face the possibility of letting their team down. Peer pressure is a wonderful motivator! When it's announced that there will be a game during class the following day, students prepare, rather than face the possibility of peer disapproval. Games can be played even with very large groups. Simply create more teams! Don't be afraid to ask for a student volunteer to help by determining which team signals readiness to answer first, or to keep score. If you play a board game during class, plan ahead to purchase or produce the requisite number of games.

8

A word to the wise: Winning is an even more powerful motivator when the instructor provides prizes for the winning team. Prizes need not be expensive: for example, a sticker, a gold-painted tongue depressor, apples, a bag of hard candy, pens you've acquired at convention booths. Local hospitals may be delighted to provide you with items they use as recruitment tools.

Several television game-show formats have found favor with nursing faculty and students. It's possible to create transparencies for the overhead projector to simulate game-show boards, for example:

list categories above each column

10	10	10	10	10	10
20	20	20	20	20	20
30	30	30	30	30	30
40	40	40	40	40	40
50	50	50	50	50	50

Write clues for each category, making sure that each becomes harder as you ascend the point scale. Divide students into teams. The team chooses a point value, the instructor gives the corresponding clue, and teams signal to be the first to answer. The game can be played with as few as three or four categories, for a short version. The short version allows the instructor to combine several activities in one class.

Watching the game show on TV before playing for the first time in class is advised. Students who watch the game shows are sticklers when it comes to the rules.

Computer-Assisted Instruction

Computer-assisted instruction (CAI) and CD-ROM programs promote active involvement in learning and provide self-paced instruction. CAI for nursing comes in several formats: drill and practice, usually used for practicing medication calculation problems; tutorials that give information and then ask questions to reinforce learning; and simulations that provide clinical case studies fostering integration of theory and practice. A simulation offers decision-making opportunities in a safe setting as the learner uses the nursing process.

Several programs mentioned in this manual are tutorials: for example, *Patient's/Resident's Rights; Violence in the Healthcare Setting; Prevention and Intervention,* and *Developing Multicultural Sensitivity.*

These programs might be used as a substitute for, and an adjunct to, textbook readings or lecture. When tutorials are menu-driven, the instructor may assign only selected parts of the program.

Other CAIs mentioned in this manual are simulations: for example, *Nursing Care of the Suicidal Client, Care of the Client Experiencing Depression, Care of the Client Experiencing Mania,* and *Medication Administration on a Psychiatric Unit.*

CAI is easily integrated into the course. The process is similar to making a decision about using a film or video. First, preview the material. Preview carefully. Some authors write feedback for each option a student chooses. The student knows immediately whether the option was correct or incorrect. Correct answers are usually reinforced, and incorrect answers are explained. Many students enjoy choosing incorrect answers, telling faculty, "I learn a lot by finding out why certain actions are incorrect." This format seems most useful to novices.

Other authors provide intermittent feedback. Using this format, the student may enter a decision, and receive the feedback, "Your response has been noted." Then, later in the course of the program, the student may learn that, at some former point, an incorrect decision was made. This format seems better suited to advanced learners.

Some programs have a scoring mechanism that can be used to record the numbers of questions the student answers correctly and the numbers answered incorrectly. Students should be advised if the instructor plans to survey or record the scores. The student will be alerted not to purposely choose incorrect answers. Some programs feature a posttest, and the possibility of recording scores for instructor retrieval. The use of a posttest allows students to learn as the program is used, to choose correct or incorrect answers as they prefer, and then take the posttest.

If, as you interact with the software, you realize the program is not appropriate for your students, with the exception of one or two small segments, don't despair. You may still be able to assign the program by giving students an errata sheet. Simply tell the students what you want them to know that's different from what the program presents. For instance, suicide precautions may differ from agency to agency or region to region. Explain to the learners, that although the program presents certain material, in the facilities in which they'll be practicing, the following protocol is observed. . . .

Although CAI simulations may be used in a variety of ways, one of the most useful is to assign the program to be used as a method of promoting integration after readings and classroom presentations are completed.

Use in the classroom: Although we generally think of a use ratio of one student to one computer, students often like to work in pairs, discussing as they progress through the program. CAI can also be used in the classroom with small groups of viewers by using a computer, a projection panel and an overhead projector, or a computer projector.

Interactive Video Disk and CD-ROM Technologies

The interactive video disk (IVD) is the delight of instructors and students alike. It combines full-motion color video and computer graphics and text. The interactive video program *Therapeutic Communication* is best assigned as one would assign readings in a textbook. This is true of the CD-ROM program *Uppers, Downers, All-Arounders,* a program on drugs of abuse. It is unrealistic to expect a learner to view many IVDs and CD-ROM programs at one sitting. A "map" explains the structure of *Therapeutic Communication,* and a user's guide accompanies the program. These features assist the instructor in determining "chapters" for possible use. The instructor should preview the program and make specific assignments. Giving learners step-by-step directions about how to access the required sections is helpful.

Writing to Learn Exercises

Some schools have adopted *Writing Across the Curriculum* or *Writing to Think/Learn.* This requires that students be given the opportunity to write for 5 or more minutes during each class. The topics should be assigned by the instructor and should be relevant to the day's material. The product of the writing opportunity should be handed in. Some faculty give each written paragraph points ranging from 1 to 5 toward the final grade; others read the submissions, but may not give a grade. If class time permits, samples may be read by authors and discussed by the class before they are submitted.

Examples of topics for in-class writing exercises:
- What would you like to learn from this course?
- Complete the sentence, "What I learned in today's class that surprised me most is . . ."
- Complete the sentence, "The thing I least understood in today's class is . . ."
- What is the essential difference between . . . and . . .?
- What is the relationship between . . . and . . .?

Advantages of in-class writing:
- encourages thinking about the topic;
- allows the faculty to assess student abilities early in the semester and make referrals for remediation, if necessary;
- provides the instructor with valuable feedback for some topics about the effectiveness of his or her teaching.

If points are given toward the final grade:
- Free writing can motivate students to organize what they are learning in class and in clinical.
- Free writing encourages attendance, since only the students present may receive credit for their work

Role Playing

It's important that introductions and summaries be used whenever role playing takes place. Faculty cannot assume learners understand what the role playing is meant to accomplish. For example, learners may be told that role playing is, in fact, behavioral rehearsal. Behavioral rehearsal is a way to become more proficient in interpersonal skills. Communication skills, like the technical skills of nursing, are improved through practice. Behavioral rehearsal "primes" learners for future situations. It increases our repertoire of possible effective responses.

Role players may be selected by asking for volunteers or by drawing lots. Because some individuals are hesitant to participate, it's helpful to allow participants to "pass" if participants are selected by lots. Another method is to divide the class into teams, and to allow the teams to select players. The facilitator can empathize, saying, "Role playing involves a willingness to take risks, to 'expose' yourself and your skills to the scrutiny of others. We can promise that if you take this risk, we will make our feedback constructive."

Before beginning the role play, the faculty facilitator should set the stage by explaining where the action takes place. After the scene has been adequately played out, stop the play and call for discussion. Several questions should be planned in advance. Other points may arise spontaneously out of the interaction between participants. Be sure the audience offers feedback to the players. The facilitator should not assume the role of authority. When the feedback given has been predominantly negative, the facilitator may ask, "What were the positive things . . . in this role play?"

If a player becomes blocked, ask the audience what might be said. When a response is given, invite the student to come forward and try the new response with the "client." The group soon learns that the facilitator will not let the stress become unbearable, and will become more willing to risk.

At the close of the role play and discussion, summarize the learning, thank the players, and end with a round of applause.

Guest Speakers

Guest speakers can be a valuable resource. Simply be sure you have given the speaker a good idea of what you wish the speaker to discuss, the student outcomes you desire, and the amount of time the speaker will have. It's wise to follow a phone call with a written summary of what you discussed. It's easy for a speaker to forget the details of a conversation and nice to have a written copy to turn to when preparation time comes.

Introduction

Once the presentation is over, don't forget to thank the speaker and encourage students to also write a note or thank you card to thank speakers and be sure they understand the value of their contribution to you and to future nurses.

Collaborative Learning

Nursing is not practiced in isolation; rather it is often a collaborative effort. If your graduates are expected to work with health care and nursing teams, instructors will need to provide opportunities for collaborative learning. Advantages of collaborative learning include preparation for the real world; development of cooperation and planning skills; leadership development; and better relationships within the class. Collaborative learning can be facilitated by making the task concrete and specific; matching the task and the size of the group (i.e.; large task, large group; setting time limits and giving deadlines; keeping groups apprised of the time remaining; and sharing the outcomes of group work).

STUDENT EVALUATION OF THE COURSE

Each student should have the opportunity to anonymously evaluate the course content and teaching strategies at midterm and at the conclusion of the course. For short courses, seeking feedback at midterm may not be practical. One possible approach to obtaining feedback is to devise a number of statements and have the students use a Likert-type scale to give opinions. At a minimum, you will probably wish to seek feedback about the relevance of course objectives, the fairness of grading criteria, as well as the teaching strategies learners are finding most helpful. Be sure to give learners space to amplify or explain and to write comments about topics you may not have included. Giving learners the opportunity to provide you with feedback at midterm allows you to make subtle changes, if necessary.

EVALUATION OF STUDENTS

Evaluation of theoretical concepts can be accomplished by paper-and-pencil testing. It is hoped the Test Bank in this instructor's manual will be helpful in revitalizing your department's testing resources.

Clinical appraisal is somewhat more complicated. Most courses stipulate that in order to pass the course, a satisfactory grade in both theory and clinical performance must be attained. For a student to attain a satisfactory clinical grade, given several assignments, stipulate that a grade of satisfactory (or C) must be attained for each. For example, the student will achieve a grade of satisfactory when the student:

- completes clinical objectives weekly;
- submits a daily journal that complies with the requirements listed in the course outline;
- achieves a satisfactory grade on
  - the process recording
  - the client assessment
  - the nursing process paper
  - the progress notes;
- has accrued no more than two clinical incident reports.

Clinical incident reports are filed if, during clinical laboratory, an incident occurs demonstrating
- the student's failure to implement safe care;
- lack of basic knowledge;
- poor judgment;
- omission of procedures or medical orders;
- placement of the client in psychological jeopardy.

Examples of such incidents include, but are not limited to
- violating policies of the hospital or the contract between the hospital and the college or university;
- ignoring basic rules of safety or common sense;
- using a grossly nontherapeutic approach such as arguing with a delusional client, exploiting a client, laughing at a client, behaving seductively, and so on, as evidenced in the journal, the process recordings, or during direct observation by instructor or staff;
- arranging meetings with clients outside clinical hours;
- ignoring instructions of faculty or staff;
- omitting ordered treatments or medications.

Use of a Practical Examination

Faculty may wish to consider a summative practical examination in addition to the traditional final examination. One teaching team has developed a series of trigger videos.

Faculty scripted several situations showing each of the following: anxiety, anger, depression, delusional thought content, denial of an alcohol or drug problem. Trigger segments were tested with nurses and non-nurses to ensure reliability of content. Five trigger situations, one from each category, are selected for each final examination. (The same examination is not given to successive groups, since students may exchange information. Mixing the segments provides many different examinations.) The examination is conducted during class time. All students are given paper and sit facing the video screen. The first trigger segment is played, and students write a therapeutic response. Segments are played with appropriate pauses for answers to be written, until all five are completed. Then, the five segments are replayed

11

without pause. The replay negates the possibility that a student could accuse faculty of unfairness. In reality, a student could ask a client to repeat what was said. The replay affords this same opportunity.

Use of a Clinical Appraisal Tool

Many teaching teams have developed clinical appraisal tools to make clinical grading as objective as possible. The areas to be assessed usually reflect the organizing concepts of the course or program. Often, the tool is written in terms of the standard to be attained, allowing the rater to simply check whether or not the learner has achieved competence. For example, when the nursing process is used as an organizing concept, items on the clinical appraisal form might be worded as follows:
- Collects data from client, health team, and written records to assess the basic needs of clients
- Performs a complete psychosocial and mental status assessment on a selected client
- On the basis of data analysis and interpretation, identifies nursing diagnoses of high priority for selected clients
- Establishes client centered goals for the identified nursing diagnoses
- Establishes outcome criteria for the goals
- Identifies individualized nursing interventions to meet client goals
- Implements nursing interventions and carries out medical and nursing orders with guidance
- Evaluates goal attainment by comparing data with identified outcome criteria
- Includes the client and health team in determining progress toward goals
- Revises the care plan as needed
- When using nursing roles as an organizing concept, appraisal items might include statements such as the following:

In the role of caregiver:
- Acts to prevent error, accident, physical or psychological injury when carrying out nursing interventions
- Establishes boundaries of the nurse-client relationship
- Establishes a supportive/therapeutic relationship with one or more clients

- Avoids stereotyping
- Behaves in a nonjudgmental manner
- Encourages client to express self without expressing own bias
- Provides environment in which clients' values, beliefs, and customs are accepted
- Structures time and activity with clients
- Identifies and supports healthy aspects of behavior and personality in assigned clients
- Encourages client participation in meeting basic needs
- Identifies client need for information
- Devises, implements, and evaluates effectiveness of a teaching plan
- Adjusts client priorities for nursing intervention as client situation changes

In the role of manager:
- Completes care within a designated time frame
- Communicates appropriate information to the health team and faculty member
- Interacts with health team in a collegial way

In the role of member of the profession:
- Practices according to legal standards of state
- Practices according to ethical standards of profession
- Provides client with privacy, confidentiality
- Identifies own learning needs
- Prepares for hospital experience according to course guidelines
- Changes behavior as a result of instructor guidance

Whenever the student is rated as not being competent, it's helpful to include explanatory examples from anecdotal notes to support the rating. This practice lessens the student's tendency to believe the instructor is being arbitrary or capricious.

FINAL THOUGHTS

Enjoy the opportunity of opening the door to a new facet of nursing for your students. The relationship you develop with each of them in many ways parallels the relationships they will be developing with clients. To provide nurture to clients, students need to have the experience of being nurtured and valued. You have a unique opportunity!

1 Mental Health and Mental Illness

THOUGHTS ABOUT TEACHING THE TOPIC

The instructor will probably devote an hour or less to this material, and will probably emphasize (1) the mental health–mental illness continuum; (2) the mental health assessment, using both the factors that influence mental health and the five criteria of mental health; and (3) the importance of becoming conversant with *DSM-IV-TR*.

The learning activities found on the Evolve website will assist students to operationalize this general knowledge. Activities can be used in class or assigned as independent work.

KEY TERMS AND CONCEPTS

iologically based mental illnesses, 6
clinical epidemiology, 5
Diagnostic and Statistical Manual of Mental Disorders (DSM-IV-TR), 3
epidemiology, 4
mental disorders, 3
mental health, 2
mental illness, 2
myths and misconceptions (regarding mental illness), 3
prevalence rate, 6

psychiatry's definition of normal (mental health), 3
psychobiological disorder, 6

OBJECTIVES

After studying this chapter, the reader will be able to
1. Assess his or her own mental health using the seven signs of mental health identified in this chapter (Table 1-1 and Figure 1-1).
2. Summarize factors that can affect the mental health of an individual and the ways that these factors influence conducting a holistic nursing assessment.
3. Discuss some dynamic factors (including social climate, politics, myths, and biases) that contribute to making a clear-cut definition of mental health elusive.
4. Explain how epidemiological studies can improve medical and nursing care.
5. Demonstrate how the *DSM-IV-TR* multiaxial system can influence a clinician to consider a broad range of information before making a *DSM-IV-TR* diagnosis.
6. Compare and contrast a *DSM-IV-TR* diagnosis with a nursing diagnosis.
7. Give examples from his or her own culture of how consideration of norms and other cultural influences can affect making an accurate *DSM-IV-TR* diagnosis.

CHAPTER OUTLINE	TEACHING STRATEGIES
Concepts of Mental Health and Illness	The validity of several concepts is explored, beginning with the idea that mental illness is what a culture regards as unacceptable and that mentally ill individuals are those who violate social norms. This is shown to be an inadequate definition by pointing out that political dissidents are not necessarily mentally ill. Another misconception to be discussed is that a healthy person must be logical and rational, with the point being made that each of us has irrational dreams and experiences irrational emotions. All human behavior lies somewhere along a continuum of mental health and mental illness. Mentally healthy persons are those who are in harmony with themselves and their environment. Such individuals may possess medical deviation or disease as long as this does not impair reasoning, judgment, intellectual capacity and the ability to make harmonious personal and social adaptations. Instead of a definition of mental health, traits possessed by the mentally healthy are identified as happiness, control over behavior, appraisal of reality, effectiveness in work, and a healthy self-concept. The misconception that mental illness is incurable or treatment is unsuccessful is refuted by contrasting people with cardiovascular disease with people with mental illness.
Epidemiology of Mental Disorders	The epidemiology of mental disorders may be defined as the quantitative study of the distribution of mental disorders in human populations. Three levels of investigation are noted: descriptive, analytic, and experimental.

Continued

13

CHAPTER OUTLINE	TEACHING STRATEGIES
Applications of Epidemiology	Clinical epidemiology is briefly explained as a broad field that addresses what happens to people with illnesses who are seen by providers of clinical care.
Prevalence	Prevalence rate is explained as the proportion of a population with a mental disorder at a given time. Table 1-2 gives the prevalence of selected psychiatric disorders in the United States.
Mental Illness and the Mental Health Continuum	The most prevalent and disabling mental disorders have strong biological influences, e.g., schizophrenia, bipolar disorder, major depression, obsessive-compulsive and panic disorders, posttraumatic stress disorder, and autism. Nurses are cautioned to remember that we do not treat diseases; rather we care holistically for people. Factors that affect a person's mental health include support systems, family influences, developmental events, cultural or subcultural beliefs and values, health practices, and negative influences impinging upon one's life. Each must be evaluated and factored into a plan of care. Figure 1-3 identifies some influences that can affect a person's mental health.

Medical Diagnosis and Nursing Diagnosis of Mental Illness

Medical Diagnoses and the *DSM-IV-TR*	In the *Diagnostic and Statistical Manual of Mental Disorders (DSM-IV-TR)*, each mental disorder is conceptualized as a clinically significant behavioral or psychological syndrome or pattern that occurs in an individual and is associated with present distress or disability or with a significantly increased risk of suffering death, pain, disability, or an important loss of freedom. *DSM-IV-TR* supports accurate diagnostic assessment by providing information about culturally diverse populations.
The *DSM-IV-TR* in Culturally Diverse Populations	Special efforts have been made in the *DSM-IV-TR* to incorporate an awareness that the manual is used in culturally diverse populations in the U.S. and internationally. Clinicians evaluate individuals from numerous ethnic groups and cultural backgrounds. Diagnostics assessment can be especially challenging when a clinician from one ethnic or cultural group uses the *DSM-IV-TR* classification to evaluate an individual from a different ethnic or cultural group.
The *DSM-IV-TR* Multiaxial System	The *DSM-IV-TR* axis system requires the clinician to consider a broad range of information about the individual by employing a multiaxial system: Axis I refers to the collection of signs and symptoms that together constitute a particular disorder; axis II refers to personality disorders and mental retardation; axis III refers to general medical conditions relevant to the mental disorder; axis IV reports psychosocial and environmental problems; and axis V is a global assessment of functioning during the preceding year, rated on a scale of 1 to 100, ranging from persistent danger of self-harm to superior functioning. Readers are cautioned that labeling can have harmful effects on the individual and family, and that cultural and social bias can influence psychiatric diagnosis.
Nursing Diagnoses and the *DSM-IV-TR*	Nursing diagnosis is described as a clinical judgment about individual, family, or community responses to actual or potential health problems and life processes. A nursing diagnosis provides the framework for identifying appropriate nursing interventions for dealing with the phenomena a client with a mental health disorder is experiencing.
Introduction to Culture and Mental Illness	In determining the mental health or mental illness of an individual, we must consider the norms and influence of culture. Cultures differ in their views of mental illness and the behavior categorized as mental illness. Although some disorders such as bipolar disorder and schizophrenia are found throughout the world, other syndromes are culture bound (e.g., running amok, pibloktoq, and anorexia nervosa). *DSM-IV-TR* provides information about cultural variations for each of the clinical disorders, a description of culture-bound syndromes, and an outline of cultural formulations for evaluating and reporting the impact of the individual's cultural context.

14

2 Relevant Theories and Therapies for Nursing Practice

THOUGHTS ABOUT TEACHING THE TOPIC

When students have completed a growth and development course prior to the psychiatric nursing course, a review of personality theories by reading may be sufficient. It's wise, however, to offer a self-paced activity or a match exercise and remind students that they are responsible for the content, whether or not it is included in a lecture. The chapter's explanation of therapies is succinct, yet it is sufficient in detail to permit learners to grasp the material. However, because learners have a limited frame of reference for therapies, most would rather explore what those in the field think rather than discuss or debate among themselves. Use of a film, followed by a discussion, may help learners grasp the basic concepts of therapy.

KEY TERMS AND CONCEPTS

aversion therapy, 29
behavioral therapy, 27
cognitive therapy, 26
conditioning, 21
conscious, 16
countertransference, 25
defense mechanisms, 17
ego, 17
id, 16
interpersonal psychotherapy (IPT), 26
milieu therapy, 30
modeling, 27
operant conditioning, 22
positive reinforcement, 22
preconscious, 16
psychodynamic psychotherapy, 25
reinforcer, 22
security operations, 18
short-term dynamic psychotherapy, 26
superego, 17
systematic desensitization, 29
transference, 25
unconscious, 16

OBJECTIVES

After studying this chapter, the reader will be able to
1. Compare and contrast the developmental stages defined by Freud and Erikson.
2. Evaluate the premises behind the various therapeutic models discussed in this chapter.
3. Identify ways that each theorist contributes to the nurse's ability to assess a client's behaviors.
4. Drawing on clinical experience, provide the following:
   a. An example of how a client's irrational beliefs influenced behavior.
   b. An example of countertransference in your relationship with a client.
   c. An example of the use of behavior modification with a client.
5. Identify Peplau's expectation of the nurse-patient relationship.
6. Clarify the difference between the art and the science of nursing.
7. Choose the one therapeutic model that would be most useful, if there were an issue that needed to be resolved.

CHAPTER OUTLINE	TEACHING STRATEGIES
Major Theories of Personality	The contributions of Freud, Erikson, Sullivan, Peplau, and Maslow are summarized.
Psychodynamic Theories **Freud's Psychoanalytic Theory**	Freud, founder of psychoanalysis, developed a complex theoretical formulation to explain the human personality. It includes a topography with the following levels of awareness: 1. Conscious—intellectual, emotional, and interpersonal aspects of behavior in awareness at a given time or easily remembered; uses logic and operates on the reality principle 2. Preconscious—experiences, thoughts, feelings, or desires not in immediate awareness, but able to be recalled 3. Unconscious—memories, thoughts, feelings, or wishes not available to the conscious mind, having been repressed; not logical; operates on the pleasure principle

Continued

Personality structure is described as three categories of experience:

1. Id—source of drives and instincts; includes genetic inheritance; reflexes, wishes; reservoir of psychic energy; uses pleasure principle and primary process thinking
2. Ego—distinguishes between reality and what's in the mind; integrates demands of reality, id, and superego; uses secondary process thinking
3. Superego—internal representative of values, ideals, and moral standards of society; strives for perfection

Freud suggested that ego defense mechanisms are developed to reduce anxiety by denying, falsifying, or distorting reality to prevent conscious awareness of threatening feelings. These mechanisms operate unconsciously.

He further wrote that the individual proceeds through a series of psychosexual stages of development from infancy to adulthood. Each stage (except latency) refers to the bodily zone that produces the main source of gratification during the stage. Each stage has its own conflict to be resolved:

1. Oral—0 to 1 year: weaning
2. Anal—1 to 3 years: toilet training
3. Phallic—3 to 6 years: oedipal conflict
4. Latency—6 to 12 years: hides sexuality from disapproving adults
5. Genital—12 to 20 years: genital sexuality

Sullivan's Interpersonal Theory

Sullivan's interpersonal theory focused on interpersonal processes observed in a social framework. Major aspects of his theory deal with anxiety and the self-system. Anxiety can be transmitted interpersonally via empathetic linkage and it can be described. Behaviors resulting from anxiety can be observed, and security operations such as selective inattention and dissociation are measures used to reduce it. Sullivan identifies three components of the self-system: the good-me, representing the part of the personality that develops in response to rewarding appraisals of others; the bad-me that develops in response to anxiety-producing appraisals from others; and the not-me that results from dissociating overwhelming feelings of horror, dread, and loathing.

Behavioral Theories
Pavlov's Classical Conditioning Theory

Pavlov hypothesized that the psychic component was a learned association between two events: the presence of experimental apparatus and the serving of meat (in dogs). He formalized his observations of behaviors in dogs in a theory of classic conditioning or respondent conditioning.

Watson's Behaviorism Theory

James B. Watson was an American psychologist who developed the school of thought referred to as behaviorism. He was strongly influenced by Pavlov's conditioning principles and began to apply these principles to human beings.

Skinner's Operant Conditioning Theory

B. F. Skinner represents the second wave of behavioral theorists and is recognized as one of the prime movers behind the behavioral movement. He labeled the most important aspect of his theory operant conditioning. Skinner believed that a person performs a behavior and experiences a consequence as a result of performing the behavior. Positive reinforcement increases the likelihood that the behavior will be repeated. Negative consequences produce a deterrent effect on behavior.

Biological Theories

A biological model of mental illness focuses on neurological, chemical, biological, and genetic issues and seeks to understand how the body and brain interact to create emotions, memories, and perceptual experiences. The recognition that psychiatric illnesses are as much physical in origin as diabetes and coronary heart disease serves to decrease the stigma surrounding psychiatric illnesses.

Nursing Theories

Peplau and the Therapeutic Relationship

Peplau, influenced by Sullivan's interpersonal theory, developed the first systematic theoretical framework for psychiatric nursing, the one-to-one nurse-patient relationship. Her theory is mainly concerned with the processes by which the nurse helps patients make positive changes in their health care status and well-being. Peplau identified stages of the nurse-patient relationship and used process recording to assist her students to hone their communication relationship skills. She describes skills that the psychiatric nurse will use including observation, interpretation, and intervention

Peplau also believed that nurses working with psychiatric patients need to have an awareness of their own behavior. She believed this self-awareness for the nurse is essential in order to keep the focus on the client.

Peplau spent a lifetime illuminating the science and art of professional nursing practice, which has had a profound effect on the nursing profession, nursing science, and the clinical practice of psychiatric nursing.

Traditional Therapeutic Approaches

Classical Psychoanalysis

Classical psychoanalysis, among the least practiced therapies and the most expensive, calls for protracted one-on-one therapy with an analyst. It makes use of free association and working through transference to uncover unconscious feelings and thoughts that interfere with the client's life. The client is more active than the therapist.

Psychodynamic and Psychoanalytic Psychotherapy

Uses the tools of psychoanalysis (free association, dream analysis, transference, countertransference), but the therapist is more active in the process and the duration of therapy is usually shorter.

Short-Term Dynamic Psychotherapy

Used to treat relatively healthy clients who have a circumscribed area of difficulty and who are willing to change. Usually 10 to 25 sessions are involved. Both client and therapist actively participate. Assessment is rapid and early. Goals are concrete and focused on lessening the client's worst symptoms, helping the client understand what is going on in his or her life, and enabling him or her to cope better. Interpretations are directed toward present life circumstances. Some positive transference is fostered to encourage the client to follow the therapist's suggestions.

Interpersonal Psychotherapy

This therapy focuses on reassurance, clarification of feeling states, and improvement in interpersonal communication and interpersonal skills. The therapist identifies the nature of the problem and selects strategies for use. Four types of problem areas have been identified: grief, role disputes, role transition, and interpersonal deficit.

Cognitive Therapy

Is active, directive, time-limited. Cognitive therapy is based on the rationale that individual affect and behavior are determined by the way in which the individual's cognitions structure the world. The therapist helps client identify, reality-test, and correct distorted conceptualizations and dysfunctional beliefs. The client learns to think more realistically and adaptively, thus reducing symptoms.

Behavioral Therapy

Is based on learning theory. Maladaptive behavior can be unlearned and adaptive behavior learned. Useful techniques include modeling, operant conditioning, systematic desensitization, and aversion.

Modeling

In modeling, the therapist provides a role model for specific identified behaviors, and the client learns through imitation.

Continued

Chapter 2   Relevant Theories and Therapies for Nursing Practice

CHAPTER OUTLINE	TEACHING STRATEGIES
Operant Conditioning	Operant conditioning is the basis for behavior modification and uses positive reinforcement to increase desired behaviors.
Systematic Desensitization	Systematic desensitization is another form of behavior modification therapy that involves the development of behavioral tasks customized to the clients' specific fears; these tasks are presented to the client while he or she is using learned relaxation techniques.

The process involves four steps:
1. The client's fear is broken down into its components by exploring the particular stimulus cues the client presents.
2. The client is incrementally exposed to the fear.
3. Clients are instructed how to design their own hierarchies of fear.
4. Clients practice these techniques every day.

Aversion Therapy	Aversion therapy, which is akin to punishment, is used widely to treat such behaviors as alcoholism, sexual deviation, shoplifting and others. Three paradigms for using aversive techniques are:

- Pairing of a maladaptive behavior with a noxious stimulus, so that anxiety or fear becomes associated with the once-pleasurable stimulus
- Punishment
- Avoidance training

Milieu Therapy	This therapy establishes a safe, supportive environment with an emphasis on group and social interaction. Rules are mediated by peer pressure; the staff view the clients as responsible humans; clients are involved in goal setting; clients have freedom of movement; there are informal client-staff relationships; and interdisciplinary staff participation.
Additional Therapies	There are other therapeutic approaches that you will be introduced later in the book. Crisis intervention, group therapy, and family therapy are examples.

18

Chapter 2   Relevant Theories and Therapies for Nursing
Practice

3 Biological Basis for Understanding Psychotropic Drugs

THOUGHTS ABOUT TEACHING THE TOPIC

Some of the material presented in this chapter reviews material learned in the anatomy and physiology course. The authors use this basic material to promote understanding of the possible disturbances associated with each of the groups of major mental disorders, and go on to look at the fact that pharmacological treatment is directed at suspected transmitter-receptor problems. Side effects and adverse effects are often related to blockade of various neurotransmitters. A major task of the instructor is to help the student realize that learning what occurs with the increase and decrease of each transmitter will simplify understanding of psychotropic drug action and side effects, since one will not have to memorize a list for each drug. Learning activities that help the learner associate drug name, action classification, and side effects can be very helpful.

KEY TERMS AND CONCEPTS

acetylcholine, 51
antagonists, 50
antianxiety or anxiolytic drugs, 57
anticholinesterase drugs, 59
atypical antipsychotic drugs, 51
atypical or novel antidepressants, 57
basal ganglia, 44
circadian rhythms,37
γ-aminobutyric acid (GABA), 47
hypnotic, 57
limbic system, 42
lithium, 53
mood-stabilizing drug, 53
monoamine oxidase (MAO), 56
monoamine oxidase inhibitors (MAOIs), 56
neurons, 38
neurotransmitter, 38
pharmacodynamics, 48
pharmacokinetics, 48
receptors, 39
reticular activating system (RAS), 42
reuptake, 39
selective serotonin reuptake inhibitors (SSRIs), 55
standard (first-generation) antipsychotic drugs, 50
synapse, 38
therapeutic index, 53
typical or standard antidepressants, 54

OBJECTIVES

After studying this chapter, the reader will be able to

1. Discuss at least eight functions of the brain and the way these functions can be altered by psychotropic drugs.
2. Describe how a neurotransmitter functions as a neuromessenger.
3. Draw the three major areas of the brain and identify at least three functions of each.
4. Identify how specific brain functions are altered in certain mental disorders (e.g., depression, anxiety, schizophrenia).
5. Describe how the use of imaging techniques can be helpful for understanding mental illness.
6. Apply to a medication teaching plan the knowledge gained from this chapter that the blockage of dopamine at the receptor site can result in motor abnormalities and hyperprolactinemia.
7. Describe the result of blockage of the muscarinic receptors and the α_1 receptors by the standard neuroleptic drugs.
8. Contrast and compare the side-effect profiles of the standard antipsychotics with those of (a) clozapine and (b) risperidone.
9. Briefly identify the main neurotransmitters that are affected by the following psychotropic drugs:
   (a) Standard (first-generation) antipsychotics
   (b) Tricyclic antidepressants
   (c) Selective serotonin reuptake inhibitors
   (d) Monoamine oxidase inhibitors
   (e) Antianxiety agents (benzodiazepines, buspirone)
   (f) Anticholinesterase drugs
10. Apply to a medication teaching plan the knowledge of why a person taking a monoamine oxidase inhibitor would have special dietary and drug restrictions.
11. Identify specific cautions you might incorporate into your medication teaching plan with regard to the following:
    (a) Herbal medicine
    (b) Genetic pharmacology (variations in effects and therapeutic actions of medications among different ethnic groups)

Continued

19

This chapter presents basic neurochemistry serving as the underpinning of normal mental function, in preparation for understanding the use of psychotropic drugs in the treatment of mental illnesses. Implied in the biological approach is that while the origins of psychiatric illnesses may be determined by multiple factors, there will eventually be an alteration in cerebral function that accounts for the disturbances in the client's behavioral and mental experiences. These alterations can be treated with psychotropic drugs, just as other biological problems are treated with drugs.

Structure and Function of the Brain

Functions of the Brain

Brain functions include monitoring changes in the external world; monitoring the composition of body fluids; regulating contractions of skeletal muscles; regulating internal organs; initiating and regulating basic drives—hunger, thirst, sex, aggressive self-protection; conscious sensation; memory; thought; mood (affect); language; regulating the sleep cycle. The author mentions ways in which psychiatric illness and its treatments alter each of these functions, as summarized below.

Function	Alteration
Monitoring external world	Altered sensory experiences (hallucinations, illusions)
Control over skeletal muscles	Movement disturbances (extrapyramidal symptoms), respiratory alterations, slurred speech
Regulating internal organs	Blood pressure variations dependent upon autonomic nervous system; anxiety activates parasympathetic nerves; hormonal effects such as menstrual cycle disturbances; corticotropin-releasing hormone (CRH) effect on general response to stress
Regulating basic drives	Over- or undereating, loss of sexual drive
Regulating sleep cycle	Sleep disturbance as a symptom of psychological distress, hypervigilance, drowsiness
Mood	Affected by circadian variations and neurotransmitter secretion (especially serotonin and norepinephrine)
Conscious experience	Inability to focus stream of consciousness or interpret external world, distorted thought patterns (loose associations), distorted speech (word salad), delusions
Memory	Inability to retain or recall past experience; cognitive disorders; learning disorders

Cellular Composition of the Brain

Neurons are specialized cells in the central nervous system (CNS), each having a cell body, an axon, and a dendrite. Each neuron carries out three types of physiological actions: they respond to stimuli, conduct electrical impulses, and release neurotransmitters. Conduction of electrical impulses involves self-propagating changes in membrane permeability allowing inward flow of sodium ions followed by outward flow of potassium ions, changing polarity, and creating an electrical charge along the length of the membrane. When the impulse reaches the end of the neuron, a neurotransmitter is released from the axon terminal. The neurotransmitter spreads across the synapse and attaches to a receptor on the surface of

Chapter 3   Biological Basis for Understanding
Psychotropic Drugs

the next neuron. Then it detaches and is either destroyed or taken back into the cell from which it was originally released (reuptake), where it may be reused or destroyed.

Organization of the Nervous System

The explanation of a neuron releasing a specific transmitter that stimulates or inhibits a postsynaptic membrane receptor and acts via negative feedback on a presynaptic receptor is accurate, but incomplete. Neurons release more than one chemical at a time (e.g., neuropeptides that may initiate long-term changes in the postsynaptic cells is a topic of investigation). Neuron development and responsiveness are also affected by chemicals brought by the blood (e.g., steroid hormones, as evidenced by psychosis resulting from hypersecretion of cortisol in Cushing's disease and use of prednisone to treat chronic inflammatory disease).

Brainstem

The brainstem regulates internal organs, is responsible for vital functions, and is the initial processing center for sensory information that is sent to the cerebral cortex. The reticular activating system (RAS) of the brainstem regulates sleep-wakefulness, and, by reaching into the limbic system of the cerebrum, affects the ability of the cerebrum to carry out conscious mental activity. The mesolimbic and mesocortical pathways project into the limbic system and seem to have a role in modulating the emotional value of sensory material.

Cerebellum

The cerebellum regulates skeletal muscle coordination and the maintenance of equilibrium.

Cerebrum

The cerebrum is responsible for mental activities, conscious perception, emotional states, memory, control of skeletal muscles for willful movement, language, and communication. The cerebral cortex is responsible for conscious sensation and initiation of movement. Basal ganglia, areas of integrating gray matter within the cerebrum, are involved in movement regulation, and the amygdala and hippocampus are involved in the emotions, learning, memory, and basic drives. As a consequence, drugs used to treat emotional disturbances may cause movement disorders, and drugs used to treat movement disorders may cause emotional changes.

Imaging techniques are used to visualize brain structure. Structural techniques—computed tomography (CT) and magnetic resonance imaging (MRI)—scans can identify gross anatomical changes in the brain. Functional imaging techniques—positron emission tomography (PET) and single photon emission computed tomography (SPECT) scans—identify physiological and biochemical changes in live tissue. Functional scans suggest the frontal cortex as the site of impairment in people with schizophrenia and people with obsessive-compulsive disorder (OCD), and the prefrontal cortex as the site of impairment in individuals with depression. It is presently thought that the limbic system (with its group of structures that includes parts of the frontal cortex, the basal ganglia, and brainstem) is a major locus of psychological activity. Within these areas, monoamine transmitters (norepinephrine, dopamine, serotonin), acetylcholine, γ-aminobutyric acid (GABA), glutamate, CRH, and endorphin are found and may provide targets for pharmacological treatment.

Disturbances of Mental Function

Some mental disturbances are related to certain drugs (e.g., LSD), excess levels of hormones (e.g., cortisol), infection (e.g., AIDS), or physical trauma (e.g., strokes). Others are of unknown etiology but may well be related to genetic factors. The incidence of both thought and mood disorders is higher in relatives of people with these diseases than in the general population. Neurotransmitters that have most consistently been linked to mental activity are norepinephrine, dopamine, serotonin, GABA, glutamate, and CRH. A particular transmitter is

Continued

21

often used by different neurons to carry out quite different functions; thus alterations in transmitter activity can affect more than one area of brain activity. Alterations in mental status, whether arising from disease or medication, are often accompanied by changes in basic drives, sleep patterns, body movement, and autonomic functions.

Mechanisms of Action of Psychotropic Drugs

Important concepts: pharmacodynamics—refers to the actions of the drug on the person (large-scale and molecular); pharmacokinetics—refers to the actions of the person on the drug (absorption, excretion, etc.).

An ideal psychotropic drug would relieve mental disturbance without inducing untoward mental or physical effects.

Most psychotropic drugs act by either increasing or decreasing the activity of certain transmitter-receptor systems.

Specific transmitter-receptor systems are targets for drug action.

Antipsychotic Drugs
Standard First-Generation Antipsychotics

These include the phenothiazines, thioxanthenes, butyrophenones, and so on. These drugs are strong antagonists of the D_2 receptors for dopamine. Blocking dopamine reduces the positive symptoms of schizophrenia such as delusions and hallucinations. These drugs also act as antagonists at muscarinic receptors for acetylcholine, α_1 receptors for norepinephrine, and H_1 receptors for histamine. Major side effects of these drugs arise from receptor-blocking activity: dopamine blockade gives rise to motor disturbances, including parkinsonism, akinesia, akathisia, dyskinesia, and tardive dyskinesia. Involuntary motor movement can be monitored via the abnormal involuntary movement scale (AIMS). Muscarinic receptor blockage leads to anticholinergic effects such as blurred vision, dry mouth, constipation, and urinary hesitancy. Blockade of α_1 receptors for norepinephrine is responsible for vasodilation and a consequent orthostatic hypotension, and for ejaculatory failure as well. Blockade of H_1 receptors contributes to sedation and substantial weight gain.

Atypical Antipsychotics

These cause few to no extrapyramidal symptoms. They also target the negative symptoms of schizophrenia as well as the positive symptoms. The difference in motor disturbances results due to their binding dopamine receptors in the limbic system preferentially over those in the basal ganglia. They are also antagonists at the 5-hydroxytryptamine α_2 (5-HTα_2) receptors for serotonin, which may explain their efficacy in treating the negative symptoms of schizophrenia.

Clozapine

May induce agranulocytosis, so frequent white blood cell (WBC) counts are required. It may also induce convulsions in a small percentage of clients. Common side effects are drowsiness, hypersalivation, tachycardia, and dizziness. Danger of agranulocytosis removes it from first-line usage.

Risperidone

Reduces delusions and hallucinations. Blocks α_1 and H_1 receptors and can cause orthostatic hypotension and sedation.

Quetiapine

Broad receptor binding profile produces sedation and weight gain along with symptoms associated with muscarinic and α_1 blockade. Extrapyramidal symptoms are few.

Other Atypical Antipsychotics
Olanzapine

Same profile as clozapine but without agranulocytosis. Major disadvantage is weight gain.

Ziprasidone

A serotonin-norepinephrine reuptake inhibitor. The major side effects are hypotension and sedation. One major safety concern is prolongation of the QT_c interval, which can be fatal if a client has a history of cardiac arrhythmia.

Aripiprazole

A unique atypical known as a dopamine system stabilizer. Side effects include sedation, hypotension, and anticholinergic effects.

Mood Stabilizers
Lithium

The mechanism of action is unknown but is probably related to affecting electrical conductivity in neurons. It may interact with sodium and potassium at the cell membrane to stabilize electrical activity. Such a mechanism of action would explain its ability to induce cardiac dysrhythmias, convulsions, and tremor. Lithium can also create fluid balance disturbances. For these reasons it has a low therapeutic index (ratio of lethal dose to effective dose) and requires close monitoring of serum lithium level.

Antiepileptic Drugs

These alter electrical conductivity in membranes and reduce the firing rate of very-high-frequency neurons in the brain. This action may account for their use in reducing mood swings in bipolar clients. Drugs in this group include carbamazepine (Tegretol), divalproex sodium (Depakote), and clonazepam (Klonopin), which has strong sedating properties.

Carbamazepine

Carbamazepine (Tegretol) is structurally similar to the tricyclic antidepressants. It treats unipolar depression. It is particularly effective in conditions such as trigeminal neuralgia. The efficacy of the drug as an analgesic may be related to its ability to reduce the firing rate of overexcited neurons as well as to its ability to calm the accompanying psychological agitation associated with the pain. Some common side effects include nausea, sedation, and ataxia. The therapeutic blood level is monitored regularly.

Divalproex

Divalproex (Depakote) is an anticonvulsant. It is structurally different from other anticonvulsants and psychiatric drugs. It is effective in treating manic depression. Common side effects include hair loss, tremor, weight gain and sedation. A baseline of liver function tests and CBC are done before an individual is started on this medication and periodically. Monitoring of the therapeutic blood level is done regularly as well.

Other Agents

Other anticonvulsants used as mood stabilizers are lamotrigine (Lamictal), gabapentin (Neurontin), and topiramate (Topamax). Clonazepam (Klonopin) is structurally a benzodiazepine, a type of antianxiety medication. It has strong sedating properties, which may account for its ability to calm a patient in the manic phase of a bipolar disorder. It may be used with lithium to increase the time between mood cycles, and it may also be used as part of a multiple-drug regimen to treat clients who show a mixture of anxious and depressive symptoms concomitantly. The serious drawback with clonazepam is that clients can develop tolerance and dependence. Baseline lab studies include CBC, liver function, and renal function tests.

Antidepressant Drugs

Evidence points to the cause of depression as a transmission deficiency of norepinephrine or serotonin or both within the limbic system.

Typical or Standard Antidepressants

Amitriptyline, imipramine, and nortriptyline—tricyclic antidepressants (TCAs)—act primarily by blocking reuptake of norepinephrine and, to a lesser degree, serotonin; thus norepinephrine is not degraded by monoamine oxidase (MAO), and more stays at the synapse. TCAs block muscarinic receptors, giving anticholinergic effects. Some TCAs block H_1 receptors in the brain, producing drowsiness.

Continued

23

CHAPTER OUTLINE	TEACHING STRATEGIES
Selective Serotonin Reuptake Inhibitors	Fluoxetine, sertraline, paroxetine, and citalopram block the reuptake of serotonin with little or no effect on the other monoamine transmitters. These drugs have less ability to block muscarinic and H_1 receptors than do the tricyclics (TCAs).
Monoamine Oxidase Inhibitors	Phenelzine and tranylcypromine: Monoamine neurotransmitters, as well as any monoamine food substance or drug, are degraded by the enzyme MAO. These drugs act by inhibiting the enzyme MAO, interfering with the destruction of monoamine neurotransmitters and increasing the synaptic level of the transmitters. In the presence of MAO inhibitors (MAOIs), tyramine is not destroyed in the liver, resulting in hypertensive crisis. Thus when MAOIs are taken, the client must observe a tyramine-free diet.
Atypical or Novel Antidepressants	Trazodone is a weak antagonist of muscarinic receptors so produces few anticholinergic effects. However, it blocks α_1 and H_1 receptors, causing orthostatic hypotension and sedation.
	Nefazodone is a relative of trazodone. It exerts no α_1 and H_1 receptor blockade. Venlafaxine blocks reuptake of both norepinephrine and serotonin, but does not block muscarinic, α_1, or H_1 receptors. It may produce feelings of anxiety, nausea, vomiting, and dizziness. Mirtazapine acts on $5\text{-}HT_2$ and α_2 presynaptic norepinephrine receptors, accounting for its antidepressant effect. Side effects of sedation, weight gain, dry mouth, and constipation are related to its actions as an antagonist at H_1 and muscarinic receptors. Bupropion has as its major side effects headache, insomnia, nausea, and restlessness.
Antianxiety or Anxiolytic Drugs	GABA exerts an inhibitory effect on neurons in many parts of the brain. Drugs that enhance this effect exert a sedative-hypnotic action on brain function and reduce anxiety.
Benzodiazepines	Diazepam, clonazepam, and alprazolam bind to specific receptors adjacent to GABA receptors. Benzodiazepine binding at sites adjacent to GABA binding allows GABA to inhibit more forcefully than it would if binding alone. Benzodiazepine potentiation of GABA accounts for its use as an anticonvulsant and its efficacy in reducing neuronal overexcitement in alcohol withdrawal. These drugs can also interfere with motor ability, attention, and judgment.
Buspirone	Buspirone reduces anxiety without strong sedative-hypnotic effects. Its action is unclear, but it may block presynaptic $5\text{-}HT_1$ receptors, preventing negative feedback and allowing more transmitter to be released.
Antidepression Treatment of Conditions Associated with Anxiety	Antidepressants have been found to be useful in the treatment of anxiety disorders: imipramine to treat panic attack, selective serotonin reuptake inhibitors (SSRIs) for OCD, and sertraline for social phobias.
Treatment of Attention Deficit Hyperactivity Disorder	Psychostimulant drugs such as methylphenidate and amphetamines show efficacy in these conditions.
Drug Treatment for Alzheimer's Disease	Much of the memory loss of Alzheimer's disease has been attributed to dysfunction of neurons that secrete acetylcholine. The anticholinesterase drugs tacrine and donepezil work by inactivating the enzyme that destroys acetylcholine.
Herbal Medicine	Today, many individuals believe that herbal medications or supplements are safer and have fewer side effects because they are "natural." Herbs are thought to be less costly than traditional medicines.
	During an intake assessment and ongoing interviews with clients, the nurse should include a nonjudgmental set of questions about the client's use of herbs or other supplements in order to have a holistic view of the client's health and treatment status.

24

4 Psychiatric Mental Health Nursing and Managed Care Issues

THOUGHTS ABOUT TEACHING THE TOPIC

This chapter presents a brief overview of what professional psychiatric nurses do, gives a brief history of the evolution of psychiatric nursing, alerts readers to current issues in managed care, and suggests future trends. Helping students gain an overview of the work of the psychiatric nurse and the levels of practice is fundamental to the course. An explanation of the role of the case manager should be given and a look at future trends in psychiatric health care skills should be a concentration in this course.

KEY TERMS AND CONCEPTS

advanced practice registered nurse—psychiatric mental health (APRN-PMH), 65
basic level registered nurse, 65
case management, 67
client advocate, 69
community nursing center, 66
evidence-based practice, 65
health maintenance organizations, 66
managed behavioral health care organizations (MBHOs), 66
managed care, 66
Nursing Interventions Classification (NIC), 64
Nursing Outcomes Classification (NOC), 64

phenomena of concern, 64
preferred provider organizations, 66
psychiatric nursing, 64
telehealth, 68

OBJECTIVES

After studying this chapter, the reader will be able to
1. Define psychiatric mental health nursing and discuss the client population served by the psychiatric nurse.
2. Explain the reasons for using standardized classification systems (North American Nursing Diagnosis Association, Nursing Interventions Classification, Nursing Outcomes Classification) in psychiatric nursing practice.
3. Compare and contrast the nursing actions of the basic level psychiatric nurse with those of the advanced level psychiatric nurse.
4. Describe recent developments that have increased the biological emphasis in psychiatric mental health nursing.
5. Discuss the impact of managed care on psychiatric nursing roles.
6. Explore emerging roles for the future of psychiatric nursing related to scientific and social trends.
7. Explain how Forchuk's case management model incorporates elements of Peplau's theory.

CHAPTER OUTLINE	TEACHING STRATEGIES
What Is Psychiatric Mental Health Nursing?	The American Nurses Association (ANA), American Psychiatric Nurses Association (APNA), and International Society of Psychiatric-Mental Health Nurses (ISPN) define who diagnoses and treats human responses to actual or potential mental health problems. Psychiatric nurses use both primary sources (client interview and client observation) and secondary sources (chart; family, friends, others; staff) to make assessments, nursing diagnoses, and to care plans.
Levels of Psychiatric Mental Health Clinical Nursing Practice	Levels of psychiatric mental health nursing clinical practice are differentiated by educational preparation, professional experience, and certification.
Basic Level	A psychiatric mental health registered nurse holds a baccalaureate in nursing and may become certified. Certification demonstrates that the nurse has met the profession's standards of knowledge and experience in the specialty. Name is followed by RNC (registered nurse clinician).

Continued

25

| CHAPTER OUTLINE | TEACHING STRATEGIES |

Advanced Level

An advanced practice registered nurse–psychiatric mental health (APRN-PMH) will have preparation at the master's degree or higher level in psychiatric nursing.

An advanced practice registered nurse–psychiatric mental health, certified specialist (RNCS) indicates certified advanced practice in the specialty by either a clinical nurse specialist or nurse practitioner.

What Do Psychiatric Nurses Do?

According to ANA Standards of Practice, basic level psychiatric mental health RNs focus on the following:
- Counseling, including crisis intervention
- Managing the therapeutic milieu
- Assisting client with self-care activities
- Administering and monitoring psychobiological treatments
- Teaching health, including psychoeducation
  Psychiatric rehabilitation
  Telehealth
  Community-based care, outreach activities
- Providing culturally relevant health promotion and disease prevention
- Case management
  Advocacy

Advanced level psychiatric mental health advanced practice RNs provide the following:
- All interventions practiced by RNs at the basic level
- Psychotherapy—individual, group, family, and other selected therapeutic treatments
- Pharmacological management (by prescribing drugs in accordance with state's nurse practice act)
- Consultation-liaison activities
  Complementary interventions
  Clinical supervisory activities
  Expanded advocacy activities

Recent Issues Affecting Psychiatric Mental Health Nursing

New understanding of neurophysiology and neuroanatomy of the brain has come about with new imaging techniques. There is evidence that many of the most serious mental disorders are psychobiological. Treatment emphasis is on psychopharmacology. The nurse is cautioned to remember that psychosocial nurses need to continue to grow in their capacity to help people with the quality of their lives through psychoeducational approaches, clarification of verbal content, alternation of environment stimuli, family systems intervention, and the classic application of the therapeutic nurse-client relationship.

Mental Health and Managed Care

Managed care attempts to provide high-quality care for less cost than previously and with more accountability to the payer. New strategies have evolved: preadmission reviews, continuing treatment authorizations, concurrent reviews, screen design to determine the appropriateness of treatment plans. The cornerstone of managed care is capitation, whereby a fixed amount of money is allocated to provide all aspects of needed health care for a client. Three common forms of managed care plans are health maintenance organizations (HMOs), preferred provider organizations (PPOs), and point of service plans (POSs). The managed behavioral health care organization (MBHO) is the term applied to managed care for mental health and substance abuse disorders. A problem seen by many is that HMOs experience maximum profit when services are limited; thus a subtle pressure against treatment is exerted. Individuals may have difficulty finding and accessing services, services may be denied, follow-up may be limited, coordination among providers and lack of continuity may be experienced. A positive aspect of managed care is the new services that have come about: extended office hours, telephone triage, and telehealth services.

26

Variability of nursing activity is based on setting and geographical location, but both the basic practice nurse and the advanced practice nurse can assume a number of roles in the MBHO, namely, clinical care manager or case manager; assessment, evaluation triage and referral nurse; client and family educator; risk manager, chief quality officer, and utilization review nurse; marketing and development specialist; corporate executive.

Future Challenges and Roles for Nurses

Future trends for psychiatric nursing indicate the need to strengthen current roles and to develop novel approaches to patient care. Psychiatric illnesses are expected to contribute 11% to 15% of the world's diseases in this century; therefore, there will be an increased need for psychiatric clinicians.

Shorter hospital stays have increased the need for community-based support for people with mental illnesses. Nurses are increasingly involved in providing primary and preventive care in community settings, including urban, rural, and school-based clinics. Another focus is on the population with prolonged mental illness, intervening with acute exacerbations, stabilization, and rehabilitative care. Astute assessment and evaluation skills are needed.

As community care continues to dominate psychiatric nursing, nurses will need to enhance their case management skills. As case managers, psychiatric nurses will find an increased need for care of individuals in home care for the elderly, children, and adolescents. Also, community nursing centers will continue to survive to serve low-income and uninsured people as long as they can secure funding.

Three more trends will affect the future of psychiatric nursing: the aging of the population, increasing cultural diversity, and ever-expanding technology. The number of elderly Americans with Alzheimer's disease and other dementias will require skilled nursing care in institutions. The healthier elderly will need services at home, in retirement communities, or in assisted living facilities.

It is projected that by the year 2050, the majority of the population will be people of color, and nurses will need to be sensitive to the different cultural needs of the population that they will serve.

Psychiatric nurses will also need to remain current with technology advances that can shape their practice. There will be an increased need for nurses to understand research and help promote and propose research areas that will address prevention of mental illness and early treatment and intervention as new methodologies become available.

Technology is also important in areas of nurse's communication, patient care, and patient teaching. The Internet and telehealth can provide individuals with health lines to care from a totally new perspective. This will mean that psychiatric nurses must remain current and become more active in providing patient care in new and innovative ways.

Finally, the psychiatric nurse will have an advocacy role in protecting the rights of clients with psychiatric disabilities. This role needs to continue to evolve. The nurse must be vigilant about local and national legislation affecting health care to identify potential detrimental effects on the mentally ill.

We know that mental health care looks much different today than it did a half century ago. We have more and better services for more individuals, but we also know that we still have individuals who do not receive decent mental health care. As concerned professionals, we need to continue to make required improvements toward the goal of serving those who are in need of mental health care in local, rural, and remote geographical areas.

27

5 Mental Health Nursing in Acute Care Settings

THOUGHTS ABOUT TEACHING THE TOPIC

Some instructors assign this chapter early, sometimes as part of the course orientation. It provides excellent information about what to expect in the inpatient setting. Topics covered in the chapter may be easily interwoven into the orientation. The use of vignettes can help students better understand the topics presented.

KEY TERMS AND CONCEPTS

OBJECTIVES

After studying this chapter, the reader will be able to
1. Analyze the psychiatric hospital experience from the client's perspective.
2. Explain how the mental health team collaborates to plan and implement care for the hospitalized client.
3. Describe the role of the nurse as advocate and provider of care for the client.
4. Explain the interrelationships among the managed care system, treatment planning, and the role of the case manager.
5. Discuss the managerial and coordinating roles of nursing on an inpatient acute care unit.
6. Discuss the process for preparing clients to return to the community for ongoing care.

CHAPTER OUTLINE	TEACHING STRATEGIES
Admission and Goals	Admission to an acute care setting is usually reserved for those conditions that require immediate assessment, stabilization, and symptom management. Most psychiatric health care inpatient settings today are found in a general hospital or at psychiatric hospitals, which provide only mental health services. Current criteria for admission include: the patient's clear danger to self or others; the client's inability to care for self and is therefore in danger of decompensation or is facing harmful consequences of an inadequate treatment capability for a mental disorder.
	Therefore, goals for acute psychiatric hospitalization include: prevention of self-harm or harm by others; stabilization of crisis with a return to the community; utilizing medication adjustment, partial hospitalization programs or another intensive daily service for patient re-stabilization.
Rights of the Hospitalized Client	Although hospitalized, the client retains rights as a citizen. Statements of rights are usually posted prominently on the unit, contained in client handbooks, and included in unit policy and procedure manuals. Specific rights are summarized in Box 5-1. Students are referred to agency client handbooks and unit policy and procedure manuals.
Interdisciplinary Teamwork and Care Management	Care planning and implementation are the responsibility of the interdisciplinary team of nurse, social worker, counselor, psychologist, occupational and activities therapists, psychiatrist, medical doctor, pharmacist, and mental health workers. Nurses frequently convene and lead planning meetings. With so many disciplines needing to make assessments, timing becomes an important issue. The first to assess are usually the intake worker, nurse, and psychiatrist. When the team meets initially, a plan of care is developed, often by individualizing or customizing a standard plan or critical pathway. Specific assessments, interventions, treatments, and outcomes are delineated along a designated timeline. The plan is monitored and facilitated by a specific caregiver or case manager.

28

CHAPTER OUTLINE	TEACHING STRATEGIES
Psychiatric Case Management	Case managers are defined as client advocates who interact with and assess clients and family, coordinate services appropriate to the client, monitor the delivery of services, and evaluate the outcome for the client. Case managers communicate with the client's insurer and provide the treatment team with guidance regarding the availability of resources. Appropriate care focuses on rapid assessment and stabilization, as well as discharge planning and follow-up within an integrated system. See the vignettes in the text for further examples.
Nursing on the Inpatient Unit **Management**	The management of daily unit functioning is assumed by nurses even when a program manager or clinical coordinator exists. (Programmatic staff services include social services, activities, occupational therapy [OT], and specialized counseling services.) The nurse manager is responsible for unit safety, effectiveness of delivery of services, and integration of services of the treatment team.
Therapeutic Strategies	Psychiatric nurses implement a major portion of the treatment plan, using formal and informal contacts. Counseling skills provide the basis for many nursing interventions.
MILIEU **Group Activities**	Experienced mental health nurses conduct specific, structured activities involving the therapeutic community, special groups, or families (e.g., goal-setting and goal-review meetings, community meetings, psychoeducational groups, and groups for creative expression).
Management of Milieu	Nurses are responsible for maintaining the milieu by monitoring and keeping communication open and constructively honest, involving clients in some decisions and explaining decisions that must be left to the staff, explaining and enforcing unit limits and rules.
Safety	Nurses are responsible for vigilance regarding safety hazards; preventing and responding to fire; supervising the unit system for maintaining knowledge of whereabouts of every client at all times; safety checks, both periodic and constant; sharp objects control; flow of visitors and objects onto the unit; prevention of illegal drug use; prevention of illicit sexual activity; prevention and containment of violence; prevention of elopement.
Documentation	Documentation is the responsibility of the entire team. The system of documentation chosen must meet professional standards, and legal, reimbursement, and accreditation requirements; and it must lend itself to retrieval for quality assurance (QA), utilization review, and research.
Psychopharmacological **Responsibilities**	Nurses are responsible for safe administration and monitoring of medications. Administering medications prn is the responsibility of the nurse who weighs client requests, does team planning, and attempts to use alternative coping strategies, using nursing judgment regarding timing and client behavior.
Crisis Management	Nurses anticipate, prevent, and manage emergencies and crises of a medical or behavioral nature on the unit. Medical crisis management calls for rapid assessment of common medical emergencies, cardiopulmonary resuscitation (CPR) skills, and use of basic emergency equipment. Behavioral crisis management requires rapid assessment, early intervention, and organized response to behavioral crises, such as violence or suicide attempts.
Preparation for Discharge **to the Community**	Nurses help clients and clients' families learn coping skills that will help them avert future crises and hospitalization. Discharge planning begins at admission and seeks a seamless transition from hospital to community.
Policy Review and Revision	Nurses participate in decisions about the care system and working environment, addressing issues such as scheduling activities, work schedules, assignments, expanding professional practice, and safety.

29

6 Mental Health Nursing in Community Settings

THOUGHTS ABOUT TEACHING THE TOPIC

Psychiatric nursing faculty teaching in associate degree programs often have more inpatient psychiatric nursing experience than community nursing experience. As a result, faculty may need to investigate opportunities for student experience in the community.

Alternatives to inpatient experiences may not be available in great numbers, but still can be used by assigning selected students to observe and participate to the extent permitted by the agency. Students who are assigned to these experiences should understand that they are expected to share their observations with classmates in structured discussions. Community-based nurses may be reluctant to take on the role of preceptor to students in addition to the duties of their busy practice world. The simplicity of expectations associated with the role can be reinforced by holding a short preceptor preparation workshop. In many educational settings the preceptors cannot be paid, and many settings may not even offer tuition benefits. Thus, it is helpful to the process of obtaining and retaining preceptors to offer as many social amenities as possible (e.g., letters of appointment as unpaid adjunct faculty, personal notes of thanks, letters of appreciation to be placed in personnel files, refreshments served at meetings, etc).

Since time may not permit in-depth classroom exploration of local mental health resources, the process of students independently learning about the resources of the community should be encouraged.

KEY TERMS AND CONCEPTS

barriers to treatment, 95
continuum of psychiatric mental health treatment, 90
deinstitutionalization, 86
ethical dilemmas, 95
seriously mentally ill, 86

OBJECTIVES

After studying this chapter, the reader will be able to
1. Explain the evolution of the community mental health movement.
2. Identify elements of the nursing assessment that are critically important to the success of community treatment.
3. Distinguish between the hospital and community settings with regard to characteristics, goals of treatment, and nursing interventions.
4. Compare and contrast the roles of the nurse in community mental health according to the nurse's educational preparation.
5. Explain the role of the nurse as the biopsychosocial care manager in the multidisciplinary team.
6. Discuss the continuum of psychiatric treatment.
7. Describe the role of the psychiatric nurse in four specific settings: partial hospitalization program; psychiatric home care; assertive community treatment; and community mental health center.
8. Identify two resources to assist the community psychiatric nurse in resolving ethical dilemmas.
9. Discuss barriers to mental health treatment.

CHAPTER OUTLINE	TEACHING STRATEGIES
Context for Psychiatric Nursing in the Community	The Community Mental Health Centers Act of 1963 heralded the era of deinstitutionalization. Federal entitlement programs (Social Security Disability, Supplemental Security Income [SSI], Medicare, Medicaid, housing assistance, food stamps) proliferated, making it possible for mentally ill individuals to live outside a hospital. Additional impetus was given to the expansion of community-based care in the 1980s, when President Carter's Commission on Mental Health highlighted the needs of the underserved chronically mentally ill. The term *transinstitutionalization* was coined to describe the process of providing institutional services in settings outside the institution. Recent research suggests that psychiatric nursing care is provided in increasingly diverse settings, including the criminal justice setting, school-based clinics, crisis centers, shelters, chemical dependency program offices, nursing homes, industry, churches, etc.
Aspects of Community Nursing	Psychiatric nursing is markedly different in the community than in hospital settings. It requires the nurse to know about many community resources, to be flexible in problem solving with client and family, and to assess support systems and

30

	living needs. The nurse is a guest in the environment of the client who requests consultation. Transition to the community setting is an acculturation process involving value clarification. Helpful personal characteristics are reviewed. The goal is to empower the client and support self-management to the extent possible given the client's disability.
Psychiatric Nursing Assessment Strategies	Assessment in the community requires enhanced understanding of the client's ability to cope with the demands of living in the community. The nurse will assess the client's needs in areas such as his or her ability to access community resources independently; financial circumstances, including ability to afford treatment and to purchase medication; availability of safe, affordable housing; access to activity; ability to afford and prepare nutritious food; and legal entanglements. Individual characteristics such as culture and language may require use of an interpreter or cultural consultant.
Psychiatric Nursing Intervention Strategies	In hospital settings, the focus of care is on stabilization and is determined by the staff. In community settings, treatment goals and interventions are negotiated, not imposed. Interventions are often directed not only at symptoms but toward facilitation of access to, and continuation of support for, basic needs such as housing and food. The nurse, instead of working with hospital staff, works with community resource people, such as the police, clergy, and landlord. The use of case management helps to achieve positive outcomes.
Roles and Functions of the Community Psychiatric Nurse	The roles and functions of the community psychiatric nurse are fluid, but to some extent dependent upon level of preparation. Advanced practice nurses function more independently; they have consultative skills, usually have prescriptive authority, and often have hospital privileges.
Member of Multidisciplinary Community Practice Team	Psychiatric mental health nurses were identified in 1963 as core members of the multidisciplinary team. Increasingly, advanced practice nurses are assuming multidisciplinary team leadership—a role once reserved for psychiatrists.
Biopsychosocial Care Manager	A role that is increasingly fulfilled by nurses is that of biopsychosocial care manager. This role includes coordination of mental health, physical health, social service, educational service, medication management, and vocational aspects of care and the services required. Care management is essential to cost-effective care.
Community Settings	As the financial, health care, regulatory, cultural, and population changes, so do the roles and settings of psychiatric nurses. Nurses are providing primary mental health care at therapeutic day care centers, partial hospitalization programs, and shelters. There are also newer environments for care including forensic settings and drug and alcohol treatment centers where psychiatric nurses are caring for clients. Mobile mental health units have been developed, and a growing number of communities and mental health programs are collaborating with other health or community services to provide integrated approaches to treatment. Technology is also contributing to the changes in community settings by providing services such as telephone crisis counseling, telephone outreach, and even the Internet to enhance access to mental health services. The services that the psychiatric nurse can provide include counseling, promotion of self-care activities, psychobiological interventions, health teaching, and case management.
Partial Hospitalization Program	Partial hospitalization programs (PHPs) offer short-term intensive treatment and education for clients. The client is receiving care for a part of the day and then is able to remain living in the community for part of the day.
	The criteria for referral to a PAP can include a need to prevent hospitalization or as a step-down from acute inpatient treatment. The client usually attends a PHP

Continued

31

for 5 or 6 hours daily. Some programs operate 7 days per week, and clients will attend the PHP for approximately 1 month. Some of the goals the multidisciplinary team may identify for clients are: clients to be able to identify their medications, and clients to be able to identify triggers to a relapse of their disease symptoms. Client goals can also include work toward self-control and client perception of support from health care providers. Have the student utilize the vignettes in the text to explore in more detail some of the nursing skills utilized by psychiatric nurses in PHP programs.

Psychiatric Home Care

Home care improves the potential for clients who are homebound or who would otherwise avoid care to receive treatment. To make contact with suspicious or reclusive clients, however, the nurse may need to be accompanied by a relative or friend of the client. It is noted that, in the home, the client is in charge and the nurse must use nonauthoritarian strategies such as persuasion and negotiation to intervene. Utilize the text vignettes to help students become more familiar with home care psychiatric nursing.

Assertive Community Treatment

Assertive Community Treatment (ACT) teams or mobile treatment teams work with the mentally ill clients who cannot effectively use traditional services. Patients can be referred from inpatient or outpatient facilities where the health care workers find a pattern of repeated hospitalization for severe symptoms along with an inability to participate in more traditional treatments. Treatment is delivered in many sites such as a fast food restaurant or other community sites. The outcomes related to nursing care on an ACT team may include client avoids alcohol and recreational drugs and performs treatment regimen as prescribed. Clients will also need to use health services congruent with their needs and will exhibit reality-based thinking. Again, utilize the vignettes in the text to help students understand the role of the psychiatric nurse as a member of the ACT team.

Community Mental Health Center

Created in the 1960s, community mental health centers provide a wide range of services for those who have no access to private care. These services are enumerated in the text.

Ethical Issues

Ethical dilemmas are common in disciplines that care for the vulnerable and disenfranchised. There is often dissonance between what is best for the individual and what is best for the community. The role of the nurse is to act, as far as possible, in the best interests of the client and of society. Boards of nursing or professional nursing organizations can be used as a resource by the individual practitioners concerning dilemmas that arise related to issues of client care and ethical dilemmas.

Future Issues

The current health care environment is offering a variety of services to the mentally ill client, but there are some mentally ill individuals who are still not receiving the mental health care that they need. There remain barriers to care such as the stigma of mental illness, and geographic financial and systems factors that impede access to psychiatric care.

To meet the needs of the mentally ill individuals in this country, educators need to increase the focus on leadership development include principles of home health nursing, increase content on gerontology, and introduce basic community health concepts. This will enable RNs who choose to work in the community psychiatric nursing field to work closely with primary health care practitioners, the community members and agencies, and be better equipped to utilize creative sites and services to meet the needs of psychiatric mental health clients who need the mental health services in community settings.

7 Culturally Relevant Mental Health Nursing

Instructors should become familiar with the various cultures represented in their locale and be able to discuss their characteristics in terms of the concepts used in this chapter. One way of helping learners operationalize the concepts associated with cultural diversity is to compile several short vignettes with questions for classroom discussion.

Concepts introduced in this chapter relate to worldview, and associated assessment and intervention techniques that can be reinforced by considering the dynamics of caring for a diverse number of clients with diverse beliefs and values.

KEY TERMS AND CONCEPTS

acculturation, 108
assimilation, 108
bicultural, 108
cultural awareness, 110
cultural broker, 106
cultural competence, 110
cultural desire, 112
cultural encounters, 111
cultural imposition, 105
cultural knowledge, 110
cultural pain, 111
cultural skill, 111
culturally relevant nursing, 99
culture, 100
culture shock, 109
culture-bound syndromes, 107
Eastern tradition, 101
enculturation, 103

ethnicity, 100
ethnocentrism, 105
ethnopharmacology, 108
generalizations, 111
immigrants, 108
indigenous cultures, 102
intraethnic diversity, 111
limited English proficiency, 106
minority, 100
preserve-accommodate-restructure framework, 112
race, 100
refugee, 109
somatization, 106
stereotyping, 111
Western tradition, 101
worldview, 100

OBJECTIVES

After studying this chapter, the reader will be able to
1. Describe the importance of culturally relevant care in mental health nursing practice.
2. Discuss potential problems in applying American or Western psychological theory to clients of other cultures.
3. Compare and contrast American nursing beliefs, values, and practices with the beliefs, values, and practices of clients from diverse cultures.
4. Perform a culturally sensitive assessment, including an assessment for risk factors and barriers to quality mental health care that culturally diverse clients frequently encounter.
5. Develop a culturally appropriate nursing care plan for clients of diverse cultures.

CHAPTER OUTLINE	TEACHING STRATEGIES
Culture, Race, Ethnicity, and Minority Status	Mental health nurses need to practice relevant nursing if they are to meet th needs of their culturally diverse clients. Care for culturally diverse clients must be congruent with the needs of the client's values, beliefs, and practices. Therefore, the psychiatric nurse must have an understanding of the definitions and interrelationships of culture, race, ethnicity, and minority status.
	In the text, culture is described as the shared beliefs values, and practices that guide a group's members in patterned ways of thinking and acting. Cultural groups can be ethnic, religious, geographic, socioeconomic, occupational, etc. Each has cultural beliefs that guide the groups' members. The norms help members make sense of the world around them and help them make appropriate decisions

Continued

33

Chapter 7   Culturally Relevant Mental Health Nursing

	as to how they should relate and act. Therefore, culture helps develop what is "normal" and "abnormal," and thus it also helps to describe mental health and mental illness for a particular culture.
	Minority is more related to economic and social standing, whereas race is used to categorize people in social and political ways rather than in a biological mode.
	The benefit of categorizing groups of people into racial/ethnic categories helps the government know the needs of its citizens, but this system has some problems. Therefore, in order for mental health nurses to make good decisions about treatment for mental health patients, it is better to focus on ethnicity rather than on race.
Demographic Shifts	Presently 25% of the U.S. population self-identifies with one of the federally defined minority groups. The United States is becoming more diverse. With these changes, every mental health nurse will care for culturally diverse clients in daily practice. Therefore, mental health nurses need to provide culturally relevant care to all clients to prevent an increase in mental health care disparities.
Worldviews and Mental Health Nursing	Western science and European-American norms for mental health have grown out of a long history, the history of Western civilization. However, many people of the world have very different philosophical histories and traditions. The Eastern cultures of Asia are based on the philosophical thought of Chinese and Indian philosophers, and the spiritual traditions of Confucianism, Buddhism, and Taoism. Therefore, traditions have inspired different views of what it means "to be a person."
	Mental health nurses must recognize that nursing theories and methods are themselves part of a cultural tradition. When a nurse understands that many of the concepts and methods of care found in psychiatric mental health nursing are based in Western cultural care ideals, the nurse is beginning the process of becoming culturally competent.
Culture and Mental Health	According to the ANA, good nursing care adapts care to the client's cultural needs and preferences. Diverse cultures evolved from three worldviews. They are not static, they change and adjust, but usually very slowly. Members of the cultural group are introduced to the culture's worldview, beliefs, values, and practices in a process called enculturation. Members learn from living within the culture, what is "right" and "wrong." The individual is free to make choices, but the choices are limited by cultural expectations.
	Deviance from cultural expectations is considered, by others within the culture, to be a problem. Often mental health is seen as the degree to which a person fulfills the expectations of the culture. But the same thoughts and behaviors that are considered mentally healthy in one culture can be considered illness in another.
	Nurses must not impose their personal values and judgments onto patients (ethnocentrism, or the belief that one's own group is superior). Clients need to be given appropriate mental health care that will address their needs and be mindful of culturally diverse differences that each client can present.
Barriers to Quality Mental Health Services	The first part of the chapter focused on the impact of culture on mental health and illness in a theoretical way. This section focuses on providing care to culturally diverse clients.
Communication Barriers	Communication is a key to mental health care. Providing clients with interpreter services to meet their communication needs is important to assure that clients are receiving adequate care. The interpreter should be, as much as possible, matched in gender, age, social status, and religion as the client. This can help the inter-

Chapter 7   Culturally Relevant Mental Health Nursing

preter to not only translate the language, interpret nonverbal communication, but also help the nurse understand the client's culture through a cultural broker.

Misdiagnosis

Misdiagnosis can be an unfortunate outcome when inappropriate instruments are used to diagnose mental illness. Instruments need to be made for specific cultural groups so that cultural differences are utilized to diagnosis mental health disease.

When the body and mind are considered as one in a specific culture, utilizing a tool to interpret mental illness in a client from a different culture can result in a misdiagnosis. Therefore some cross-cultural mental heath experts are skeptical about using the *Diagnostic and Statistical Manual of Mental Disorders (DSM-IV-TR)* criteria fro diagnosing mental illness in culturally diverse populations, since criteria are based on predominately white American samples.

Some examples in the text of culture-bound illnesses include ghost illness, hwa-byung, or neurasthenia. These illness cannot be found in the *DSM-IV-TR* but are prominent in certain cultural groups.

Ethnic Variation in Pharmacodynamics

The third clinical practice issue addressed here is the pharmacodynamics of variations in drug metabolism. There is a growing realization that many drugs vary in their action and effect along genetic-ethnic lines. These genetic variations in drug metabolism are documented for several classifications of drugs, including antidepressants and antipsychotics.

Ethnopharmacology investigates these ethnic variations in drug pharmacokinetics. Making dosage variations in patients from different ethnic backgrounds is not enough to assure appropriate dosing and treatment.

Mental health nurses need to be aware that there are ethnic variations in drug metabolism so that they can recommend appropriate measures to assure effective treatment for clients with tolerable side effects.

Culturally Diverse Populations at Risk

Some of the challenges that diverse populations of mental health clients face can include issues related to the experience of being an immigrant, the socioeconomic disadvantages of minority status, and the severe stigma associated with mental health problems that is found in some cultural groups.

Immigrant Status

As immigrants, individuals face many unknowns upon arrival to this country. There are barriers to work; language barriers; their cultural traditions and values, which once provided them with stability, are challenged by new cultural norms. During the period of adjustment to a new country, many immigrants find that the hope they first felt on arrival has turned to anxiety and depression.

The acculturation process may take several generations or may be more quickly realized. Some individuals may become bicultural, whereas others suffer culture shock, not being able to adapt to new norms readily. Many families find that children adapt to a new cultural norm more easily than do adults. This sets the stage for intergenerational conflict.

Refugees are a special kind of immigrant. Refugees have left their homeland to escape intolerable conditions and would have preferred to stay in their own culture if that had been possible. Many refugees feel imposed upon. Many from Southeast Asia, Central America, and Africa have been traumatized by war, genocide, torture, and other catastrophic events. The trauma and loss make them vulnerable to posttraumatic stress disorder.

Continued

35

Minority Status

In the United States, the incidence of various types of mental health disorders among cultural and racial minority groups is similar to that of white Americans, if the poor and other vulnerable populations within the minority groups are excluded. The higher incidence of mental health problems in minority groups is related to poverty, not ethnicity.

People who live in poverty are two to three times more likely to develop mental illness than those who live above the poverty line. Poverty is highly associated with other disadvantages, such as scarce educational and economic opportunities, which in turn are associated with substance abuse and violent crime.

People from cultural minorities report that they have perceived bias from health care providers which was culturally uncomfortable, making them less likely to seek medical services in the future.

Stigma of Mental Illness

Many individuals in all sectors of American society associate mental health problems with moral weakness. In some cultural groups, the view is that mental illness is a failure of the family, which can bring shame and stigma as a result.

Culturally Competent Care

This chapter describes why the nursing needs of culturally diverse client populations may be different from the needs the nurse might otherwise assume. The cultural aspect of mental health care cannot be ignored if a nurse will provide holistic care. How do nurses provide culturally competent care? Care should include attitudes and behaviors that enable a nurse to work effectively within the client's cultural context, according to the Office of Minority Health. Culturally competent care goes beyond culturally sensitive care; it adapts care to the client's cultural needs and preferences.

Campinha-Bacote recommends a blueprint with the Process of Cultural Competence in the Delivery of Health Care Model. In this blueprint, nurses view themselves as becoming culturally competent rather than being culturally competent. Nurses remain open to learning rather than considering themselves as a culturally competent expert. The five constructs below are a part of the model.

Cultural Awareness

This construct indicates that the nurse is committed to "cultural humility," a lifetime commitment to self-evaluation and critique regarding one's level of cultural awareness. Through cultural awareness, the nurse recognizes that during an encounter with a patient, three cultures intersect: the culture of the client, the culture of the nurse, and the culture of the setting. In the nurse's role as a client advocate, the nurse negotiates and advocates on behalf of the client's cultural needs and preferences.

Cultural Knowledge

Nurses enhance their cultural knowledge by attending cultural events and programs, forging friendships with members of diverse cultural groups, and attend in-services at which members of diverse groups talk about their cultural norms. Nurses can also use Internet sources, such as the Evolve website, to enhance their knowledge level.

Resources and guides can include worldview, beliefs and values, nonverbal communication patterns, etiquette norms, family roles and psychosocial norms, cultural views about mental health and illness, and patterns related to health and illness.

Cultural Encounters

According to Campinha-Bacote multiple cultural encounters with diverse clients deters nurses from stereotyping. Each person is a unique blend of the many cultures that a person belongs to. The nurse comes to know that although there are patterns that characterize a culture, members of the culture adhere to the culture's norms in diverse ways. The best source of information about a client's culture is the client.

Chapter 7   Culturally Relevant Mental Health Nursing

CHAPTER OUTLINE	TEACHING STRATEGIES
Cultural Skill	Cultural skill is the ability to perform a cultural assessment in a sensitive way. The first step is to assure meaningful communication. Utilization of an interpreter, if needed, should be engaged. The nurse has many various cultural assessment tools that are available to help give an accurate assessment of the client's mental health.
	Areas that deserve special attention during a client mental health assessment include: ethnicity and religious affiliation, spiritual practices, degree of proficiency with speaking/reading English, dietary patterns, attitudes about pain and experiences with pain, attitudes about and experiences with Western medicines, and other cultural considerations.
	The nurse must develop a therapeutic plan that is mutually agreeable, culturally acceptable, and potentially capable of producing positive outcomes. Leininger suggests a preserve-accommodate-restructure framework for care planning. This framework helps the nurse preserve the aspects of the client's culture that promotes health and well-being. The nurse also utilizes accommodation and restructuring to help clients establish a plan of care to provide the best outcome possible for the client.
Cultural Desire	Cultural desire prompts the nurses to have a genuine concern for client's welfare, and a willingness to listen until they truly understand the client's viewpoint. Cultural desire inspires openness and flexibility in applying nursing principles to meet the client's cultural needs.

8 Legal and Ethical Guidelines for Safe Practice

THOUGHTS ABOUT TEACHING THE TOPIC

Learners often find it difficult to simply read information about legal and ethical issues. Clarification via classroom discussion is frequently necessary. Further discussion in clinical conference will help in operationalizing concepts. Some learners find it easier to learn basic facts in an interactional format; for them computer-assisted instruction may be useful for portions of the content. You may also want to include case studies that encompass a patient who is hospitalized involuntarily.

KEY TERMS AND CONCEPTS

assault, 128
autonomy, 116
battery, 128
beneficence, 116
bioethics, 116
child abuse reporting statutes, 126
civil rights, 118
commitment, 120
conditional release, 121
confidentiality, 119
defamation of character, 127
discharge, 121
duty to warn, 125
elder abuse reporting statutes, 127
ethical dilemma, 116
ethics, 116
false imprisonment, 128
fidelity, 116
implied consent, 123
informed consent, 122
intentional tort, 128
involuntary admission, 120
involuntary outpatient commitment, 120
justice, 116

least restrictive alternative doctrine, 119
negligence, 129
punitive damages, 128
right to privacy, 125
right to refuse treatment, 122
right to treatment, 121
social norms, 117
tort, 127
veracity, 116
voluntary admission, 120
writ of habeas corpus, 119

OBJECTIVES

After studying this chapter, the reader will be able to

1. Compare and contrast the terms *ethics* and *bioethics,* and identify five principles of bioethics.
2. Discuss at least five client rights that come under the Patient's Bill of Rights.
3. Give examples of the client's (a) right to treatment, (b) right to refuse treatment, and (c) right to informed consent.
4. Identify the steps nurses are advised to take if they suspect negligence or illegal activity on the part of a professional colleague or peer.
5. Apply legal considerations of client privilege (a) after a client has died, (b) if the client tests positive for human immunodeficiency virus, or (c) if the client's employer states a "need to know."
6. Provide explanations for situations in which health care professionals have a duty to break client confidentiality.
7. Discuss a client's civil rights and how they pertain to restraint and seclusion.
8. Develop an awareness of the balance between the client's rights and the rights of society with respect to the following legal concepts relevant in nursing and psychiatric nursing: (a) duty to intervene, (b) documentation and charting, and (c) confidentiality.

CHAPTER OUTLINE	TEACHING STRATEGIES
Ethical Concepts	Ethics is the study of philosophical beliefs about what is considered right or wrong in a society. Bioethics is a term used in relation to ethical dilemmas surrounding client care.
	Five principles of bioethics are defined: beneficence, autonomy, justice, fidelity, and veracity. Resources that can help nurses resolve ethical dilemmas include legal advice, ANA code of ethics, nurse practice acts, hospital and organizational

	policies, patients' Bill of Rights, colleagues, clergy, as well as examination of one's own ideals and morals.
Mental Illness and the Social Norm	What constitutes desirable or acceptable behavior is decided by the society that establishes the norms. Methods of changing behavior are also decided by the society.
	The question is raised whether behavior modification and psychotropic drugs that alter behavior and thought processes are contrary to society's norms of freedom of expression.
Responsibilities of the Therapeutic Relationship	From an ethical perspective, the therapist has legal and ethical obligations to the client and society: not to abuse the power that can exist in the relationship, to demonstrate fidelity, to observe confidentiality, and to develop self-awareness.
Mental Health Laws	These laws are concerned with protecting the public safety and the rights of the individual client and are legislated at the state level.
Civil Rights	Mentally ill individuals are guaranteed the same rights under federal and state laws as any other citizen. Determination of legal competency may be necessary and is performed in the courts. A legal guardian will be appointed for the person whose mental illness renders him or her incompetent. It is essential for the nurse to know state laws regarding care and treatment of the mentally ill and to be familiar with policies of the agency in which he or she works.
SPECIFIC CLIENT RIGHTS	
Client Consent	This must be obtained for specific therapies and treatments and for participation in experiments or research.
Communication	Clients have the right to communicate fully and privately with those outside the facility, to access phones and mail, and to receive unopened correspondence.
Freedom from Harm	This prohibits abuse and neglect, overuse of medication, unnecessary physical restraint, and isolation for staff convenience or as punishment.
Dignity and Respect	This prohibits disrespectful staff behavior, and discrimination on the basis of ethnicity, gender, age, disability, or religion.
Confidentiality	Records are confidential and cannot be released without consent; no photos may be taken without consent. Discussions about clients are never held in public places.
Participation in Plan of Care	Clients have a right to a care plan that involves them in decision making and that is regularly reviewed. Clients have the right to be informed of benefits, risks, and side effects of all medications and treatment used and must give informed consent to the treatment to be used.
Admission, Commitment, and Discharge Procedures	
Due Process in Civil Commitment	Clients have a right to due process in civil commitment. All clients have the privilege of the writ of habeas corpus and the right to the least restrictive treatment.
Admission to the Hospital	Admission laws vary from state to state. Each nurse must become aware of the laws in his or her state. Admission status does not determine whether clients are capable of making informed decisions about health care, so involuntarily admitted clients may be capable of consenting to treatment. Both types of commitments give clients the right to retain freedom from unreasonable bodily restraints and the right to refuse medications.

Continued

Chapter 8   Legal and Ethical Guidelines for Safe Practice

Voluntary Admission

Sought by the client or client guardian through written application to the facility.

Involuntary Admission (Commitment)

Admission that is made without the client's consent. It is necessary when a person is a danger to self or others, is in need of psychiatric treatment, or is unable to meet his or her own basic needs. Three types of commitment procedures are commonly available: judicial, administrative, and agency. Involuntary hospitalization can be categorized by the nature and purpose of the admission: emergency, observational or temporary, indeterminate or extended stays.

Release from the Hospital

This depends on the client's admission status. Voluntary clients can demand and receive release.

Conditional Release

Conditional release usually requires outpatient treatment for a period of time.

Discharge

Discharge is unconditional release.

Client's Rights Under the Law
Right to Treatment

Federal law entitles any client hospitalized in a public hospital to treatment. Further treatment must be in a humane environment, by qualified and sufficient staff, and with an individualized plan of care.

Right to Refuse Treatment

A competent client may refuse treatment or withdraw consent for treatment at any time. However, the right to refuse treatment with psychotropic drugs is less clear. Forcible administration of medication is justified when the need to protect the public outweighs the possibility of harm to the medicated individual. A number of cases were reviewed to show the complexity of translating legal policy into legal standard.

Right to Informed Consent

A client has the right to determine what will be done with his or her body and must agree to invasive tests or treatments. When a client accepts medication, consent is implied.

Rights Surrounding Involuntary Commitment and Psychiatric Advance Directives

Clients concerned that they may be subject to involuntary psychiatric commitment can prepare an advance psychiatric directive document that will express their treatment choices.

Rights Regarding Restraint and Seclusion

These are authorized when a client's behavior is physically harmful to the client or others; when behavior presents a danger to the facility; when less restrictive measures are insufficient to protect the client or others; to decrease sensory overstimulation; or when the client requests a controlled environment. Restraint or seclusion is permitted only on the written order of a physician, for a specified time-limited period, with regular review and documentation of the client's condition. Any extension of the original order must be reauthorized. Restraints must be removed when client behavior indicates it is safe. While restrained the client must be protected from all sources of harm. Documentation must include specific ways in which client needs were met during restraint or seclusion. Restraint can never be used as punishment or for convenience of staff. The least restrictive means of restraint for the shortest possible duration is the rule.

Maintenance of Client Confidentiality
Ethical Considerations

The ANA code for nursing states a nurse safeguards the client's right to privacy by protecting information of a confidential nature. Breeches of confidentiality have ethical and legal ramifications.

Legal Considerations

The client's right to have treatment and medical records kept confidential is legally protected. Generally, the nurse's legal duty to maintain confidentiality is to act to protect the client's right to privacy. The legal privilege of confidentiality is legis-

	lated, so if it has not been legislated for nurses in a particular state, the nurse must respond to a court's inquiries regarding client disclosures even if the information implicates the client in a crime. Nurses must know the laws in their state relating to privileged communication and warning of infectious disease exposure.
Health Insurance Portability and Accountability Act	The psychiatric client's right to have treatment and medical records kept confidential is legally protected. The Health Insurance Portability and Accountability Act of 1996 (HIPAA) privacy rule states that you may not, without the client's consent, disclose information obtained from the client or information in the medical record to anyone except those necessary for implementation of a client's treatment plan.
Client's Employer	The nurse may not release information to the client's employer without the client's consent.
Rights After Death	The rule is: do not divulge information after a person's death that could not have been legally shared before the death.
Client Privilege and Human Immunodeficiency Virus Status	State laws vary. Nurses must understand the laws in their state.
Exceptions to the Rule **Duty to Warn and Protect Third Parties**	Nurses must know the state law regarding the necessity for therapists to warn and protect a third party if a client is dangerous or making threats against the party.
Child and Elder Abuse Reporting Statutes	All states and the District of Columbia have child abuse reporting statutes. Many require nurses to report cases of suspected child abuse. Many states have elder abuse reporting statutes, most of which require RNs and others to report cases of elder abuse.
Tort Law Applied to Psychiatric Settings	Torts are civil wrongs for which money damages are collected from the wrongdoer by the injured party.
Common Liability Issues **Protection of Clients**	Common legal issues relate to failure to protect the safety of clients. Examples: injury, miscommunication, medication errors, abuse of the therapist-client relationship, and misdiagnosis.
Defamation of Character	Can be charged if confidential information is divulged that results in harm to the client's reputation (e.g., confidentiality of HIV status of a client is breached).
Supervisory Liability	May be incurred if nursing duties are delegated to persons who cannot safely perform the duties.
Short-Staffing Issues	Short staffing has raised client safety concerns. Nurses should report short staffing using the agency procedure and should be careful not to work outside the scope of employment.
Intentional Torts	These require a voluntary act with intent to bring about a physical consequence, and include assault; battery; and false imprisonment. Many liability insurance policies do not cover intentional torts.
Assault and Battery	An assault is an act resulting in a person's apprehension of an immediate harmful or offensive touching (battery). In an assault there is no physical contact. Battery is actual unconsented touching.
False Imprisonment	False imprisonment is an act with the intent to confine a person to a specific area.

Continued

41

Chapter 8   Legal and Ethical Guidelines for Safe Practice

Punitive Damages	Moneys are awarded to an injured party in an intentional tort action to punish the defendant.
Violence	Employers are rarely held responsible for employee injuries due to violent client behavior. Nurses have the responsibility to protect themselves by setting policies that create a safe environment, using good judgment about placing themselves in a potentially violent situation, calling security or law enforcement for support as necessary. The nursing assessment of potential for violence should be documented. Under certain circumstances, the nurse's duty includes protection of third parties based upon the duty to warn.
Negligence	This is an act or omission that breaches a duty of care and is responsible for injury to another person. Elements required to prove negligence are duty, breach of duty, cause in fact, proximate cause, and damages.
Determination of a Standard of Care	Standards of care differ from minimal state requirements for licensure. Standards of care are determined in a number of ways: the standard exercised by other nurses with the same degree of skill or knowledge in similar circumstances, statements written by professional organizations, hospital policies and procedures.
Guidelines for Nurses Who Suspect Negligence	Nurses have a legal duty to report risks of harm to clients; document clear and accurate evidence before accusing and communicate concern directly to the person involved. If risky behavior continues, communicate to a supervisor; if the supervisor fails to act, report concerns to a person at the next higher level.
Duty to Intervene and Duty to Report	A nurse has a duty to intervene to protect the client: by checking when a doctor's order should be clarified or changed; by leaving the client in the safe hands of another professional; by reporting impaired or incompetent colleagues; or by reporting abusive behavior. In such cases, the nurse should follow agency policies and communicate using the chain of command.
Unethical or Illegal	Specific behaviors requiring the nurse to exercise the duty to intervene and the duty to report include diversion of drugs, sexual misconduct with clients, impairment due to substance abuse, and abusive behavior.
Documentation of Care **Purpose of Medical Records**	The purpose of a medical record is to provide accurate and complete information about the care and treatment of the client and to give health care personnel responsible for that care a means of communicating with each other. Accuracy and timeliness are vital.
Facility Use of Medical Records	In addition to providing information to caregivers, the record can be used for quality improvement and risk management purposes.
Medical Records as Evidence	The chart is a recording of data and opinions made in the normal course of the client's hospital care. It is considered good evidence because it is presumed to be true, honest, and untainted by memory lapses. Medical records are used as evidence in personal injury cases to determine the extent of client pain and suffering, to determine extent of injury in abuse cases, in workers' compensation cases, police investigations, conservatorship proceedings, competency hearings, commitment procedures, professional and hospital negligence cases, etc.
Nursing Guidelines for Computerized Charting	Guidelines state that documentation should be accurate, descriptive, factual (as opposed to opinion), legible, timely, complete, and unchanged. Computerized charting makes it important to understand how to protect the confidentiality of records (e.g., entering only the records for which there is authorization, and using passwords appropriately).

Assessment Strategies and the Nursing Process

THOUGHTS ABOUT TEACHING THE TOPIC

Since learners should be familiar with the nursing process by this time, the instructor will not need to spend a great deal of time reviewing basic information. If lecture time is to be devoted to this topic, a review of diagnoses often used in psychiatric nursing could be helpful. Opportunities to write nursing diagnoses and outcome criteria should be provided to ensure that each student understands the components and structure of each element before beginning clinical work. One method involves the use of vignettes to give practice in formulating diagnoses and writing outcome criteria. (One such critical-thinking exercise is included at the end of the textbook chapter.) Work may be structured to be individual or performed in small groups.

The instructor may also wish to emphasize the similarities and differences in assessment for psychiatric nursing. For example, the use of the client history and mental and emotional status as assessment strategies is quite different from the data-gathering tools for most clients with medical-surgical problems.

KEY TERMS AND CONCEPTS

counseling, 148
evidence-based practice (EBP), 147
health teaching, 149
mental status examination (MSE), 141
milieu therapy, 149
Nursing Interventions Classification (NIC), 146
Nursing Outcomes Classification (NOC), 146
outcome criteria, 146
psychosocial assessment, 142
self-care activities, 149

OBJECTIVES

After studying this chapter, the reader will be able to
1. Conduct a mental status examination of a classmate.
2. Perform a psychosocial assessment of a client agreed upon with your instructor.
3. Explain three principles the nurse follows in planning actions to reach agreed-upon outcome criteria.
4. Construct a plan of care for a client with a mental health problem.
5. Identify three advanced practice psychiatric nursing interventions.
6. Demonstrate one of the basic nursing interventions (with your instructor's guidance) and evaluate your care using your stated outcome criteria.
7. Contrast and compare the differences and similarities among the Nursing Interventions Classification, Nursing Outcomes Classification, and evidence-based nursing practice.

CHAPTER OUTLINE	TEACHING STRATEGIES
Standard I. Assessment	A mental status examination (MSE) and the assessment of a client's psychosocial status are a part of any nursing assessment, along with assessment of the client's physical health. The MSE and psychosocial assessment are not limited to psychiatric clients. Initial assessment clarifies the client's immediate needs; ongoing assessment enlarges the database and identifies new problems. Time given for assessment interview ranges from a single short interview in an emergency to many interviews. Purposes of the psychiatric assessment are as follows:

Establish rapport
Obtain understanding of current problem
Assess person's current level of psychological functioning
Identify goals
Perform MSE
Identify behaviors, beliefs, or areas of client life to be modified to effect positive change
Formulate a plan of care

Primary source for data collection is the client. Secondary sources include family, friends, neighbors, police, health caregivers, medical records.

Continued

43

Personal Considerations

Both the client and the nurse bring to their relationship their total background experiences. These include cultural beliefs and biases, religious attitudes, educational background, and occupational and life experiences, as well as attitudes regarding sexual roles. Therefore, it is important for nurses, through examining their personal beliefs and clarifying their values, to be aware of their biases and values and not feel compelled to impose their personal beliefs on others. This process of self-monitoring is part of professional behavior.

Assisting a person toward optimal functioning is accomplished through three levels of intervention: primary (preventive), secondary (treatment), and tertiary (rehabilitative). Underlying premises: individuals have the right to decide their destiny and be involved in decision making; nursing intervention is designed to assist individuals to meet their own needs or to solve their own problems. The ultimate goal of all nursing action is to assist individuals to maximize their independent level of functioning.

During the initial interview the nurse and client are strangers. Both experience anxiety, although for different reasons. Both bring to the relationship their total background experiences. Nurses need to examine personal beliefs and clarify their values so as not to impose them on others. Countertransference issues may play a role in the nurse's perceptions. (Countertransference is the nurse's reactions to a client that are based on the nurse's unconscious needs, conflicts, problems, or view of the world.) Experience and supervision help separate out bias.

If, during the assessment interview, the client becomes defensive or upset regarding any topic, the nurse can acknowledge that the topic makes the client uncomfortable and suggest discussing it when the client is more comfortable. Recognize that increased anxiety is "data."

Age Consideration

A thorough physical examination must be completed before any medical diagnosis is made because a number of physical conditions mimic psychiatric disorders. See Box 9-1 for examples.

Assessment of an Elderly Client

Be aware of physical limitations: a sensory, motor, or medical condition that could cause increased anxiety, stress, or physical discomfort for the client. Make accommodations at the beginning of the interview when possible.

Assessment of Children

Useful tools include storytelling, dolls, drawing, and games to promote disclosure.

Assessment of an Adolescent Client

Adolescents are particularly concerned about confidentiality; however, threats of suicide or homicide, use of illegal drugs, or issues of abuse cannot be kept confidential. The HEADSSS Interview (Box 9-2) is a structured tool useful in identifying risk factors.

Psychiatric Nursing Assessment

Gathering Data

Use of a standardized nursing assessment tool facilitates the assessment process. Too rigid application of the tool decreases spontaneity. Learners are advised to maintain an informal style, using clarification, focusing, and exploration of pertinent data. Basic components of the psychiatric nursing assessment include client history, consisting of the presenting problem, current lifestyle, and life in general (subjective data); and the mental and emotional status (objective data). The nurse attempts to identify client strengths and weaknesses, usual coping strategies, cultural beliefs and practices that may affect implementing traditional treatment, and spiritual beliefs or practices integral to client lifestyle. At the conclusion of the assessment, it is useful to summarize pertinent data with the client. And make the client aware of what will happen next.

44

CHAPTER OUTLINE	TEACHING STRATEGIES
Special Note on Spiritual and Cultural Assessment	It is important for nurses to support spiritual aspects of care, just as they do biophysical elements. Carson & Koenig highlight the necessity for mental health nurses and allied clinical staff to be conscious that their clients may have spiritual and religious needs. See text for questions that can be incorporated into the client assessment.
Cultural and Social Assessment	Because nurses are increasingly faced with caring for culturally diverse populations, there is an increasing need for nursing assessment, nursing diagnoses and subsequent care to be planned around unique cultural health care beliefs, values, and practices. See text for questions that you can incorporate into your client assessment.
Verifying Data	Data obtained from the client should be validated with secondary sources whenever possible. Family view is of particular importance. Examples are provided of other validating sources and what can be learned from them.
Using Rating Scales	Rating scales are used for evaluation and monitoring. Table 9–1 lists several in common use today.
Standard II. Nursing Diagnosis Formulating a Nursing Diagnosis	A nursing diagnosis has three structural components: 1. Problem (unmet need). The nursing diagnostic title states what should change. 2. Etiology (probable cause). Is linked to the diagnostic title with the words "related to." Identifies the causes the nurse can treat through nursing interventions. 3. Supporting data (signs and symptoms). State what the condition is presently like and validate the diagnosis. The author provides a critical thinking exercise on page 152 where students can practice formulating nursing diagnoses.
Standard III. Outcome Criteria Determining Outcomes	Outcomes are the measurable behaviors or situations that should be realistic and obtainable. Outcome criteria are the hoped-for outcomes that reflect the maximal level of client health that can realistically be reached by nursing intervention. The Nursing Outcomes Classification (NOC) is mentioned as a source of standardized outcomes based on research and clinical practice. Goals should be realistic and acceptable to both client and nurse and should be stated in observable/measurable terms. They should also indicate client outcomes, include specific time for achievement, be short and specific, and be written in positive terms.
Standard IV. Planning	Consists of identifying nursing interventions that will help meet the outcome criteria and are appropriate to the client's level of functioning. Interventions are written for each goal. Interventions should be seen as instructions of all people working with the client. Interventions need to be safe, appropriate, evidence-based, and individualized. Nursing Interventions Classification (NIC) is a research-based standardized language of approximately 500 interventions nurses can use to plan care.
Standard V. Implementation	Seven areas of intervention are at the basic level of nursing: counseling, milieu therapy, promotion of self-care, psychobiological interventions, health teaching, case management, and health promotion and health maintenance.

Continued

45

	Advanced practice interventions include psychotherapy, prescriptive authority and treatment, and consultation.
Counseling	Calls for use of basic techniques of therapeutic communication. Interventions include reinforcing healthy patterns of behavior; employing problem-solving, interviewing and communication skills; crisis intervention; stress management; relaxation techniques; conflict resolution; and behavior modification.
Milieu Therapy	Includes providing for client safety and comfort, setting limits, reteaching activities that meet client physical and mental health needs.
Promotion of Self-Care Activities	Nurses assist the client in assuming personal responsibility for activities of daily living (ADLs) with the aim of improving the client's functional status.
Psychobiological Interventions	An important nursing function is administration of medication and the attendant responsibilities of observing therapeutic and untoward effects, monitoring therapeutic blood levels, and teaching client and family about the drug.
Health Teaching	Includes identifying health education needs and teaching basic principles of physical and mental health.
Case Management	A case manager coordinates health services among a variety of agencies, depending upon the client's needs and resources. Case management can be done by a variety of individuals including: nurses, social workers, and others.
Health Promotion and Health Maintenance	Psychiatric-mental health nurses employ a variety of health promotion and disease prevention strategies. The text provides a thorough list of factors that will be considered when working with the individual client to reach their optimum level of wellness.
Advanced Practice Interventions Psychotherapy	The advanced practice registered nurse in psychiatric-mental health nursing (APRN-PMH) is educationally and clinically prepared to conduct individual, group, and family psychotherapy, as well as other therapeutic treatments for clients with a variety of mental health disorders.
Prescriptive Authority	The APRN-PMH is educated and clinically prepared to prescribe psychopharmacological agents in accordance with state and federal laws and regulations.
Consultation	The APRN-PMH consults with other clinicians to provide services for clients and effect change within the system.
Standard VI. Evaluation	Evaluation is an ongoing process throughout all phases of the nursing process.
Evaluating Outcome Criteria	The three possible outcomes when goals are evaluated are goal met, goal not met, goal partially met. Client behaviors should be recorded as evidence.
Documentation	Reasons for documentation are reviewed. The various charting methods are reviewed in Table 9-3.

10 Developing Therapeutic Relationships

THOUGHTS ABOUT TEACHING THE TOPIC

The nurse-client relationship is the medium through which the nursing process is implemented. Understanding the purpose of a nurse-client relationship, the characteristics of a therapeutic relationship, and the phases through which it will progress are important considerations. The importance of student understanding of values as determinants of behavior cannot be understated. Developing this self-awareness is an ongoing process, which can be supported by the instructor who encourages students to identify values, prompting their actions during clinical conferences and in a journal.

KEY TERMS AND CONCEPTS

confidentiality, 165
contract, 164
countertransference, 159
empathy, 157
genuineness, 157
intimate relationship, 156
orientation phase, 164
social relationship, 156
termination phase, 167
therapeutic encounter, 163
therapeutic relationship, 156
transference, 159
values, 162
values clarification, 162
working phase, 165

OBJECTIVES

After studying this chapter, the reader will be able to

1. Contrast and compare the purpose, focus, communications styles, and goals for (a) a social relationship, (b) an intimate relationship, and (c) a therapeutic relationship.
2. Define and discuss the role of empathy, genuineness, and positive regard on the part of the nurse in a nurse-client relationship.
3. Identify two attitudes and four actions that may reflect the nurse's positive regard for a client.
4. Analyze what is meant by boundaries and the influence of transference and countertransference on boundary blurring.
5. Contrast and compare the three phases of the nurse-client relationship.
6. Role-play how you would address the four areas of concern during your first interview with a client.
7. Explore aspects that foster a therapeutic nurse-client relationship and those that are inherent in a nontherapeutic nursing interactive process as identified in the research of Forchuk and associates (2000).
8. Describe four testing behaviors a client may demonstrate and discuss possible nursing interventions for each behavior.

CHAPTER OUTLINE	TEACHING STRATEGIES
Therapeutic Versus Other Types of Relationships	A therapeutic relationship incorporating principles of mental health nursing is clearly defined and different from other types of relationships. It has specific goals such as facilitating communication of distressing thoughts and feelings; assisting clients with problem solving to help facilitate ADLs; helping clients examine self-defeating behaviors and test alternatives; and promoting self-care and independence.
Social Relationships	These relationships are primarily initiated for the purpose of friendship, socialization, enjoyment, or task accomplishment. Characteristics include mutually met needs and superficial communication. Communication techniques include giving advice and meeting dependency needs. Little evaluation of the interaction occurs.
Intimate Relationships	These occur between two individuals who have an emotional commitment to each other. Each reacts naturally to the other. Mutual needs are met; personal information, intimate desires, and fantasies are shared. Short- and long-range goals are usually mutual.

Continued

47

CHAPTER OUTLINE	**TEACHING STRATEGIES**

Therapeutic Relationships

These focus on client needs rather than nurse needs. Client issues, problems, and concerns are explored and potential solutions are discussed. New coping skills develop and behavioral change is encouraged. The nurse uses communication skills, understanding of human behavior, knowledge of the stages and phenomena occurring in a therapeutic relationship, and personal strengths to enhance client growth. Nurses' roles include teacher, counselor, socializing agent, liaison, etc.

Factors That Enhance Growth in Others

The following factors are considered crucial in effective helpers: genuineness, empathy, and positive regard.

Genuineness

Explained by Rogers as congruence, genuineness is awareness of feelings as they arise in the relationship and the ability to communicate them when appropriate. Genuineness, or congruence, would be demonstrated by not hiding behind the role of nurse, by listening to and communicating without distorting others' messages, and by being clear and concrete.

Empathy

The ability to see things from the other person's perspective, to experience what the other is feeling, and to communicate this understanding, which denotes acceptance. It is not to be confused with sympathy, which has more to do with compassion and pity. *Sympathy is not objective; empathy is objective.*

Positive Regard

Implying respect is the ability to view another as being worthy of being cared about, and as someone who has strengths and achievement potential. Attitudes and actions that convey positive regard are willingness to work with clients to help them develop their own resources, attending, and suspending value judgments.

Attitudes

One attitude through which a nurse might convey respect is willingness to work with the client.

Actions

Some actions that manifest an attitude of respect are attending, suspending value judgments, and helping clients develop their own resources.

Helping Clients Develop Resources

Involves being aware of clients' strengths, encouraging them to use their own resources and to work at their highest level of functioning. It conveys respect for the client, minimizes helplessness and dependency, and validates potential for change.

Establishing Boundaries

Separating the client's needs from the nurse's needs is how the nurse role and the client role are differentiated. However, boundaries may blur when the relationship slips into a social context and when the nurse's behavior reflects getting self-needs met at the expense of client needs. Resultant actions include overhelping, controlling, and narcissism (i.e., finding weakness, helplessness, and illness in clients in order to feel helpful).

Transference

A process whereby a client unconsciously and inappropriately displaces onto individuals in his or her current life (therapist) those patterns of behavior and emotional reactions that originated with significant figures from childhood. Occurs in all relationships; however, it is intensified in relationships of authority. Examples of transference are desire for affection and respect, gratification of dependency needs, hostility, competitiveness, and jealousy.

Countertransference

The opposite of transference occurs when the therapist displaces onto the client positive or negative feelings caused by people in the therapist's past. Examples include overidentification with the client, power struggles, and competitiveness with the client. Working through transference and countertransference issues is crucial to professional growth of the nurse and positive change in the client, and is best dealt with by use of supervision by an experienced professional.

48

CHAPTER OUTLINE	TEACHING STRATEGIES
Self-Check on Boundary Issues	Readers are encouraged to be reflective about relationships with clients and others and to use a process similar to the self-test found in Figure 10–1.
Understanding Self and Others **Values**	These are abstract standards representing an ideal. Values influence choices and provide a framework for life goals. They are largely culturally oriented, and are formed through the example of others (modeling). Nurses will be required to plan and implement care for clients having values that differ from the nurse's own values; therefore, nurses must have self-awareness regarding their own values and sensitivity to the values of others.
Values Clarification	This is a process of helping people to understand and build their value system. A value may result from one of seven subprocesses, in an emotional, cognitive, or behavioral framework: Prizing one's beliefs and behaviors (emotional) 1. Cherishing the value 2. Publicly affirming the value when appropriate. Choosing one's beliefs and behaviors (cognitive) 3. Choosing the value from alternatives 4. Choosing the value after consideration of consequences 5. Choosing the value freely Acting on one's beliefs (behavioral) 6. Acting in accordance with the value 7. Acting on the value with a pattern, consistency, and repetition
Phases of the Nurse-Client **Relationship**	In the professional helping relationship, relevant behaviors include accountability, focus on client needs, clinical competence, and supervision to validate performance quality. An abbreviated or limited relationship is referred to as a therapeutic encounter. The nurse-client relationship is the medium through which the nursing process is implemented. There are four phases: preorientation, orientation, working, and termination.
Preorientation Phase	This phase involves the thoughts and feelings the nurse experiences prior to the first clinical session and planning for the first interaction with clients. Several student concerns are discussed, such as fear of physical harm and fear of saying the wrong thing.
Orientation Phase	The second phase ranges from a few meetings to a longer term, especially with chronically mentally ill clients. Initially, each interacts according to his or her background, standards, values, and experiences. Initial emphasis is on establishing trust. Four issues are addressed: (1) parameters of the relationship (i.e., purpose of the meetings); (2) a formal or informal contract (i.e., an agreement on specific places, times, dates, duration of meetings, and goals for meetings); (3) confidentiality (i.e., the information the client shares with the nurse will be shared with the treatment team, but not with others with no need to know); (4) termination (i.e., the client should know the date of termination if the relationship is not open-ended). During this phase the nurse will need to be aware of transference-countertransference issues; respond therapeutically to client "testing" behaviors; promote an atmosphere of trust; foster client articulation of problems; and establish mutually agreed-upon goals.

Continued

49

Establishing Trust

A major emphasis during the first few encounters with the client is providing an atmosphere in which trust can grow.

Working Phase

In the third phase, tasks include maintaining the relationship; gathering further data; promoting clients' problem-solving skills, self-esteem, and use of language; facilitating behavioral change; overcoming resistance behaviors; evaluating problems and goals, and redefining them as necessary; and fostering practice of alternative adaptive behaviors. Unconscious motivation and needs may cause the client to experience intense emotions and prompt client behaviors such as acting out anger inappropriately, withdrawing, intellectualizing, manipulating, and denying. Transference and countertransference may be experienced.

Termination Phase

The final stage of the relationship arouses strong feelings in both client and nurse that need to be recognized and worked through, and which will provide an excellent learning experience for both client and nurse. This is a time for summarizing goals, reviewing situations that occurred, and evaluating progress.

What Hinders and What Helps the Nurse-Client Relationship

The work of Forchuk and others tells us the importance of consistent, regular, and private interactions with clients in developing therapeutic relationships. The following behaviors were inherent in a mutually satisfying relationship: consistency, pacing, listening, positive initial impressions, promoting client comfort and balancing control, trust on the part of the client, and active participation by the client in the relationship. The specific behaviors that hampered development of positive relationships were inconsistency, unavailability, lack of self-awareness on the part of the nurse, and negative feelings on the part of the nurse.

11 The Clinical Interview and Communication Skills

THOUGHTS ABOUT TEACHING THE TOPIC

An essential task of the instructor is to help the student communicate effectively. The more active the learner, the more easily the objectives seem to be operationalized. Thus, independent study and readings may be used for initial learning, to be followed by in-class activities such as role playing, the analysis of filmed material, or analysis and discussion of process recordings.

Faculty often find that, in a group, reinforcing use of therapeutic communication is more effective than dwelling on nontherapeutic student choices. Dramatizations, as in films, videos, or role playing, followed by discussion, allow the learner to identify principles and analyze interactions. Written exercises and process recordings also allow learners to identify techniques and consider their effectiveness.

The element of interactivity makes computer-assisted instruction and interactive video ideal media for teaching and reinforcing therapeutic communication techniques. The learner can work independently at his or her own pace without the fear of revealing lack of knowledge.

If students will be using a journal and submitting it to the instructor, be sure to point out that this is one avenue for obtaining the supervision discussed in the chapter.

KEY TERMS AND CONCEPTS

active listening, 186
clarifying techniques, 189
clinical supervision, 173
cultural filters, 185
double messages, 180
double-bind messages, 181
excessive questioning, 190
exploring, 189
feedback, 178
giving advice, 192
giving approval, 192
nonverbal behaviors, 180
nonverbal communication, 180
obstructive (nontherapeutic) techniques, 185
paralinguistics, 183
paraphrasing, 189

process recordings, 174
reflecting, 189
restating, 189
silence, 186
therapeutic (helpful) techniques, 185
verbal communication, 179
"why" questions, 193

OBJECTIVES

After studying this chapter, the reader will be able to
1. Identify and give rationales for suggested (a) setting, (b) seating, and (c) beginning of the nurse-client interaction.
2. Explain to a classmate the importance of clinical supervision and how it works.
3. Identify four client behaviors a nurse can anticipate and discuss possible nursing interventions for each behavior.
4. Identify three personal factors that can impede accurate communication.
5. Identify two environmental factors that can impede accurate communication.
6. Give a personal example of a recent complementary exchange and a recent symmetrical exchange and explain how the relationship affected the quality of the communication.
7. Discuss the differences between verbal and nonverbal communication and identify five areas of nonverbal communication.
8. Identify two attending behaviors that the nurse might focus on to increase communication skills.
9. Relate potential problems that can arise when nurses are insensitive to cultural differences in clients' communication styles.
10. Compare and contrast the range of nonverbal and verbal behaviors of different cultural groups in the areas of (a) communication style, (b) eye contact, and (c) touch. Give examples.
11. Demonstrate the use of four techniques that can enhance communication, highlighting what makes them effective.
12. Demonstrate the use of four techniques that can obstruct communication, highlighting what makes them ineffective.

Continued

Chapter 11   The Clinical Interview and Communication Skills

CHAPTER OUTLINE	TEACHING STRATEGIES
The Clinical Interview	The clinical interview is a systematic attempt to understand those problems in clients' lives that interfere with meeting their goals and to help them improve their skills or learn alternative ways of dealing effectively with their problems. The content and direction of the clinical interview are decided by the client. The client leads. The nurse employs communication skills and active listening, observes how congruent the content is with the process, and provides the opportunity for the client to reach specific goals.
How to Begin the Interview	Setting—A setting that enhances feelings of security is best. Strive for relative privacy.
	Seating—Seating should be arranged so that conversation can take place in normal tones and eye contact can be comfortably maintained, or avoided, by placing chairs at a 90- or 120-degree angle, or side by side. Avoid a desk "barrier" between nurse and client. The door should be accessible to both.
	Introductions—Nurses tell the client who they are, their school name, the purpose of meeting, and how long and when they will meet. They ask how the client would like to be addressed. Confidentiality should be addressed at some point.
	How to start—After introductions, give the client the lead by using an open-ended statement. Facilitate communication using general leads, statements of acceptance, and other therapeutic techniques.
	Tactics to avoid—Avoid arguing, minimizing the client's problem, praising, giving false reassurance, interpreting or speculating on dynamics, probing, joining in if client verbally attacks a significant person in his or her life, criticism of a staff member, and "selling" the client on treatment.
	Helpful guidelines—Speak briefly; say nothing when you don't know what to say; when in doubt, focus on feelings; avoid giving advice and relying on questions; note nonverbal cues; and keep the focus on the client.
Clinical Supervision and Process Recordings	Working with a supervisor to examine one's interactions, obtain insights, and devise effective strategies for dealing with clinical issues enhances a nurse's professional growth and minimizes burnout. Clinical supervision methods can include analyzing a videotape, audiotape, or process recording of an interaction.
What to Do in Response to Specific Client Behaviors	Reading about what to do in response to certain client behaviors, such as crying, asking the nurse to keep a secret, threatening to commit suicide, and leaving the interview, can be very helpful to new nurses. This information is given in Table 11–2.
Communication	The idea of "saying the wrong thing" is explored, and the reader is urged to learn communication skills and apply them with concern and respect.
The Communication Process	Communication is the process of sending a message to one or more persons. Berlo's model explains the communication process and identifies:

The stimulus—reason for beginning communication;
The sender—initiates the interpersonal contact;
The message—the information sent;
The media—how the information is sent (auditory, tactile, smell, or any combination of these);
The receiver—receives and interprets the message;
The feedback—receiver's response to the sender.

Factors That Affect Communication

Factors that can distort sending and receiving messages include the following: personal factors, which include emotional, social, and cognitive factors, such as mood, previous experience, cultural differences, knowledge levels, and language use; environmental factors, which include physical and societal factors, such as noise, lack of privacy, uncomfortable surroundings, presence of others, and expectations of others; and relationship factors, which refer to whether the participants are equal Peplau's principles to guide communication during the nurse-client interview are clarity and continuity.

Verbal Communication

Verbal communication consists of all words a person speaks. When we speak, we communicate beliefs and values, perceptions and meanings; convey interest and understanding or insult and judgment; convey messages clearly or convey conflicting or implied messages; convey clear, honest feelings or disguised, distorted feelings. Words have different meanings for different people (e.g., the word "trip" may produce a number of different mental images).

Nonverbal Communication

Nonverbal communication consists of behaviors displayed by an individual to express thoughts or feelings (e.g., tone of voice, manner, facial expression, body posture, eye contact, eye cast, hand gestures, sighs, fidgeting, and yawning). Interpretation of nonverbal communication depends on culture, class, gender, age, sexual orientation, and spiritual norms.

Interaction of Verbal and Nonverbal Communication

The verbal message is considered the content; the nonverbal message is considered the process. It is desirable for verbal and nonverbal messages to be congruent. If the verbal message is not reinforced or is contradicted by the nonverbal message, the message is confusing. Such an occurrence is called a double or mixed message.

Negotiating Cultural Communication Barriers

Whenever interacting with culturally diverse clients, nurses should be aware of the cultural meanings of certain verbal and nonverbal communications if therapeutic alliances are to be formed.

Communication styles—Intensity, high affect, and use of gestures mark the communication style of clients who are from Hispanic, French, and Italian cultures. Calm, low affect, and sparse gestures mark the communication style of Asian Americans, German Americans, and British Americans. Guarded, selective communication is common among African American clients.

Eye contact—Culture dictates comfort or lack of comfort with direct eye contact. For example, Hispanic, Japanese, and Native American cultures call for avoiding eye contact as a sign of respect. Chinese culture considers it polite to look to one side or gaze around. In some Arab cultures, a woman making eye contact with a man may imply sexual interest or promiscuity. Direct eye contact is employed in German, Russian, French, British, and many African American cultures.

Touch—Response to touch is often culturally defined. In general, people from Hispanic, Italian, French, and Russian cultural backgrounds are accustomed to touch. German, Swedish, and British Americans practice little touching. Chinese Americans may not want to be touched by strangers. Japanese may shake hands but a pat on the back is unacceptable. In India, men may shake hands with other men but not with women. Nurses must be sensitive and open to learning about culturally specific nonverbal behavior. Students should be cautioned to know the agency policy regarding touch, as many agencies have a "no touch" policy.

Continued

53

Effective Communication Skills

Use of Silence

Use of silence can be a significant means of influencing, and being influenced by others. Possible meanings of a client's silence include emotional blocking, unreadiness to disclose, anger or hostility, insult, and acknowledgment of nurse's lack of cultural sensitivity. The nurse's silence can indicate willingness to let the client set the pace, can communicate strength and support as a client regains composure, or can provide an opportunity to think.

Active Listening

Active listening includes observing client's nonverbal behaviors, listening to and understanding client's verbal message, listening to and understanding the person in the context of the social setting of his or her life, and listening for inconsistencies or things the client says that need clarification. Ability to listen is affected by cultural filters that influence when to listen and what to ignore. These filters introduce cultural bias into our listening. Active listening helps clients use their abilities to solve problems, clarify thinking, and link ideas. It also enhances client self-esteem.

Clarifying Techniques

Use of clarifying techniques allows the nurse to seek verification from the client regarding the nurse's interpretation of the client's messages.

Paraphrasing—Paraphrasing is restating the basic content of a message using different words.

Restating—Restating is repeating the same key words the client has just spoken.

Reflecting—Reflecting takes the form of a question or simple statement, conveying the nurse's observations of the client when sensitive issues are discussed.

Exploring—Exploring is asking the client to tell you more; to describe or give an example.

Degree of Openness

Questions or statements can be classified as open-ended, focused, or closed-ended, and may be placed along a continuum of openness. Three variables influence placement on the continuum of openness: the degree to which the verbalization produces spontaneous and lengthy response, the degree to which the verbalization does not limit the client's answer set, and the degree to which the verbalization opens up a moderately resistant client.

Open-ended questions require more than one-word answers. Open-ended questions are valuable as opening phrases of any interview and work well with resistant or guarded clients.

Closed-ended questions ask for specific information and limit the client's freedom to give lengthy answers.

Obstructive Techniques to Monitor and Minimize

Asking Excessive Questions

Especially closed-ended questions; they put the nurse in the role of interrogator. This conveys lack of respect for and insensitivity to client needs.

Giving Approval or Disapproval

Giving approval or disapproval usually involves a value comment that may easily be misinterpreted by the client. The client may see the behavior as a way to please the nurse, and continue it for that reason, rather than of his or her own volition.

Advising

Advising is rarely helpful to clients; it interferes with their ability to make personal decisions and may undermine client confidence. Instead, seek the client's opinion regarding actions he or she can take.

Asking "Why" Questions

Often imply criticism, and can lead to rationalization. Instead, ask the client what is happening.

Chapter 11   The Clinical Interview and Communication Skills

12 Understanding Stress and Holistic Approaches to Stress Management

THOUGHTS ABOUT TEACHING THE TOPIC

The instructor may choose to spend time emphasizing and clarifying concepts discussed in the chapter concerning the relationship of stress and altered physiological function, the relationship of stress and anxiety, and the nurse's role in helping the client identify stressors and develop healthy approaches to coping with stress. Students often bring up examples from their personal lives.

The instructor may also wish to have students explore the relationship between stress and nurse burnout.

KEY TERMS AND CONCEPTS

assertiveness training, 207
Benson's relaxation techniques, 204
biofeedback, 206
cognitive reframing, 206
coping styles, 202
distress, 198
eustress, 198
guided imagery, 205
humor, 207
journal keeping, 206
meditation, 204
physical stressors, 200
progressive muscle relaxation (PMR), 206
psychological stressors, 200
psychoneuroimmunology (PNI), 198
restructuring and setting priorities, 206

OBJECTIVES

After studying this chapter, the reader will be able to
1. Recognize the short- and long-term physiological consequences of stress.
2. Contrast and compare Cannon's (fight-or-flight), Selye's (general adaptation syndrome), and psychoneuroimmunological models of stress.
3. Identify the relationship between stress and anxiety.
4. Analyze and give examples of the ways in which culture can affect a person's perception of and reaction to stress.
5. Assess life change units in a client's life using the Life-Changing Events Questionnaire.
6. Differentiate among four categories of coping and give at least two examples of each.
7. Teach a classmate or client two simple behavioral techniques to help lower stress and anxiety.
8. Explain how cognitive techniques can help lower a person's level of stress.

CHAPTER OUTLINE	TEACHING STRATEGIES
Acute and Long-Term Effects of Stress: General Adaptation Theory	Stress is a universal experience. Selye initially defined stress as the nonspecific result of any demand upon the body, and expanded Cannon's theory of stress with his formulation of the general adaptation syndrome (GAS). GAS occurs in two stages: (1) an initial adaptive response (fight or flight), or acute stress, and (2) the eventual maladaptive consequences of prolonged stress. Later, Selye distinguished between distress, which is destructive to health, and eustress, which is beneficial stress that motivates energy.
Stressors	Two categories of stressors exist: (1) physical, exemplified by environmental conditions such as cold, trauma, excessive heat and physical conditions such as infection, hemorrhage, hunger, or pain; (2) psychological, exemplified by divorce, job loss, unmanageable debt, death of a loved one, retirement, marriage, unexpected success.
	Researchers have found that the perception of a recent life event determines the person's reactions to it.
Mediating Factors	Mediating factors include age, sex, culture, life experiences, life style, and social support. Self-help groups are a means of providing social support. Ideally, high-quality social support should be provided since research tells us it is linked with high satisfaction. High-quality support relationships are free from conflict and negative interactions; they are close, confiding, and reciprocal. Low-quality support relationships may negatively affect a person's coping effectiveness in a crisis.

Continued

55

CHAPTER OUTLINE	TEACHING STRATEGIES
Culture	Culture plays a role in determining what is considered dangerous, how to manage violations of social code, what reactions are permissible in given experiences, how a stressful event is appraised, and how emotion generated by the event should be expressed. Culture plays a role in how people experience stressors in their lives and what interventions will be useful. The majority of Asian, African, and Central American peoples express subjective distress in somatic terms, rendering psychological interpretations less useful.
Spirituality and Prayerfulness	Religious and spiritual beliefs are helpful for many people coping with stress. Studies have demonstrated that spiritual practices can enhance the immune system and sense of well-being.
Assessing Stress and Coping Styles Measuring Stress	The Recent Life-Changing Events Questionnaire is available for self-rating. Recent findings suggest that life stress over the last 35 years has increased markedly. Other findings note there is a gender difference in the way in which certain factors such as finances are rated.
Assessing Coping Styles	Rahe identifies four categories of coping styles that people use as stress buffers: (1) health-sustaining habits, (2) life satisfactions, (3) social supports, (4) response to stress. Nurses evaluate these to identify areas to target for improvement. Coping strategies include psychological defense mechanisms, psychophysiological defenses that are in our awareness (e.g., headache) or out of awareness (hypertension or depression).
Holistic Approaches to Stress Management	Benefits of stress reduction include altering the course of medical conditions such as hypertension; decreasing need for medications such as antihypertensives; diminishing or eliminating the need for unhealthy behaviors such as smoking; increasing cognitive functions such as learning, breaking up static patterns of thinking to allow creative perceptions of events; and increasing sense of well-being via endorphin release.
Behavioral Approaches	Cognitive behavioral methods are the most effective ways to reduce stress. Behavioral methods include a number of relaxation techniques.
Relaxation Techniques	Benson's relaxation technique allows clients to switch from the sympathetic mode of autonomic arousal to the parasympathetic mode of relaxation, and can be learned with practice. Relaxation techniques should be used with physician approval as they may not be appropriate for use by depressed, hallucinating, or delusional clients, or by those in severe pain.
Meditation	This is mind training to develop greater calm, increased relaxation, and the ability to access inner resources for both healing and operating more effectively in the world.
Guided Imagery	This is used in conjunction with the relaxation response. A person is led to envision images that are calming and health enhancing. Imagery techniques are useful for pain relief; and for reducing levels of cortisol, epinephrine, and catecholamines, thus supporting the immune system and producing β-endorphins (which increase the pain threshold and enhance lymphocyte proliferation).
Breathing Exercises	Learning abdominal breathing can be helpful in the modification of stress and anxiety reactions.

Chapter 12   Understanding Stress and Holistic
Approaches to Stress Management

Behavioral Techniques Requiring Special Training

Therapeutic Touch (TT)   This technique employs the steps of centering, scanning, and rebalancing to manipulate a client's energy fields, usually for the purpose of pain relief or promotion of healing.

Muscle Relaxation and Exercise   Yoga can reduce stress and relieve muscle tension and pain. Another technique, called progressive muscle relaxation (PMR), achieves deep relaxation by systematically tensing and releasing various muscle groups.

Biofeedback   This technique uses sensitive instrumentation that gives a person information on his or her physiological functions such as brain waves, skin temperature, blood pressure, etc., to help the individual gain control over what had been considered involuntary functions.

Cognitive Approaches

Journal Keeping and Writing   Keeping an informal diary of daily events and activities helps identify sources of daily stress. The individual can then take measures to modify or eliminate the stressors.

Priority Restructuring   Once stressful events have been identified, the individual can shift the balance from stress-producing events to stress-reducing activities. Adding daily pleasant events has a positive effect on the immune system.

Cognitive Reframing   This includes restructuring of irrational beliefs and replacing worried self-statements with more positive self-statements. Essentially, reframing is reassessing a situation. Restructuring a disturbing event to one that is less disturbing gives the client a sense of control, reduces sympathetic nervous system stimulation, and, in turn, reduces secretion of cortisol and catecholamines.

Assertiveness Training   Involves learning behavior that allows one to stand up for one's rights without violating the rights of others. Four formulas for assertive communication are (1) simple assertion via a direct statement; (2) empathic assertion, showing understanding of the other's feelings and assertively stating what one needs; (3) nonaccusingly describing the situation, stating one's feelings about the situation, and asking for change; (4) confrontational assertion.

More Effective Stress Reducers   Music, pets, and exercise: Benefits of each are reviewed.

13 Understanding Anxiety and Anxiety Defenses

THOUGHTS ABOUT TEACHING THE TOPIC

Because the material in this chapter is fundamental to understanding human behavior, the instructor will probably spend time emphasizing and clarifying the universality of anxiety, assessment of levels of anxiety, the use of defense mechanisms, and nursing interventions appropriate for each level of anxiety.

Discussion of personal experiences with one's own anxiety and of contacts with anxious individuals often serves to establish the foundation. Written exercises such as mini–case studies or instructor-made videotapes can help students identify defense mechanisms and compare and contrast levels of anxiety. Once the student can correctly assess the level of anxiety experienced by the client, planning nursing intervention seems to follow logically.

KEY TERMS AND CONCEPTS

acting-out behaviors, 219
acute (state) anxiety, 213
altruism, 217
anxiety, 212
chronic (trait) anxiety, 213
denial, 220
devaluation, 219
displacement, 218
dissociation, 219
fear, 213
humor, 218
idealization, 219
mild anxiety, 213
moderate anxiety, 213
normal anxiety, 213
panic level of anxiety, 215
passive aggression, 218
projection, 219
psychotic denial, 220
rationalization, 218
reaction formation, 218
repression, 218
severe anxiety, 214
somatization, 218
splitting, 219
sublimation, 218
suppression, 218
undoing, 218

OBJECTIVES

After studying this chapter, the reader will be able to

1. Explore the difference between normal anxiety, acute anxiety, and chronic anxiety.
2. Contrast and compare the four levels of anxiety in relation to perceptual field, ability to learn, and physical and other defining characteristics.
3. Summarize five properties of the defense mechanisms.
4. Define and give at least two clinical examples of defense mechanisms in each of the following categories: most healthy, intermediate, and immature.

CHAPTER OUTLINE	TEACHING STRATEGIES
About Anxiety	Anxiety is a universal human experience. Dysfunctional behavior is often a defense against anxiety. Anxiety, a feeling of apprehension, uneasiness, uncertainty, or dread resulting from a real or perceived threat whose actual source is unknown or unrecognized, can be differentiated from fear. Fear is a reaction to a specific danger. The body, however, reacts in similar ways physiologically to both fear and anxiety
	Normal anxiety provides the energy to carry out tasks involved with living and striving toward goals (e.g., studying, beginning work on time, working toward a promotion). Acute anxiety, or state anxiety, is precipitated by imminent loss or change threatening the individual's sense of security. Chronic anxiety, or trait anxiety, is anxiety that one has lived with for a long time.

Levels of Anxiety

Mild Anxiety

Occurs in the normal experience of everyday living. Ability to perceive is in sharp focus and problem solving becomes more effective. Slight discomfort, restlessness, or mild tension-relieving behaviors may be observed.

Moderate Anxiety

Perceptual field narrows; some details are excluded from observation. Selective inattention may be experienced. Problem-solving ability is reduced, and may be improved in the presence of a supportive person. Physical symptoms include tension, pounding heart, increased pulse and respiration rate, diaphoresis, and mild somatic symptoms.

Severe Anxiety

Perceptual field is greatly reduced. Learning and problem solving are not possible, and the person may appear dazed and confused, experience a sense of doom, and have intensified somatic complaints.

Panic Level of Anxiety

Results in markedly disturbed behavior, inability to process environmental stimuli, and possible loss of touch with reality. Hallucinations may be experienced. Physical behavior may be erratic, uncoordinated, and impulsive. Automatic behaviors are used to reduce and relieve anxiety.

Interventions

Mild to Moderate Levels of Anxiety

The nurse can help the client focus and solve problems with the use of specific communication techniques. Other helpful interventions include providing a calm presence, recognition of the person's distress, and willingness to listen.

Counselors of clients with mild to moderate anxiety help clients focus and problem-solve by using communication techniques such as open-ended questions, broad openings, and clarification seeking. Counselors maintain a calm presence; they recognize the person's distress and show willingness to listen.

Severe to Panic Levels of Anxiety

A person with a severe to panic level of anxiety is unable to solve problems, may not fully understand what is happening, and may not be in control of his or her actions. The nurse is concerned about client safety and the safety of others. Physical needs (fluids, rest) must be met to prevent exhaustion. A quiet environment is best, and medications and restraints may be used after less restrictive interventions have failed. Themes in conversation may be identified.

Counselors communicate via firm, short, simple statements; point out reality if there are distortions; reduce environmental stimuli; provide a safe environment; and meet physical needs.

The Nurse's Response

Nurses work with people in high-stress situations: severe to panic levels in emergency rooms and intensive care units, mild to moderate levels in other settings. Such work is uncomfortable and intimidating; it requires self-awareness and professional supervision.

Defenses Against Anxiety

Defense mechanisms are automatic psychological processes that protect the individual against anxiety and from the awareness of internal or external dangers or stressors. These relief behaviors are used by everyone to lower anxiety, maintain ego function, and protect the sense of self. Maladaptive use may lead to distortions in reality and self-deception. Five important properties of defense mechanisms are (1) defenses are a major means of managing conflict and affect; (2) defenses are relatively unconscious; (3) defenses are discrete; (4) defenses are reversible; (5) defenses are adaptive as well as maladaptive.

Continued

59

Chapter 13   Understanding Anxiety and Anxiety Defenses

CHAPTER OUTLINE	TEACHING STRATEGIES
Most Healthy Defenses	Altruism—Emotional conflicts and stressors are dealt with by working with others
	Sublimation—The unconscious process of substituting constructive and socially acceptable activity for strong impulses that are not acceptable
	Humor—A way of dealing with stress or emotional conflicts using amusing or ironic aspects of the conflict or stressors
	Suppression—The conscious denial of disturbing situations or feelings
Intermediate Defenses	Repression—The exclusion of unwanted experiences or emotions from the conscious awareness; also the cornerstone of the defense mechanisms
	Displacement—Placing emotions associated with a particular person, object, or situation onto another person, object, or situation that is nonthreatening
	Reaction formation—Overcompensation
	Somatization—The transfer of anxiety from the psychological to a physical symptom that has no organic cause
	Undoing—Making up for an argument with someone by giving a gift to "undo"
	Rationalization—Justifying illogical or unreasonable ideas, actions, or feelings by developing acceptable explanations that satisfy the teller as well as the listener
Immature Defenses	Passive aggression—Dealing with emotional conflict or stressors by indirectly and unassertively expressing aggression toward others
	Acting out behaviors—Dealing with emotional conflicts or stressors by actions rather than reflections or feelings
	Dissociation—Feeling unattached to self, others, or environment
	Devaluation—Giving negative value to self or others to try to appear "good" and reduce stress and anxiety
	Idealization—Emotional stressors are dealt with by idealizing or exaggerating another's qualities
	Splitting—Inability to integrate positive and negative attributes to another at the same time; the all or nothing way of dealing with stressors; prevalent in individuals with borderline personality disorder
	Projection—Placing one's own negative attributes onto another person, object, or situation; also called "blaming" or "scapegoating"
	Denial—Escaping from unpleasant realities by ignoring their existence; a hallmark defense mechanism in alcohol or drug addicted individuals ("I can stop drinking or taking drugs anytime I want to.")
Case Study and Nursing Care Plan: Severe Level of Anxiety	Takes the reader through use of the nursing process with a client in a very realistic situation.

60

14 Anxiety Disorders

THOUGHTS ABOUT TEACHING THE TOPIC

It is helpful to students to review each of the disorders and then, via discussion and questioning, to focus on similarities and differences among the disorders. When time is limited, faculty may wish to assign chapters on the anxiety disorders and the somatoform and dissociative disorders together. When the topics are combined, the focus in classroom activities can be on commonly used nursing diagnoses and interventions.

KEY TERMS AND CONCEPTS

acute stress disorder, 236
agoraphobia, 233
anxiolytic drugs, 246
behavioral therapy, 244
cognitive restructuring, 244
cognitive therapy, 244
cognitive-behavioral therapy, 244
compulsions, 234
flashbacks, 236
flooding, 244
generalized anxiety disorder (GAD), 235
modeling, 244
obsessions, 234
panic attack, 232
panic disorder, 232
phobia, 234
posttraumatic stress disorder (PTSD), 236

relaxation training, 244
response prevention, 244
social anxiety disorder, 234
social phobia, 234
specific phobias, 234
systematic desensitization, 244
thought stopping, 244

OBJECTIVES

After studying this chapter, the reader will be able to

1. Identify genetic, biological, psychological, and cultural factors leading to anxiety disorders.
2. Describe clinical manifestations of each anxiety disorder.
3. Formulate four appropriate nursing diagnoses that can be used in treating a person with an anxiety disorder.
4. Name three defense mechanisms commonly found in clients with anxiety disorders.
5. Describe feelings that may be experienced by nurses caring for clients with anxiety disorders.
6. Propose realistic outcome criteria for a client with (a) generalized anxiety disorder, (b) panic disorder, and (c) posttraumatic stress disorder.
7. Describe five basic nursing interventions used with clients with anxiety disorders.
8. Discuss three classes of medication appropriate for anxiety disorders.
9. Define two advanced practice interventions for anxiety disorders.

CHAPTER OUTLINE	TEACHING STRATEGIES
	Anxiety is a normal response to threatening situations. It becomes pathological when it interferes with adaptive behavior, causes physical symptoms, or exceeds a tolerable level. Individuals with anxiety disorders use rigid, repetitive, and ineffective behaviors to try to control anxiety.
Prevalence	Anxiety disorders are the most common of all psychiatric disorders in the United States, affecting up to 13.3% of the population. People may have more than one anxiety disorder. Women are affected more than men.
Comorbidity	Anxiety disorders and depression occur together frequently. *DSM-IV-TR* criteria for mixed anxiety-depressive disorder are given, although the criteria are still being researched. Other frequent comorbid disorders include substance abuse, somatization, and other anxiety disorders.

Continued

61

Theory
Genetic Correlates

Anxiety disorders tend to run in families. There is evidence of specific genetic contributions that increase a person's susceptibility to specific anxiety disorders. However, no anxiety disorder has been proved to be the result of a specific gene.

Biological Findings

General anxiety and panic disorder—One theory suggests that aberrant production of a substance that interferes with benzodiazepine binding to receptors or altered receptor sensitivity interfering with proper benzodiazepine receptor function is involved. A biological basis for panic is supported by research.

Phobias—Social phobias may well be related to noradrenergic dysfunction.

Obsessive-compulsive disorder—Neuroimaging techniques point to orbitofrontal-limbic-basal ganglia circuit dysfunction, whereas neurochemistry points to serotonin dysregulation.

Posttraumatic stress disorder (PTSD)—A number of theories exist, including one suggesting that extreme stress is associated with damaging effects to the brain.

Cultural Considerations

Manifestations of anxiety differ from culture to culture. Culture-bound illnesses must be differentiated from anxiety disorders. In some cultures, anxiety is expressed through somatic symptoms; in others, cognitive symptoms predominate.

Clinical Picture
Panic Disorder

Recurrent, unexpected panic attacks of sudden onset are a clinical symptom of this disorder. Physical symptoms of sympathetic arousal are accompanied by terror, limited perceptual field, and severe personality disorganization.

Panic Disorder with Agoraphobia

Clinical picture for this disorder is recurrent panic attacks accompanied by fear of being in an environment or situation from which escape might be difficult or embarrassing or in which help may not be available (e.g., being alone outside; being home alone; traveling in a car, bus, or plane; being on a bridge or in an elevator).

Simple Agoraphobia

Simple agoraphobia is fear of being in an environment or situation from which escape might be difficult (as listed above).

Phobias

Phobias are persistent, irrational fears of a specific object, activity, or situation that lead to a desire for avoidance or actual avoidance of the specific object or situation. *Specific phobias* are provoked by a specific object (e.g., a dog or spider) or situation (e.g., a storm); they are common and usually do not cause much difficulty because people can avoid the situation/object. *Social phobia,* or social anxiety disorder, is provoked by exposure to a social situation or a performance situation and can cause great difficulty.

Obsessive-Compulsive Disorder

Obsessions are thoughts, impulses, or images that persist and recur and that cannot be dismissed from the mind. *Compulsions* are ritualistic behaviors that an individual feels driven to perform to reduce anxiety. They can be seen separately but usually co-exist.

Generalized Anxiety Disorder

This is characterized by the presence of excessive anxiety or worry lasting for 6 months or longer; symptoms can include poor concentration, tension, sleep disturbance, and restlessness.

Posttraumatic Stress Disorder

PTSD involves reexperiencing of a highly traumatic event involving actual or threatened death or serious injury to self or others to which the person responded with intense fear or helplessness. Symptoms usually begin within 3 months after the traumatic incident and include flashbacks, persistent avoidance of stimuli associated with the trauma, numbness, or detachment, and increased arousal.

Acute Stress Disorder	This occurs within 1 month after exposure to a highly traumatic event, such as described for PTSD. Individual must display three dissociative symptoms during or after the event (e.g., numbness, detachment, derealization, depersonalization, or dissociative amnesia.
Substance-Induced Anxiety Disorder	Symptoms of anxiety, panic attacks, obsessions, and compulsions that develop with the use of a substance or within a month of stopping use.
Anxiety Due to Medical Condition	Symptoms of anxiety are sometimes the physiological result of a medical condition such as pheochromocytoma, cardiac dysrhythmias, hyperthyroidism, etc.
Application of the Nursing Process Assessment	
Overall Symptoms of Anxiety	Clients prone to anxiety disorders are encountered in a variety of community settings. Assessment will usually involve determining if the anxiety is from a secondary source (medical condition) or a primary source (anxiety disorder). Symptoms specific to various anxiety disorders include panic attacks, phobias, obsessions, and compulsions.
Defenses Used in Anxiety Disorders	Defense mechanisms associated with the various anxiety disorders are detailed in Table 14-7. A preliminary screening test for anxiety disorders is shown in Box 14-1. The Hamilton Rating Scale for Anxiety is often used (Table 14-8); for example: feeling like one is going to die or having a sense of impending doom; having narrowed perceptions and difficulty concentrating or problem-solving; increased vital signs, muscle tension, dilated pupils; complaints of palpitations, urinary frequency or urgency, nausea, tight throat; complaints of fatigue, insomnia, irritability, disorganization.
Self-Assessment	Nurse's feelings may include tension or anxiety, frustration, anger, being overwhelmed, fatigue, desire to withdraw, and guilt related to having negative feelings.
Assessment Guidelines	(1) Physical and neurological examinations will help determine if anxiety is primary or secondary. (2) Assess for potential for self-harm and suicide. (3) Do a psychosocial assessment to identify problems that should be addressed by counseling. (4) Note that cultural differences can affect the way in which anxiety is manifested.
Nursing Diagnosis	Useful diagnoses include, but are not limited to *anxiety, ineffective coping, disturbed thought processes, chronic low self-esteem, situational low self-esteem, powerlessness, deficient diversional activity, social isolation, ineffective role performance, ineffective health maintenance, disturbed sleep pattern, self-care deficit, imbalanced nutrition,* and *impaired skin integrity.*
Outcome Criteria	Useful outcome criteria describe the client's state or situation that is expected to be influenced by nursing interventions. Nursing Outcomes Classification (NOC) is suggested as a resource. Examples of outcomes for anxiety control include the following: client will monitor intensity of anxiety, eliminate precursors of anxiety, seek information to reduce anxiety, plan successful coping strategies, use relaxation techniques, report adequate sleep, report decrease in frequency of episodes, etc.
Planning	Planning usually involves selecting interventions that can be implemented in a community setting, since clients with anxiety disorders are not usually hospitalized in an inpatient psychiatric unit.
	Clients with mild or moderate anxiety should be encouraged to be involved in planning, whereas for clients with severe anxiety, the nurse will need to be more directive.

Continued

63

Intervention

Overall guidelines for interventions(Nurses need to (1) identify community resources that can offer the client effective therapy, (2) identify community support groups for people with anxiety disorders, (3) assess need for interventions for families and significant others, (4) provide thorough teaching when medications are used.

Counseling

To assist clients to improve or regain coping abilities, counseling is often combined with other cognitive and behavioral therapies.

Cognitive therapy—Assumes that cognitive errors made by the client produce negative beliefs that persist. Counseling calls for the nurse to assist the client to identify these thoughts and negative beliefs and to appraise the situation realistically.

Cognitive restructuring—This therapy calls for the nurse to assist a client to identify automatic negative anxiety-arousing thoughts and negative self-talk, discover the basis for the thoughts, and to assist the client to appraise the situation realistically and replace automatic thoughts and negative self-talk with realistic thinking.

Cognitive-behavioral therapy—Uses a variety of approaches such as psychoeducational methods, continuous panic self-monitoring, breathing retraining, development of anxiety management skills, and in vivo exposure to feared stimuli.

Relaxation training—Teaching muscle relaxation will result in reduction of tension and anxiety.

Modeling—Shows client how an individual copes effectively and expects the client to imitate the adaptive behavior.

Systematic desensitization—Graduated exposure gradually introduces the client to a phobic object or situation in a predetermined sequence of least to most frightening. Teaches the client to use a relaxation technique for anxiety management.

Flooding (implosion therapy)—Extinguishes anxiety as a conditioned response by exposing a client to a large amount of the stimulus he or she finds undesirable.

Response prevention—The individual who would reduce anxiety by performing a ritual is not permitted to perform the ritual.

Thought stopping—A technique calling for the client to shout "STOP" or snap a rubber band on the wrist whenever an obsessive thought begins. This helps the client dismiss the thought.

Milieu Therapy

If the client with an anxiety disorder does require hospitalization, the environment should be structured to offer safety and predictability, should have activities to shift the client's focus from his or her anxiety and symptoms, and should provide therapeutic interactions.

Promotion of Self-Care Activities

Clients with anxiety disorders can usually meet their own basic physical needs. Self-care activities most likely to be affected are discussed below.

Nutrition and Fluid Intake

For clients with OCD who are involved with their rituals to the exclusion of all else, nutrition and fluid intake could be affected. Assess weight and encourage intake.

Personal Hygiene and Grooming

Excessive neatness, rituals associated with bathing and grooming, and indecision are common among clients with phobias and OCD. Skin integrity may be a problem when rituals involve washing.

Elimination

Clients with OCD may suppress urges to void and defecate.

Sleep

Anxious clients often have difficulty sleeping. Clients with GAD, PTSD, and stress disorder may have nightmares.

Psychobiological Interventions
Antidepressants

Selective serotonin reuptake inhibitors (SSRIs) are the first-line treatment for anxiety disorder. They are more prevalent than the TCAs because of their more rapid onset of action and fewer problematic side effects. Monoamine oxidase inhibitors (MAOIs) are reserved for treatment-resistant conditions because of the life-threatening risks from hypertensive crisis. With MAOIs, there are many dietary restrictions as well which can also lead to difficulties for clients. Also effective for treatment of anxiety is Venlafaxine (Effexor) which is a SNRI.

Antidepressants have the secondary value of treating comorbid depressive disorders in clients but should be used with caution because of untoward effects if the client suffers from another psychiatric or alcohol and other drug disorder which can be adversely affected by the antidepressants.

Anxiolytics

These reduce anxiety to allow clients to participate in therapies directed at underlying problems. Benzodiazepines may be prescribed for short periods of time only because they are habituating. Accumulation of active metabolites can lead to increased sedation, decreased cognitive function, and ataxia. Buspirone is a nonbenzodiazepine and does not cause dependence. It may take 2 to 4 weeks for full effects to become apparent.

Other Classes of Medication

The β-blockers are useful for treatment of social anxiety disorder and panic disorder. Antihistamines: Hydroxyzine (Atarax, Vistaril) relieves symptoms of anxiety but produces no dependence, tolerance, or intoxication.

Integrative Therapy

Consumers are using a wide number of herbs and dietary supplements to relieve stress. Caution is urged because herbs and dietary supplements are not subjected to rigorous testing. Kava kava is one herb that studies show may have considerable promise as a treatment for anxiety.

Evaluation

Identified outcomes serve as a basis for evaluation. In general, evaluation will focus on whether or not there is reduced anxiety, recognition of symptoms as anxiety-related, reduced incidence of symptoms, performance of self-care activities, maintenance of satisfying interpersonal relationships, assumption of usual roles, and use of adaptive coping strategies.

15 Somatoform and Dissociative Disorders

THOUGHTS ABOUT TEACHING THE TOPIC

The use of the nursing process is similar for clients with the various somatoform disorders; thus, emphasizing the similarities seems to work well for students. The lecturer might focus on providing a brief clinical picture of each disorder. Learners might list nursing diagnoses commonly used and then develop a generic care plan using these diagnoses. The same approach may be used for dissociative disorders.

Because many learners will work in the medical-surgical area, exploration of feelings about working with a client who has many physical complaints unsubstantiated by diagnostic tests may be a useful strategy.

KEY TERMS AND OBJECTIVES

alternate personality (alter) or subpersonality, 267
body dysmorphic disorder, 259
conversion disorder, 259
depersonalization disorder, 265
dissociative amnesia, 265
dissociative disorders, 264
dissociative fugue, 266
dissociative identity disorder (DID), 266
factitious disorder, 253
hypochondriasis, 258
la belle indifférence, 259
malingering, 253
pain disorder, 259

psychosomatic illness, 253
secondary gains, 260
somatization, 253
somatization disorder, 258
somatoform disorders, 252

OBJECTIVES

After studying this chapter, the reader will be able to
1. Compare and contrast essential characteristics of the somatoform and the dissociative disorders.
2. Differentiate symptoms of somatoform disorders from (a) malingering, (b) factitious disorder, and (c) psychosomatic illness.
3. Give a clinical example of what would be found in each of the somatoform disorders.
4. Describe five psychosocial interventions that would be appropriate for a client with somatic complaints.
5. Plan interventions for a client with conversion disorder who is receiving a great deal of secondary gain from his or her "blindness." Include self-care and family teaching.
6. Explain the key symptoms of the four dissociative disorders.
7. Compare and contrast dissociative amnesia and dissociative fugue.
8. Identify three specialized elements in the assessment of a client with a dissociative disorder.

CHAPTER OUTLINE	TEACHING STRATEGIES

SOMATOFORM DISORDERS
Prevalence and Comorbidity

Prevalence for each disorder, when known, is listed in Table 15-1. Substance abuse may be comorbid with somatoform pain disorder.

Theory

Somatization is defined as the expression of psychological stress through physical symptoms. Somatoform disorders are characterized by the following:

1. Complaints of physical symptoms not explainable by physiological tests.
2. Psychological factors and conflicts seem important in initiating, exacerbating, and maintaining the disturbance.
3. The client's inability to control the symptom voluntarily.
4. Symptoms that are not intentionally produced (as in malingering or factitious disorder).

No clear etiology exists for somatoform disorders.

Biological Factors

Unexplained physical symptoms (somatization disorder and hypochondriasis) can arise from faulty perceptions and incorrect assessments of bodily sensations associated with attention deficits and cognitive impairments. Somatoform pain disorder may be associated with abnormalities in brain chemical balance or structural abnormalities of sensory or limbic systems. Serotonin and endorphin deficiency may affect incoming pain signals, while serotonin deficiency may be a factor in body dysmorphic disorder. Conversion disorder may be associated with CNS arousal disturbances, and cytokine system dysregulation may be associated with symptoms such as fatigue and anorexia.

Genetic Factors

Somatization disorders tend to run in families, according to twin studies and studies of first-degree female relatives of clients with somatization disorder.

Cultural Factors

Type and frequency of somatic symptoms varies across cultures. Somatization disorder, rarely seen in American men, is common in cultures that permit men to use physical symptoms to deal with stress. Conversion is seen more often among low socioeconomic populations.

Psychoanalytic Theory

This theory holds that psychogenic pain, illness, and loss of function are related to a repressed conflict and a transformation of anxiety into a physical symptom. In conversion disorder, the symptom is symbolically related to the conflict. Psychoanalytic theory suggests hypochondriasis is related to anger, aggression, or hostility, with origins in past losses, and is expressed as a need for help and concern from others. In body dysmorphic disorder, some theorists believe the special meaning attached to a part of the body is traceable to an event during an early developmental stage and that the individual makes use of repression, symbolization, and projection.

Behavioral Theory

This theory suggests somatoform symptoms are learned ways of communicating helplessness, which allows the individual to manipulate others. The symptoms are reinforced by attention, obtaining financial gain, and avoiding certain activities the individual dislikes.

Cognitive Theory

Cognitive theory holds that the client with hypochondriasis focuses on body sensations, misinterprets their meanings, and then becomes alarmed by them.

DSM-IV-TR Criteria and the Clinical Picture of Somatoform Disorders

Somatization Disorder

History of many physical complaints beginning before age 30, occurring over a period of years (resulting in seeking treatment), and impaired social, occupational, or other functioning are the clinical symptoms of somatization disorder.

Hypochondriasis

This involves preoccupation with having a serious disease, or with fear of having a serious disease, that lasts for over 6 months, causing impaired social or occupational functioning; despite appropriate medical tests and reassurance, the preoccupation persists

Pain Disorder

Pain disorders involve pain in one or more anatomical sites of sufficient severity to cause distress, require clinical attention, and cause impaired social or occupational functioning.

Body Dysmorphic Disorder

BDD involves preoccupation with an imagined defect in appearance, causing significant distress and impairment in social or occupational functioning.

Conversion Disorder

This disorder is characterized by the presence of one or more symptoms suggestive of a neurological disorder that cannot be explained by a known neurological, medical, or cultural-bound symptom. Psychological factors such as stress or conflicts

Continued

67

are associated with onset or exacerbation of the symptom(s). Clients with conversion disorder may sometimes display indifference to their condition, an attitude called la belle indifférence.

Application of the Nursing Process
Assessment

Overall Assessment

Perform routine assessment, plus the following.

Symptoms and Unmet Needs

Collect data about nature, location, onset, character, and duration of symptoms or loss of function. Assess affect for lack of concern. Assess for dramatic presentation, ideas about symptoms, and workups that have been performed, results of workups, and resistance to suggestion that symptoms are psychogenic. Note alterations in rest, comfort, activity, and self-care.

Voluntary Control of Symptoms

Somatoform symptoms are not under the individual's voluntary control, whereas symptoms associated with malingering and factitious disorders are under voluntary control.

Secondary Gains

These include getting out of usual responsibilities, getting attention, and manipulating others as a result of the symptoms.

Cognitive Style

Assessing a client's cognitive style may help distinguish between hypochondriasis (has more anxiety about symptoms and shows obsessive attention to details) and somatization disorder (client is often rambling and vague).

Ability to Communicate Feelings
and Emotional Needs

The ability to communicate feelings and emotional needs is often poor in clients with somatoform disorders. The client's chief means of communicating emotional needs may be his or her somatic symptoms.

Dependence on Medication

Dependence on medication to relieve pain or anxiety or to induce sleep needs to be assessed in clients with somatoform disorders. Dependence develops quickly. If treatment has been sought from a number of physicians, substance misuse may occur.

Self-Assessment

Nurse's feelings include anger, helplessness, finding the client difficult and unsatisfying to work with, and perplexity that a client who has no physical basis for symptoms is being treated on a medical unit.

Assessment Guidelines

Assessment should include questions to determine: a history of any similar episodes, prior visits to multiple physicians, instances of abuse as a child, and relevant psychosocial distress issues.

Nursing Diagnosis

Common NANDA diagnoses include *ineffective coping, impaired social interaction, powerlessness, ineffective role performance, interrupted family processes, ineffective sexuality pattern, chronic low self-esteem, situational low self-esteem, spiritual distress, self-care deficit, disturbed sleep pattern,* and *risk for caregiver role strain.*

Outcome Criteria

Outcome criteria and goals should be realistic and attainable and structured in small steps to help staff and client see that progress is being made. For example: will learn more adaptive skills to get needs met as evidenced by replacing reliance on anxiolytics through use of alternative coping strategies such as assertive communication and relaxation techniques; will improve social interaction by establishing and completing a contract to attend a specified number of social or diversional activities daily; will demonstrate improved self-esteem as evidenced by making realistic appraisals of strengths and weaknesses.

Planning	Nursing interventions should focus initially on establishing a helping relationship, given the client's resistance to the concept that no physical cause for the symptom exists and the client tendency to go from caregiver to caregiver.
Intervention	Interventions usually take place in the home or clinic setting.
Basic Level Interventions	The nurse attempts to help the client improve functioning through the development of effective coping strategies.
Promotion of Self-Care	Use matter-of-fact approach to support highest level of self-care of which the client is capable.
Health Teaching	Clients using somatization may need basic information about how the body functions as part of cognitive restructuring. Other coping skills that may be taught include relaxation skills, assertiveness training, biofeedback, and physical exercise.
Case Management	"Doctor shopping" is a common practice of clients with somatoform disorders. Having a case manager may help client avoid this by giving the client someone to whom to relate.
Psychobiological Interventions	Monitor benzodiazepines closely as clients may use them unreliably. Antidepressants, especially the SSRIs, are showing the greatest promise.
Advanced Practice Interventions	Advanced practice nurses use various types of psychotherapy or consultation with primary care providers.
Evaluation	Evaluations often reveal that goals and outcomes are only partially met. This should be considered a positive finding when one considers the amount of resistance to change these clients often exhibit.
DISSOCIATIVE DISORDERS	Dissociative disorders involve disruption of the usually integrated mental functions of consciousness, memory, and identity or perception of environment (e.g., depersonalization disorder involves feeling detached or disconnected from mind or body; a client whose ability to integrate memories is impaired has dissociative amnesia; a client unable to maintain his or her identity may develop a dissociative fugue or dissociative identity disorder.
Prevalence	No known data.
Comorbidity	Mood disorders and substance-related disorders are commonly associated with all of the dissociative disorders. In addition, dissociated amnesia also may be present with conversion disorder or personality disorder. Dissociative fugue may co-occur with PTSD. Clients with DID may also have PTSD, borderline personality disorder, sexual disorders, eating disorders, or sleep disorders. Dersonalization disorder may occur with hypochondriasis, anxiety disorder, or personality disorder.
Theory **Biological Factors**	The development of the limbic system may be faulty, allowing experiences to be detached from memory. Early trauma and lack of attachment may affect neurotransmitter availability. Depersonalization has a possible neurological link as evidenced by its occurrence with epilepsy, brain tumors, and schizophrenia.
Genetic Factors	Dissociative identity disorder is more common among first-degree relatives of individuals with the disorder than among the population at large.
Cultural Factors	In some cultures, culture-bound disorders look remarkably like dissociative disorders.
	Care must be taken to consider the client's culture when making the diagnosis.

Continued

Chapter 15 Somatoform and Dissociative Disorders

Psychosocial Factors

Learning theory suggests dissociative disorders are learned methods for avoiding stress and anxiety, and that the more often "tuning out" is used, the more likely it is to become automatic. All dissociative disorders are believed to be linked with traumatic life events. Abused individuals, for example, may learn to use dissociation to defend against feeling pain and to avoid remembering.

***DSM-IV-TR* and the Clinical Picture of Dissociative Disorders**

Depersonalization Disorder

In this disorder, a persistent or recurrent alteration in perception of the self to the extent that the sense of one's own reality is temporarily lost occurs, while reality-testing ability remains intact. The individual may feel mechanical, dreamy, or detached from the body.

Dissociative Amnesia

This is the inability to recall important personal information of a traumatic or stressful nature. It is more pervasive than forgetfulness. Two types exist: localized and selective.

Dissociative Fugue

Dissociative fugue is the inability to recall identity and information about the past accompanied by travel away from the customary locale.

Dissociative Identity Disorder (DID)

DID is characterized by the presence of two or more distinct alternative or sub-personality states that recurrently take control of behavior. Each subpersonality has its own pattern of perceiving, relating to, and thinking about self and the environment.

Application of the Nursing Process

Assessment

For a diagnosis of dissociative disorder to be made, medical and neurological status, substance abuse, and coexistence of other psychiatric disorders must be ruled out.

Overall Assessment

Should include each of the following:

Identity and Memory

Look for clues to multiple personality—gaps in memory, use of third person when communicating, blackouts, etc.—when assessing client's identity and memory.

Client History

Look for differing sets of memories about childhood, incidents of finding strange clothing in closets, and new belongings the client can't remember buying in assessment of client's history.

Mood

Depression often triggers clients to seek help. Mood shifts may signal DID. Fugue and amnesia victims may seem indifferent or perplexed.

Use of Alcohol and Other Drugs

Dissociative episodes may be associated with drug and alcohol use. Ask specific questions to assess use and abuse.

Impact on Client and Family

Families often find it difficult to accept the erratic behavior of the client with a dissociative disorder. Amnesic clients are often quite dysfunctional. Fugue clients may function well in undemanding occupational and social situations. Clients with DID often have family and occupational problems.

Suicide Risk

Thoughts of suicide are not uncommon when a client's life has been substantially disrupted; therefore, the client's suicide risk must be assessed.

CHAPTER OUTLINE	TEACHING STRATEGIES
Self-Assessment	Nurse's feelings include skepticism, frustration, anger, inadequacy, fatigue, and hypervigilance.
Nursing Diagnosis	Diagnoses often seen include *disturbed personal identity, ineffective coping, anxiety, ineffective role performance, interrupted family processes, risk for self-directed violence, risk for other-directed violence, social isolation, disturbed body image, chronic low self-esteem, powerlessness,* and *disturbed sleep pattern.*
Outcome Criteria	An example of outcome criteria is the following: Client will demonstrate ability to integrate identity and memory as evidenced by describing who he or she is, describing feelings about events in the past, and reporting absence of depersonalization episodes.
Planning	Planning is highly individualized since client needs can be very different. A rule of thumb is, plan for safety first.
Intervention **Basic Level Interventions**	These are detailed in Table 15-7 and include ensuring client safety; providing nondemanding, simple routine; encouraging client to do things for him- or herself; assisting with decision making as necessary, not flooding client with data regarding past events; providing support; helping client see consequences of using dissociation to cope with stress; teaching stress-reducing methods, etc.
Milieu Therapy	High anxiety and crises may occur necessitating hospitalization. Close observation and suicide precautions may be required to meet safety and security needs. The environment should be quiet, simple, structured, and supportive.
Health Teaching	Prevention of dissociative episodes can be taught. The client learns to identify triggers to dissociation, and to develop a plan to interrupt the dissociation by singing, playing an instrument, talking to someone, icing the hands, etc. Daily journal writing puts the client in touch with feelings and provides concrete examples of overcoming triggers to dissociation.
Psychobiological Interventions	There is no evidence that medication of any type has been therapeutic. Antidepressants are the most useful because many with DID have mood disorder.
Advanced Practice Interventions	Therapies used by the advanced practice nurse to treat individuals with dissociative disorders include cognitive-behavioral therapy and psychodynamic psychotherapy. Cognitive-behavioral group therapy has been successful for female sexual assault survivors.
Evaluation	Treatment is considered successful when outcomes are met and when client safety has been maintained, anxiety has been alleviated, conflicts have been explored, new coping strategies permit optimal function, and stress is handled adaptively.

71

16 Personality Disorders

THOUGHTS ABOUT TEACHING THE TOPIC

Students may have had little experience in relating to individuals with PDs. The behaviors demonstrated by these clients are among the most difficult for novices to deal with therapeutically. It's helpful for students to have an opportunity to operationalize intervention strategies in a safe environment via use of role playing or case studies before working with a client. Role playing can be used to demonstrate manipulation, impulsiveness, splitting, devaluation of others, suspiciousness, blaming and accusing others, and demanding behaviors.

KEY TERMS AND CONCEPTS

antisocial personality disorder, 282
avoidant personality disorder, 284
borderline personality disorder, 282
dependent personality disorder, 284
dialectical behavior therapy (DBT), 295
entitlement, 282
histrionic personality disorder, 282
manipulative, 282
narcissistic personality disorder, 284
obsessive-compulsive personality disorder, 285
paranoid personality disorder, 280

personality, 275
personality disorder (PD), 276
schizoid personality disorder, 280
schizotypal personality disorder, 280
splitting, 279

OBJECTIVES

After studying this chapter, the reader will be able to
1. Analyze the interaction of biological determinants and psychodynamic factors in the etiology of personality disorders.
2. Identify the three clusters of personality disorders.
3. Describe the main characteristic of one personality disorder from each cluster and give an example.
4. Formulate two nursing diagnoses for cluster B personality disorders.
5. Discuss the nature and importance of crisis intervention for people with personality disorders.
6. Describe the feelings that are experienced by nurses and others when working with people with personality disorders.
7. Discuss two realistic nursing outcomes for clients with borderline personality disorder.
8. Plan basic interventions for an impulsive, aggressive, or manipulative client.

CHAPTER OUTLINE	TEACHING STRATEGIES
	Personality disorders (PDs) involve long-term and repetitive use of maladaptive and often self-defeating behaviors. People with PD do not recognize their symptoms as uncomfortable; thus they do not seek treatment unless a severe crisis occurs. All PDs have four characteristics in common: (1) inflexible and maladaptive response to stress; (2) disability in working and loving; (3) ability to evoke interpersonal conflict; (4) capacity to frustrate others. People with PD tend to be perceived as aggravating and demanding by health care workers, so the potential for value judgments is high and effective care is at risk.
Prevalence and Comorbidity	In the general population, is 10% to 15%, depending on severity. Personality disorders are predisposing factors for many other psychiatric disorders and may coexist with depression, panic disorder, substance use disorder, eating disorder, anxiety disorder, PTSD, somatization, and impulse control disorders.
Theory	It's unlikely that there is a single cause for a discrete personality disorder.
Biological Determinants	Schizotypal PD occurs more frequently in nonpsychotic first-degree relatives of schizophrenics than in control families. Paranoid PD occurs more frequently in relatives with major depression than in controls. Antisocial behavior is more related to genetic factors than environment.
Chronic Trauma	Repeated cycles of trauma may reorganize the brain's cortical map, cognitive and behavioral development, and the unconscious. Later, clients may act out a forgotten history, disconnect from emotions, and develop fear of others. They are unable to attach

72

adaptively to others and seem unable to perceive cues others give them about how to do so. Thus manipulation and power struggles are the norm in all relationships with a person with PD. Stress experienced by the person with PD is thought to beget a more efficient neurochemical system for rekindling an inner experience of crisis.

Psychosocial Factors

Issues include use of repression, suppression, undoing, and consolidation to explain PDs. The goal of psychodynamic therapy is to form a relationship that can correct past experiences.

***DSM-IV-TR* and the Clinical Picture of Cluster A Disorders (Odd or Eccentric)**

Characteristics of clients with the various cluster A disorders are listed below.

Paranoid Personality Disorder

Characteristics: suspicious of others; fear others will exploit, harm, or deceive them; fear of confiding in others (fear personal information will be used against them); misread compliments as manipulation; hypervigilant; prone to counterattack; hostile; and aloof.

Psychotic episodes may occur in times of stress. Nurses should give straightforward explanations of tests, history taking, and procedures, side effects of drugs, changes in treatment plan, and possible further procedures, to counteract client fear.

Schizoid Personality Disorder

Characteristics: avoids close relationships, is socially isolated, has poor occupational functioning, and appears cold, aloof, and detached. Social awareness is lacking and relationships generate fear and confusion in the client. Nurses should strive for simplification and clarity to help decrease client anxiety.

Schizotypal Personality Disorder

Characteristics: ideas of reference; magical thinking or odd beliefs; perceptual distortions; vague, stereotyped speech; frightened, suspicious, blunted affect; distant and strained social relationships. These clients tend to be frightened and suspicious in social situations. Explanations can ease their anxiety.

***DSM-IV-TR* and the Clinical Picture of Cluster B Disorders (Dramatic, Emotional, Erratic)**

The clinical characteristics of clients with cluster B disorders follow.

Antisocial Personality Disorder

Characteristics: has superficial charm, violates rights of others, exploits others, lies, cheats, lacks guilt or remorse, is impulsive, acts out, and lacks empathy. As clients these individuals are extremely manipulative and aggressive. Nurses must establish and adhere to a plan of care, and maintain clear boundaries if they are to minimize client manipulation and acting out.

Borderline Personality Disorder

Characteristics: unstable, intense relationships; identity disturbances; impulsivity; self-mutilation; rapid mood shifts; chronic emptiness; intense fear of abandonment; splitting; and anger. A major defense is splitting (alternating between idealizing and devaluing). Self-mutilation and suicide-prone behavior are often-used impulsive self-destructive behaviors. Anger is intense and pervasive and help with anger management is an important intervention. Relationship building, safety, and limit setting are other foci.

Histrionic Personality Disorder

Characteristics: center of attention; flamboyant; seductive or provocative behaviors; shallow, rapidly shifting emotions; dramatic expression of emotions; overly concerned with impressing others; exaggerates degree of intimacy with others; self-aggrandizing; preoccupied with own appearance. Experience depression when admiration of others is not given. Suicide gestures may result in client entry into the health care system. A thorough assessment of suicide potential must be undertaken, and support offered in the form of clear parameters of psychotherapy.

Narcissistic Personality Disorder

Characteristics: grandiosity, fantasies of power or brilliance, need to be admired, sense of entitlement, arrogant, patronizing, rude, overestimates self and underestimates others. This behavior covers a fragile ego. In health care setting demand the best of everything. When client is corrected, when boundaries are

Continued

73

defined, or when limits are set on client's behavior, client feels humiliated, degraded, and empty. To lower anxiety the client may launch a counterattack. The nurse should gently help the client identify attempts to seek and become perfect, exhibit grandiose behavior, and sense of entitlement.

DSM-IV-TR and the Clinical Picture of Cluster C Disorders (Anxious, Fearful)

Characteristics found in clients with cluster C disorders follow.

Avoidant Personality Disorder

Characteristics: social inhibition, feelings of inadequacy, hypersensitivity to criticism, preoccupation with fear of rejection and criticism, and self perceived to be socially inept.

Low self-esteem and hypersensitivity grow as support networks decrease. Demands of workplace often overwhelming. Project that caregivers will harm them through disapproval and perceive rejection where none exists. Nurses can teach socialization skills, provide positive feedback, and build self-esteem.

Dependent Personality Disorder

Characteristics: inability to make daily decisions without advice and reassurance, need of others to be responsible for important areas of life, anxious and helpless when alone, and submissive. Solicit care taking by clinging. Fear abandonment if they are too competent. Experience anxiety and may have co-existing depression.

Obsessive-Compulsive Personality Disorder

Characteristics: preoccupied with rules, perfectionistic, too busy to have friends, rigid control, and superficial relationships. Complains about others' inefficiencies and gives others directions.

Application of the Nursing Process

Assessment

Assessment Tools

The Minnesota Multiphasic Personality Inventory (MMPI) is useful to evaluate personality.

Assessment of History

The nurse should seek information about the medical history; suicidal or homicidal ideation; current use of medications and other substances, food, and money; involvement with the courts; current or past physical, sexual, or emotional abuse; as well as seek information about the client's current level of crisis and dysfunctional coping styles.

Self-Assessment

The nurse may experience intense feelings of confusion, helplessness, anger, and frustration. The client may attempt to manipulate or disparage the nurse, create conflict via splitting or faction forming. Support and supervision for the nurse are essential.

Nursing Diagnosis

Useful diagnoses include *ineffective coping, anxiety, risk for other-directed violence, risk for self-directed violence,* and *impaired social interaction, social isolation, fear, disturbed thought processes, defensive coping, self-mutilation, chronic low self-esteem, ineffective therapeutic regimen management.*

Outcome Criteria

Realistic goal setting is important, because change occurs so slowly. Small steps are necessary. Examples include minimizing self-destructive or aggressive behavior; reducing the effect of manipulative behaviors; linking consequences to both functional and dysfunctional behaviors; initiating functional alternatives to prevent a crisis; ongoing management of anger, anxiety, shame, and happiness.

Planning

Clients with personality disorder are usually admitted to psychiatric institutions for reasons other than their personality disorder. Most often seen are borderline and antisocial clients. The former are impulsive, suicidal, self-mutilating, aggressive, manipulative, and even psychotic, under stress. The latter are manipulative, aggressive, and impulsive.

Intervention

When clients blame and attack others, the nurse needs to understand the context—that the attacks spring from feeling threatened. The nurse must orient the client to reality whenever the client imputes malevolent intentions to the nurse or others and reassure the client that even though the caregiver has been insulted or threatened, the client will still be helped and protected. The nurse must explain how people, systems, families, and relationships work and acknowledge shortcomings and limitations.

Communication Guidelines

Nurses enhance their ability to be therapeutic when they are able to use authenticity and trustworthiness, are able to set limits, and learn to deal with manipulation.

Milieu Therapy

Goal of milieu therapy is affect management within a group context. Nurses must help clients verbalize feelings rather than act them out.

Psychobiological Interventions

Antipsychotics may be useful for brief periods to control agitation, rage, and brief psychotic episodes. Antidepressants may be useful for clients with borderline PD. Medication compliance is usually an important issue as clients with PD are fearful about taking something over which they have no control.

Case Management

Case management is geared toward reducing the necessity for hospitalization.

Evaluation

Caregiver should not measure personal self-esteem based on client's ability to change, since the ability to change is severely limited in clients with PD.

Some students, especially those who are visually oriented, find using a concept map helpful in learning. Following is a concept map for PDs.

Concept Map: Personality Disorders

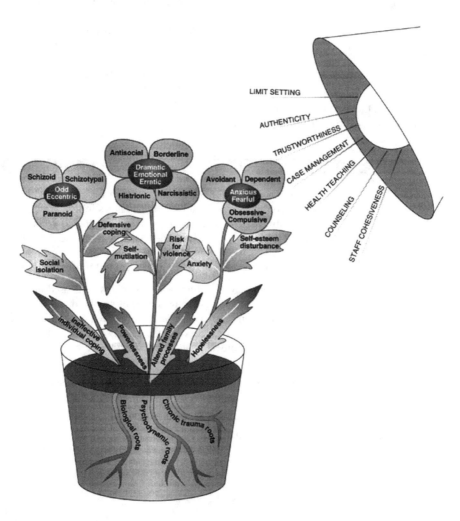

17 Eating Disorders

THOUGHTS ABOUT TEACHING THE TOPIC

Films on anorexia nervosa, bulimia nervosa, and obesity caused by compulsive eating are excellent vehicles for assisting learners to meet chapter objectives and for promoting discussion.

Because caring for clients with eating disorders requires considerable nursing skill, behavioral rehearsals in the form of role playing can help prepare learners for common, recurrent clinical situations. Since it is often difficult for the normal-weight individual who has no eating problems to empathize with a client with an eating disorder, role playing can be helpful in raising awareness.

KEY TERMS AND CONCEPTS

anorexia nervosa, 299
binge eating disorder, 300
bulimia nervosa, 299
cognitive distortions, 309
ideal body weight, 308

OBJECTIVES

After studying this chapter, the reader will be able to
1. Discuss the four theories of eating disorder discussed in this chapter.
2. Compare and contrast the signs and symptoms (clinical picture) of anorexia nervosa and bulimia nervosa.
3. Identify three life-threatening conditions, stated in terms of nursing diagnoses, for a client with an eating disorder.
4. Identify three realistic outcome criteria for (a) a client with anorexia nervosa and (b) a client with bulimia nervosa.
5. Recognize which therapeutic interventions are appropriate for the acute phase of anorexia nervosa and which are appropriate for the long-term phase of treatment.
6. Explain the basic premise of cognitive-behavioral therapy in the treatment of anorexia nervosa and bulimia nervosa.
7. Empathize with and describe in the reader's own words the possible thoughts and feelings of a young anorectic girl during the acute phase of her illness.
8. Distinguish between the needs of and treatment(s) for clients with acute bulimia and bulimic individuals in long-term therapy.
9. Differentiate between the long-term prognosis of anorexia nervosa, bulimia nervosa, and binge eating disorder.

CHAPTER OUTLINE	TEACHING STRATEGIES
Prevalence	Lifetime prevalence of anorexia nervosa for women is about 0.5%. The prevalence of bulimia nervosa for women ranges from 1% to 3%. Female athletes, especially where thinness is emphasized, have demonstrated an increase in eating disorders, and male body builders have demonstrated an increase in anorexia nervosa. Males with eating disorders tend to have later onset and be involved in a sport or occupation in which weight control is associated with performance.
Comorbidity	Major depressive disorder or dysthymia is diagnosed in 50% to 75% of clients with eating disorders. The incidence of bipolar disorder may be as high as 13%. Obsessive-compulsive disorder is common among clients with bulimia nervosa. Other comorbid disorders include anxiety disorder, substance abuse disorder, and personality disorder. In addition, a history of sexual abuse is more common in those with eating disorders than in the general population.
Theory	The eating disorders are actually separate entities as they do not have a common cause, common pathology, or common treatment.
Neurobiological and Neuroendocrine Models	A number of theories exist: an eating disorder causes depression or is a variant of a depressive disorder; biological relatives of clients with eating disorders show increased frequency of depression; neuroendocrine abnormalities have been doc-

CHAPTER OUTLINE	TEACHING STRATEGIES

	umented in clients with eating disorders; cholecystokinin is at low levels in bulimics. These theories and findings may help explain the drive toward dieting, hunger, preoccupation with food, and tendency toward binge eating.
Psychological Models	Psychological theories explore issues of control in anorexia and affective instability and poor impulse control in bulimia.
Sociocultural Models	Sociocultural models and theory consider our present societal ideal of being thin and the influence of role conflict. In societies where women have social-role choices, the incidence of eating disorders increases; eating disorders do not flourish in male-dominated societies where women are forced into stereotypical nurturing roles. In modernizing countries such as China, anorectic behavior may grow out of spiritual or ascetic values.
Genetic Models	These theories explore genetic vulnerabilities as a basis for predisposing people to eating disorders. A twin study showed a 56% concordance rate for monozygotic twins for anorexia nervosa.
ANOREXIA NERVOSA **Application of the Nursing Process** **Assessment** **Overall Assessment**	The client with anorexia nervosa often enters the health care system via admission to the ICU with electrolyte imbalance. The nurse should assess for lanugo; low blood pressure, pulse, and temperature consistent with malnutrition; poor hydration. Explore client perception of the problem; eating habits and history of dieting; methods used to achieve control; value attached to specific weight; shape; interpersonal and social functioning; mental status. Table 17–1 contains further information.
Self-Assessment	The nurse often has difficulty relating empathetically to the client who "chooses" to engage in behaviors that put life at risk. Giving encouragement may cross the line to authoritarianism and a parental role. Frustration is experienced as the client resists weight gain.
Assessment Guidelines	The client and family will need to be assessed in order to provide ongoing monitoring, teaching, and support to help address the issues of physical and psychological health and ongoing treatment for the eating disorder.
Nursing Diagnosis	Useful diagnoses include *imbalanced nutrition: less than body requirements; decreased cardiac output, risk for injury, disturbed body image, anxiety, chronic low self-esteem, deficient knowledge, ineffective coping, powerlessness;* and *hopelessness.*
Outcome Criteria	Examples of outcome criteria include the following: client will normalize eating patterns, as evidenced by eating 75% of three meals per day plus two snacks; client will achieve 85% to 90% of ideal body weight; client will demonstrate improved self-acceptance as evidenced by verbal and nonverbal data; client will participate in long-term treatment to prevent relapse, etc.
Planning	Type of treatment is partly determined by severity of weight loss. Another factor to consider is the experienced disruption of the client's life. Outpatient therapy is the mainstay of treatment, but hospital admission may be required if an anorectic client is below 75% of ideal body weight and is medically unstable. Brief hospitalization can address only acute complications such as electrolyte imbalance, dysrhythmias, limited weight restoration, and acute psychiatric symptoms such as depression. The refeeding syndrome is a severe, and potentially catastrophic, complication in which the demands the replenished circulatory system place on the nutritionally depleted cardiac mass result in cardiovascular collapse.

Continued

77

Intervention

Basic Level Interventions:
Acute Care

Typical admission is for a crisis state. The nurse is challenged to establish trust in a very short time and monitor the eating pattern as well.

Milieu Therapy

Focus is on establishing more adaptive behavioral patterns including normalization of eating. This includes precise mealtimes, adherence to selected menu, observation during and following meals, regularly scheduled weighing, and client privileges correlated with weight gain and treatment plan compliance. To ensure there is no self-induced vomiting, close monitoring of bathroom use after meals and after visits is necessary.

Counseling

The basic level nurse on an inpatient unit will focus on issues that are important to the patient, dependent on the assessment. Any acute psychiatric symptoms such as suicidal ideation are addressed immediately, and a weight restoration program is begun. The treatment goal is set at 90% of ideal body weight, the weight at which most women menstruate. As clients begin the weight-restoration program they will participate in milieu therapy, attend individual and group psychotherapy along with nutritional counseling. Cognitive therapy addresses distortions of thinking.

Health Teaching

Self-care activities are an important part of the plan. Activities include learning constructive coping skills, improving social skills, and developing problem-solving and decision-making skills. Eating out in a restaurant is practiced; preparing a meal and eating forbidden foods are also explored.

Advanced Practice Interventions:
Long-Term Treatment

One to 6 years is common. Foci are on weight maintenance and achievement of a sense of self-worth and self-acceptance not exclusively based on appearance; achieving a balance between dependence and independence; and improving communication within families. A combination of individual, group, couples, and family therapy gives the best chance for successful outcomes.

Psychotherapy

Whatever the treatment setting, the goals of treatment remain the same: weight restoration with normalization of eating habits and beginning treatment of psychological, interpersonal, and social issues that are integral to the experience of the client. In the acute weight restoration phase, interventions are determined by the unstable weight and a cognitive behavioral approach is necessary. Critical pathways are useful for hospitalized clients and those treated via a psychiatric home care program.

Psychopharmacology

SSRIs have been reported to improve the rate of weight gain and reduce relapse. Olanzapine has been reported to decrease agitation and resistance to treatment.

Evaluation

Goals are daily guides to reaching successful outcomes and must be continually reevaluated for appropriateness.

BULIMIA NERVOSA

DSM-IV-TR subtypes the disorder as purging and nonpurging types.

Application of the Nursing Process
Assessment
Overall Assessment

Clients with bulimia nervosa often do not appear physically or emotionally ill. Weight is usually at or slightly below ideal body weight. Inspect for enlarged parotid glands, dental erosion, and caries if client has induced vomiting. History may reveal poor impulse control, compulsivity, chaotic interpersonal relationships. Client is sensitive to others' perceptions of her illness, and may experience shame and feeling out of control.

Self-Assessment

Building trust with the client is essential, but is difficult because the nurse often feels the client is not being honest when she does not report actively bingeing or purging (due to feelings of shame).

78

Nursing Diagnosis	Useful diagnoses include *risk for injury, decreased cardiac output, disturbed body image, powerlessness, chronic low self-esteem, anxiety, ineffective coping.* Problems resulting from purging are a first priority because electrolyte and fluid balance and cardiac function are affected.
Outcome Criteria	Examples of outcomes include the following: client will refrain from binge eating; will abstain from purging; will demonstrate new skills for managing stress, anxiety, shame; will be free of self-directed harm, etc.
Planning	General hospital admission is reserved for life-threatening complications such as fluid and electrolyte imbalance. Admission to an inpatient psychiatric unit for severe psychiatric symptoms (i.e., acute suicidal risk) provides short-term care. Referrals are provided for continued outpatient treatment.
Intervention **Basic Level Interventions:** **Acute Care**	A medically compromised client will be referred to an inpatient setting where they can participate in cognitive-behavioral model of treatment which is highly effective for the treatment of bulimia. Therapy will help the client restructure eating to interrupt the cycle of eating and purging to begin to incorporate more normalized eating habits. The client receives education, support and therapy for the bulimia and for comorbid disorders such as substance dependence and depression.
Milieu Therapy	Structured to interrupt the binge-purge cycles via observation during and after meals to prevent purging; normalization of eating; and appropriate exercise.
Counseling	Clients with bulimia are usually more ego-dystonic and therefore will more readily establish a therapeutic alliance with the nurse. This alliance allows the basic level nurse, along with other members of the interdisciplinary team to provide services and give the client necessary feedback regarding distorted beliefs.
Health Teaching	Client learns how to cope with challenges such as eating out.
Advanced Practice Interventions: Long-Term Treatment **Psychotherapy**	Cognitive-behavioral therapy is most effective. Reduction in purging by session 6 predicts a successful outcome. Focus is on changing dysfunctional attitudes to ones of self-acceptance and correcting faulty perceptions of weight and shape. The client needs to help to change faulty perceptions and be able to treat comorbid disorders at the same time.
Psychopharmacology	Antidepressants, especially SSRIs, may be useful.
Evaluation	Evaluation is accomplished by comparing desired outcomes to the actual outcomes.
BINGE EATING DISORDER	Binge eating disorder refers to obesity associated with binge eating that serves the function of mood regulation. Goal of treatment is modification of disordered eating and control of depressive symptoms, resulting in a more appropriate weight. Not all obesity is the result of binge eating. Cognitive-behavioral therapy is the most promising. The usefulness of SSRIs is being studied.

79

THOUGHTS ABOUT TEACHING THE TOPIC

Although nearly everyone has experienced a low mood, most learners cannot conceptualize the depth and breadth of the experience of depression. Learning activities to sensitize students include first-person accounts of depression, books and articles about the experience of depression, and films and videotapes portraying depressed individuals.

KEY TERMS AND CONCEPTS

anergia, 331
anhedonia, 331
dysthymic disorder (DD), 328
hypersomnia, 336
light therapy, 352
major depressive disorder (MDD), 327
mood, 328
novel antidepressants, 344
psychomotor agitation, 334
psychomotor retardation, 334
selective serotonin reuptake inhibitors (SSRIs), 343
St. John's wort, 352
transcranial magnetic stimulation (TMS), 352
tricyclic antidepressants (TCAs), 345
vegetative signs of depression, 334

OBJECTIVES

After studying this chapter, the reader will be able to
1. Compare and contrast major depressive disorder with dysthymia.
2. Discuss the links between the stress model of depression and the biological model of depression.
3. Assess behaviors in a depressed individual at the reader's clinical site with regard to each of the following areas: (a) affect, (b) thought processes, (c) feelings, (d) physical behavior, and (e) communication.
4. Formulate five nursing diagnoses for a client who is depressed and include outcome criteria.
5. Name unrealistic expectations that a nurse may have while working with a depressed person and compare them with the reader's personal reactions.
6. Role-play six principles of communication that are useful with depressed clients.
7. Evaluate the advantages of the selective serotonin reuptake inhibitors over the tricyclic antidepressants.
8. Explain the unique attributes of two of the newer atypical antidepressants for use in specific circumstances.
9. Write a medication teaching plan for clients taking the tricyclic antidepressants, including (a) adverse effects, (b) toxic reactions, and (c) other drugs that can trigger an adverse reaction.
10. Discuss two common adverse reactions to the monoamine oxidase inhibitors, state one serious toxic reaction, and identify the appropriate medical intervention.
11. Write a medication teaching plan for a client taking a monoamine oxidase inhibitor, including foods and drugs that are contraindicated.
12. Describe the types of depression for which electroconvulsive therapy is most helpful.

CHAPTER OUTLINE	TEACHING STRATEGIES
Prevalence	The lifetime prevalence for a major depressive episode is 17%. Most studies find that major depressive disorder (MDD) is twice as common in women as in men. The prevalence rates for MDD appear unrelated to ethnicity, education, income or marital status. Dysthymic disorder (DD) occurs in about 5.1% of the population during their lifetime.
Children and Adolescents	Major depressive disorder is said to occur in up to 18% of preadolescents.
Elderly	Depression in the elderly is a major health problem. Among the elderly, prevalence differs related to living arrangement: 3.5% for those in the community up to 15% to 20% for those in nursing homes.

Comorbidity

A depressive syndrome frequently accompanies other psychiatric disorders such as schizophrenia, substance abuse, eating disorders, anxiety disorders, and personality disorders. Depression is high among people with a medical disorder.

Depressive Disorders and Clinical Presentations

Major Depressive Disorder

Severe emotional, cognitive, behavioral, and physical symptoms of depression, with a history of one or more major depressive episodes and no history of manic or hypomanic episodes, characterize major depressive disorders. At least 60% can expect to have a second episode.

Dysthymia

Mild to moderate symptoms of depression experienced over most of the day, more days than not, for at least 2 years, would be diagnosed as dysthymia. Hospitalization is rarely necessary. Age of onset: from early childhood to early adulthood.

Subtypes

Major depressions may be diagnosed with a specifier, such as psychotic features, catatonic features, melancholic features, postpartum onset, seasonal features (seasonal affective disorder, or SAD), or atypical features.

Theory
Biological Theories
Genetic Factors

Twin studies show that genetics plays a role in development of depressive disorders. Identical twins have a fivefold greater concordance rate than dizygotic twins.

Biochemical Factors

Depression is probably a biologically heterogeneous disorder, the result of various neurotransmitter (e.g., serotonin, norepinephrine, acetylcholine, dopamine) abnormalities. However, medical treatment is often successful.

Alterations in Hormonal Regulation

Research into the relationship of depression and hyperactivity of the limbic-hypothalamic-pituitary-adrenal axis is ongoing. The dexamethasone suppression test lends some credence to this theory.

Sleep Abnormalities

May be evident in up to 90% of hospitalized clients during a major depressive episode. People prone to depression tend to have a premature loss of deep slow-wave sleep and REM latency. Clients without REM latency seem to respond poorly to tricyclic antidepressants.

Psychodynamic Influences and Life Events

Psychosocial stressors and interpersonal events appear to trigger certain neurophysical and neurochemical changes in the brain. Early life trauma may result in long-term hyperactivity of the CNS corticotropin-releasing factor and norepinephrine systems with a neurotoxic effect on the hippocampus. These changes could cause sensitization to even mild stress in adulthood and predispose to major depression.

Cognitive Theory

This theory suggests depression is the product of irrational or illogical thinking and negative processing of information. Beck's cognitive triad includes these: a negative, deprecating view of self; a pessimistic view of the world; and the belief that negative reinforcement will continue in the future. The goal of cognitive therapy is to change the way clients think by assisting them to identify and test negative cognition, develop alternative thinking patterns, and rehearse new cognitive and behavioral responses.

Learned Helplessness

Seligman suggests that although anxiety is the initial response to a stressful situation, anxiety is replaced by depression if the person feels that the self has no control over the outcome of the situation. A person who believes that an undesired

Continued

Chapter 18   Mood Disorders: Depression

event is his or her fault and that nothing can be done to change it is prone to depression. A behavioral approach helps individuals gain a sense of control and mastery by teaching new and more effective coping skills and ways to increase self-confidence.

Application of the Nursing Process

Assessment

Overall Assessment

Goldberg suggests evaluating depressive symptoms, then assessing possible cause and past episodes.

Assessment Tools

A number of standardized screening tools are available: the Beck Depression Inventory, the Hamilton Depression Scale, the Zung Depression Scale, the Geriatric Depression Scale, etc.

Safety First: Assessment of Suicide Potential

Evaluate for suicidal or homicidal ideation. About 10% to 15% of depressed people eventually commit suicide. Questions are given to assist the nurse to assess suicidal tendency.

Key Findings

Include depressed mood; anhedonia; anxiety; psychomotor retardation; poor memory and concentration; dwelling on perceived faults and failures; delusions of being punished or of being a terrible person; feelings of worthlessness, helplessness, guilt, and anger; and vegetative signs (change in bowel habits, eating habits, sleep disturbances, and disinterest in sex).

Areas to Assess

Affect

Sadness, dejection, and hopelessness are reflected. Posture is slumped. Eye contact is poor. Bouts of weeping may occur or client may be unable to cry. Anhedonia is present.

Thought Processes

Assessment of suicidal ideation is the highest priority. Delusions of being punished for bad deeds or being a terrible person are common, as is trouble concentrating or thinking. Judgment is poor, indecisiveness is common, and memory is impaired.

Feelings

Anxiety, worthlessness, guilt, anger, hopelessness, and helplessness are experienced. Themes of inadequacy and incompetence are repeated relentlessly. Guilt is seen in rumination over present and past failings. Delusional belief that one is being punished by God for terrible sins is common. Helplessness is evidenced by inability to carry out even simple tasks. Hopelessness is present and has been identified as having the following attributes: negative expectations for the future, loss of control over future outcomes, passive acceptance of the futility of planning to achieve goals, and emotional negativism, as expressed in despair, despondency, or depression. Anger and irritability are outcomes of feelings of helplessness. Anger in depression is often expressed inappropriately in property destruction, hurtful verbal attacks, or physical aggression toward others or self.

Physical Behavior

Lethargy and fatigue can result in psychomotor retardation, which can range from slowed movement to complete inactivity and incontinence. Psychomotor agitation may be seen in other clients. Grooming and personal hygiene are often neglected. Vegetative signs of depression are universal. Changes in eating patterns are common, with anorexia occurring in 60% to 70% of people with depression. Sleep pattern disturbances are a cardinal sign of depression. Terminal insomnia is prevalent, but some experience hypersomnia. Change in bowel habits is common, with constipation seen in clients with psychomotor retardation, and diarrhea sometimes occurring in clients with psychomotor agitation. Loss of libido usually occurs, with males sometimes experiencing impotence.

Chapter 18   Mood Disorders: Depression

CHAPTER OUTLINE	TEACHING STRATEGIES
	Communication: Slow speech is common. Comprehension is slowed, with muteness possible. More time is needed by the client to compose a reply.
Self-Assessment	Nurse's feelings and self-assessment: Depressed clients often reject the overtures of the nurse and others. Clients are resistant to change and do not appear to respond to nursing interventions. Nurses experience frustration, hopelessness, and annoyance. Nurses can alter these responses by recognizing unrealistic expectations they have for self or client, identifying feelings they are experiencing that originate with the client, and understanding the part that neurotransmitters play in the precipitation and maintenance of a depressed mood.
Unrealistic Expectations of Self	Nurses often expect more of themselves and the client than they or the client can produce. This leads to feelings of anxiety, hurt, anger, helplessness, and incompetence. Expectations need to be made conscious and worked through with peers or supervisors.
Client Feelings Experienced by the Nurse	Although the feelings originate in the client, the nurse may experience (via empathy) intense feelings of anxiety, frustration, annoyance, and helplessness. The nurse can discuss these feelings with peers and supervisors to separate personal feelings from those originating in the client. Unless feelings are dealt with, the nurse is likely to withdraw from the client.
Assessment Guidelines	Always evaluate the client's risk for harm to self or others. Also important are a thorough physical and neurological exam. The client's history, current medications, and evaluation for other psychiatric disorders is also important. The nurse must assess family and significant other support to help with education and referrals.
Nursing Diagnosis	Useful diagnoses include *risk for self-directed violence, disturbed thought processes; chronic low self esteem, powerlessness, spiritual distress, impaired social interaction, activity intolerance, imbalanced nutrition: less than body requirements, constipation, disturbed sleep pattern, ineffective coping,* and *interrupted family processes, ineffective role performance, risk for impaired parent/infant/child attachment,* etc.
Outcome Criteria	Outcome criteria and short-term goals are individualized for each client. A sample of NOC outcome criteria provides examples.
Planning	Interventions are designed to produce behaviors that meet outcome criteria.
Intervention	Three phases in treatment and recovery from major depression are conceptualized as 1. The acute phase (6 to 12 weeks)—psychiatric management and initial treatment 2. The continuation phase (4 to 9 months)—treatment continues to prevent relapse 3. The maintenance phase (1 or more years)—continuation of antidepressants to prevent relapse
Basic Level Interventions	Addresses counseling, health teaching, self-care activities, and milieu management.
Counseling and Communication Strategies	Depressed clients may be unable to carry on conversations with the nurse and the nurse may become anxious as a result. The nurse must realize that sitting in silence communicates caring. Communication guidelines: Use technique of making observations; use simple, concrete words; allow time for client to respond; listen for covert messages and ask about suicide plans; avoid platitudes. Counseling

Continued

Chapter 18   Mood Disorders: Depression

guidelines: help clients question underlying assumptions and beliefs and consider alternative explanations; work with clients to identify cognitive distortions that encourage negative self-appraisal; encourage activities that raise self-esteem (developing problem-solving skills, coping skills, and assertiveness); encourage exercise (e.g., running, weightlifting); encourage formation of supportive relationships; provide referrals to religious or spiritual resources as needed.

Health Teaching

Helping clients and families to understand that depression is a medical illness is the goal. The biological symptoms of depression should be explained, along with teaching about medications. Predischarge counseling should include clarification of interpersonal stresses and discussion of measures to reduce tension for the family system. Possible use of aftercare facilities can be explored.

Self-Care Activities

Client should be assisted with self-care activities as necessary.

Milieu Therapy

Hospitalization is necessary for acutely suicidal clients, to regulate medication or, when indicated, to provide a course of ECT. Milieu protocols for client safety are useful. During the continuation and maintenance phases, people find that various short-term therapies are useful for dealing with the presence and aftermath of the episode. Support groups may also be helpful.

Advanced Practice Interventions
Psychotherapy

Nurses may conduct short-term therapies, which have produced good results. Interpersonal psychotherapy (IPT) focuses on the role of dysfunctional interpersonal relationships in precipitating and perpetuating depression. Cognitive behavior therapy teaches the connection between thoughts and feelings, the negative thoughts typical of depression, and the reframing of thinking. The behavioral component may be used to teach depressed clients effective social and coping skills. Group treatment and interactive group therapy may also be helpful.

Psychopharmacology

A combination of specific psychotherapies and antidepressants has been found to be superior to either alone.

What Antidepressants Can Do

Antidepressants can positively alter poor self-concept, degree of withdrawal, vegetative symptoms, and activity level. Target symptoms include sleep disturbance, appetite disturbance, fatigue, decreased sex drive, psychomotor retardation or agitation, diurnal variations, impaired concentration or forgetfulness, and anhedonia. It may be necessary to take antidepressants for 1 to 3 weeks or longer before response is shown.

Factors Considered in Choosing a Specific Antidepressant

Primary considerations are: side effects profile, ease of administration, history of past response, safety and medical considerations, and specific subtype of depression. Secondary considerations are: neurotransmitter specificity, family history of response, blood level considerations, and cost.

Psychopharmacological and Other Somatic Treatments

First-line agents are considered to be SSRIs, novel antidepressants, and tricyclic antidepressants. Second-line agents are MAOIs and ECT.

Selective Serotonin Reuptake Inhibitors

Are recommended as first-line therapy in all depressions except psychotic depression, melancholic depression, or mild depression. They have a low incidence of anticholinergic side effects, low cardiotoxicity, and faster onset of action than tricyclics. Client compliance is better than with other antidepressants. SSRIs are prescribed with success for several anxiety disorders and for some clients with dysphoric disorder. Common side effects include mild anticholinergic effects (dry mouth, blurred vision, urinary retention), agitation, sleep disturbance, tremor,

84

anorgasmia, headache. Autonomic reactions are dry mouth, sweating, weight change, mild nausea, and loose bowel movements. Serious side effects include central serotonin syndrome (CSS), as evidenced by abdominal pain, diarrhea, sweating, fever, tachycardia, elevated blood pressure (BP), delirium, myoclonus, irritability, hyperpyrexia, cardiovascular shock. Risk is great if given concurrently with an MAOI, so a time gap should exist between medications.

New Atypical (Novel) Antidepressants

There are many newer antidepressants and more continue to be released. Cymbalta is the newest of these novel antidepressants. The novel antidepressants affect reuptake of different neurotransmitters. They do not have similar effects nor do they have the same side effect profiles. See Table 18-11 and 18-12 for more details about each of these novel antidepressants. Drug monographs for each of the newer antidepressants can be found on the Evolve website.

Alprazolam (Xanax) is effective for mild to moderate depression with anxious features. It has few side effects, but can be habituating.

Tricyclic Antidepressants

The TCAs act by inhibiting reuptake of norepinephrine and serotonin by the presynaptic neurons in the CNS, and require 10 to 14 days or longer to act. Treatment is started with low doses and increased. Therapy is continued 6 to 12 months to prevent early relapse. Common side effects include anticholinergic effects such as dry mouth, blurred vision, tachycardia, orthostatic hypotension, constipation, urinary retention, esophageal reflux. Serious side effects are cardiac dysrhythmias, tachycardia, myocardial infarction, heart block. Adverse drug interactions may occur when TCAs are taken concurrently with MAOIs, phenothiazines, barbiturates, disulfiram, oral contraceptives, anticoagulants, benzodiazepines, alcohol, nicotine, and some antihypertensives. Contraindications are recent myocardial infarction, narrow-angle glaucoma, seizures, pregnancy. Administering the total daily dose at night is beneficial as their sedative effects will aid sleep, and minor side effects will occur during sleep when the client is unaware of them (fosters compliance). Areas for the nurse to discuss with client and family are detailed in Box 18-5.

Monoamine Oxidase Inhibitors

These are effective treatment for atypical depression and several anxiety disorders when dietary restriction of tyramine is observed. Common side effects include orthostatic hypotension, weight gain, edema, change in heart rate and rhythm, constipation, urinary hesitancy, vertigo, hypomanic or manic behavior, insomnia, weakness, fatigue. Adverse reactions are an increase in BP with possible stroke; hyperpyrexia; convulsions and death in the presence of tyramine-containing foods. Contraindications include cerebrovascular accident; congestive heart failure; hypertension; liver disease; foods containing tyramine, tryptophan, and dopamine; surgery in 10 to 14 days; children under 16. Box 18-7 can be used as a teaching guide for clients and families.

Electroconvulsive Therapy

This therapy is given when a rapid, definitive response is needed to prevent suicide; extreme agitation or stupor occurs; risks of other treatment outweigh risks of ECT; there is poor response to drugs; or when a client prefers it. It is useful for major depressions and manic clients who are rapid cyclers. The procedure requires informed consent. Client preparation is similar to preoperative preparation; post-treatment is similar to care of unconscious client. Potential side effects include confusion, disorientation, short-term memory loss.

Integrative Approaches for Depression

Nurses should be knowledgeable about these therapies in order to give information to clients.

Continued

85

CHAPTER OUTLINE	TEACHING STRATEGIES
Light Therapy	Light therapy successfully treats seasonal affective disorders. It is probably effective because of the influence of light on melatonin. It is delivered by a special balanced light slanted toward a client's face for a total of 30 minutes daily.
St. John's Wort	This is a plant product found to be somewhat effective for mildly to moderately depressed individuals. It interacts with a number of substances and drugs and may produce CSS and hypertensive crisis when tyramine is ingested.
Exercise	Exercise is effective against mild depression.
Transcranial Magnetic Stimulation	This integrative approach is a new technology that exposes the cerebral cortices to an electromagnetic field. There is no seizure induction. More research is indicated to evaluate its effectiveness.
Future of Treatment	There is a great need for more early detection, interventions, achievement of remission, prevention of progression, and integration of neuroscience and behavioral science.
Evaluation	Evaluation is based on outcome criteria and goals. Outcomes often relate to thought processes, self-esteem, and social interactions because these are problematic in people who are depressed.

19 Mood Disorders: Bipolar

THOUGHTS ABOUT TEACHING THE TOPIC

Few students can imagine the hyperactivity, rapid mood swings, grandiosity, and disorganization of the manic client. Since nursing interventions and decisions are difficult to execute when students are meeting their first manic client, behavioral rehearsals in the classroom are helpful. After students read the material, several "rehearsal" possibilities (which can be "mixed and matched") exist:

- Create a series of role plays.
- Create trigger situations on video using essentially the same type of situations as for role plays.
- Assign students to use a computer simulation.

KEY TERMS AND CONCEPTS

OBJECTIVES

After studying this chapter, the reader will be able to

1. Assess a manic client's (a) mood, (b) behavior, and (c) thought processes and be alert to possible dysfunction.
2. Formulate three nursing diagnoses appropriate for a manic client and include supporting data.
3. Explain the rationale behind five methods of communication that may be used with a manic client.
4. Teach a classmate at least four expected side effects of lithium therapy.
5. Distinguish between signs of early and severe lithium toxicity.
6. Write a medication care plan specifying five areas of client teaching regarding lithium carbonate.
7. Contrast and compare basic clinical conditions that may respond better to anticonvulsant therapy with those that may respond better to lithium therapy.
8. Evaluate specific indications for the use of seclusion for a manic client.
9. Defend the use of electroconvulsive therapy for a client in specific situations.
10. Review with a bipolar client at least three of the items presented in the psychoeducation teaching plan (Box 19-2).
11. Distinguish between the focus of treatment for a person in the acute manic phase and that for a person in the continuation or maintenance phase of a bipolar I disorder.

CHAPTER OUTLINE	TEACHING STRATEGIES
Prevalence	Bipolar disorder is a chronic mood syndrome which manifests in recurring mood episodes. Bipolar disorders include bipolar I disorder—at least one episode of mania alternating with major depression; bipolar II disorder—hypomanic episodes alternating with major depression; cyclothymia—hypomanic episodes alternating with minor depressive episodes (at least 2 years in duration). Periods of normal functioning may alternate with periods of illness. There is no cure so clients and families require support and education to reduce relapse and increase quality of life. Lifetime prevalence of bipolar I disorder is about 0.8% to 1.0% of the population.
Comorbidity	Substance use disorders commonly co-exist with bipolar disorder. Other associated disorders include personality disorders, anxiety disorders, anorexia nervosa, bulimia nervosa, and attention deficit hyperactivity disorder.
Theory	Bipolar disorders are thought to have different features one from the other.

Continued

87

**Biological Theories
Genetic Factors**

The rate of bipolar disorders in relatives can be as high as 5 to 10 times over rates found in the general population. Twin studies and studies of relatives of people with bipolar disorder point to genetic transmission as well.

Neurobiological Factors

Mood disorders are likely the result of complex interactions between neurotransmitters and hormones.

Neuroendocrine Factors

The hypothalamic-pituitary-thyroid adrenal axis (HPTA) is an area that is being studied in individuals with mood disorders. Hypothyroidism has been associated with mood disorders.

Neuroanatomical Factors

The regions of the prefrontal cortex and medial temporal lobe have been implicated in pathophysiology of bipolar disorders as have the neurocircuits surrounding these areas.

Sociological Findings

Bipolar disorders may be more prevalent in the upper socioeconomic classes.

**Psychological
Influences**

Psychosocial factors may play a role in precipitation of manic episodes; more study is required.

**Application of the Nursing Process
Assessment**

Early diagnosis and treatment can help individuals avoid suicide, alcohol, substance abuse, marital/work problems and development of medical comorbidity.

**Assessment of the
Characteristics of Mania**

The most common characteristics of mania include mood, behavior, thought processes, and cognitive functioning.

Assessing Level of Mood

The euphoric mood associated with bipolar illness is unstable. Overjoyous mood may alternate with irritability and belligerence. The person laughs, jokes, talks with uninhibited familiarity, is enthusiastic, concocts elaborate schemes to get rich and acquire unlimited power. The person may give away money and gifts, have lavish parties, and spend money freely.

Assessing Behavior

During mania, the client starts many projects, but finishes few. He or she is hyperactive, moving rapidly from one place to another. There may be indiscriminate spending, foolish business ventures, great generosity. He or she may be sexually indiscreet, manipulative, faultfinding, profane, and adept at exploiting the vulnerabilities of others. The person is often too busy to sleep, eat, or rest. Nonstop physical activity and lack of sleep and food can lead to physical exhaustion and even death, if untreated. Colorful, inappropriate, even bizarre dress, and overdone makeup are seen. The manic client is highly distractible and has poor concentration. After mania, the person often emerges startled and confused by the shambles of his or her life.

Assessing Thought Processes

Flight of ideas—accelerated speech with abrupt changes of topic usually based on understandable associations or plays on words—is common.

Rapid speech, verbosity (sometimes circumstantial), jokes, puns, and sexually explicit, vulgar, loud language may manifest. Themes revolve around grandiosity, extraordinary sexual prowess, brilliant ability, and great artistic talents. Grandiose delusions of persecution may be seen. The person has poor concentration and attention span, and is distractible. At the farthest point on the continuum, speech may show clang associations—the stringing together of words because of the way they sound (rhyming). Speech may become disorganized and incoherent.

CHAPTER OUTLINE	TEACHING STRATEGIES
Self-Assessment	The manic client elicits numerous intense emotions on the part of the nurse: frustration, anger, embarrassment, and fear, to name a few. Fatigue is common. The client is out of control and resists being controlled through the use of humor, manipulation, power struggles, and aggressive demanding behavior. Manic clients are masterful at pointing out staff faults and in splitting staff. Setting and maintaining limits is difficult, but essential.
Assessment Guidelines	Six important points are spelled out in the assessment alert: (1) assess danger to client or others; (2) protect client from consequences of overgenerosity; (3) assess for need for hospitalization; (4) assess medical status; (5) assess for co-existing conditions needing special intervention; and (6) assess client and family understanding of bipolar disorder, medications, support groups, etc.
Nursing Diagnosis	Risk for injury is often the priority nursing diagnosis. Table 19–2 lists other useful diagnoses including *risk for self-directed violence, risk for other-directed violence, disturbed thought processes, ineffective coping, defensive coping, impaired verbal communication, impaired social interaction, deficient fluid volume, imbalanced nutrition: less than body requirements, constipation, disturbed sleep pattern, self-care deficit, interrupted family processes, caregiver role strain.*
Outcome Criteria **Phase I: Acute Phase (Acute Mania)**	Client will be free of injury—cardiac status stable, well hydrated, free of abrasions. Client will report absence of delusions, racing thoughts. Client will have balanced sleep-rest-activity pattern. Outcomes depend upon nursing diagnoses and the phase of the illness the client is experiencing.
Phase II: Continuation of Treatment Phase	Client will demonstrate adherence to medication regimen. Client and family will participate in psychoeducational classes, etc.
Phase III: Maintenance Treatment Phase	Client and family are aware of prodromal signs of escalating mood or depression. Client participates in ongoing supportive modality, etc.
Planning	Planning is geared toward the phase of treatment as well as co-occurring issues such as risk of violence or suicide, family crisis, etc.
Acute Phase	During the acute phase, measures are taken to medically stabilize the client while maintaining client safety. Nursing care is geared toward lowering physical activity, increasing food and fluids, ensuring sleep, alleviating bowel or bladder problems, and intervening with self-care needs and medication management. Seclusion or ECT may be part of the plan.
Continuation Phase	During the continuation phase, the focus is on maintaining medication compliance and preventing relapse. Client and family psychoeducation is a must. The need for communication skills training and problem-solving skills is evaluated and referrals are made to community programs, groups, and support groups.
Maintenance Phase	During the maintenance phase, the goal is to continue to prevent relapse and limit the duration and severity of future episodes.
Intervention	Establishment of a therapeutic alliance is critical. Many clients minimize the consequences of their behaviors or deny the seriousness of the disease. Some are reluctant to give up the euphoria of the disorder. Medication noncompliance is a major cause of relapse.
Acute Phase	During the acute phase of treatment, the hospital is the safest place to provide external controls on destructive behavior and provide medical stabilization. Unique approaches to communication and to providing safety are offered in Table 19-3.

Continued

89

Psychopharmacology: Mood Stabilizers

Lithium is the antimanic drug of choice used as a mood stabilizer. It is effective in reducing elation, grandiosity, flight of ideas, irritability, manipulativeness, and anxiety. To a lesser extent it controls insomnia, agitation, distractibility, and threatening or assaultive behavior. Initially, an antipsychotic drug may be given to treat acute mania to prevent exhaustion and coronary collapse. An alternative is to initiate treatment with lithium and benzodiazepines to address insomnia and hyperactivity. Physical workup is necessary before beginning therapy to assess client ability to tolerate drug. Dosages of 300 to 600 mg (three times a day) may be needed to reach a maintenance level of 0.4 to 1.3 mEq/L. At serum levels of about 1.5 mEq/L, early signs of toxicity can occur. Severe toxicity requiring emergency measures can be seen at levels of 2.0 to 2.5 mEq/L.

Adverse reactions are associated with serum levels of 2.0 mEq/L or above. Blood levels are drawn weekly or biweekly until the therapeutic level is reached. After that levels are checked every month. After 6 months to 1 year of stability, levels are checked every 3 months.

Maintenance therapy: Relapse occurs within several weeks of stopping lithium. Clients should take lithium for 9 to 12 months after an episode. Others continue on the drug indefinitely. When lithium is to be discontinued, the dose must be gradually tapered. Risks of long-term lithium therapy include hypothyroidism and inability to concentrate urine; thus periodic thyroid and renal tests are called for.

Contraindications: Prior to beginning therapy, a medical evaluation is necessary. It should include renal function test, thyroid status, and evaluation for dementia or neurological disorders. Contraindications include cardiovascular disease, pregnancy or breast-feeding, renal or thyroid disease, brain damage, myasthenia gravis, and children under 12 years old.

Antiepileptic drugs are useful for clients who do not respond to lithium or who cannot tolerate lithium. Conditions under which anticonvulsant use may be preferable are listed in the chapter.

Carbamazepine (Tegretol) may be used in conjunction with lithium or separately. Works well with rapid cyclers and with those manifesting paranoid thinking. Blood level monitoring is called for.

Valproate sodium (Depakene) and divalproex sodium (Depakote) are also useful for rapid cycling and with those manifesting dysphoric symptoms.

Lamotrigine and gabapentin may be useful for clients' refractory to other therapy. See Table 19-5 for dose range and concerns of the AEDs.

Anxiolytics: Clonazepam and lorazepam are effective in managing psychomotor agitation seen in mania.

Electroconvulsive Therapy

May be used to treat severe manic behavior, especially in treatment-resistant individuals.

Milieu Therapy: Seclusion

Control during the acute hyperactive phase nearly always includes treatment with an antipsychotic such as haloperidol or chlorpromazine. Seclusion may be necessary to reduce overwhelming environmental stimuli, protect client from injuring self or others, prevent destruction of property. Seclusion or restraint requires consent of the client except during an emergency, and must have the written order of a physician. It can be used only when other less restrictive measures have failed. Observation and care to be given while the client is in seclusion are agency specific. Careful documentation according to agency protocol is necessary.

CHAPTER OUTLINE	TEACHING STRATEGIES
Continuation Phase	The goal is to prevent relapse. The phase usually lasts 4 to 9 months. Client needs determine the community resources to be used (e.g., day hospital, home visits, etc.).
Health Teaching	Focuses on information about bipolar illness, the importance of medication compliance, symptoms of impending episodes, and the importance of regularization of sleep patterns, meals, exercise.
Maintenance Phase	Medication follow-up and compliance, day hospitalization or home visits, and family support are all part of this phase, which is aimed at preventing recurrence.
Psychotherapeutic Approaches	Psychotherapy can help people work through strained interpersonal relationships, marriage and family problems, academic and occupational problems, and legal or social difficulties. Cognitive-behavioral therapy (CBT) has been found to be effective. Psychotherapy is important in encouraging medication compliance. One study showed clients treated with CBT more often took medication as prescribed than did clients who were not in therapy.
Support Groups	Support groups are of benefit to client and family. Groups include Depression and Bipolar Support Alliance, National Mental Health Association, National Alliance for the Mentally Ill, and Manic-Depressive Association.
Evaluation	Outcome criteria dictate the frequency of evaluation of short-term goals. Whenever goals remain unmet, preventing factors are analyzed.

Chapter 19   Mood Disorders: Bipolar

20 The Schizophrenias

THOUGHTS ABOUT TEACHING THE TOPIC

Although the establishment of a trusting relationship is essential to any nurse-client relationship, it seems difficult for students to establish a relationship with schizophrenic clients. The client's anxiety about relating, along with withdrawal and suspiciousness, makes establishing relationships difficult. Students can be helped to empathize with the client through a classroom activity called a "trust walk."

Students can profit from opportunities to identify and assess the numerous symptoms of schizophrenia. Strategies that may be helpful include the following:
- using role playing situations during class;
- creating trigger videos to be shown, responded to, and discussed in class;
- distributing a crossword puzzle to students or using it as a classroom game.

Integrating theory and practice, using all phases of the nursing process when caring for schizophrenic clients, can be fostered by
- computer-assisted instructional programs;
- independent viewing of selected films, using an instructor-prepared film guide with questions that are answered and submitted to the instructor for review;
- using films in class and discussion content.

Learning the considerable number of neuroleptic medications may be promoted by assigning Psychotropic Medication Administration: Outpatient Clinic, a CAI in which learners make assessments and decisions about psychiatric clients taking various medications (neuroleptics, antidepressants, lithium).

KEY TERMS AND CONCEPTS

acute dystonia, 408
affect, 388
akathisia, 408
ambivalence, 388
associative looseness, 388
atypical (novel) antipsychotics, 404
autism, 388
automatic obedience, 394
blocking, 415
clang association, 393
cognitive symptoms, 395
concrete thinking, 392

conventional (traditional) antipsychotics, 404
delusions of being controlled, 392
delusions, 391
depersonalization, 394
derealization, 394
echolalia, 393
echopraxia, 393
extrapyramidal side effects (EPSs), 405
hallucinations, 393
ideas of reference, 413
illusions, 393
negative symptoms, 394
negativism, 394
neologisms, 393
neuroleptic malignant syndrome (NMS), 410
paranoia, 412
positive symptoms, 391
pseudoparkinsonism, 408
stereotyped behaviors, 394
stupor, 394
tardive dyskinesia (TD), 410
thought broadcasting, 392
thought insertion, 392
thought withdrawal, 392
waxy flexibility, 394
word salad, 393

OBJECTIVES

After studying this chapter, the reader will be able to
1. Describe the progression of symptoms from the prepsychotic phase (prodromal symptoms) to the acute phase of schizophrenia.
2. Discuss at least three of the neurobiologic-anatomical-nongenetic findings that indicate that schizophrenia is a neurological disease.
3. Differentiate between the positive and negative symptoms of schizophrenia with regard to (a) their response to traditional and atypical antipsychotic medications, (b) their effect on quality of life, and (c) their significance for the prognosis of the disease.
4. Formulate three nursing diagnoses that are appropriate for a person with schizophrenia.
5. Discuss how to deal with common reactions a nurse may experience while working with a schizophrenic client.
6. Role-play with a classmate interventions for a client who is hallucinating, delusional, and exhibiting looseness of associations.

7. Develop a teaching plan for a client with schizophrenia who is taking a traditional antipsychotic drug, such as haloperidol (Haldol).
8. Compare and contrast the properties of the conventional (traditional) with the newer atypical antipsychotic drugs in the following areas: (a) target symptoms, (b) indications for use, (c) adverse effects and toxic effects, (d) need for client and family teaching and follow-up, and (e) cost.
9. Identify the effective strategies of individual, group, and family therapies that are most useful for clients with schizophrenia and their families.
10. Differentiate among the three phases of schizophrenia in terms of symptoms, focus of care, and intervention needs.
11. Apply the key elements of a teaching plan for a client with schizophrenia and a family member to the nursing care of one client with schizophrenia.
12. Analyze the different approaches to the care of a client with paranoid schizophrenia and a client with disorganized schizophrenia.

CHAPTER OUTLINE	TEACHING STRATEGIES
Epidemiology	The lifetime prevalence of schizophrenia is 1% worldwide. Typical age of onset is during the late teens and early twenties. Men and women are equally represented but there are some differences.
Comorbidity	Substance abuse disorders occur in approximately 40% to 50% of individuals with schizophrenia. It is associated with negative outcomes such as incarceration, violence, suicide, and HIV infection. Nicotine dependence may be as high as 80% to 90%. Other comorbid disorders include depressive symptoms, anxiety disorders, and psychosis-induced polydipsia.
Theory	Schizophrenia most likely occurs as a result of a combination of factors including: genetic and nongenetic factors (e.g., viral infection, birth injuries, nutritional factors).
Neurobiological Findings Dopamine Hypothesis	The dopamine hypothesis states excess dopamine is responsible for psychotic symptoms. This theory was based on the knowledge that antipsychotic drugs block some dopamine receptors, limiting the activity of dopamine and reducing psychotic symptoms. Other drugs (e.g., amphetamines), increase activity of dopamine and can simulate symptoms of paranoid schizophrenia in a nonschizophrenic client.
Alternative Biochemical Hypotheses	The role of other neurotransmitter systems (norepinephrine, serotonin, glutamate, GABA, neuropeptides, and neuromedullary substances) are being studied. Newer drugs target serotonin and norepinephrine and may provide more information about causation. Phencyclidine use induces a schizophrenia-like state. This observation has renewed interest in the NMDA receptor complex and the possible role of glutamate in schizophrenia.
Genetic Findings	Genetic vulnerability seems likely. Schizophrenia and schizophrenia-like symptoms occur at an increased rate among relatives of schizophrenic clients.
Neuroanatomical Findings	Studies suggest schizophrenia is a disorder of brain circuits. Structural cerebral abnormalities could cause circuit disruptions. Findings suggest that possible brain abnormalities might be enlarged lateral ventricles, cortical atrophy, third ventricle dilation, ventricular asymmetry, cerebellar atrophy, and frontal lobe atrophy. PET scans suggest reduced frontal lobe activity.
Nongenetic Risk Factors	Birth and pregnancy complications (e.g., viral infection, poor nutrition, exposure to toxins) place individuals at increased risk for developing schizophrenia as adults. Although there is no indication that stress causes schizophrenia, stress may

Continued

93

precipitate it in a vulnerable individual. Other risk factors include birth during the winter, birth in an urban area, low socioeconomic status.

Application of the Nursing Process
Assessment
***DSM-IV-TR* Criteria**
for Schizophrenia

Around 1908 Bleuler coined the term *schizophrenia* and referred to four fundamental signs: affect (flat, inappropriate emotions); associative looseness (jumbled, illogical thinking); autism (thinking not bound to reality); and ambivalence (simultaneously holding two opposing emotions, ideas, or wishes). *DSM-IV-TR* provides diagnostic criteria for all subtypes of schizophrenia: paranoid, catatonic, disorganized, undifferentiated, residual.

Course of the Disease

The course of the disease usually involves recurrent acute exacerbations of psychosis. It can be presented in three phases: the acute phase, the maintenance phase, and the stabilization phase.

Prepsychotic Early Symptoms

These begin 1 month to 1 year before the first psychotic episode and include increased anxiety; evidence of a thought disorder, such as poor concentration; inability to keep out intrusive thoughts; attaching symbolic meaning to ordinary events; and misinterpretation of others' actions or words. In the latter part of this phase, the client may experience emotional and physical withdrawal, hallucinations, delusions, odd mannerisms, preoccupation with religion, neologisms, preoccupation with homosexual themes.

Treatment-Relevant Dimensions
of Schizophrenia

A client with abrupt onset of symptoms with good premorbid functioning usually has a more favorable prognosis than a person with a slow onset over a period of 2 or 3 years. Childhood history of withdrawal, seclusive, eccentric, and tense behavior are unfavorable diagnostic signs. The younger the client is at onset, the more discouraging the prognosis.

Positive Symptoms

Florid psychotic symptoms such as hallucinations, delusions, bizarre behavior, and paranoia. Positive symptoms are associated with acute onset; normal premorbid functioning and normal functioning during remissions; normal CT scans; and favorable response to antipsychotics.

Alterations in Thinking

Delusions: fixed false beliefs (with themes of ideas of reference, persecution, grandiosity, unusual bodily function, jealousy, being controlled). About 75% of schizophrenic clients experience delusions at some time during their illness. Other common delusions include: thought broadcasting (the belief that one's thoughts can be heard by others), thought insertion (the belief that thoughts of others are being inserted into one's mind), thought withdrawal (the belief that thoughts have been removed from one's mind), and delusions of being controlled (belief that one's body or mind is controlled by an outside agency).

Concrete thinking: impaired ability to use abstract concepts. Interpretation is literal.

Alterations in Speech

Associative looseness: loosely associated, haphazard, illogical, confused speech that can sometimes be decoded.

Neologisms: newly coined words having meaning only for the client.

Echolalia: pathological repeating of another's words.

Clang association: meaningless rhyming of words.

Word salad: mixture of words meaningless to the listener.

CHAPTER OUTLINE	TEACHING STRATEGIES
Alterations in Perception	Hallucinations are sensory perceptions for which there is no external stimulus. Auditory hallucinations are most common among schizophrenics. Voices may tell the client what to do (commanding) or speak to or about him or her (usually derogatory). Behavioral indications of the presence of auditory hallucinations include tilting head as if listening and answering back. Hallucinations may also be visual, olfactory, gustatory, or tactile.
	Personal boundary difficulties may also be referred to as loss of ego boundaries. Examples include (1) depersonalization—feeling that the person has lost his or her identity or that the body has changed, and (2) derealization—false perception that the environment has changed.
Alterations in Behavior	Bizarre behaviors take the form of stilted rigid demeanor, eccentric dress or grooming, and rituals.
	Extreme motor agitation—running about in response to inner or outer stimuli.
	Stereotyped behaviors—motor patterns that have become mechanical and purposeless.
	Automatic obedience—performing commands in a robotlike fashion.
	Waxy flexibility—excessive maintenance of a posture for long periods of time.
	Stupor—remaining motionless and unresponsive.
	Negativism—active negativism involves the client doing the opposite of what is suggested; passive negativism involves not doing the things one is expected to do such as getting out of bed, eating, etc.
	Agitated behavior—related to difficulty with impulse control; because of cognitive deterioration, clients lack social sensitivity and may act out impulsively.
Negative Symptoms	Apathy, lack of motivation, anhedonia, poor social functioning, and poverty of thought are associated with insidious onset; premorbid history of emotional problems; chronic deterioration; CT scan showing atrophy; and poor response to antipsychotic therapy.
	These are the symptoms that most interfere with adjustment and ability to survive such as ability to initiate and maintain relationships, initiate and maintain conversation, hold a job, make decisions, maintain adequate hygiene and grooming.
	Negative symptoms include poverty of speech or speech content, thought blocking, anergia, anhedonia, avolition, affective blunting (minimal emotional response), inappropriate affect (incongruent response), or bizarre affect (grimacing, giggling, etc.).
Cognitive Symptoms	Represent a major disability associated with schizophrenia. Cognitive impairment involves difficulty with attention, memory, problem solving, and decision making.
Depressive and Other Mood Symptoms	Depression recognition during assessment is crucial because depression affects a majority of people with schizophrenia; may herald a psychotic relapse; increase the likelihood of substance abuse, suicide, or it may be associated with impaired functioning.
Self-Assessment	The intensity of the client's emotions can evoke intense, uncomfortable, and frightening emotions in staff. If feelings are not worked through, feelings of helplessness can increase anxiety. Defensive behaviors may emerge to thwart client progress and undermine nurse self-esteem. Slow client progress can lead to frustration. Team evaluation of progress can assist with this.

Continued

95

Assessment Guidelines

It is important to assess if the client has had a medical workup, including the presence of psychosis. Also assess if client is dependent on alcohol or other drugs. Is the individual experiencing hallucinations or delusions and assess if the client's belief system is founded in reality. Be sure to be alert for co-occurring disorders such as depression, anxiety, substance dependency or a history of violence and ask if the client taking medications and is he or she adhering to the medication regimen as prescribed?

It is also important is to assess the support for the client (e.g., family, significant others) and assess the client's global functioning.

Nursing Diagnosis

Useful nursing diagnoses include *disturbed thought processes, disturbed sensory perception, impaired verbal communication, ineffective coping, imbalanced nutrition: less than body requirements, risk for self-directed violence, risk for other-directed violence, activity intolerance, constipation, incontinence, impaired physical mobility, self-care deficit, compromised family coping, disabled family coping, chronic low self-esteem, and risk for loneliness, social isolation, impaired parenting, caregiver role strain.*

Outcome Criteria

Desired outcomes vary with the phase of the illness.

Phase I (Acute)

The acute phase essentially involves crisis intervention with client safety and medical stabilization as the overall goal. If the client is at risk for violence to self or others, initial outcome criteria would address safety issues (i.e., "Client will remain safe while hospitalized"). Another appropriate focus would be on outcomes that reflect improvement in intensity and frequency of hallucinations, delusions, and increasing ability to test reality accurately.

Phase II (Maintenance) and Phase III (Stablilization)

Outcome criteria will focus on helping the client to adhere to medication regimens, to understand the nature of the illness, and to participate in psychoeducational activities for client and family.

Planning

Planning appropriate interventions is guided by the phase of the illness.

Acute Phase

Often requires hospitalization for stabilization. The treatment team will identify long-term care needs, identify and provide appropriate referrals for follow-up and support. Discharge planning must consider living arrangements, economic resources, social supports, family relationships, and vulnerability to stress.

Maintenance and Stabilization Phases

Foci include client and family education; skills training; building relapse prevention skills; and identifying need for social, interpersonal, coping, and vocational skills.

Intervention
Basic Level Interventions

Interventions are geared to the phase of the illness. In the acute phase, interventions are focused on symptom stabilization and safety and usually include medication; supportive and directive communication; limit setting; and psychiatric, medical, and neurological evaluation. Hospitalization is reserved for situations in which partial hospitalization or day treatment is ineffective or unavailable.

Phase II and III interventions include psychoeducation about the disease, medication, side effect management, cognitive and social skills enhancement, identifying signs of relapse, attention to self-care deficits. Stress minimization is of concern. Helping client reduce vulnerability to relapse will include providing information about maintaining a regular sleep pattern; reducing alcohol, drug, and caffeine intake; keeping in touch with supportive family and friends; staying active; having a daily or weekly schedule; taking medication regularly. Attention should be given to client strengths and healthy functioning.

Milieu Therapy

Clients with schizophrenia improve more on a structured hospital unit rather than in an open environment. A therapeutic milieu provides safety, useful activities, resources for resolving conflicts, and opportunities for learning social and vocational skills.

Activities

During the acute phase, a structured milieu is more advantageous to the client than the freedom of an open unit. Participation in activity groups decreases withdrawal, promotes motivation, modifies aggression, and increases social competence. Involvement in activity groups results in increased self-concept scores.

Safety

In the acute phase, the risk for violence usually stems from hallucinations or delusions. Attempts should be made to use the least restrictive method of coping with violence (e.g., initially use verbal intervention, followed by medication, and lastly seclusion or restraint).

Counseling: Communications Guidelines

Be familiar with principles for dealing with hallucinations, delusions, and associative looseness. Use a nonthreatening and nonjudgmental manner. Speak simply, using a louder voice. Use client's name. Box 20-3 identifies other strategies.

Hallucinations

Intervention requires knowledge of the content of the hallucinations.

Delusions

Rely on empathy. Clarify the reality of client's experience. Do not focus on delusional content. Do not use logic to refute delusion and do not argue. Clarifying misinterpretations is useful. Spend time with client in reality-based activities.

Associative Looseness

Loose associations mirror client thoughts. Don't pretend to understand when you can't. Tell client you're having difficulty understanding, placing the problem with yourself (i.e., "I'm having difficulty understanding what you're saying" instead of "You're not making sense"). Look for and mention recurring themes. Emphasize what's going on in the environment and involve client in simple reality-based activities. Tell client when you do understand, reinforcing clear communication.

Client and Family Health Teaching

Topics include the illness; how stress and medication affect the illness; problem-solving skills; coping strategies to deal with symptoms; sources of ongoing support; symptoms of relapse; and the type of environment most supportive for client.

Case Management

Case management allows effective monitoring of client progress. Alternatives to hospitalization include partial hospitalization, halfway houses, and day treatment programs. Self-help community groups may also be useful.

Advanced Practice Interventions

Psychotherapy

While medication maintenance has been shown to be the single most important factor in prevention of relapse, a combination of medication and psychosocial interventions lowers the relapse rate even further. Client concerns that can be addressed are relationship problems, family concerns, depression, losses, and medication.

Individual Therapy

Supportive therapy is the modality found to be most helpful. Skills training to enhance social functioning, cognitive rehabilitation to improve information-processing skills, and cognitive content therapy to change abnormal thoughts or responses to hallucinations through coping strategies are also useful.

Group Therapy

May be used to develop interpersonal skills, resolve community problems, and teach use of community supports. Medication groups can help clients deal with

Continued

97

side effects, alert staff to potential adverse or toxic effects, minimize isolation, and increase compliance.

Family Therapy

Further reduces relapse rate when a psychoeducational approach is used. This format expands clients' and relatives' social networks, expands problem-solving capacity, and lowers emotional overinvolvement of families.

Psychopharmacology

Antipsychotics allow client management in the community as well as in the hospital. Noncompliance with medications usually precedes relapse. Maintenance is required for 1 year after one episode, 2 years after two episodes, and probably lifelong after three episodes.

Atypical Antipsychotics

These drugs can diminish the negative symptoms (as well as the positive symptoms) and include clozapine, risperidone, olanzapine, quetiapine, ziprasidone, and aripiprazole, the newest of the antipsychotic agents, all of which have a good side effect profile. These drugs cause few or no extrapyramidal symptoms or tardive dyskinesia and may improve neurocognitive defects associated with schizophrenia. Use of clozapine, however, carries the risk of agranulocytosis. All tend to promote weight gain and are more expensive than the older drugs.

Conventional (Traditional) Antipsychotics

Target D_2 receptors. These drugs relieve the positive symptoms of schizophrenia and include the phenothiazines, thioxanthenes, butyrophenones, dibenzoxazepines, and dihydroindolones.

Selection is often made on the basis of major side effects. Extrapyramidal effects, such as dystonia, akathisia, and pseudoparkinsonism, are treated by lowering dose and prescribing antiparkinsonian drugs such as trihexyphenidyl (Artane), benztropine (Cogentin), or diphenhydramine (Benedryl). Anticholinergic side effects include dry mouth, urinary retention, constipation, and blurred vision. Sedation, orthostatic hypotension, lowered seizure threshold, and agranulocytosis are other side effects.

All standard antipsychotics can cause tardive dyskinesia (TD), which typically involves involuntary tonic muscular spasms of the tongue, lips, fingers, toes, jaw, neck, trunk, and pelvis. The drugs must be discontinued, but no cure for TD exists. Assessment is performed using the Abnormal Involuntary Movement Scale.

Neuroleptic malignant syndrome occurs in less than 1% of those taking standard antipsychotics, is potentially fatal, and is characterized by lowered level of consciousness, increased muscle tone, and autonomic dysfunction (including fever, hypertension, tachycardia, tachypnea, diaphoresis, and drooling). Agranulocytosis, also a serious side effect, can be fatal.

Adjuncts to Antipsychotic Drug Therapy

Antidepressants may be ordered for coexisting depression.

Antimanic agents may be useful for suppressing episodic violence and may help alleviate comorbid depression.

Benzodiazepines may be ordered during the acute phase to reduce agitation.

When to Change an Antipsychotic Regimen

Change should be considered when the current regimen is ineffective, supplemental medications are needed, side effects are intolerable.

Specific Nursing Interventions for Paranoid, Catatonic, and Disorganized Schizophrenia

CHAPTER OUTLINE	TEACHING STRATEGIES
Paranoia	Paranoia is characterized by intense and strongly defended irrational suspicion. Projection is the most common defense mechanism used by paranoid clients. These clients usually feel frightened, lonely, and helpless. The paranoid facade is a defense against painful feelings.
Counseling: Communication Guidelines	Paranoid clients are unable to trust others and are guarded, tense, reserved, and aloof. They often adopt a superior, hostile, and sarcastic attitude to distance others. They may disparage others and dwell on others' shortcomings. Staff must not react with anxiety or client rejection. Frequent discussion with peers and clinical supervision are helpful.
	Readers are referred to the communication card.
Self-Care Needs	These are usually minimal. Nutrition may be problematic if client is suspicious that food has been tampered with. If this is the case, provide food in unopened containers. Suspicion may also interfere with sleep.
Milieu Needs	Risk for violence is present because the client may respond with hostility or aggression to hallucinations or delusions. Homosexual urges may also be projected onto the environment.
Catatonia: Withdrawn Phase	The essential feature of catatonia is abnormal motor behavior. Onset is usually abrupt and the prognosis favorable. In the withdrawn phase the client may demonstrate posturing, waxy flexibility, stereotyped behavior, extreme negativism or automatic obedience, echolalia, and echopraxia.
Counseling: Communication Guidelines	Clients may actually appear comatose and mute. Although seemingly unaware of the environment, the client is aware and may remember events accurately at a later date. Readers are referred to the communication card.
Self-Care Needs	When a client is extremely withdrawn, physical needs take priority. The client may need complete care, including hand or tube feeding, incontinence care, and passive exercise, as well as assistance with hygiene, dressing, and grooming.
Milieu Needs	The continuum from decreased spontaneous movement to complete stupor is described and waxy flexibility explained. Readers are cautioned that the client may move from stupor to an outburst of gross motor activity prompted by hallucinations, delusions, or neurotransmitter changes.
Catatonia: Excited Phase **Counseling: Communication Guidelines**	During the excited phase, the person talks or shouts continually. Verbalizations may be incoherent. Staff communication should be clear and directed. The major concern is safety of client and others.
Self-Care Needs	Client may exhibit gross hyperactivity (running, striking out, etc.). Exhaustion and collapse, as well as safety, are the primary concerns. IM administration of antipsychotic medication is usual. Provision of nutrition, fluids, and rest are of high priority. The client may be destructive and aggressive in response to hallucinations or delusions. The reader is referred to the CD-ROM.
Disorganized Schizophrenia	The most regressed and socially impaired clients carry this diagnosis. They show grossly inappropriate affect, bizarre mannerisms, grimaces, giggles, incoherent speech, blocking, and extreme social withdrawal. Onset is often early and insidious. The prognosis is often poor, the client being able to live only in a structured and well-supervised setting.

Continued

99

Counseling: Communication Guidelines

These clients experience persistent and severe perceptual problems and frequently display looseness of associations, incoherence, clang association, word salad, and blocking.

Self-Care Needs

Clients need much help grooming as clients have no awareness of social expectations. They are often too disorganized to carry out ADLs.

Milieu Needs

These highly regressed clients exhibit primitive behaviors that require a structured and protective milieu.

Undifferentiated Schizophrenia

This illness is characterized by active signs of the disorder, but with symptoms that do not clearly fall into one specific category. It often has an early and insidious onset with disability remaining fairly stable over time.

Residual Type of Schizophrenia

The client no longer has active-phase symptoms but evidences two or more residual symptoms (such as lack of initiative, marked social withdrawal, impaired role function, speech deficits, odd beliefs, magical thinking, and unusual perceptual events).

Evaluation

Evaluation is based on established outcomes. Goals may need to be revised to become more realistic and attainable. Client input may shed light on reasons desired behaviors have not occurred.

21 | Cognitive Disorders

THOUGHTS ABOUT TEACHING THE TOPIC

Although teaching students the nursing care for cognitively impaired clients has long been considered part of psychiatric nursing, it's likely that the material may be better placed in other courses. For example, delirium is more often encountered on acute medical-surgical units, in the ICU, or on a chemical detoxification unit than on a "psych" floor.

Clients with dementia are more often encountered in long-term residential care settings, in adult day care, or in the home. The challenge for the psychiatric nursing instructor will be to arrange clinical observations or experiences to give learners contact with the cognitively impaired client at the time the theory is presented. The placement on the unit of material deserves special consideration. Faculty usually prefers not to break the continuity of the experience on the psychiatric unit.

KEY TERMS AND CONCEPTS

agnosia, 433
agraphia, 436
Alzheimer's disease, 431
amnestic disorder, 424
aphasia, 433
apraxia, 433
cognitive disorders, 423
confabulation, 433
delirium, 423
dementia, 424
hallucinations, 426
hypermetamorphosis, 436
hyperorality, 436
hypervigilance, 427

illusions, 426
perseveration, 433
primary dementia, 431
pseudodementia, 433
secondary dementia, 431
sundowning, 425

OBJECTIVES

After studying this chapter, the reader will be able to
1. Compare and contrast the clinical picture of delirium with the clinical picture of dementia.
2. Discuss three critical needs of a person with delirium, stated in terms of nursing diagnoses.
3. Identify three outcomes for clients with delirium.
4. Summarize the essential somatic and psychotherapeutic interventions for a client with delirium.
5. Compare and contrast the signs and symptoms occurring in the four stages of Alzheimer's disease.
6. Give an example of the following symptoms assessed during the progression of Alzheimer's disease: (a) amnesia (b) apraxia, (c) agnosia, and (d) aphasia.
7. Formulate at least three nursing diagnoses suitable for a client with Alzheimer's disease and define two outcomes for each.
8. Formulate a teaching plan for a caregiver of a client with Alzheimer's disease, including interventions for (a) communication, (b) health maintenance, and (c) safe environment.
9. Compose a list of appropriate referrals in the community for persons with Alzheimer's and their families. Include telephone numbers for at least one support group, hotline, source of further information, and caregiver respite service.

CHAPTER OUTLINE	TEACHING STRATEGIES
Prevalence	Delirium is characterized by a disturbance of consciousness and a change in cognition, such as impaired attention span, disorientation, and confusion, that develop over a short period of time and fluctuates throughout the day. It is always secondary to another condition. It is transient and recovery occurs when the cause is corrected. Delirium can affect up to half of all hospitalized and elderly medically ill people at any one time, and up to 60% of nursing home residents aged 75 years or older may be delirious at any one time. Dementia develops more slowly and is characterized by multiple cognitive deficits, including memory impairment. In a majority of the cases, dementias are primary, progressive, and irreversible. Alzheimer's disease accounts for 60% to 80% of all dementias in the

Continued

United States. Amnestic disorder is characterized by loss of both short- and long-term memory. Other cognitive impairments are not present. Amnestic disorders are always secondary to another condition.

DELIRIUM

Nurses encounter delirium on medical-surgical units. Postoperative delirium, drugs, cerebrovascular disease, and CHF are common causes. It is more often seen in the elderly and is also seen in children with fever and in terminally ill clients. Delirium results in disturbances in consciousness and cognitive difficulties, typically thinking, memory, attention, and perception. Delirium fluctuates in intensity. Mild delirium tends to become more pronounced in the evening (sundowning). Nursing concerns center on assisting with proper health management to eradicate the underlying cause, preventing physical harm due to confusion, aggression, or electrolyte and fluid imbalance, and using supportive measures to relieve distress.

Application of the Nursing Process
Assessment
Overall Assessment

Note duration of onset (often abrupt) and orientation to time, place, and person. Ability to focus is usually impaired. There are fluctuating levels of consciousness (usually worse at night and early morning). The Mini-Mental State Examination is a useful tool. Assessment should include cognitive and perceptual ability, physical needs, and mood and behavior.

Cognitive and Perceptual
Disturbances

Cognitive disturbances are distractibility, attention deficits, and difficulty remembering recent events. Perceptual disturbances include illusions and visual and tactile hallucinations, which cause increased anxiety.

Physical Safety

Physical safety is primary. Delirious clients wander, pull out lines and catheters, and climb out of bed over side rails. Clients who cannot recognize and interpret reality are usually highly anxious. Make physical environment as simple and clear as possible; elevate head of bed slightly; use eyeglasses, hearing aids, and adequate lighting to help maintain orientation. Clocks and calendars may be helpful. Spending time with the client when not engaged in a technical nursing intervention is helpful.

Bacteriological Safety

Skin breakdown is possible due to self-care deficits, poor nutrition, bed rest, and incontinence.

Biophysical Safety

Observe for autonomic signs of tachycardia, sweating, flushed face, dilated pupils, elevated BP; report them. Note sleep-wake cycles, level of consciousness, hypervigilance, and effects of medications.

Moods and Physical Behaviors

Mood often is labile—the individual may swing dramatically from euphoria to apathy to anger. Physical behaviors are usually congruent with the mood of the moment, with confusion and fear being common.

Self-Assessment

Feeling challenged by the magnitude of the client symptoms is common. Feeling negative may occur when the delirium is secondary to substance use or abuse.

Assessment Guidelines

There are eleven Assessment Guideline steps to help the nurses assess patient's delirium, beginning with levels of consciousness, which is key in delirium.

Nursing Diagnosis

Useful diagnoses include *risk for injury, deficient fluid volume, disturbed sleep pattern, impaired verbal communication, acute confusion, fear, self-care deficit, impaired social interaction,* and *disturbed sensory perception.*

Intervention

Management involves treating the underlying organic causes. Carefully titrated doses of antipsychotic or antianxiety medication may be called for. Nursing care

102

	involves careful supervision by nursing staff; encouragement of one or two significant others to stay with the client; use of eyeglasses and hearing aids to support accurate sensory input; simple, direct communication; reorientation via communication; clocks and calendars; frequent explanations; a calm approach.
Evaluation	Evaluation is performed by using planned outcomes. Short-term goals are particularly important: Is client oriented? Are tubes intact? Is anxiety level decreased from panic to moderate or low?
DEMENTIA: ALZHEIMER'S DISEASE	Dementia develops more slowly and is characterized by multiple cognitive deficits that include memory impairment. A primary dementia is irreversible. Reversible cases are usually secondary to other processes (e.g., tumors, trauma, infections, toxic disturbances, vitamin deficiencies), which, when treated, allow the dementia to improve. Some secondary dementias, such as HIV encephalopathy, are progressive.
	Examples of primary dementias include Alzheimer's disease, Pick's disease, multi-infarct dementias. There is no cure. Primary dementias are progressive. The person shows a progressive decline in ADLs, memory, and personality disorganization. Alzheimer's disease attacks indiscriminately, striking men and women, black and white, rich or poor.
Theory	The cause of Alzheimer's disease is unknown, but several etiological hypotheses exist.
Pathological Findings **Alzheimer's Tangles**	β-amyloid protein deposits are found in the brain of the client with Alzheimer's disease (AD). Neurofibrillary tangles form in the hippocampus, the area of the brain responsible for short-term memory and emotions. Neuritic plaques are cores of degenerated neuron material that are found. Granulovascular degeneration, filling brain cells with fluid and granular material, is also noted.
Genetic Findings	Family members of people with dementia of the Alzheimer type have a higher risk of acquiring the disease than the general population. At least four genes are involved in the transmission of AD.
Nongenetic Findings	Risk factors include increasing age, Down syndrome, and head injury. Folic acid deficiency and elevated homocysteine levels may also be risk factors.
Neurochemical Changes	A possible culprit is reduced level of acetyltransferase (needed to synthesize the neurotransmitter acetylcholine).
Application of the Nursing Process **Assessment** **Overall Assessment**	Clients may deny early memory loss and compensate by using social graces. Later, denial, confabulation, perseveration, and avoidance of answering questions are noted as defensive maneuvers, and the symptoms of aphasia, apraxia, agnosia, memory impairment, and disturbances in executive functioning develop.
Diagnostic Tests for Dementia	The diagnosis of AD is made after all other possibilities have been ruled out via diagnostic testing. CT, PET, and other scans reveal brain atrophy and rule out neoplasms. Complete physical examinations and neurological examinations are necessary. Depression and other illnesses may cause pseudodementia and must be investigated.

Continued

Chapter 21 Cognitive Disorders

Assessment for Stage of the Disease

Stage 1: Mild Alzheimer's Disease

Loss of ability is insidious. The person loses energy, drive, initiative, and has difficulty learning new things. Personality and social skills remain intact. Doing the marketing or managing finances shows impairment.

Stage 2: Moderate Alzheimer's Disease

Deterioration is evident. The person can't remember addresses or dates. Hygiene and self-care are affected; mood becomes labile; and driving judgment poor. He or she denies deterioration and withdraws.

Stage 3: Moderate to Severe Alzheimer's Disease

The person is not able to identify familiar objects or people (severe agnosia). He or she needs repeated instructions for the simplest of tasks (advanced apraxia), and may become incontinent and require total care. Agitation, violence, or paranoid delusions may be seen. He or she wanders. Some criteria for nursing home placement include wandering; danger to self or others; incontinence; and interfering with sleep or health of others.

Stage 4: Late Alzheimer's Disease

Agraphia (inability to read and write), hyperorality (putting everything in the mouth), blunting of emotions, visual agnosia (inability to recognize objects), and hypermetamorphosis (touching everything in sight) are common. Ability to talk and walk is lost and coma and stupor follow.

Self-Assessment

Understanding the process of the disease is helpful to the nurse contending with the client's confusion, psychotic states, and violent and aggressive behavior. Staff burnout is helped by setting realistic client goals, avoiding the hopeless stance, and involving staff in research.

Assessment Guidelines

There are nine steps of guidelines for dementia, beginning with an assessment to help identify the underlying cause of the dementia. Then, explore how well the family is prepared and educated about the progress of the particular dementia that their family member is experiencing. See text for the specific guidelines.

Nursing Diagnosis

Client safety is of paramount importance as wandering, falls, accidents, ingestions of noxious substances and seizures may occur. Useful diagnoses include *risk for injury, impaired verbal communication, impaired environmental interpretation syndrome, impaired memory, chronic confusion, ineffective coping, self-care deficit,* and *disturbed sensory perception.* For the family, consider *caregiver role strain* and *anticipatory grieving.*

Outcome Criteria

Outcome criteria must be identified for each nursing diagnosis (e.g., *risk for injury:* client will remain safe in the hospital or at home; *self-care deficit:* client will participate in self-care at optimal level; *impaired environmental interpretation syndrome:* client will remain nonaggressive when experiencing paranoid ideation; *caregiver role strain:* family members will name two organizations within their area that can offer support, or family will state they have outside help that allows them to take personal time for themselves).

Planning

Is geared toward the client's immediate needs and caregiver needs, including useful community resources.

Intervention

The nurse's attitude of unconditional positive regard is the single most effective tool in caring for clients with dementia. It promotes cooperation, reduces catastrophic outbreaks, and increases family members' satisfaction with care. Management of depression, hallucinations, delusions, agitation, insomnia, and wandering is important. Staff should facilitate the highest level of functioning of which the client is capable. Supportive intervention with the family who are losing a loved one to dementia is critical.

Counseling: Communication Guidelines	Provide only one visual clue at a time, know that client may lack understanding of assigned task, remember that relevant information is retained best, break tasks into small steps, give only one instruction at a time, and report, record, and document all data. Other guidelines are given in Table 21–7.
Health Teaching	Health teaching and support for families are vital components of care for the family of clients with dementia. Families need information about communicating with the client and structuring for self-care activities, as well as where to get information, support, and legal and financial guidance. (Computer Line and Alzheimer's Association are two resources.)
Support	The Alzheimer's Association is a national umbrella agency that provides various forms of assistance to persons with the disease and their families. Although many families manage the care of their loved one through death, other families need help along the way. There are many factors that family members need help with. The Alzheimer's Association can provide families with information about locating and return of missing people with AD, housekeeping, home health aids, prevention of caregiver emotional and physical fatigue, how and when to place the ill member, and legal and financial matters.
	Assisting clients to cope with their environment is the basis of nursing therapy. Safety, activities that increase socialization, and planning for minimization of fatigue are important considerations.
Psychopharmacology	
Cognitive Impairment	Various drugs are in use to address the cognitive impairment associated with AD. Tacrine (THA, Cognex), a cholinesterase inhibitor, may delay Alzheimer's progress, but has a high incidence of liver side effects. Donepezil (Aricept) inhibits acetylcholine breakdown and appears to slow deterioration in cognitive function but without the liver toxicity attributed to tacrine. Rivastigmine (Exelon), a brain-selective acetylcholinesterase inhibitor, and galantamine (Reminyl), a reversible cholinesterase inhibitor, are newer drugs. Memantine (Namenda), a drug that works by affecting NMDA receptors, was approved for use in the United States in October 2003 and became available to doctors, patients, and pharmacies in January 2004. A vaccine designed to clear the brain of β-amyloid plaques is currently being tested.
Behavioral Symptoms	Problems often seen are hallucinations, paranoia. agitation, and verbal or physical aggression. Small doses of antipsychotics, benzodiazepines, and buspirone may be ordered. SSRIs may be used to treat depression, which is very common.
Alternative and Complementary Treatments	A number of herbal drugs are currently under investigation. Caution is advised since "herbal," or "all natural," does not necessarily mean safe.
Evaluation	Goals will need to be altered as the client's condition deteriorates. Frequent evaluation and reformulation of outcome criteria and short-term goals help diminish staff and family frustration.

105

22 Crisis

THOUGHTS ABOUT TEACHING THE TOPIC

The basic concepts necessary to understand crisis theory and crisis intervention are contained in this chapter. The instructor will emphasize

- classification of crises;
- characteristics of crises having relevance for nurses;
- impact of crisis intervention on clients in crisis;
- goals for clients in crisis: return to precrisis state, client safety, and reducing anxiety;
- emotional reactions and common problems faced by beginning practitioners.

When lecture time is very limited, the instructor may elect to discuss crisis intervention theory using examples and situations drawn from the chapters on family violence and rape trauma.

KEY TERMS AND CONCEPTS

adventitious crisis, 459
crisis intervention, 457
critical incident stress debriefing (CISD), 465
maturational crisis, 458
phases of crisis, 459
primary care, 465
secondary care, 465
situational crisis, 458
tertiary care, 465

OBJECTIVES

After studying this chapter, the reader will be able to

1. Differentiate among the three types of crisis discussed in this chapter and give an example of each from the reader's own experience.
2. Delineate at least six aspects of crisis that have relevance for nurses involved in crisis intervention.
3. Develop a handout including areas to assess during crisis, with at least two sample questions for each area.
4. Discuss four common problems in the nurse-client relationship that are frequently encountered by beginning nurses when starting crisis intervention and discuss at least two interventions for each problem.
5. Compare and contrast the differences among primary, secondary, and tertiary intervention, including appropriate intervention strategies.
6. Explain to a classmate four potential crisis situations, common in the hospital setting, that a client may face and give concrete examples of how they can be minimized.
7. Make a list of at least five resources in the community that could be used as referrals for a person in crisis.

CHAPTER OUTLINE	TEACHING STRATEGIES
	Crises are acute, time-limited occurrences experienced as overwhelming emotional reactions to a situation: perhaps a developmental event, societal event or cultural event. Crisis is not a pathological state; rather, it is a struggle for equilibrium and adjustment when problems are perceived as insolvable. A crisis presents a danger to personality organization and a potential opportunity for personality growth. The experience of violence in our society is increasing, as evidenced by family violence, school shootings, bombings, road rage, etc.
Comorbidity	A psychological crisis refers to an individual's inability to solve a problem. Factors that limit problem solving include the number of other stressful life events with which the individual is dealing, the presence of unresolved losses, concurrent psychiatric disorder, concurrent medical problems, excessive pain or fatigue, and the quality and quantity of a person's usual coping skills.
Theory	Lindemann was an early crisis theorist, and crisis theory was further developed by Caplan. Aguilera and Mesnick have set the standard for crisis work by nurses.

106

Types of Crisis
Maturational Crisis

Occurs when a person arrives at a new, predictable stage of development where formerly used coping styles are no longer appropriate. An example is the passage from school-age child to adolescent or from adolescent to adult. Temporary disequilibrium ensues. If support systems and adequate role models are absent, successful resolution may be difficult or may not occur at all. If alcohol or drugs interrupt progression through maturational stages the result may be diminished coping skills (i.e., skill development is arrested at the age at which substance abuse began).

Situational Crisis

Involves a critical life problem and arises from an external source (e.g., job loss, death of a loved one, abortion, job change, change in financial status, divorce, pregnancy, severe illness). The stressful event involves a loss or change that threatens a person's self-concept and self-esteem.

Adventitious Crisis

An unplanned, accidental event that is not part of everyday life. The event may be a natural disaster (such as a flood, fire, or earthquake), a national disaster (such as war or a riot), or a crime of violence (such as a bombing, rape, murder, spousal or child abuse). Studies have shown a critical need for psychological first aid and debriefing for persons of all ages after any adventitious crisis.

Phases of Crisis
Phase 1

Crisis event stimulates anxiety, which stimulates use of problem-solving techniques and defense mechanisms to lower the anxiety.

Phase 2

If usual defensive response fails, anxiety continues to rise and individual becomes disorganized. Trial-and-error problem solving begins in an effort to restore balance.

Phase 3

If trial-and-error attempts fail, anxiety escalates and person mobilizes automatic relief behaviors such as withdrawal and flight.

Phase 4

If problem remains unsolved and anxiety continues at severe or panic level, serious personality disorganization occurs (e.g., confusion, immobilization, violence against others, suicide attempts, aimless running and shouting).

Aspects of Crisis That Have Relevance for Nurses

There are specific aspects of crisis theory that are basic to crisis intervention. See Box 22-1 for details.

Application of the Nursing Process
Assessment
Overall Assessment

Equilibrium may be adversely affected by (1) unrealistic perception of the precipitating event, (2) inadequate situational supports, (3) inadequate coping mechanisms. Assessment should include determining need for external controls due to suicidal or homicidal ideation (Have you considered killing yourself or someone else since this problem began?), perception of the precipitating event, situational supports, and personal coping skills.

Assessing the Client's Perception of the Precipitating Event

Clear definition of the problem is necessary for resolution. Sample questions:

- Has anything upsetting happened to you within the past few days or weeks? What was happening in your life before you started feeling this way?
- What leads you to seek help now?
- Describe how you are feeling right now.
- How does this problem affect your life? Your future? What would need to be done to resolve this situation?

Continued

107

Assessing Situational Supports

It is necessary to determine resources available to the person. If resources are not available, the nurse acts as a temporary support system while relationships with individuals or community groups are established. Questions to ask:
- With whom do you live?
- To whom do you talk when you feel overwhelmed?
- Who is available to help you?
- Where do you go to worship? Where do you go to school? During past difficult times who did you want most to help you? Who is most helpful?

Assessing Personal Coping Skills

The individual's level of anxiety should be assessed. It is necessary to determine whether client has exhausted all coping resources and whether hospitalization is required. Questions include the following:
- Have you thought of killing yourself or someone else? If yes, have you thought of how you would do this?
- What things help you to feel better?
- What did you try this time? What was different this time?
- What helped you through difficult times in the past?
- What do you think might happen now?

Self-Assessment

The nurse must self-monitor feelings to ensure that he or she is not preventing expression of painful feelings by the client. Problems faced by beginning practitioners include the following:
- need to be needed;
- unrealistic goals;
- difficulty dealing with issue of suicide;
- difficulty terminating.

Nurses working in disaster situations may become overwhelmed by witnessing catastrophic events. They, too, need support and debriefing.

Assessment Guidelines

There are six guidelines indicated in the text including identifying whether the client's response to the crisis warrants psychiatric treatment, and identifying whether the client was able to identify precipitating factors. The other assessment factors include assessment and identification of situational supports, coping styles, religious or cultural beliefs and identification of primary, secondary, and tertiary needs of the client in crisis.

Nursing Diagnosis

Possible diagnoses include: *risk for self-directed violence, chronic low self-esteem, hopelessness, powerlessness, anxiety, acute confusion, disturbed thought processes, sleep deprivation, social isolation, risk for loneliness, impaired social interaction, ineffective coping, interrupted family processes, risk for posttrauma syndrome, rape-trauma syndrome, dysfunctional grieving,* etc.

Outcome Criteria

Criteria must be realistic and be established with the client. They must consider the client's cultural and personal values. Helping the client to return to precrisis state is always one of the most important primary considerations.

Planning

The nurse may be involved in planning for an individual (abuse), a group (suicide), or a community (disaster). Data from two questions will guide planning. (1) What is the effect of the crisis on the person's life (i.e., can he or she still work, go to school, care for family)? (2) How is the crisis affecting significant people in the client's life? As planning begins the nurse will want to help the client gain a feeling of safety and may even offer a solution to help the client understand that options are available.

108

CHAPTER OUTLINE	TEACHING STRATEGIES
Intervention	There are two basic goals: (1) client safety: external controls may be applied for protection from suicidal or homicidal urges, and (2) anxiety reduction allows for use of inner resources.
	Some important considerations: crisis intervention requires a creative, flexible approach; the client solves the problem; the client is in charge of his or her life; the client is able to make decisions; the crisis intervention relationship is between partners.
Counseling Strategies	There are three levels of nursing care in crisis intervention: primary care, secondary care, and tertiary care.
Primary	Promotes mental health and lowers the incidence of crisis. Examples: (1) evaluating stressful life events the person is experiencing to recognize potential problems; (2) teaching coping skills such as decision making, problem solving, assertiveness, and relaxation as ways to handle stress; (3) assisting in evaluation of timing of or reduction of life changes to decrease negative effects of stress.
Secondary	Establishes intervention during a crisis to prevent prolonged anxiety from diminishing personal effectiveness and personality organization. It occurs in hospitals, emergency rooms, clinics, and mental health centers.
Tertiary	Provides support for clients who have experienced a disabling crisis and are recovering. Examples of agencies providing tertiary care are rehabilitation centers, sheltered workshops, day hospitals, and outpatient clinics.
Evaluation	Evaluation compares goals with outcomes to determine effectiveness and is usually done 4 to 8 weeks after the initial interview. If the intervention has been successful, client anxiety and function should be at pre-crisis level.

23 Suicide

THOUGHTS ABOUT TEACHING THE TOPIC

Many faculty choose to co-assign this material to the unit on alterations in mood (Chapter 18). The rationale for this is that many depressed clients are considered to be suicidal, and the student must learn about both suicide precautions and no-suicide contracts in order to give care to selected clients. It is, however, necessary to make students aware that clients other than those diagnosed with affective disorder may present the risk for suicide.

Faculty should also be sensitive to the fact that students in the group may have entertained suicidal ideation or may have made suicidal attempts at one time or have family members who have. Often such as student will seek to discuss this privately with the faculty member, some for the purpose of seeking reassurance that earlier behaviors will not disqualify him or her from graduating, and others, to seek help.

KEY TERMS AND CONCEPTS

completed suicides, 473
copycat suicide, 475
lethality, 477
no-suicide contract, 481
parasuicide, 476
postvention, 480
primary intervention, 480

psychological autopsies, 475
SAD PERSONS scale, 478
secondary intervention, 480
suicidal ideation, 476
suicide, 475
suicide attempt, 476
tertiary intervention, 480

OBJECTIVES

After studying this chapter, the reader will be able to
1. Describe the profile of suicide in the United States, noting psychosocial and cultural factors that affect risk.
2. Identify three common precipitating events.
3. Name the most frequent coexisting psychiatric disorders.
4. Using the SAD PERSONS scale, explain ten risk factors to consider when assessing for suicide.
5. Describe three expected reactions a nurse may have when beginning work with suicidal clients.
6. Give examples of primary, secondary, and tertiary (postvention) interventions.
7. Describe basic level interventions that take place in the hospital or in the community.
8. Identify key elements of suicide precautions and environmental safety factors in the hospital.

CHAPTER OUTLINE	TEACHING STRATEGIES
Prevalence	Suicide is the eleventh leading cause of death in the United States. There are about 75 suicides daily. The elderly have the highest risk of suicide.
Comorbidity	Disorders that can be viewed as risk factors for suicide are depressive disorders, schizophrenia, alcohol use disorder or substance abuse, borderline and antisocial personality disorder, and panic disorder.
Theory **Biological Factors**	Twin and adoption studies suggest the presence of genetic factors in suicide. Also, low levels of the neurotransmitter serotonin are thought to play a role in an individual's decision to commit suicide. There is a pattern identifying suicide behavior in families as well. And physical illness is considered an important factor in 11% to 15% of suicides.
Psychosocial Factors	Freud originally theorized that suicide resulted from aggression turned inward. Karl Menninger added to Freud's base by describing three parts of suicidal hostility: the wish to kill, the wish to be killed, and the wish to die. Beck identified a central emotional factor underlying suicide intent as hopelessness.

110

The suicidal persons most likely to act out their fantasies are those who have suffered a loss of love, suffered a narcissistic injury, experienced overwhelming moods like rage or guilt, or identify with a suicide victim.

Cultural Factors

Cultural factors include religious beliefs, family values, and attitude toward death. All of these have an impact on suicide. Generally in the United States, European Americans have twice the suicide rate of minority groups; the exception to this is Native Americans, whose suicide rate is equal to European Americans.

Application of the Nursing Process

The process of suicide risk assessment is based on identification of specific risk factors, psychosocial and medical history, and interaction with the interviewer. The nurse usually completes this assessment in conjunction with a physician or another clinician. Not all clients with suicidal ideation really want to die.

Assessment
Verbal and Nonverbal Clues

Clues are usually sent out to supportive people. An example of overt verbalization is, "Life isn't worth living anymore." A covert verbalization would be, "You won't have to bother with me much longer." Most often it is a relief for people contemplating suicide to talk to someone about their despair. Asking specific questions is appropriate for the nurse (e.g., "Are you experiencing thoughts of suicide?" "Do you have a plan for committing suicide?" If yes, "What is your plan?").

Behavioral clues include writing farewell notes and giving away prized possessions. Somatic clues include sleep disturbance, weight loss, and focus on somatic symptoms in lieu of psychological pain; emotional clues include social withdrawal, feelings of hopelessness, and complaints of exhaustion.

Lethality of Suicide Plan

Three main elements to consider are (1) specificity of details of the plan (the more details included in the plan, the higher the risk); (2) lethality of proposed method (i.e., how quickly the person would die using the method(high-risk methods include using a gun, jumping off a high place, hanging, inhaling carbon monoxide, and staging a car crash; low-risk methods include wrist slashing, ingesting pills); and (3) availability of means (if the means are available, the risk is greater than when one still has to secure the means).

Lethality of the method indicates how quickly a person would die by the method is classified as higher or lower risk. These are also termed "hard" methods (gun, jumping off a high place, hanging, carbon monoxide poisoning, staging a car crash) or "soft" methods (slashing one's wrists, inhaling natural gas, or ingesting pills.)

Assessment Tools

The SAD PERSONS scale is used to evaluate 10 major risk factors for suicide potential. The higher the score, the greater the risk and the greater the need for hospitalization.

Self Assessment

Universal reactions include (1) anxiety related to latent suicidal inclination in self or feelings of personal rejection by the client, (2) irritation associated with believing client is trying to get attention, (3) avoidance in response to feelings of helplessness, and (4) denial of seriousness of the suicidal ideation as way of avoiding experiencing feelings aroused by the suicidal person.

Assessment Guidelines

These include assessing a client's risk factors, history of suicide attempts, assessment of medical or psychiatric diagnoses. Other significant factors include sudden changes in mood, relevant support system or if significant others report changes in behavior such as withdrawal, preoccupation, silence, and remorse.

Continued

111

Nursing Diagnosis

Useful diagnoses include *risk for self-directed violence, ineffective coping, ineffective or compromised family coping, disabled family coping, hopelessness, powerlessness, social isolation, spiritual distress, risk for loneliness, chronic low self-esteem, deficient knowledge.*

Outcome Criteria

Goals should be consistent with the suicidal person's perceptions and ability to achieve the goals. Outcomes and goals for the nursing diagnosis *risk for violence: self-directed* are nearly always of concern (e.g., client expresses feelings, maintains connectedness in relationships, seeks help when feeling self-destructive, does not require treatment for suicide gestures or attempts). The reader is also referred to NOC.

Planning

The plan of care for suicidal client is based upon the assessment of risk factors.

Intervention
Levels of Intervention

Primary intervention—Activities that provide support, information, and education to avoid situations that could become serious.

Secondary intervention—Treatment of the actual suicidal crisis; client ambivalence is an important tool for the nurse.

Tertiary intervention (or postvention)—Interventions with family and friends of a person who has either committed suicide or recently attempted suicide and interventions with a person who has recently attempted suicide are geared toward minimizing the traumatic aftereffects of the suicide or attempt.

Basic Level Interventions

NIC offers the following topics pertinent to the care of the suicidal client: *suicide prevention, hope instillation, coping enhancement, self-esteem enhancement, family mobilization,* and *support system enhancement.*

Milieu Therapy with Suicide Precautions

Placing a suicidal person in a controlled hospital environment can provide structure and control, and can give the person time to evaluate his or her situation with professional staff. Monitoring of suicidal intent and extent of hopelessness should be ongoing. Hospitalization can provide time for the individual to reestablish relationships and make contact with appropriate community agencies.

Counseling

Is practiced in the community, in hospitals, on telephone hotlines. Counseling requires warmth, sensitivity, interest, concern, and consistency on the part of the helping person. It must include establishment of a personal relationship with the suicidal person, encouragement of more realistic problem-solving behaviors, and reaffirmation of hope. Counselors should (1) remain calm and listen, (2) deal directly with the topic of suicide, (3) encourage problem solving and positive actions, (4) get assistance from other resources, (5) convey to the person: the crisis is temporary, unbearable pain can be survived, help is available, you are not alone.

Health Teaching

The nurse teaches the client about the psychiatric diagnosis, medications, age-related crises, community resources, coping skills and communication skills, especially the expression of anger. The text lists a variety of intervention programs.

Case Management

Reconnecting clients with family or significant supportive friends can have a major impact on the client's recovery and referrals to community services are essential.

Psychobiological Interventions

SSRIs provide an alternative to hospitalization. Suicide possibility increases with extreme anxiety and lack of sleep. Anxiolytics may be necessary, but medication for more than 1 to 3 days should not be supplied at any one time and follow-up plans must be made. Co-existing psychiatric conditions should be treated. ECT should be considered if the client is seriously depressed and highly suicidal, since its effects are more immediate than those of antidepressants.

Advanced Practice Interventions

There are several types of psychotherapy that are used for treatment of suicidal clients. See text for more details. The APRN can also provide clinical supervision for direct care staff. The APRN can also provide aftercare for the client and consultation in the inpatient and outpatient, ER or forensic settings.

Survivors of Completed Suicide: Postvention

For friends and family of a suicide victim, postvention should be instituted within 72 hours and be continued through at least the first anniversary of the death. Confusion, stigma, isolation from supports, anger at the deceased, and guilt are issues to be resolved. Posttraumatic loss debriefing, a seven-stage process, can help initiate an adaptive grief process. Self-help groups for families of individuals who have committed suicide can be of considerable help.

Staff should have the opportunity to work through self-blame, guilt, anger, and loss of self-esteem associated with caring for a client who commits suicide.

Evaluation

Be aware that sudden behavioral changes can signal suicidal intent, especially when depression is lifting, and that anniversaries of losses are difficult times. Evaluation is focused on outcome criteria established during the planning phase.

113

24 Anger and Aggression

THOUGHTS ABOUT TEACHING THE TOPIC

It seems logical to begin by giving learners strategies to deescalate impending aggression and protocols to use when actual aggression takes place. Role playing verbal interventions is helpful, and practicing physical interventions is essential. Emphasizing the fact that fear is a normal response to dealing with an aggressive client can be reassuring to beginning students. Discussion of feelings should be followed by reassurance that team intervention increases safety for both clients and staff. Information about the use of seclusion and restraint usually accompanies the information on aggression.

KEY TERMS AND CONCEPTS

aggression, 490
anger, 490
deescalation techniques, 496
restraint, 496
seclusion, 496

OBJECTIVES

After studying this chapter, the reader will be able to
1. Compare and contrast three theories that explore the nature of aggression.
2. Compare and contrast interventions for a client with healthy coping skills with those for a client with marginal coping behaviors.
3. Explain why behavioral and cognitive-behavioral techniques are useful modalities for anger management.
4. Apply at least four principles of deescalation with a moderately angry client.
5. Describe four criteria for the use of seclusion or restraint over verbal intervention.
6. Role-play with classmates by using understandable but unhelpful responses to anger and aggression in clients; discuss how these responses can affect nursing interventions.

CHAPTER OUTLINE	TEACHING STRATEGIES
	Anger and aggression are difficult targets for nursing intervention, particularly if their focus is the nurse, because they imply threat and elicit emotional and personal responses. Anger is an emotional response to the perception of frustration of desires, threat to one's needs, or challenge. Aggression is harsh physical or verbal action that reflects rage, hostility, and potential for physical or verbal destructiveness. Anger and aggression are the last two stages of a response that begins with feelings of vulnerability followed by uneasiness. Intervention in the early stages is desirable.
Prevalence	Anger and aggression are considered universal emotions and can be identified across cultures via facial expression. Both are responses to threat or loss of control. The health care environment readily causes feelings of lack of control in clients. Aggression and violence are usually a result of unchecked escalation of anger. There is evidence that checks on aggression may be less available now than they have been, leading to an increased incidence of violence. Rates for suicides, homicides, and domestic violence give insight into the prevalence of violence in general.
	The Centers for Disease Control and Prevention reported over 50,000 deaths from suicide and homicide in 2001. The leading cause of death for those 15 to 34 years of age is homicide. NIOSH reported a rate of assaults of hospital workers of 8.3 assaults per 10,000 workers in 1999. Violence is most frequent in psychiatric units, ERs, waiting rooms, and geriatric units.
Comorbidity	A correlation has been found between quickness to anger and hyperactivity and attention deficits and impulsivity in male children. In adults, incidence of anger is higher in the presence of unipolar depression, PTSD, mania, personality disorders, and Tourette's disease. Anger and hostility are also risk factors for cardiovascular disease and CVA.

114

CHAPTER OUTLINE	TEACHING STRATEGIES
Theory	
Another Look at an Old Theory	Drive and instinct theories led to the view that anger was an innate driving force sometimes essential to survival and harmful if repressed. Later research has shown that expression of anger is not always beneficial and can lead to increased anger and negative physiological changes such as cardiac reactivity. Repression of anger, however, is shown to lead to essential hypertension in women and is associated with immunological problems in both sexes. Anger management techniques have been shown to be beneficial.
Behavioral Theory Base	Children learn aggression by imitating others and by repeating behavior that has been rewarded. Anger and aggression learned in the family and from TV watching have two intrinsic rewards: keeping the angry person in control while intimidating others, and providing relief of pent-up distress. Research by Bandura suggests that emotional arousal has an increased probability of expression as aggression when the context is predisposed to aggression. Milieu therapy has found that rigid intolerance of affect and an authoritarian style by nurses have been associated with assault.
Cognitive Theory Base	Cognitions drive anger. When individuals appraise events as threatening, the cognition leads to the emotional and physiological arousal necessary to take action. For example, clients kept waiting without explanation may interpret this as neglect and lack of respect. Anger escalates when cognitions such as "They have no right to treat me as a non-person" follow. Initial feelings such as fear, hurt, humiliation, or powerlessness may generate anger as a response to "being made to feel this way." Nurses tend to respond to client anger according to the interpretation given to the client's anger and their self-appraised ability to manage the situation. Those with high self-efficacy moved to help the client. Others showed a decreased ability to problem-solve.
Neurobiology of Anger and Aggression	
Brain Abnormalities	Many neurological conditions are associated with anger and aggression (e.g., Alzheimer's disease, temporal lobe epilepsy, traumatic brain injury, brain tumors).
Serotonin	A relationship between low levels of serotonin and impulsive aggression has been shown in studies.
Genetic and Environmental Factors	Research findings indicate that violence is a function of both genetics and childhood environment. Some are more biologically predisposed than others.
Application of the Nursing Process	
Assessment	
Overall Assessment	It is important to identify anxiety before it escalates to anger and aggression. Expressions of anxiety and anger look quite similar: increased rate and volume of speech, increased demands, irritability, frowning, redness of face, pacing, twisting hands, or clenching and unclenching of fists. Assessment should include taking an accurate history of the client's background, usual coping skills, and perception of the issue. Clients' perceptions often provide a useful point of intervention.
Self-Assessment	The nurse's ability to intervene safely in situations of anger and violence depends on self-awareness. Nurses' responses to angry clients can escalate along a continuum similar to that of clients. The more a nursing intervention is prompted by emotion, the less likely it is to be therapeutic. The phenomenon of emotional contagion is explained. Nurses' responses reflect norms from their families of origin, personal issues, and situational events. In addition to self-assessment, techniques

Continued

115

such as deep breathing, muscle relaxation, empathetic interpretation of clients' distress, and review of intervention strategies can be helpful.

Assessment Guidelines

The simple best predictor of future violence is a history of violence. See text for other important assessment guidelines.

Nursing Diagnosis

Three especially useful diagnoses are *ineffective coping, risk for self-directed violence,* and *risk for other-directed violence. Ineffective coping* is useful for individuals who have adequate day-to-day coping skills, but are overwhelmed by the stresses of illness or hospitalization. Clients may have a pattern of maladaptive coping that is marginally effective and consists of strategies that have been developed to meet unusual or extraordinary situations such as abusive families. Ideally intervention aborts the development of aggression. If anger is not resolved, the diagnoses of *risk for self-directed violence* or *risk for other-directed violence* may become relevant.

Outcome Criteria

Outcome criteria from NOC for aggression self-control are listed in Table 24-1 as examples.

Planning

Planning interventions necessitate having a sound assessment and determining what the situation calls for from among alternatives such as psychotherapeutic approaches to teach the client new skills for handling anger or immediate intervention to prevent overt violence via deescalation techniques, restraints or seclusion, or psychopharmacy.

Intervention

Basing Interventions on Stages of the Violence Cycle

Preassaultive Stage: Verbal Deescalation Approaches

- The client becomes increasingly agitated.
- The staff needs to be educated.
- The better educated the staff, the less chance for injury.
- Verbal interventions include:
  - Analyze the client and situation.
  - Use verbal techniques of deescalation.
  - Demonstrate respect for the client's personal space.
  - Interact with the client.
  - Invest time in the process.
  - Pay attention to the environment.
  - Assure your safety.

Assaultive Stage: Restraint, Medication, Seclusion

If the client progresses to the assaultive stage, the staff must respond quickly and as a team. It is advisable, to use five members of the team or more as indicated. One leader speaks with the client and instructs members of the team. The intervention usually requires physical restraints and seclusion of the client. The goal of the use of seclusion and restraints is safety of the client and others.

Seclusion and physical restraints cannot be used without a physician's order and are used only after exhaustion of all other intervention alternatives have failed. The client must have 24-hour one-on-one observation. And the circumstances for physical restraint include: client is a clear and present danger to self or others, client has been legally detained for involuntary treatment, or client requests seclusion or restraints for his or her own safety.

Postassaultive Stage

Processing with the client is an important part of the therapeutic process but only after the client no longer requires seclusion and restraints. This allows the client to learn from the situation, to identify the stressors that precipitated the behavior, and to plan alternative ways of responding in the future.

CHAPTER OUTLINE	TEACHING STRATEGIES
Return to Baseline: Critical Incident Debriefing	The staff processing of a critical incident is essential to ensure that quality care was provided to the client, and the staff have an opportunity to examine their responses to the client. Several questions to be answered are included in the text.
Documentation of a Violent Episode	There are several areas that are essential to document in situations where violence was either averted or actually occurred. The nurse must document the assessment of the behaviors that occurred during the preassaultive stage, the nursing interventions and the client's responses and evaluation of the interventions used. Details should be included. See text for list of areas to document.
General Hospital Settings **Angry Clients with Healthy Coping Who Are Overwhelmed**	Interventions are aimed at collaborating with the client to find ways to reestablish or substitute similar means for dealing with the overwhelming situation. The nurse acknowledges the client's distress, validates it as understandable, and indicates willingness to search for solutions. Validation cannot occur unless nurses recognize their own self-protective responses to angry clients to prevent negative cycles of staff-client conflict. If the client is unable to communicate the source of the anger, the nurse can often make an accurate guess. Naming the feeling can lead to dissipation of anger by helping the client feel understood.
Angry Clients with Marginal Coping Skills	Clients with marginal coping skills need different interventions than clients with basically healthy coping skills. They often achieve feelings of control or mastery via the use of anger and intimidation. Clients with chemical dependence and clients with personality styles that externalize blame are examples of clients who become angry at staff for not providing relief from discomfort or anxiety. Intervention requires a respectful approach that establishes a sense of mutual collaboration. The nurse can maintain respect by remembering that clients are doing the best they can, clients want to improve, and client behaviors make sense within their worldview. Other interventions: provide comfort items before they are requested to build rapport; be clear about what you can and can't do; offer distractions (such as magazines, games); provide predictable interactions with staff.
	When verbal abuse occurs, three interventions can be used. (1) Leave the room when abuse begins, stating you will return in a specific amount of time (e.g., 20 minutes). Be matter-of-fact. The alternative is to break off conversation and eye contact and finish the procedure before leaving the room. (2) Attend positively to nonabusive communication by the client. (3) Schedule regular frequent contacts with client, giving attention that is not contingent on client's behavior.
Inpatient Psychiatric Settings	Not all psychiatric clients are violent. Aggression appears to be correlated less with certain disorders than with client characteristics. The best predictors of violence are previous violent behavior and impulsivity. Conflict with staff and interactions with staff that involve limit setting are common reasons for violence. Limit-setting styles of nurses that are belittling or that provide solutions without options are more likely to precipitate anger than are platitudes, providing solutions with options, affective involvement without options, and affective involvement with options. Studies show that cognitive therapy can be helpful.
Clients with Cognitive Deficits	Clients with cognitive deficits (e.g., clients with Alzheimer's disease, multi-infarct dementia, brain injury) are at risk for acting aggressively. Interventions include reality orientation; orientation aids such as calendars and clocks; simplified environment; a calm, unhurried approach; and identification of antecedents of anxiety. Validation therapy may be used to calm clients when reality orientation is not effective. Validation involves the client's describing the current situation and the nurse's commenting on what appears to be underlying the distress.

Continued

117

Sedation is often not the best solution because it may further cloud the client's sensorium, making disorientation worse.

Deescalating techniques are commonsense principles such as maintaining calmness; assessing the situation, identifying stressors and what client considers to be his or her need; using a calm voice and nonthreatening nonverbal communication, being empathetic, genuine, and honest; maintaining a large personal space; not arguing, giving options.

Evaluation

An evaluation provides information about whether outcome criteria have been met. See Table 24-1 for specific outcome criteria.

Concept Map

Some students, especially those who are visually oriented, find use of a concept map is helpful in learning. On the following page is a concept map for aggression.

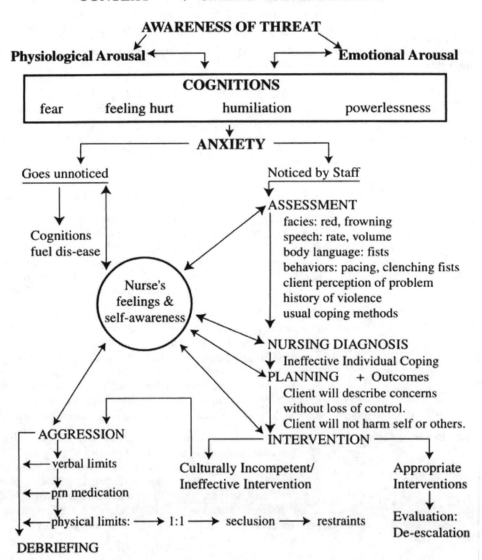

25 Family Violence

THOUGHTS ABOUT TEACHING THE TOPIC

The authors explore family violence in this chapter, thereby providing the instructor with a variety of examples to help students operationalize crisis theory. Because individual states have specific laws regarding the reporting of abuse, instructors may wish to review the provisions of the law as part of this unit of material.

For many students this material evokes strong emotions. Be prepared for this in classroom discussions. Because some students have experienced family violence, it is wise to have an established referral system with student services or an outside agency.

KEY TERMS AND CONCEPTS

acute battering stage, 510
crisis situation, 510
economic maltreatment, 511
emotional violence, 511
escalation-deescalation, 510
family violence, 508
health care record, 517
honeymoon stage, 510
neglect, 511
perpetrators, 508
physical violence, 510
primary prevention, 520
safety plan, 521
secondary prevention, 520
sexual violence, 510
shelters or safe houses, 521
tension-building stage, 510
tertiary prevention, 521
vulnerable person, 509

OBJECTIVES

After studying this chapter, the reader will be able to
1. Discuss the epidemiological theory of violence in terms of stresses on the perpetrator, vulnerable person, and environment that could escalate anxiety to the point at which violence becomes the relief behavior.
2. Contrast and compare three characteristics of perpetrators with three characteristics of a vulnerable person.
3. Name three indicators of (a) physical violence, (b) sexual violence, (c) neglect, and (d) emotional violence.
4. Describe four areas to assess when interviewing a person who has experienced family violence.
5. Formulate four nursing diagnoses for the survivor of violence and list supporting data from the assessment.
6. Write out a safety plan, including the essential elements, for an abused spouse.
7. Compare and contrast primary, secondary, and tertiary levels of intervention, giving two examples of intervention for each level.
8. Identify two common emotional responses the nurse might experience when faced with a person subjected to family violence.
9. Describe at least three possible referrals for a violent family (child, adult, elder abuse) and write down the telephone numbers of the corresponding agencies in the community.
10. Name and discuss three psychotherapeutic modalities that are useful in working with violent families.

CHAPTER OUTLINE	TEACHING STRATEGIES
Prevalence	True prevalence is unknown because of underreporting and variability of reporting methods. It has been estimated that half of all Americans have experienced violence in their families. It is estimated that approximately 20% to 30% of the women in this country will experience domestic violence during their lives, and that 2 million older Americans are victims of physical, psychological, or other forms of abuse and neglect. Violence can occur in gay and lesbian relationships.
Comorbidity	The secondary effects of violence, such as anxiety, depression, and suicide, are health care issues that can last a lifetime. Social factors that reinforce violence include the wide acceptance of hitting children; increasingly violent movies, video games, Internet sites, and comic books; the violent themes in rap music, and the increase in pornography.

Continued

119

CHAPTER OUTLINE	TEACHING STRATEGIES

Theory

Family violence refers to physical injury to or causing mental anguish by one family member against another, or the deprivation of essential services by a caregiver.

Conditions for Violence

Perpetrator

Someone who initiates (perpetrates) violence considers personal needs more important than the needs of others. Propensity for violence is rooted in childhood and is manifested by lack of self-regard and inability to assume adult roles. A perpetrator may be a female responding to a violent spouse; a younger woman married to a frail older man; a teenager being violent toward a parent; or a violent male. Violent males believe in male domination; act out to feel in control and powerful; are jealous; monitor and restrict activities of vulnerable persons; control family finances; are prone to being abusive when intoxicated; are remorseful, act childlike, and yearn to be nurtured following violent episodes. Both male and female perpetrators perceive themselves as having poor social skills. Their relationships with significant others are usually enmeshed and codependent.

Vulnerable Person

The vulnerable person is the one who is abused. Pregnancy increases the risk of violence. Violence also escalates when the wife makes a move toward independence. The risk for violence is greatest when the spouse attempts to leave the relationship. Children are most likely to be abused if they are under 3 years old, perceived as "different," remind the parents of someone they do not like, are the product of an unwanted pregnancy, or do not meet parental fantasy expectations. Adolescents are also at risk for abuse, at least as frequently as children. Older adults are particularly vulnerable when in poor mental or physical health, or are disruptive. Abused elderly may be either male or female being cared for by a spouse or child who was a victim of abuse.

Crisis Situation

A crisis situation is an event that puts stress on the family with a violent member. Social isolation contributes to ineffective coping during a crisis situation.

Cycle of Violence

The cycle of violence that alternates with periods of safety, hope, and trust, is described in terms of escalation and deescalation. Four stages have been identified. (1) Tension-building stage: includes minor incidents such as pushing and verbal abuse. The vulnerable person does NOT tell the perpetrator that abuse is unacceptable. The abuser rationalizes that abuse is acceptable; the abused person minimizes importance of incidents and may blame self. (2) Acute battering stage: a perpetrator releases built-up tension by beating a vulnerable person; the victim depersonalizes the incident. Both perpetrator and victim are in shock. (3) Honeymoon stage: perpetrator feels remorse and acts in kindly, loving ways by apologizing or bringing gifts; victim believes promises and apologies, and drops criminal charges. (4) Tension-building stage: abuse reoccurs and cycle begins again.

Types of Maltreatment

Five types of maltreatment have been identified: (1) Physical violence includes battering and physical endangerment (reckless behavior toward a vulnerable person). (2) Sexual violence (i.e., any sexual approach or act, explicit or implicit, toward a child), which is usually perpetrated by father or stepfather, is abuse. The sexual abuse of adults is usually referred to as sexual assault or rape. (3) Emotional violence involves infliction of mental anguish (e.g., terrorizing, demeaning, showing hostility, ignoring, withholding affection, threatening abandonment). (4) Neglect can be physical (health care), developmental (nurturing), or educational (deprivation). (5) Economic maltreatment involves using another's resources without permission, for one's own personal gain.

120

Application of the Nursing Process
Assessment

Overall Assessment	Nurses will see persons experiencing violence in every health care setting. Complaints may be vague and need exploration. Assessments should include a history of sexual abuse, family violence, and drug use or abuse, and should be conducted with only the nurse and client present.
Interview Process and Setting	Assessment requires privacy and interviewer tact in questioning. The following techniques are useful: Sit near client; establish rapport; reassure client that he or she did nothing wrong; allow client to tell story without interruption; be non-judgmental. In verbal approaches, use open-ended techniques if possible, such as, "Tell me what happened to you," "What happens when you do something wrong?" "Describe how you discipline your child." Determine need for further help by assessing violence indicators, levels of anxiety and coping responses, family coping patterns, support systems, suicide potential, and drug and alcohol use. Once trust has been established, openness and directness about the situation can strengthen the relationship.
Self-Assessment	Working with those experiencing violence gives rise to strong emotions on the part of the nurse. Professional or peer supervision is a necessary part of dealing with these responses.
Assessing Types of Maltreatment	
Physical Violence	Overt signs of battering include bruises; scars; burns; wounds around head, face, chest, arms, abdomen, back, buttocks, and genitalia; injuries in various stages of healing. Covert minor complaints often heard include "accidents," "back trouble," "falls." Sexual abuse may be suspected with bruising or injury around genitalia, and presence of urinary tract infection. Also be suspicious if explanations do not fit the injury; client minimizes the seriousness of the injury; a child under 6 months has bruises; or respiratory problems are present in young child (may suggest "shaken-baby syndrome"). Ask clients directly, but in a nonthreatening way, whether the injury has been caused by someone close to them. Observe nonverbal response for hesitation or lack of eye contact. Then ask specific questions about the last time abuse occurred, how often it happens, in what ways the client is hurt.
Sexual Violence	Victims often display various psychopathologies, including depression. Remember sexual abuse of boys appears to be common, but underreported, underrecognized, and untreated.
Emotional Violence	Wherever physical or sexual violence is occurring, emotional violence occurs. It may also exist alone, when low self-esteem, anguish, and isolation are instilled in place of love and acceptance.
Neglect	Signs include appearing undernourished, dirty, and poorly clothed. Inadequate medical care is a form of neglect.
Economic Maltreatment	Failure to provide for the needs of the victim even when adequate funds are available.
Assessing Level of Anxiety and Coping Responses	Nurses should note nonverbal responses, hesitation, lack of eye contact, vague statements, vigilance, inability to relax, sleep deprivation, physical signs of chronic stress. Note defensiveness about loved ones, even if they perpetrate violence.
Assessing Family Coping Patterns	Nurses should show a willingness to listen and avoid use of a judgmental tone. Living with children and older adults in the same household can cause frustration, stress, and anger.

Continued

121

Assessing Support Systems	Is client in a dependent position, relying on perpetrator for basic needs? Is client isolated from others?
Assessing Suicide Potential	Suicide may seem the only answer for one who feels trapped in a relationship that she is desperate to leave. Suicide threats by a perpetrator may be used to manipulate victim: "If you leave, I'll kill myself."
Assessing Homicide Potential	A vulnerable person is at greater risk for homicide if there is a gun in the home; when alcohol or drugs are used; if the perpetrator has been violent previously; or when the perpetrator is jealous and obsessive about the relationship and tries to control all of victim's daily activities. Inquire whether the client feels safe about going home.
Assessing Drug and Alcohol Use	A person experiencing violence may self-medicate. If a battered person presents in an intoxicated state, allow him or her to become sober before making a referral. A client should not be discharged to her spouse.
Maintaining Accurate Records	For legal reasons records should contain an accurate, detailed history; descriptions of findings; verbatim statements of who caused injury and when injury occurred; a body map to indicate information about injuries; photos; physical evidence of sexual abuse acquired by carefully following legal protocols.
Assessment Guidelines	During the assessment and counseling, maintain an interested and empathetic manner. Refrain from displaying emotional extremes and follow the eight guideline questions in the text.
Nursing Diagnosis	Diagnoses are focused on the underlying causes and symptoms of family violence. Useful diagnoses include *risk for injury, anxiety, fear; ineffective coping, disabled family coping, powerlessness, caregiver role strain, chronic low self-esteem, interrupted family processes, impaired parenting.* Pain related to physical injury would take a high priority.
Outcome Criteria	The NOC classification is used to identify criteria for abuse cessation.
Planning	Plans should center on client safety, and should also take into consideration the needs of the abuser if he or she seems willing to learn violence-free alternatives to aggression.
Intervention	Nurses are mandated reporters of child and elder abuse or neglect. Many states require reporting of violence against women, and many have marital rape statutes. A reasonable basis for suspecting maltreatment is all that is required. Immunity from criminal or civil liability is provided when reporting is mandated. The importance of considering cultural issues that may affect response to violence and to interventions is stressed. In situations in which translation is required, the translator should NOT be a member of the victim's family.
	Primary intervention consists of measures taken to prevent the occurrence of family violence, and includes reducing stress and increasing social support and coping skills. Secondary prevention involves early intervention in abusive situations. Tertiary prevention involves the rehabilitative process, and support for survivors.
Basic Level Interventions **Counseling**	Counseling involves crisis intervention and promotion of growth. The role of the nurse is to support the victim, counsel about safety (having a plan for escape and use of a safe house), and facilitate access to other resources as appropriate.
Case Management	This includes coordination of community, medical, criminal justice, and social systems to provide comprehensive services for the family.

122

CHAPTER OUTLINE	TEACHING STRATEGIES
Milieu Therapy	Interventions are geared toward stabilizing the home situation and maintaining a violence-free environment. It often involves providing economic support or job opportunities, social support from public health nurse, social worker, etc., and family therapy.
Self-Care Activities	The goal is empowerment. Examples include provision of referral numbers for other agencies, legal, counseling, vocational counseling, parenting resources, etc.
Health Teaching	Teaching topics include normal developmental and physiological changes (explanation is geared to helping the family members gain a more positive view of the victim and the crisis situation), coping skills, risk factors for violence, and parenting skills. Candidates for special attention are new parents whose behavior toward an infant is rejecting, hostile, or indifferent; teenage parents; retarded parents; parents who grew up watching their mother being beaten.
Advanced Practice Interventions	An advanced practice nurse carries out some type of psychotherapy after the crisis intervention, when the situation is less chaotic. It is aimed at empowerment, communication, validation, support, and respect for individual autonomy.
Individual Therapy	This is aimed at helping the victim recognize feelings about experiencing violence, about self, and about options. For the perpetrator who meets criteria for intermittent explosive disorder, therapy is most effective if court-ordered. Nurse therapists working with perpetrators have a duty to warn potential victims.
Family Therapy	If violence is recent and both partners agree to be involved, family therapy may be used. Desired outcomes: perpetrator will recognize inner states of anger and use alternative coping strategies; family members will listen to each other and communicate openly.
Group Therapy	Provides assurances that one is not alone and that positive change is possible. Self-help groups are also helpful for many people. Nurses engaged in therapy with perpetrators have a duty to warn potential victims.
Evaluation	Evaluation of brief interventions can be based on whether the survivor acknowledges the violence and is willing to accept intervention or is removed from the violent situation. Evaluation of long-term processes should note reduction in incidence of violence and healthier coping patterns.

123

26 Sexual Assault

THOUGHTS ABOUT TEACHING THE TOPIC

Since the majority of learners are female, and many have not received other information about rape and rape prevention, this session may serve a dual purpose: teaching how to care for a rape victim and how to protect oneself against rape. On the other hand, one or more members of the group may have been victims of rape. If this is the case, the instructor may need to be prepared for expression of strong feelings, and may need to refer the student to health services for counseling.

Many instructors find using audiovisual materials to provide discussion triggers helpful. Students often respond best when beginning the discussion by being asked to list the concrete measures the emergency department nurse should take to perform an assessment or to preserve evidence during the examination. Mini–role-playing situations can evolve out of the discussion.

KEY TERMS AND CONCEPTS

acquaintance or date rape, 531
acute phase, 532
blame, 538
compound reaction, 536
controlled style of coping, 535
expressed style of coping, 534
long-term reorganization phase, 533
rape-trauma syndrome, 531
silent reaction, 537
spousal or marital rape, 531

OBJECTIVES

After studying this chapter, the reader will be able to
1. Define sexual assault (rape).
2. Discuss the reasons that rapes go unreported.
3. Distinguish between the acute and long-term phases of the rape-trauma syndrome and identify some common reactions during each phase.
4. Identify and give examples of five areas to assess when working with a person who has been sexually assaulted.
5. Formulate two long-term outcomes and two short-term goals for the nursing diagnosis *rape-trauma syndrome*.
6. Analyze one's own thoughts and feelings regarding the myths about rape and its impact on survivors.
7. Identify six overall guidelines for nursing interventions related to sexual assault.
8. Describe the role of the sexual assault nurse examiner to a colleague.
9. Discuss the responsibilities of the nurse when a rape survivor is discharged from the emergency department, citing specific referrals in the community.
10. Develop a handout delineating the nurse's role when staffing a rape-crisis hotline.
11. Discuss the long-term psychological effects of sexual assault that might lead to a survivor's seeking psychotherapy.
12. Identify three outcome criteria that would signify successful interventions for a person who has suffered a sexual assault.

CHAPTER OUTLINE	TEACHING STRATEGIES

Sexual assault (rape) is an act of violence and nonconsensual sex is the weapon used by the perpetrator. Rape engulfs its victims in fear. After the rape the individual often carries the additional burden of shame, guilt, fear, anger, distrust, and embarrassment. One in six women and 1 in 33 men will experience an attempted or completed rape during their lifetime. A male who is raped is more likely to have physical trauma and to have been victimized by several assailants than is a female.

Theory

Types of rape include stranger rape, spousal or marital rape, and acquaintance or date rape, with the latter two being more common than stranger rape. Sexual distress as a sequela is more common among women who have been attacked by intimates, whereas fear and anxiety are more common in those assaulted by

124

strangers. Depression is common to both. Date rape has increased due to the use of drugs in conjunction with alcohol that are given to the victim. The drugs make the victim unable to ward off attackers and unable to remember details as a witness. The rape-trauma syndrome is a variant of posttraumatic stress disorder and consists of two phases, each with separate symptoms.

Acute Phase of Rape-Trauma Syndrome

This phase occurs immediately following the assault and may last for 2 weeks. Symptoms include shock, numbness, disbelief, disorganization in life style, cognitive impairment with confusion, poor concentration, poor decision making, and somatic symptoms. Hysteria, restlessness, crying, smiling may be noted. Denial after assault is a protective action to give the person time to prepare for reality.

Long-Term Reorganization Phase of Rape-Trauma Syndrome

This phase occurs 2 or more weeks after the rape. Nurses can help the client prepare for reactions that are likely to occur such as intrusive thoughts of event; flashbacks; dreams; insomnia; increased motor activity; anxiety; mood swings; development of fears and phobias, such as fear of indoors or outdoors, being alone, crowds, sexual activity. Intervention and support for the survivor can help prevent sequelae such as anxiety, depression, suicide, difficulties with daily functioning, interpersonal relationships, sexual dysfunction, and somatic complaints.

Application of the Nursing Process
Assessment

Nurse talks with the victim, people accompanying victim, and police to gather data. Interventions will include: treatment and documentation of injuries, treatment for sexually transmitted disease (STD), pregnancy risk evaluation and prevention, crisis intervention and arrangements for follow-up counseling, and collection of medicolegal evidence while maintaining the proper chain of evidence. Assessment should ascertain the level of client anxiety, coping mechanisms used, availability of support systems, signs and symptoms of emotional trauma, and signs and symptoms of physical trauma. A sexual assault nurse examiner or forensic nurse specialist may perform these activities.

Overall Assessment
Assessing the Level of Anxiety

Clients in severe to panic-level anxiety will be unable to problem-solve or process information. Nursing intervention should focus on lowering client anxiety to moderate or below where goals can be set and information assimilated.

Assessing Coping Mechanisms Used

The same coping skills that have helped the client before will be used in adjusting to the rape. New ways may also be developed. Behavioral responses include crying; withdrawing; smoking; wanting to talk about the event; acting hysterical; confused, disoriented, or incoherent; or even laughing or joking. These behaviors are examples of an expressed style of coping. A controlled style of coping reaction is evidenced by masked facies; calm, subdued appearance, or shocked, numb, confused appearance; distractibility; and indecisiveness. An emotional style of coping reaction is evidenced by anxiety, shock, humiliation, embarrassment, self-blame, low self-esteem, shame, guilt, and anger. If the nurse can help the client verbalize her thoughts, understanding of the client's cognitive coping mechanisms can be gained. The nurse can facilitate this with questions such as, "What do you think might help?" "What can I do to help you in this difficult time?"

Assessing Support Systems Available

Availability, size, and utility of a survivor's social support system need to be assessed. Often partners or family do not understand rape and may not be good supports. Be alert to the victim's nonverbal communication.

Continued

125

Assessing Signs and Symptoms of Emotional Trauma	The extent of psychological trauma may not be readily apparent from behavior, especially if the person uses the controlled style of coping during the acute phase of rape trauma. Conduct a nursing history. Allow the client to talk at a comfortable pace. Pose questions in nonjudgmental descriptive terms. Avoid "why" questions. If suicidal thoughts are expressed, assess what precautions are needed by asking direct questions.
Assessing Signs and Symptoms of Physical Trauma	Characteristic physical signs of rape involve injuries to face, head, neck, and extremities, which should be documented on a body map. The nurse takes a brief GYN history, including last menstrual period, likelihood of current pregnancy, and history of STD. The pelvic examination should be explained, understanding that the client may see it as another body violation. Medicolegal evidence must be collected and preserved. Explanations should be given along with support and reassurance. Consent forms must be signed for photos, pelvic examination, collection of body fluids for DNA testing, etc. Be sure to follow agency protocols to preserve evidence. HIV testing may be advised. Pregnancy prophylaxis and STD prevention may be undertaken.
Self-Assessment	A nurse's attitude, belief in myths about rape, and preconceived judgments can influence the care given to rape victims. Nurses must examine their feelings about abortion because a client might choose to abort a fetus produced as a result of rape.
Assessment Guidelines	There is a list of suggested methods to assess the client of sexual assault in the text. The guidelines help the nurse to assess psychological trauma, level of anxiety, physical trauma, support systems and how to encourage the client to share the traumatic experience. Documentation of assessment data is also addressed in the guidelines.
Nursing Diagnosis	*Rape-trauma syndrome, rape-trauma syndrome: compound reaction, and rape-trauma syndrome: silent reaction* are useful diagnoses. All three include an acute phase of disorganization and a long-term phase of reorganization. Rape-trauma syndrome: compound reaction includes reliance on alcohol or other drugs or reactivated symptoms of previous physical or psychiatric illness; rape-trauma syndrome: silent reaction applies when the individual is unable to describe or discuss the rape but manifests other behaviors such as change in relationships with men, nightmares, phobic reactions, or marked changes in sexual behavior.
Outcome Criteria	Outcome identification—Examples of short-term survivor's goals: will begin to express feelings about assault before leaving the emergency department; will speak to community-based rape victim advocate before leaving the emergency department; will keep follow-up appointment, etc. Examples of goals for long-term reorganization phase: will discuss need for follow-up crisis counseling and other support; will state that the acuteness of memory of the rape is less vivid and less frightening by 3 to 5 months; will state that physical symptoms have subsided within 3 to 5 months.
Planning	Since individuals are mainly treated in the ER, treatment must include follow-up support and care.

126

CHAPTER OUTLINE	TEACHING STRATEGIES

Intervention

Rape is considered an acute adventitious crisis. A return to previous level of functioning requires mourning losses, experiencing anger, and working through fears.

Basic Level Interventions
Counseling

The survivor may be too traumatized, ashamed, or afraid to come to the hospital, but may use a telephone hotline instead. Cultural definitions of what constitutes rape may also affect decision to come to the hospital.

Hispanic females, acculturated in marianismo (ennoblement of female chastity) may view selves as tainted by rape. African American women may find support groups more helpful than individual therapy.

Nurses' attitudes have important therapeutic effects. Provide nonjudgmental care and maximum emotional support. Confidentiality is crucial. Listen and let victim talk. Feeling understood allows client to feel more in control of the situation. Help client separate issues of vulnerability from blame. Focusing on one's behavior, which is controllable, allows survivor to believe that similar experiences can be avoided in the future. If the survivor consents, involve her support systems and discuss with her the nature and trauma of sexual assault and the delayed reactions that may occur. Social support moderates somatic symptoms.

Promotion of Self-Care Activities

Give referral information and follow-up instructions verbally and in writing. Anxiety is likely to affect the amount of verbal information the client can retain.

Case Management

Caring for survivors needs to include physical and psychological care. Survivors may seek help from medical professionals rather than from mental health professionals because medical treatment is more socially acceptable. Outpatient nurses can make a more focused assessment and referral if they are aware of the stigma clients may feel. Reassessment should take place in person or by phone within 24 to 48 hours. Follow-up visits for assessment and necessary treatment should occur at 2, 4, and 6 weeks after the initial evaluation. Clients should be assessed for psychological progress as well as the presence of sexually transmitted disease and pregnancy.

Advanced Practice Interventions
Survivor

The survivor is likely to benefit from individual therapy, group therapy, or support group to alleviate emotional trauma such as fears, phobias, nightmares, or flashbacks. Some survivors are susceptible to psychotic episodes or emotional disturbances so severe that hospitalization is necessary. Depression and suicidal ideation are frequent sequelae.

Rapist

Therapy is essential for behavioral change to occur, but few acknowledge the need and no single method or program has been found to be totally effective for rapists.

Evaluation

Survivors are evaluated as recovered if they have an absence of signs and symptoms of PTSD (i.e., sleep well, with only a very few instances of nightmares; eat according to pre-rape pattern; are calm, relaxed, or only mildly suspicious, fearful, or restless; show minimal or no strain in relationships with family and friends; are generally positive about selves; and are free from somatic reactions).

Continued

Concept Map

Some students, especially those who are visually oriented, find use of a concept map is helpful in learning. On the following page is a concept map for rape.

Concept Map: Rape

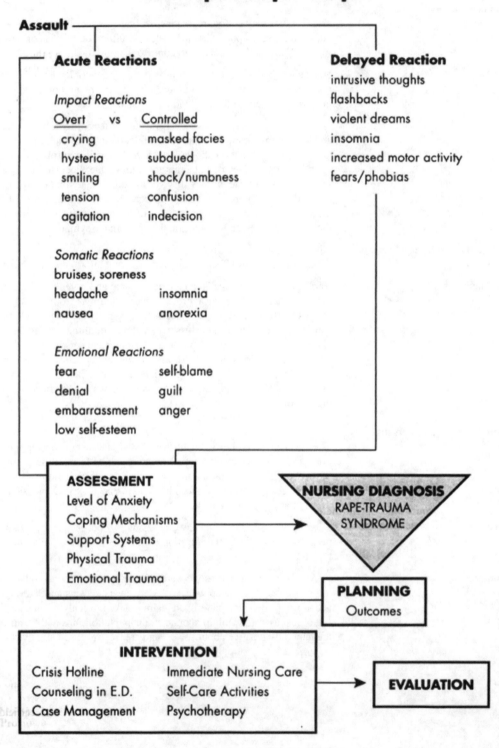

Assault

Acute Reactions

Impact Reactions

Overt	vs	Controlled
crying		masked facies
hysteria		subdued
smiling		shock/numbness
tension		confusion
agitation		indecision

Somatic Reactions
bruises, soreness
headache   insomnia
nausea   anorexia

Emotional Reactions
fear   self-blame
denial   guilt
embarrassment   anger
low self-esteem

Delayed Reaction
intrusive thoughts
flashbacks
violent dreams
insomnia
increased motor activity
fears/phobias

ASSESSMENT
Level of Anxiety
Coping Mechanisms
Support Systems
Physical Trauma
Emotional Trauma

NURSING DIAGNOSIS
RAPE-TRAUMA
SYNDROME

PLANNING
Outcomes

INTERVENTION
Crisis Hotline   Immediate Nursing Care
Counseling in E.D.   Self-Care Activities
Case Management   Psychotherapy

EVALUATION

128

27 Care of the Chemically Impaired

THOUGHTS ABOUT TEACHING THE TOPIC

Because most graduates will deal with drug- and alcohol-abusing clients in the community and in the general hospital, it's important to spend time on assessment strategies, including recognizing intoxication and impending withdrawal. Because role playing can help the learner gain both skill and empathy, this teaching-learning strategy can be very helpful, particularly as it relates to assessment and intervention techniques. Discussion of interpersonal interventions that might be necessary on the medical-surgical unit, e.g., limit setting, may also be useful. Learners should also be assisted to learn about resources available in the community to assist clients and families with substance abuse problems. It's highly advisable to arrange for student experience and observation in an alcoholism or drug treatment facility. If, however, only a few students can be given that opportunity, their experiences should be shared with the entire group during a conference or in class.

There are many videos/DVDs that can be helpful to teach students the process of addiction and recovery such as *28 Days, Bill's Story* (the story of one of the co-founders of AA), *Ray* (the story of Ray Charles). Having students view these videos and concentrating on the rehabilitation methodologies and perspectives can be valuable discussion topics for a class, clinical post conference or workshop.

KEY TERMS

addiction, 548
Al-Anon, 565
Alateen, 565
Alcoholics Anonymous (AA), 566
antagonistic effect, 549
blood alcohol level (BAL), 554
Cannabis sativa, 557
codependence, 551
dual diagnosis, 547
enabling, 560
flashbacks, 549
relapse prevention, 564
substance-abuse intervention, 563
synergistic effects, 549
tetrahydrocannabinol (THC), 557
therapeutic communities, 566
tolerance, 549
withdrawal, 549

OBJECTIVES

After studying this chapter, the reader will be able to

1. Compare and contrast the terms *substance abuse* and *substance dependence,* as defined by the *Diagnostic and Statistical Manual of Mental Disorders.*
2. Explain the difference between tolerance and withdrawal, and give a clinical definition of each.
3. Discuss four components of the assessment process to be used with a person who is chemically dependent.
4. Describe the difference between the behaviors of an alcoholic person and a nondrinker in relation to blood alcohol level.
5. Compare and contrast the symptoms seen in alcohol withdrawal and those seen in alcohol delirium.
6. List the appropriate steps to take if one observes an impaired co-worker.
7. Describe aspects of enabling behaviors and give examples.
8. Compare and contrast the signs and symptoms of intoxication, overdose, and withdrawal for cocaine and amphetamine.
9. Distinguish between the symptoms of narcotic intoxication and those of narcotic withdrawal.
10. Discuss the effects of the techno drugs ecstasy (MDMA), Rohypnol, γ-hydroxybutyric acid (GHB), and Eve (MDE).
11. Discuss treatment of a person who is withdrawing from alcohol delirium, including nursing care and pharmacological therapy.
12. Discuss the synergistic and antagonistic effects of drugs in polydrug abusers and give an example of each.
13. Formulate six nursing diagnoses that might apply to substance-abusing clients, including diagnoses in the physical, medical, and safety areas.
14. Develop three short-term outcomes relating to (a) withdrawal, (b) active treatment, and (c) health maintenance.
15. Analyze the pros and cons of the following treatments for narcotic addictions: (a) methadone or L-α-acetylmethadol, (b) therapeutic communities, and (c) self-help, abstinence-oriented programs.
16. Recognize the phenomenon of relapse as it affects substance abusers during different phases of treatment.
17. Plan steps in relapse prevention.
18. Evaluate four indications that a person is successfully recovering from substance abuse.

Continued

129

Prevalence

Studies indicate that 13.8% of American adults have had either an alcohol-dependent or alcohol abuse problem at one point in their lives. Estimate suggests that about 2.4 million of the U.S. population over age 12 need treatment for drug use disorders, and an additional 13 million people need treatment for alcohol use disorders.

Psychiatric Comorbidity

About 50% of people with a serious mental illness are dependent on or addicted to an illicit drug. The suicide risk is three to four times higher in substance abusers than in the general population. Clients with dual disorders often require longer treatment, have more crises, and respond more slowly to treatment. Common examples of dual disorders include the combinations of major depression with cocaine addiction, alcohol addiction with panic disorder, alcoholism and polydrug addiction with schizophrenia, and borderline personality disorders with episodic polydrug abuse.

Medical Comorbidity

Alcohol can affect all organ systems, but often-seen problems involve the CNS (Wernicke's encephalopathy and Korsakoff's psychosis) and the GI system (esophagitis, gastritis, pancreatitis, hepatitis, cirrhosis). Cocaine abusers may experience malnutrition, myocardial infarction, and stroke. IV drug users have a higher incidence of HIV, TB, STDs, abscesses, and bacterial endocarditis. Smoking a substance increases the incidence of respiratory problems and intranasal use predisposes to sinusitis and perforated nasal septum.

Theory

Addiction study incorporates the concepts of loss of control of substance ingestion, using drugs despite associated problems, and a tendency to relapse.

Biological Theories

Children of alcoholic parents are more likely to develop alcoholism than are children of nonalcoholic parents. Both alcohol use and drug use have recently been demonstrated to affect selected neurotransmitter systems. Alcohol and certain other drugs act on the GABA system; cocaine use is associated with deficiency in dopamine and norepinephrine.

Psychological Theories

The following are associated psychodynamic factors: intolerance for frustration and pain, lack of success in life, lack of affectionate and meaningful relationships, low self-esteem, and risk-taking propensity. A person uses substances to feel better, and over time this habitual behavior develops into an addiction.

Sociocultural Theories

There are differences in the incidence of substance abuse in various groups. In Asian cultures, the prevalence rate of alcoholism is relatively low, due in part to an often-found inability to break down acetaldehyde, an intermediate in alcohol metabolism, which produces unpleasant symptoms. Another theory correlates substance use with the degree of socioeconomic stress experienced by individuals.

Definitions
Tolerance and Withdrawal

Tolerance is the need for higher and higher doses of substances to achieve the desired effect. Withdrawal involves physiological and psychological signs and symptoms associated with stopping or reducing use of substances.

Flashbacks

Flashbacks are the transitory recurrences of perceptual disturbance reminiscent of disturbances experienced in earlier hallucinogenic intoxication.

Synergistic Effects

Synergistic effects refer to the intensification or prolongation of the effect of two or more drugs occurring when they are taken together (e.g., alcohol and a benzodiazepine).

Antagonistic Effects

Antagonistic effects refer to weakening or inhibiting the effect of one drug by using another (e.g., using cocaine and heroin together, or using naloxone (Narcan), a narcotic antagonist, to treat opiate overdose).

CHAPTER OUTLINE	TEACHING STRATEGIES

Codependence

Codependence is a cluster of behaviors that prevents one individual from taking care of his or her own needs due to preoccupation with another who is addicted to a substance.

Application of the Nursing Process
Assessment

Assessment is complex because of polydrug use, dual diagnosis, and comorbid physical illness.

Interview Guidelines

The nurse should ask questions about what is being taken (prescribed; over-the-counter; social drugs—caffeine and nicotine, alcohol, other drugs), amount, length of use, route, and drug preference. Questions should be asked in a matter-of-fact and nonjudgmental way:

- What drugs did you take before coming to the hospital?
- How did you take the drugs (route)?
- How much did you take? (For ethanol, ask about beer, wine, and liquor individually.)
- When was the last dose(s) taken?
- How long have you been using substances? When did this episode start?
- How often and how many do you use?
- What problems has substance use caused for you? Your family? Friends? Job? Health? Finances? The law?

How a person responds is significant for assessment purposes: rationalizations merit further assessment. Some will answer guardedly, being careful of what is said. Some will answer with hopelessness about being able to attain a drug-free state. Physical indicators of substance abuse should be assessed, including dilated or constricted pupils, abnormal vital signs, needle marks, tremors, and alcohol on the breath. The nurse should also take a history from family and friends and check belongings for drug paraphernalia. There is a significant link between ethanol consumption and injury. Check neurological signs, especially with comatose clients. Urine toxicology and bronchoalveolar lavage (BAL) are useful. Be alert for comorbid psychiatric impairment.

Assessing Psychological Changes

Psychological characteristics associated with substance abuse include denial, depression, anxiety, dependency, hopelessness, low self-esteem, and various psychiatric disorders. Some people with psychiatric disorders self-medicate; for these people the symptoms remain even after sobriety is achieved. On the other hand, psychological changes that occurred as a result of drinking resolve quickly. Substance-abusing people are concerned about being rejected by nurses; they may be anxious about recovering because to do so they must give up the substance they think they need to survive, and because they are concerned about failing at recovery. These concerns prompt the addict to establish a predictable defensive style using denial, projection, and rationalization, and characteristic thought processes such as all-or-none thinking and selective attention, as well as behaviors that include conflict minimization, avoidance, passivity, and manipulation.

Assessing Signs of Intoxication and Withdrawal
Central Nervous System
   Depressants

These include alcohol, benzodiazepines, barbiturates, and sedatives. Intoxication signs and symptoms include slurred speech; incoordination; ataxia; drowsiness; disinhibition of sexual and aggressive impulses; and impaired judgment, social, and occupational function, and attention and memory. Withdrawal from alcohol and CNS depressants is associated with severe morbidity and mortality, unlike withdrawal from other drugs. Multiple drug and alcohol dependencies can result in simultaneous withdrawal syndromes that present a bizarre clinical picture and may pose problems for safe withdrawal.

Continued

131

Chapter 27   Care of the Chemically Impaired

Alcohol Withdrawal

Early signs (anxiety, anorexia, insomnia, and tremor) develop within a few hours after cessation or reduction of alcohol intake, peak after 24 to 48 hours, then disappear unless the withdrawal progresses to alcohol withdrawal delirium. Other signs and symptoms include startling easily, "shaking inside," vivid nightmares, illusions, confusion, fright, elevated pulse and BP, and grand mal seizures. The client requires a kind, warm, supportive manner from the nurse; consistent and frequent orientation to time and place; and clarification of illusions.

Alcohol Withdrawal Delirium

This is a medical emergency with up to a 10% mortality rate. Delirium usually peaks after 2 to 3 days (48 to 72 hours) after cessation or reduction of intake and lasts 2 to 3 days. Features of withdrawal delirium include anxiety, insomnia, anorexia, delirium, autonomic hyperactivity (elevated pulse and BP, diaphoresis), disturbed sensorium (clouded consciousness, disorientation), perceptual disturbances (visual and tactile hallucinations), fluctuating levels of consciousness, paranoid delusions, agitation, and fever.

Central Nervous System Stimulants

These include amphetamines, cocaine, crack, caffeine, and nicotine. These stimulants accelerate normal body functioning. Common signs of abuse include pupil dilation, dryness of oronasal cavity, excessive motor activity, tachycardia, elevated BP, twitching, insomnia, anorexia, grandiosity, impaired judgment, paranoid thinking, hallucinations, hyperpyrexia, convulsions, and death. Dependence develops rapidly. Periods of "high" are followed by deep depression as the body tries to rebalance neurotransmitters.

Cocaine and Crack

Cocaine is a naturally occurring drug extracted from leaves of the coca bush. Crack is an alkalinized form of cocaine. Dependence develops rapidly. Cocaine is a schedule II substance. People who sniff cocaine develop deterioration of the nasal passages. Those who smoke the drug can incur lung damage, upper GI problems, and throat infections. IV users may experience endocarditis, heart attacks, angina, and needle-related infections such as hepatitis and HIV. Cocaine has both anesthetic and stimulant effects. As an anesthetic it blocks conduction of electrical impulses within nerve cells that transmit pain impulses. As a stimulant it produces sexual arousal and violent behavior. It produces an imbalance of dopamine and norepinephrine that may be responsible for many of the physical withdrawal symptoms: depression, paranoia, lethargy, anxiety, insomnia, nausea and vomiting, sweating and chills.

Nicotine and Caffeine

Nicotine can act as a stimulant, depressant, or tranquilizer. It is addicting. Bupropion (Wellbutrin, Zyban) has been a successful treatment for nicotine withdrawal. Caffeine is a stimulant ingested daily by many in coffee, tea, and cola drinks.

Opiates

Opiates include opium, morphine, heroin, codeine, and fentanyl and its analogue methadone and meperidine. Signs of intoxication include constricted pupils, decreased respiration and BP, drowsiness, slurred speech, psychomotor retardation, euphoria or dysphoria, and impaired attention, memory, and judgment. Overdose causes respiratory depression, coma, convulsions, and death.

Marijuana (*Cannabis sativa*)

The active ingredient in marijuana is tetrahydrocannabinol (THC), which has mixed depressant and hallucinogenic properties. Effects include detachment, relaxation, euphoria, apathy, intensification of perceptions, impaired judgment, slowed perception of time, impaired memory, and heightened sensitivity to stimuli. Overdose may cause panic reactions. Dependence is associated with lethargy, anhedonia, difficulty concentrating, and memory impairment.

Hallucinogens

Hallucinogens alter mental state within a very short period of time.

CHAPTER OUTLINE	TEACHING STRATEGIES
Lysergic Acid Diethylamide (LSD) and LSD-Like Drugs	LSD, mescaline, and psilocybin produce a "trip" characterized by slowing of time, lightheadedness, images in intense colors, and visions in sound (synesthesia). A "bad trip" may produce severe anxiety, paranoia, and terror compounded by distortions in time and distance. The best treatment for a bad trip is reassurance in a pleasant environment. Flashbacks—transitory recurrence of the drug experience—occur when a person is drug-free.
Phencyclidine Piperidine (PCP)	The route of administration of PCP plays a significant role in the severity of intoxication: symptoms appear within 1 hour of oral ingestion and within 5 minutes of IV use, sniffing, or smoking. PCP produces a blank stare, ataxia, muscle rigidity, vertical and horizontal nystagmus, and a tendency toward violence. High doses may lead to hyperthermia, chronic jerking of the extremities, hypertension, and kidney failure. Suicidal ideation should always be assessed, especially in cases of toxicity or coma. Long-term use can result in dulled thinking, lethargy, loss of impulse control, poor memory, and depression.
Inhalants	Inhalants are substances (paint, glue, cigarette lighter fluid, and propellant gases used in aerosols) that when sniffed result in intoxication.
Rave and Techno Drugs, Club Drugs, Date Rape Drugs	Drugs included in this category are ecstasy (3,4-methylenedioxy-methamphetamine, MDMA), and ketamine. Ecstasy ("Adam," "yabba," "XTC") is a substitute amphetamine representing one of a distinct category of drugs labeled entactogens. These drugs produce euphoria, increased energy, increased self-confidence, increased sociability, and some psychedelic effects. Adverse effects include hyperthermia, rhabdomyolysis, acute renal failure, hepatotoxicity, cardiovascular collapse, depression, panic attacks, and psychosis. The drugs most frequently used to facilitate sexual assault are flunitrazepam (Rohypnol), and GHB because they produce rapid disinhibition and relaxation, as well as retrograde amnesia. Alcohol potentiates the effects of these drugs.
Self-Assessment	Nurses' responses to clients who use illicit substances sometimes include disapproval, intolerance, condemnation, and belief that the client is morally weak. The manipulative behaviors sometimes used by these clients may lead the nurse to feel angry and exploited. In some areas, recreational use of drugs is so common that nurses may accept intoxication and overdose as normal phenomena. This causes the nurse to underestimate the amount of support and education the client needs. Enabling (i.e., supporting or denying the client's physical or psychological substance dependence) is highly detrimental. Enabling behaviors include encouraging denial by agreeing that the client drinks or takes drugs only socially, ignoring clues to possible dependency, demonstrating sympathy for client's reasons for abusing substances, and preaching. Nurses must attend to personal feelings that arise when they work with drug abusers if they are to be therapeutic.
Chemically Impaired Nurse	Nurses have a 32% to 50% higher rate of chemical dependency than the general population. Without intervention or treatment the problems associated with chemical dependency escalate and the potential for client harm increases. Early indicators of substance abuse problems in nurses include changing lifestyle to focus on activities that encourage substance use, showing inconsistency between statements and actions, displaying increasing irritability, projecting blame, isolating self from social contacts, deteriorating physical appearance, episodes of vaguely described illness, frequent tardiness or absences, manipulating possession of keys to narcotics, and deepening depression. When the impaired nurse is on duty, clients may complain that their pain is unrelieved by their narcotic analgesic and increases in inaccurate drug counts and vial breakage may occur.

Continued

133

Clear, accurate documentation by co-workers is vital. Once there is documentation, the nurse manager must be informed. Intervention is the responsibility of the nurse manager. If the situation persists without intervention by the nurse manager, the information needs to be taken to the next level in the chain of command. Although reporting a colleague is difficult, not reporting is an enabling behavior. Referral to a treatment program should be an option. Reports to the state board for nursing by nursing administration must contain factual documentation.

Assessment Guidelines

The assessment guidelines for chemically impaired clients include assessment of medical needs, psychological needs, family support and education and recovery motivation.

Nursing Diagnosis

The list of potential diagnoses includes, but is not limited to, *anxiety, ineffective coping; ineffective health maintenance, risk for injury, impaired verbal communication, disturbed sensory perception, hopelessness, risk for infection, impaired parenting, ineffective breathing pattern, sexual dysfunction, disturbed sleep pattern, impaired social interaction, disturbed thought processes, risk for self-directed violence, risk for other-directed violence, interrupted family processes, self-care deficit, imbalanced nutrition: less than body requirements, powerlessness, chronic low self-esteem, spiritual distress, impaired skin integrity,* etc.

Outcome Criteria
Withdrawal

Example: Remains free from injury while withdrawing; evidence of stable condition within 72 hours.

Initial and Active Drug Treatment

Example: Maintains abstinence from chemical substances, demonstrates acceptance for own behavior at end of 3 months, continues attendance for treatment and maintenance of sobriety, attends a relapse prevention program during active course of treatment, states he or she has a stable group of drug-free friends with whom to socialize at least three times weekly, etc.

Health Maintenance

Example: Demonstrates responsibility for taking care of health care needs, as evidenced by keeping appointments and adhering to medication and treatment schedules; client medical tests will demonstrate after 6 months a reduced incidence of medical complications related to substance abuse.

Planning

Abstinence is the safest treatment goal for all addicts. Planning must also address major psychological, social, and medical problems, as well as the substance-abusing behavior. Lack of interpersonal and social supports and even lack of ability to meet basic needs for shelter, food, and clothing may complicate planning.

Intervention

Aim of treatment is toward self-responsibility, not compliance. Choice of program is often influenced by cost and health insurance coverage. Outpatient programs work best for employed substance abusers who have an involved support system. People without support and structure do better in inpatient programs.

Communication Guidelines

These involve working with dysfunctional anger, manipulation, impulsiveness, and grandiosity. A warm, accepting relationship can assist the client to feel safe enough to begin looking at problems with openness and honesty. Characteristics of a counselor that facilitate work with substance abusers include knowledge of addiction, ability to form caring relationships, capacity to tolerate anxiety and depression, persistence and patience, capacity to listen, and honesty. Principles for counseling interventions include the following: expect abstinence, individualize goals and interventions, set limits on behavior and on conditions under which treatment will continue, support and redirect defenses rather than attempt to remove them, recognize that recovery is carried out in stages, and look for therapeutic leverage.

134

Chapter 27   Care of the Chemically Impaired

Intervention Strategies
Primary Prevention

Primary prevention through health teaching can impact how youngsters and adolescents choose to solve problems and relate interpersonally. Participation in groups such as scouting, school clubs, 4-H clubs, and organized church activities lowers risk for substance abuse. These activities and part time jobs develop self-confidence and self-esteem in young people. Targeting the elderly who are experiencing stressful life events can also be helpful in preventing alcohol abuse among the elderly. Primary prevention of HIV infection among the population using needles can be facilitated by needle exchange programs.

Brief Interventions

Any interaction with a substance-abusing client can be used as an opportunity for managing associated behaviors. Key interventions can be remembered by using the acronym FRAMES (*f*eedback, *r*esponsibility, *a*dvice, *m*enu [options], *e*mpathy, *s*elf-efficacy). Motivational interviewing is another technique to motivate change. Five general principles to motivate change: (1) express empathy; (2) develop discrepancy; (3) avoid argument; (4) roll with resistance; and (5) support self-efficacy.

Dual-Diagnosis Principles

The six guidelines presented in the text include issues about dual diagnosis, common treatment suggestions, and outcome expectations.

Psychotherapy

Evidence-based practice indicates that cognitive-behavioral therapy, psychodynamic and interpersonal therapies, group and family therapies, and participation in self-help groups are all effective treatment modalities. Critical issues that arise within the first 6 months of therapy include physical changes as the body adapts to functioning without the substance, needing to learn new responses to former cues to drink or use drugs, experiencing full-strength emotions instead of drug-mediated emotions, need to address family and co-worker responses to client's new behavior, need to develop coping skills to prevent relapse and ensure prolonged sobriety.

Relapse Prevention

The goal of relapse prevention is to help the person learn from relapse so that periods of sobriety can be lengthened over time and lapses and relapses are not viewed as total failure.

Self-Help Groups for Client and Family

Counseling and support should be encouraged for all families with a drug-dependent member. Groups include Al-Anon, Alateen, Adult Children of Alcoholics, Pills Anonymous, and Narcotics Anonymous.

Twelve-Step Programs

These programs have three fundamental concepts: (1) individuals with addictive disorders are powerless over their addiction, and their lives are unmanageable; (2) although individuals with addictive disorders are not responsible for their disease, they are responsible for their recovery; and (3) individuals can no longer blame people, places, and things for their addiction—they must face their problems and their feelings. Alcoholics Anonymous (AA) is the prototype for other 12-step programs such as Pills Anonymous, Narcotics Anonymous, etc. Each offers the behavioral, cognitive, and dynamic structures necessary to help a person refrain from addictive behaviors and to change and grow. Self-help groups for family members include Al-Anon, Narc-Anon, ACoA, Alateen, etc. These groups work with family issues and codependency issues.

Residential Programs

These programs are best suited for individuals who have a long history of antisocial behavior. The addict is expected to remain in the program at least 90 days and may stay a year or more in some residential communities. The goal is to effect a lifestyle change, including abstinence from drugs, development of social skills, and elimination of antisocial behavior.

Continued

135

Intensive Outpatient Programs

Clients who once were hospitalized for treatment are now treated in the community due to cost reduction necessities. A clinical pathway for an intensive outpatient program is shown.

Outpatient Drug-Free Programs and Employee Assistance Programs

These are geared to the polydrug-abusing or alcoholic client rather than to the client who is addicted to heroin. EAPs have been developed to provide delivery of mental health services in occupational settings.

Psychopharmacology
Alcohol Withdrawal Treatment

Not all people who stop drinking require management of withdrawal. Medication should not be given until symptoms of withdrawal are seen. Early symptoms are tremors, diaphoresis, rapid pulse, elevated BP, occasional tactile or visual hallucinations, Interventions include medication, as needed, for management of withdrawal symptoms (using cross-dependent sedatives); monitoring vital signs; administration of thiamine to prevent Wernicke's syndrome; correction of hypomagnesemia; maintaining fluid and electrolyte balance while avoiding overhydration. Anticonvulsants such as diazepam or phenobarbital may be used on a short-term basis to control seizures. Phenytoin is used only if the person has a history of primary seizure disorder.

Treatment of Alcoholism
Naltrexone (Trexan, Revia)

This drug is helpful to some recovering alcoholics to reduce cravings. Is also a narcotic antagonistic that blocks the euphoric effects of opioids for up to 72 hours. It has low toxicity with few side effects and is nonaddicting.

Disulfiram (Antabuse)

Taken daily, this drug is useful for preventing impulsive drinking because disulfiram with alcohol produces a severe reaction. Care must be taken to teach the client to avoid hidden sources of alcohol in food, fumes, and skin preparations.

Treatment of Opioid Addiction
Methadone (Dolophine)

This drug is a synthetic opiate. In a sufficient dosage taken daily, it blocks craving for and effects of heroin. Methadone maintenance helps keep the client out of the illegal drug culture while counseling is undertaken. Methadone is highly addicting and, when stopped, produces withdrawal. Because it is an oral drug, it reduces risk of HIV infection from needles.

Clonidine (Catapres)

This drug is a nonopioid suppressor of opioid withdrawal symptoms and when combined with naltrexone is an effective nonaddicting treatment for opioid addiction.

Buprenorphine (Subutex)

This drug is a partial opioid agonist. At low doses it blocks signs and symptoms of opioid withdrawal. Early studies suggest it suppresses heroin use.

Treatment of Nicotine Addiction

A nicotine patch provides transdermal doses of nicotine and has been shown to double long-term abstinence rates.

Evaluation

Effectiveness of treatment is judged by increasing lengths of time of abstinence, decreased denial, acceptable occupational functioning, improved family relationships, the client's ability to relate normally and comfortably with others without using drugs or alcohol, and the ability to use existing supports and skills used in treatment.

28 Severe Mental Illness: Crisis Stabilization and Rehabilitation

THOUGHTS ABOUT TEACHING THE TOPIC

Students who have been assigned to units primarily caring for acutely mentally ill clients may not have experienced an opportunity to interact with and assess a severely and persistently mentally ill individual. If possible, instructors may arrange a 1-day observation at one of the following types of facilities specializing in caring for the severely and persistently mentally ill or homeless: a day care center, a medication clinic, a mobile clinic, an outreach clinic, or a temporary shelter for the homeless. It may be possible to arrange for a student to accompany a community mental health nurse for a day. In large cities, the Veterans Administration may also have special programs and homeless shelters to deal with the needs of homeless and chronically mentally ill veterans.

KEY TERMS AND CONCEPTS

assertive community treatment (ACT), 580
cognitive interventions, 584
deinstitutionalization, 576
dual-diagnosis treatment, 579
institutionalized, 576
psychoeducation, 582
rehabilitation, 577
severe mental illness (SMI), 575
social skills training, 583
stigma, 579
supported employment, 584
vocational rehabilitation, 584

OBJECTIVES

After studying this chapter, the reader will be able to
1. Discuss the behavior and symptoms of severe mental illness as they relate to the person's daily functioning and to family and other interpersonal relationships.
2. Describe three common problems associated with severe mental illness.
3. Explain six evidence-based practices for the care of the severely mentally ill person.
4. Explain the role of the nurse in the care of the severely mentally ill person.
5. Develop an outline for a psychoeducational teaching plan for a person with severe mental illness. (Choose one of your clients or a client in a facility you use in your clinical experience.)
6. Discuss the importance of medication and adherence to the medication regimen for the severely mentally ill client.

CHAPTER OUTLINE	TEACHING STRATEGIES
Severe Mental Illness	Chronic or severe and persistent mental illness refers to a mental illness extending in time beyond the acute stage into a long-term stage that is marked by persistent impairment of functioning. Individuals with severe and persistent mental illness have different illnesses, needs, and outcomes. Often the severity and course of the illness are influenced by poverty, racism, and substance abuse. The extent of severe and persistent mental illness was easier to quantify prior to deinstitutionalization.
Older Population	Before 1975 psychiatric hospitals were the long- term residences for the severely and persistently mentally ill. Institution-caused dependency was evident in most clients, along with the symptoms of the mental illness.
Younger Population	Most younger clients have never experienced institutionalization, but rather have had only short hospitalizations. This group tends to deny illness and use recreational drugs, creating a different set of problems, including problems with the law.
Development of a Severe Mental Illness	The original problem sets in motion an erosion of basic coping mechanisms and compensatory processes. In the case of schizophrenia, a person's thought processes, ability to maintain contact with others, and ability to stay employed may deteriorate. Self-care and relations with others suffer. Interactions may be perceived as bizarre, unsatisfying, and anxiety-provoking by the client and others.

Continued

137

Poor communication causes rising tension and poor self-image. Employment may be difficult or impossible. There is unpredictability of the disease course, contributing to additional stress. Fear of relapse and avoidance of stress can cause withdrawal from life that heightens social isolation and apathy.

Careful assessment can detect early signs of exacerbation and lead to intervention that decreases the severity of the exacerbation and its disruption of the person's life. Rehabilitation addresses disabilities and inabilities to lessen or eradicate them.

Common Problems Associated with Severe Mental Illness

Access to Housing

Housing is the first need of the seriously mentally ill. Due to poor communication skills, cognitive problems, and other symptoms, people with severe mental illness become homeless. Adults with severe mental illness are increasingly using temporary homeless shelters, jails, and prisons as housing resources. Life on the street has a negative effect on an individual's self-esteem. Safe, affordable housing is critical if people with severe mental illnesses are to maintain themselves within the community.

Nonadherence to Medication Regimen

Treatment success rates tell us medications do work: e.g., bipolar disorder has an 80% treatment success rate; major depression, a 65% success rate, etc. Many reasons for medication noncompliance exist, among them cost, distressing side effects, confusion about how to take the medication. Other problems include a disparity between treatment standards and what clinicians actually prescribe, and failure to adequately monitor long-term side effects. A solution to the latter is to have clients followed by nurses or physicians rather than social workers.

Comorbid Medical Conditions

Ideally, there needs to be collaboration between the psychiatric team and the primary care provider. Multiple studies indicate there is a higher risk for certain medical disorders.

Coexisting Substance Abuse

Many individuals with severe mental illness also have substance abuse problems (dual diagnosis). Clinical implications of substance abuse among the severely mentally ill include poor medication adherence, increased suicide rates, increased violence, homelessness, worsening psychotic symptoms, increased HIV infection, increased use of institutional services.

Stigma

Studies show that individuals with mental illness expect and fear rejection, which increases their tendency to withdraw from society.

Comprehensive Community Resources

The goal of community-based health care programs is to provide broad community mental health services that will prevent psychiatric hospitalization, maintain stability in a community setting, and achieve the highest possible level of functioning. Various services include the following:

Adult outpatient services, which provide evaluation for possible psychiatric hospitalization, initiate treatment, respond to crisis calls and walk-in requests for service, and coordinate psychiatric emergency responses with hospitals, police, and other community service providers.

Day care services, which provide alternatives to 24-hour care

Case managers to serve as coordinators to ensure integration and cooperation of various elements of the system and act as advocates for clients in the system.

Regional outpatient clinics, which provide therapeutic and rehabilitative services for clients with dual diagnosis. Outreach and case management services, which provide care for seriously mentally ill clients who are homeless by sending workers into streets, parks, shelters, bus stations, beaches, and anywhere the mentally ill are found.

Overview of Nursing Interventions

Nurses use the following basic interventions with psychiatric mental health clients: crisis intervention, health teaching, psychobiological interventions, counseling, case management, milieu therapy, promotion of self-care activities, and psychiatric rehabilitation.

Case Management

Case Managers provide entrance into the system of care and coordinate a wide range of community support and rehabilitative services, including food, shelter, and clothing needs. Case managers supply crisis stabilization to prevent relapse and hospitalization.

Overview of Rehabilitation

Outcomes for rehabilitation for the severely mentally ill clients are for them to do the following:
- Retain positive coping strategies during times of stress or crisis with the aid of nurse, family, and friends.
- Maintain optimal functioning in work, home, community.
- Function in the community with minimal need for inpatient services.
- Maintain stable function between episodes of exacerbations.

Crisis Stabilization

Crisis theory and intervention can be successfully adapted with people who have long-term mental illness. Characteristics of such individuals include inadequate problem-solving ability; inadequate communication skills; low self-esteem; poor success with work, school, or family, and social relationships; inpatient or outpatient treatment for at least 2 years. While these problems exist, it is important to emphasize healthy aspects in assessment.

Potential crisis situations include (1) change in treatment approaches; (2) problems or changes with work, school, family, and anniversaries of significant or traumatic events; (3) lack of money, transportation, or problems meeting basic needs; (4) sexual relationships when the client is unsure of his or her sexual identity.

Adapting the crisis model serves to prevent temporary difficulty in functioning from progressing to severe personality disorganization, and returning the client to the previous level of functioning. Adaptations include focusing on client strengths, modifying and setting realistic goals with the client, taking a more active role in the problem-solving process, and using direct interventions such as making arrangements the person would ordinarily be able to make without assistance.

Client and Family Psychoeducation

Client and family understanding of the disease process is vital. Concerns that should be addressed include safety, communication, medication compliance, symptom and behavior management, and resources for respite and day care. Written instructions should be given in addition to oral instructions, and supportive follow-up by phone or home visits should occur to help client and family deal with the burden, stigma, and isolation related to mental illness. The psychoeducational model has five basic aims. The treatment team must (1) develop a genuine working relationship with family and other supportive persons; (2) develop a structured and stable teaching plan that meets client and family needs (e.g., medication teaching, signs of relapse, available treatment centers, available support groups); (3) minimize family tendency to be self-critical and demoralizing; (4) develop step-by-step communication and problem-solving skills; (5) help the family develop a network of involved understanding and supportive people and resources.

Continued

139

Social Skills Training and Illness Self-Management

Social skills training involves using a variety of learning techniques to teach client's discrete skills, such as independent living skills, conversation skills, dating, job seeking, affect regulation, etc. The need for these skills has increased with the success of the newer antipsychotic drugs in reducing both positive and negative symptoms of schizophrenia.

Vocational Rehabilitation Programs and Supported Employment

Studies show that clients with severe mental illness who completed a vocational rehabilitation program demonstrated significant improvement on measures of assertiveness, work behaviors, and decreased depression, and improved income and employment status.

Cognitive Interventions

Cognitive-behavioral strategies have been used to treat hallucinations, delusions, and negative symptoms. Common strategies include distraction when auditory hallucinations occur and reframing or verbally challenging delusional beliefs.

Chapter 28   Severe Mental Illness: Crisis Stabilization
and Rehabilitation

29 Psychological Needs of the Medically Ill

THOUGHTS ABOUT TEACHING THE TOPIC

This chapter will help learners gain awareness that clients on medical-surgical units are more than a collection of physical symptoms. Although certain emotional reactions are shared by a majority of clients (e.g., anxiety), the chapter helps learners see that clients' emotional responses may be much more complex. Use of videos allows learners to become aware of the intense emotions in a safe setting. Use of computer-assisted instruction allows the learner to participate in decision making, also in a safe environment.

KEY TERMS AND CONCEPTS

coping strategies, 593
holistic approach, 588
holistic assessment, 594
human rights abuses, 597
psychiatric liaison nursing, 598
quality-of-life assessment, 595
stigmatized medically ill persons, 597

OBJECTIVES

After studying this chapter, the reader will be able to
1. Describe at least two common mental health sequelae and two psychological responses to a serious medical illness.
2. Construct a *DSM-IV-TR* diagnosis for an individual who has a substance abuse problem, has severe cardiac disease, and is soon to be evicted from his apartment.
3. Defend the teaching of relaxation and coping skills by nurses.
4. Perform a psychosocial (psychological-social-spiritual) nursing assessment.
5. Assess the client's coping skills: (a) identify areas for teaching, (b) identify areas of strength.
6. Identify two instances in which a consultation with a psychiatric liaison nurse might have been useful for one of your medical-surgical patients.

CHAPTER OUTLINE	TEACHING STRATEGIES
Psychological Factors Affecting Medical Conditions	Nurses who care for physically ill clients ideally maintain a holistic view that involves an awareness of psychological, social, cultural, and spiritual issues. Usually, some time-limited crisis intervention or brief supportive counseling is sufficient to bolster the person's already adequate coping skills until the crisis is past. If short-term intervention is not enough, the nurse may need to utilize long-term interventions to meet the holistic needs of a client.
Psychological Responses to Serious Medical Illness	Some of the concerns of people, faced with a severe physical illness, include: Will I be disfigured? Will I have a long-term disability? Will I be able to function as a (wife/husband, parent, and person in society)?
Depression	Depression is a risk factor for medical noncompliance. The odds are three times greater that depressed clients will be noncompliant with medical treatment recommendations than will nondepressed clients.
Anxiety	Anxiety accompanies every illness. Verbalization is an effective outlet for anxiety, but ability to verbalize may be compromised by cultural expectations, disability, or lack of a listener. Helplessness often accompanies anxiety. Self-centeredness, characterized by unreasonable requests of caregivers, may also cover inadequacy and anxiety.
	Long-term pervasive anxiety or an anxiety disorder can be a risk factor for a medical disorder. It is important for nurses to identify and assess coexisting or resulting psychological response or disorders.

Continued

141

Substance Abuse	Long-term abuse of various substances can lead to medical complications such as hepatic conditions from ETOH use, lung disease with marijuana use, cardiac toxicity from cocaine use, etc. Or clients who are diagnosed with serious medical conditions turn to alcohol and/or other substances in order to cope with overwhelming feelings of hopelessness, fear, anxiety, depression, and/or pain.
Grief and Loss	Any type of treatment or procedure that is intended to treat a physical illness and that creates a major permanent change is accompanied by feelings of loss. Dynamics involved in coping with these feelings are similar to those operating in a person who is dealing with his or her own imminent death or the death of a loved one. Grieving involves spiritual changes, as well as emotional changes, and as such requires client spiritual assessment.
Denial	Denial may cause minimizing of symptoms such as pain or may cause the client to focus on the positive while leaving negative information about an illness unnoted. Caregivers may unwittingly collude with the person in denial by not performing complete assessments or accepting the person's subjective appraisals.
Fear of Dependency	Responses to being dependent may take the form of anger, inability to accept nurturing, and refusal of treatment. Others may fear that dependency needs will go unmet and do not express any negative feelings to caregivers. Suppressed negative feelings may gain expression as somatic complaints.
Holistic Assessment of a Client's Needs	Components of holistic assessment include a psychosocial assessment, assessment of usual coping strategies, and an overall quality-of-life assessment, including ADLs, social activities, social supports, client's perception of quality of life, feelings, pain. Religious or spiritual assessment and assessment of cultural beliefs are covered as part of the inquiry into social supports.
Psychosocial Assessment	An outline for a psychosocial assessment is given in Table 29-2.
Assessment of Usual Coping Strategies	People who undergo a life-threatening disease or chronic illness most often deal with distressing physical side effects and change in their body image. Typical concerns of clients with new colostomies and clients with breast cancer are reviewed. It is important for the nurse to know if clients have the coping strategies and social supports to help them deal with the consequences of their illness. Table 29–3 compares effective and ineffective coping behaviors.
Intervention Strategies	Useful intervention strategies for reducing stress and inducing relaxation include meditation, guided imagery, breathing exercises, progressive muscle relaxation, and biofeedback. Cognitive approaches such as journal keeping, restructuring, setting priorities and goals, cognitive reframing, and assertiveness training may be useful.
Human Rights Abuses of the Stigmatized Medically Ill	Stigmatized medically ill persons include those who are HIV positive and people who have transgender surgery or treatment. Stigmatization can result in inadequate care, undue stress, worsening of physical illness, and even death. Examples of human rights abuse include neglect in fully investigating somatic complaints in the emergency department, avoidance of contact with or refusal to care for such persons, hasty labeling with a psychiatric diagnosis, and inappropriate psychiatric admission. These situations occur more frequently in cases of persons who lack family support, those from lower socioeconomic classes, newly arrived immigrants, and those with an "unacceptable" alternative lifestyle.
Role of the Psychiatric Liaison Nurse	The psychiatric liaison nurse, a resource for staff, is a master's degree nurse with expertise in both psychiatric and medical-surgical nursing who functions as a nursing consultant in the management of psychosocial concerns and as a clinician in helping the client deal more effectively with physical and emotional problems.

Chapter 29   Psychological Needs of the Medically Ill

30 Care for the Dying and for Those Who Grieve

THOUGHTS ABOUT TEACHING THE TOPIC

Although nearly everyone has experienced a loss, many learners cannot conceptualize the depth and breadth of the experience of losing a loved one. Learning activities are designed to sensitize learners to the feelings experienced by those who are dying and those who are grieving.

Students may benefit from a one-day observation in a hospice unit or, if available, with a hospice home care nurse.

KEY TERMS AND CONCEPTS

anticipatory grief, 607
bereavement, 612
caring presence, 604
disenfranchised grief, 613
Four Gifts of Resolving Relationships, 608
grief, 612
hospice, 602
mourning, 613
palliative care, 602
public tragedies, 613

OBJECTIVES

After studying this chapter, the reader will be able to
1. Contrast and compare the goals of end-of-life care inherent in the hospice model with those of the medical model and be specific about these differences.
2. Analyze the effects of specific tasks that health care workers (nurses and social workers) can perform when working with a dying person and his or her family and loved ones.
3. Analyze how the Four Gifts of Resolving Relationships could have affected the dying experience of someone you cared for in the past and consider how it could affect your response to a dying loved one in the future.
4. Using the seven motifs as a guide, describe how a loved one of yours might confront death in terms of how this person confronts life. Which motif might the person adopt and what guidelines might be best suited to the person at the time of dying?
5. Explain how the distinction between the words *bereavement* and *mourning,* as presented in this chapter, can help to enhance the effectiveness of a holistic approach.
6. Differentiate among some of the characteristics of normal bereavement and dysfunctional grieving.
7. Explain why frameworks (models) of understanding loss through stages (Kübler-Ross, Parkes, Engel, Lindemann, Bowlby, etc.) are helpful for people but are not the focus of care.
8. Apply some of the guidelines for helping people to cope with loss of a client, friend, family member, or classmate.
9. Discuss at least seven behavioral outcomes that indicate a successful bereavement.
10. Identify situations and circumstances that could affect a person's coming to terms with loss.

CHAPTER OUTLINE	TEACHING STRATEGIES
Care for the Dying	Caring for the terminally ill challenges nurses. The hospice and palliative care movement has shown that care of the dying in America leaves much to be desired. Physical pain and client and family fears are poorly addressed. Feelings of anxiety and helplessness are pervasive.
Hospice and Palliative Care	The hospice movement, which had its beginning in England in the 1960s, began to address the needs of dying clients by seeking to effectively manage physical symptoms, especially pain, as a way of palliating the process of dying. Kübler-Ross began her work with dying clients in the United States in the late 1960s. She identified distinctive phases or cycles in our response to terminal illness—denial, anger, bargaining, depression, and acceptance—and she realized that personal growth did not cease in the last stages of life. Hospices began to appear in America. An interdisciplinary team care model was employed.

Continued

143

Palliative care is a medical specialty that grew out of the hospice movement. It seeks to address not only physical pain but also emotional, social, and spiritual pain to achieve the best possible quality of care for clients and families. Palliation focuses aggressively on comfort care. Medications and treatments may be combined in unusual ways, given in different dosages, or used for nonstandard purposes until the client obtains relief.

Hospice care is available to all, regardless of age or ability to pay. It is a benefit covered under Medicare Part A and mirrored by most commercial insurance. It is appropriate for clients in the end stages of virtually any disease, when curative therapies are no longer operational. The hospice philosophy of care is based upon the principles of client dignity and respect; treating the client and family or significant others; supporting a peaceful, pain-free death; client control and choice; viewing the client holistically; bereavement support of the family after the death.

Nursing Goals in End-of-life Care

Nursing the terminally ill requires shifts in expectations for both ourselves and our clients. A nurse's sense of competence and effectiveness often comes from helping clients get better and more independent. The terminally ill are going to grow weaker and die. It is not possible to set goals for improvement; instead, goals are focused on physical and spiritual comfort. Neither nurse nor client is in control, often resulting in feelings of inadequacy and frustration. Premourning, or grieving the loss of a person before the person has died, may take place. Shifts in orientation can help the adjustment to nursing the terminally ill.

Practice the Art of Presence

Because dying is a fundamentally personal and meaningful experience, the role of the nurse includes human presence and receptivity. The nurse's sense of competency and professionalism gained through taking action sometimes has to yield to a willingness to embrace the mystery and powerlessness of the dying process. The nurse needs excellent clinical skills but also needs to learn the skills of being present, listening attentively, allowing time for silence and time for a client to respond. The nurse must be attentive to nonverbal cues and the use of therapeutic touch. A nurse should always be aware of his or her own feelings working in hospice nursing.

Assess for Spiritual Issues

Most professional nursing associations, as well as the Joint Commission of Healthcare Organizations, call for nurses to assess client spirituality in all health care delivery settings. Nurses can explore with clients: spiritual themes such as how a client assigns meaning and value, how they experience connections and becoming, and when they have sensed a transcendent realm, or a dimension beyond the self. Spirituality is more than a religious affiliation and can be an important component that explains how and individual defines hope and healing. See Box 30-1 for spirituality assessment tools.

Provide Palliative Symptom Management

It is the client or the client's advance directives and medical proxy that define the goals of care in palliative nursing. Helping to keep the patient pain-free and comfortable during the terminal stages of their illness is a difficult but important part of symptom management.

The most commonly reported symptoms for patients with terminal illness include lack of energy, pain, lack of appetite, feeling drowsy, difficulty concentrating, feeling sad, shortness of breath, agitation, worrying, cough, nervousness, and constipation.

Palliative nurses assess for psychosocial sources of suffering, such as family discord, fears, lack of information, unacknowledged grief responses, poor coping skills and son on. The nurses must keep an active continuous assessment of the medication effects and needs of the patient. Other methods of care can include massage, aroma therapy, art and music therapy and other complementary therapies to reduce the client's suffering.

Becoming an Effective Communicator

The nurse can share medical expertise about the normal progression of the disease, the effects of medications, reasons to change drug regimens, and how to provide comfort care.

Convey Information to Enhance Competency

Information dispels myths and fears and strengthens sense of control. Information needs to be repeated, written down, and reviewed if individuals under stress are to understand and retain it.

Make Limited but Realistic Predictions

Families must live with the dual reality of impending death and continued life. Clients and families may want or dread having a timeline. A two-pronged approach can be helpful: (1) Focus on the here and now, as life is today. (2) Describe what the nurse is seeing and finding during physical examinations; paint a picture from which family members can draw their own conclusions. Comments about indicators such as pulse, color, blood pressure, weakness, appetite, and level of consciousness can guide the family to interpretations they can accept.

Counsel about Anticipatory Grieving

Anticipatory grieving, when not understood, can cause family members to withdraw prematurely from the client so as to avoid pain. The nurse can teach about the symptoms and facilitate open discussion of the client's and family's experiences. Naming the experiences and talking about them normalizes the process and makes it less frightening.

The Four Gifts of Resolving Relationships

Sharing four important "gifts" is a way of healing relationships before the person dies. The gifts are forgiveness, love, gratitude, and farewell. The individual voices or writes of resentment or hurt and willingly lets go of blame and anger. In addition, the person asks, "Is there anything I have done, or not done, for which I need to say I'm sorry?" The second gift is to express in words how we love each other. The third gift is thanking the person for what she or he has been in your life. Reminisce; listen to favorite stories; acknowledge things usually taken for granted. The fourth gift is to acknowledge the coming separation. This gives and receives permission for the death to occur.

Practicing Good Self-Care

The greater call for human-to-human presence in end-of-life nursing leads to increased vulnerability to emotional attachment. This increases the need for the nurse to be continuously attentive to self-care.

The nurse must establish an emotional balance and health and continuously rely on support of the multidisciplinary team and to practice good self-care. This invites nurses and other healthcare personnel to greater self-understanding, wisdom and compassion, and the team approach is integral to this process.

Confronting the Prospect of Dying: Seven Motifs

The only individual who can identify the needs of the dying client is the client. To provide holistic care for the dying requires getting to know about the client in a much broader context. One recent contribution to this field of research found seven distinct motifs emerging from extensive interviews with their research population. They are known as the seven cohesive patterns characterizing the ways in which participants viewed the prospect of their own death.

Also important is that an individual's death should be evaluated in light of the client's life motif and not by any one else's standard.

Continued

Chapter 30   Care for the Dying and for Those Who Grieve

The seven motifs are explained in the text:
1. Struggle: Living and Dying are a Struggle
2. Dissonance: Dying Is Not Living
3. Endurance: Triumph of Inner Strength
4. Incorporation: Belief System Accommodates Death
5. Coping: Working to Find a New Balance
6. Quest: Seeking Meaning in Dying
7. Volative: Unresolved and Unresigned

These seven motifs are a starting place to work with clients who are dying. There is a rich experience in caring for individuals who are dying. Each situation where a nurse cares for a dying individual forms a new motif in which the nurse can help the dying client die with dignity, care, and respect if the nurse will utilize the seven motifs, experience, and attentiveness to the individual needs for each client.

Care for Those Who Grieve

Loss is a part of life, and grief is the normal response to loss. Losses include loss of relationships; loss of health; loss of status or prestige; loss of security; loss of self-confidence or self-concept; symbolic losses; and change in circumstances. Bereavement is a physically painful experience.

Reactions to Bereavement

Grief refers to the subjective feelings and affect precipitated by loss. Mourning refers to the processes by which grief is resolved. Mourning involves disengaging strong emotional ties from a significant relationship and reinvesting them in a new and productive direction.

Bereavement refers to the social experience of dealing with loss of a loved one through death. For nurses to be helpful to clients, they must first examine their own feelings and the personal experience of loss. Understanding theories, models, tasks and other factors can help nurses facilitate their own grief and reduce bereavement overload.

Disenfranchised Grief

This is grief a person experiences when they incur a loss that is not and cannot be openly acknowledged, publicly mourned, or socially supported.

Grief Engendered by Public Tragedy

This is grief that involves a loss whose impact is felt broadly across a community or the general public. The loss involves a strong element of surprise and shock. Common public tragedies include: a terrorist assault, an assassination; a tornado, earthquake, flooding etc.

Frameworks for Understanding Loss

Characteristics of the grief process include shock and disbelief, sensation of somatic distress, preoccupation with the image of the deceased, guilt, anger, change in behavior (emotional turmoil, disorganization, restlessness), and reorganization of behavior directed toward a new object or activity. The process of mourning is often divided into stages (phases).

Acute Stage

Four to eight weeks in length, this stage involves shock and disbelief, developing awareness, and restitution.

Shock and Disbelief

Initially, denial is used for a few hours to a few days to buffer against intolerable pain, thus slowly allowing the person to acknowledge the reality of the death.

Development of Awareness

Denial fades and painful feelings surface. The reality of death is experienced, often accompanied by feelings of anger and guilt. Crying is common. A person unable to cry may have difficulty in successfully completing the work of mourning.

Restitution

The formal ritualistic phase of mourning, restitution brings people together in funeral rites.

CHAPTER OUTLINE	TEACHING STRATEGIES
Long-Term Stage	This stage goes on for 1 to 2 years or longer and includes experiences of sensations of somatic distress, preoccupation with the image of the deceased, and feelings of anger.
Helping People Cope with Loss	Prolonged and serious alterations in social adjustment, as well as medical disease, may develop if the phases of mourning are interrupted or if needed support is not available. Retelling the story of bereavement is therapeutic. The most helpful nursing intervention is listening. Banal advice is useless. Table 30–3 provides guidelines for helping people grieve. Table 30–4 offers guidelines for what to say to a person who is suffering loss. Box 30–4 offers guidelines to help people cope with catastrophic grief.
Unresolved and Dysfunctional Grief	A history of depression, substance abuse, or posttraumatic stress disorder can complicate grief. A number of indicators that a person may have potential for dysfunctional grieving are listed. They include factors such as level of dependency on deceased, degree of ambivalence in the relationship, age of the deceased, unresolved conflicts with the deceased, the number of previous losses, death associated with a cultural stigma or associated with violence, etc. The importance of assessment for suicide potential is mentioned.
Successful Mourning	The tasks involved in mourning are to accept the reality of the loss, to share in the process of working through the pain of grief, to adjust to an environment in which the deceased is missing, to restructure the family's relationship with the deceased, and to reinvest in other relationships and life pursuits. Resolution is accomplished when the bereaved can remember realistically both the pleasures and the disappointments of the lost loved one.

147

31 Psychiatric Forensic Nursing

THOUGHTS ABOUT TEACHING THE TOPIC

The faculty member may assign this chapter to students as a required reading. Students may spend clinical time with a basic level nurse in a correction facility or prison, or may be assigned to spend clinical time in a program where offenders are receiving treatment for alcoholism or drug addiction rather than be incarcerated.

Psychiatric forensic nursing could be taught with other lecture topics such as care of the homeless client, alcohol and other drug addiction, or with ethical legal issues in nursing.

KEY TERMS AND CONCEPTS

competence to proceed, 627
correctional mental health nursing, 625
correctional nursing, 625
criminal profiler, 628
expert witness, 627

fact witness, 627
forensic nursing, 623
legal sanity, 626
psychiatric forensic nursing, 625
victimology, 624

OBJECTIVES

After studying this chapter, the reader will be able to
1. Define forensic nursing, psychiatric forensic nursing, correctional nursing, and correctional mental health nursing.
2. Describe the nature of the nurse-client relationship in each of these nursing specialties.
3. Discuss the difference between a fact witness and an expert witness.
4. Describe the role of a sexual assault nurse examiner.
5. Discuss the significance of the terms *legal sanity* and *competence to proceed.*

CHAPTER OUTLINE	TEACHING STRATEGIES
	Nurses traditionally deal with violence in their practice. In 2002, 15% of U.S. households experienced violent or property crimes including rape/sexual assault, robbery, aggravated and simple assault, household burglary and other crimes. But only recently have many of these nurses formalized their interest in working with victims, perpetrators, and the legal system.
Definition of Forensic Nursing	Forensic nursing is an emerging specialty area of practice that combines elements of nursing science, forensic science, and the criminal justice system. Some specialties in the nursing profession are defined by the settings where the nurse practices, whereas others are defined by the population that the nurses serve. Forensic nursing is defined by the nature of the nurse-client relationship and the functions being performed.
	In 1995, the ANA recognized forensic nursing as a specialty practice area. In forensic nursing, the nurse-client relationship is predicated on the possibility that a crime has been committed.
Forensic Nursing Role Functions	The role functions within forensic nursing center on the identification, collection, documentation, and preservation of potential evidence and complement client care roles with assessment and treatment roles related to competence, risk, and dangerousness.
Working with Victim or Perpetrator	Physiological forensic nurses focus on the alleged victim, whereas psychiatric forensic nurses work with the alleged perpetrator and focus on the needs of the court.

148

Psychiatric Forensic Nursing

Psychiatric forensic nursing is defined as the psychiatric nursing assessment, evaluation, and treatment of individuals pending or following a criminal hearing or trial. The client that a forensic nurse will work for is the attorney or the court. Some of the functions are quite unique for a nurse, such as to assess a perpetrator's ability to formulate intent or assess the risk for violence and for committing additional crimes, and collection of evidence, etc. See Box 31-1 for a more detailed list.

Correctional and Correctional Mental Health Nurses

Correctional mental health nursing is defined by the location of the work or the legal status of the client. Correctional nurses face inmates that are older, sicker and remain imprisoned longer when compared with inmates of 20 years ago. Today, more inmates will suffer from chronic or infectious disease that nominates. But correctional nurses do not contribute data regarding the alleged offenses of the inmates. In fact, nurses frequently care for inmates without knowing why inmates are incarcerated because knowing would prejudice their level of care.

Correctional mental health nurses care for inmates housed in a jail's or prison's psychiatric unit or on a forensic hospital's long-term ward where persons judged as "not guilty by reason of insanity" are treated.

Some of the major differences between psychiatric forensic nursing, correctional nursing, and correctional mental health nursing are summarized in the text into the following categories: nurse-client relationships; approach of the nurse; purpose of relationship; practice setting; and examples of nursing functions.

Roles Within Psychiatric Forensic Nursing

Forensic Examiner

A forensic examiner conducts court-ordered evaluations of legal sanity or competency to proceed, responds to specific medicolegal questions requested by the court, and testifies as an expert witness in courtroom testimony.

Legal Sanity

Legal sanity is the individual's ability to determine right from wrong in reference to the act charged, the capacity to know the nature and quality of the act charged, and the capacity to form the intent to commit the crime.

Competence to Proceed

Competence to proceed is the individual's ability to proceed with a trial. It is defined as the capacity of the accused to work with a lawyer in their own defense. Since competence to proceed is a determination of mental capacity at the time of the trial and not at the time of the crime, the defendant's competency must be determined each time he or she goes to court.

Competency Therapist

Psychiatric forensic nurses working as competency therapists are responsible to assess the competence and mental disorder of an individual, conduct a forensic interview, document and complete a formal report to the court, and give expert witness testimony. The competency therapist realizes that the client is the court, not the defendant, and the work product is a competent defendant and a completed report.

Expert Witness

Most psychiatric forensic nursing roles illustrate the differences between a fact witness and an expert witness in the court system. A fact witness will testify regarding facts; what is seen or heard, performed, or documented regarding a patient's care. An expert witness, on the other hand, is recognized by the court as having a higher level of skill or expertise in a designated area of nursing.

Continued

CHAPTER OUTLINE	TEACHING STRATEGIES
Consultant to Law Enforcement Agencies	Deinstitutionalization precipitated a need for interagency cooperation between mental health agencies and law enforcement. The perpetrator's well-being is the focus of the interaction that may result in civil detention and admission to a hospital. Community mental health nurses have traditionally acted in this role.
Hostage Negotiator	Hostage negotiators are trained to work with negotiation teams to report the mental state of a perpetrator and recommend appropriate negotiation strategies. With consultants, there are fewer incidents in which hostages are killed or seriously injured by a perpetrator. The first use of a psychiatric forensic nurse as a consultant was reported in 1993. The psychiatric forensic nurse in this role is not an advocate for the perpetrator, but is an advocate for the process of hostage negotiation.
Criminal Profiler	Criminal profilers are trained to piece together all available data left at a crime scene. They use the data to describe the type of individual who would have committed a particular crime. They use a combination of behavioral and psychological indicators to piece together a reconstruction of the crime, formulate a hypothesis, develop a profile, and test it against the known data. The psychiatric forensic nurse is comfortable with the nursing process of assessment, analysis, planning, implementation, and evaluation.
Consultant to Attorneys	Psychiatric forensic nurses may be used as a resource for education and information about mental illness by either side of the courtroom. The nurse may be asked to testify regarding mental health treatment options, medications, and community resources.
Other Subspecialty Areas of Forensic Nursing	Physiological forensic nurses work as coroners or death investigators, sexual assault nurse examiners, child abuse specialists or elder abuse specialists, battered woman specialists, or legal nurse consultants.
	Basic level registered nurses can work as death investigators or as sexual assault investigators.
Professionalism in Psychiatric Forensic Nursing	Nurses who work with forensic psychiatry need to be assertive and be able to work with autonomy. It can be a difficult area of nursing to be viewed as an expert.

Chapter 31   Psychiatric Forensic Nursing

32 Disorders of Children and Adolescents

THOUGHTS ABOUT TEACHING THE TOPIC

Most instructors will spend only enough time to give learners a broad overview of nursing of clients with disorders of childhood and adolescence, since this is considered a specialty area. Nurses with associate degrees act as community resources, and are asked questions by neighbors, friends, and families. At a minimum, it is important for learners to develop a broad base of information and to be able to recognize when a child's behavior indicates that consultation with a mental health professional is warranted.

KEY TERMS AND CONCEPTS

OBJECTIVES

After studying this chapter, the reader will be able to
1. Explore what factors and influences contribute to child and adolescent mental disorders and how they relate to multimodal intervention strategies for these young clients.
2. Explain how the characteristics associated with resiliency can mitigate against etiological influences.
3. Identify characteristics of mental health in children and adolescents.
4. Discuss various components involved in constructing a holistic assessment of a child or adolescent.
5. Explore areas in the assessment of suicide that may be unique to children or adolescents.
6. Describe the clinical features and behaviors of at least three child and adolescent psychiatric disorders and identify useful intervention strategies for each.
7. Compare and contrast at least six treatment modalities for children and adolescents.
8. Formulate three nursing diagnoses, stating client outcomes with corresponding interventions, for at least three child and adolescent psychiatric disorders discussed in this chapter.

CHAPTER OUTLINE	TEACHING STRATEGIES
Prevalence	One in five U.S. children and adolescents suffers from a major mental illness. Approximately 60% of all children in out-of-home care have moderate to severe mental health problems.
Comorbidity	ADHD, a prominent comorbid condition, in emotionally disturbed children, occurs in 90% of individuals with juvenile-onset bipolar disorder, 90% of children with oppositional defiant disorder, and 50% of children with conduct disorder. Childhood depression is also associated with a high incidence of comorbidity.
Child and Adolescent Psychiatric Nurse	The inpatient care of the 1980s has been modified by managed care and budget cuts to brief treatment. The nurse must work with more acutely ill clients in a shorter time period, making it more difficult to achieve a therapeutic alliance and bring about lasting behavioral changes. The majority of children hospitalized are diagnosed with a conduct disorder; they infrequently come from an intact home. Lack of a family support system limits the nurse's ability to work on parenting issues and ensure that gains made in treatment are sustained. Much of the care of child and adolescent clients has moved from inpatient to outpatient facilities and into the community.

Continued

151

Theory

Etiology of mental illness in children and adolescents encompasses multiple factors.

Genetic Influences

Hereditary factors are implicated in autism, bipolar disorder, schizophrenia, attention deficit problems, and mental retardation. Direct genetic link is noted in Tay-Sachs disease, phenylketonuria, and fragile X syndrome.

Biochemical Factors

Alterations in neurotransmitters play a role in causing depression, mania, and ADHD. Elevated testosterone levels have been studied and may have a role in mediating response to environmental stress.

Temperament

Temperament is the style of behavior the child habitually uses to cope with the demands and expectations from the environment. It is thought to be genetically determined and may be modified by the parent-child relationship.

Social and Environmental Factors

Risk factors include severe marital discord, low socioeconomic status, large families and overcrowding, parental criminality, maternal psychiatric disorders, and foster care placement. Child abuse and stressful life events relate to increased incidence of accidental injuries, anxious children, depression, and suicidal behaviors. Traumatic life events can lead to insecure attachments, PTSD, conduct disorders, delinquency, and impaired social and cognitive function. Abused children are at risk for dissociative identity disorder (DID).

Cultural and Ethnic Factors

Culture shock and cultural conflicts related to assimilation issues put immigrant children at risk for mental and learning disorders. Differences in cultural expectations, stresses, and support or lack thereof by the dominant culture have a profound effect on development and the risk of mental, emotional, and academic problems.

Resiliency

Resilience is formed by the relationship between the child's constitutional endowment and environmental factors. Characteristics of a resilient child include temperament that adapts to environmental change, ability to form nurturing relationships with other adults when the parent is not available, ability to distance self from emotional chaos of the parent or family, good social intelligence, and ability to use problem-solving skills.

Overall Assessment
Mental Health Versus Mental Illness

A mentally disturbed child is one whose personality development is impaired, whereas a mentally healthy child progresses with only minor setbacks or difficulties.

Assessment Data

The type of data collected depends on the setting, the severity of the presenting problem, and the availability of resources. Agency policy determines which data are collected and how they are documented. In all cases the physical examination is part of the complete workup. See Box 32-1 for more details.

Data Collection

Methods of data collection include interviewing, screening, testing, observing, and interacting. Histories are taken and structured questionnaires and genograms can be used.

Interviews with children and adolescents are semistructured, to give freedom to describe current problems. Play activities are used with younger children who cannot respond to a direct approach.

Mental Status Assessment

The mental status assessment in children is similar to the adult assessment except that the developmental level is considered.

CHAPTER OUTLINE	TEACHING STRATEGIES
Developmental Assessment	Developmental assessment provides information about the child's current maturational level, which, when compared with the chronological age, identifies developmental lags and deficits. Abnormal findings are often related to stress, adjustment problems, or more serious disorders.
Suicide Risk	Areas to explore include suicidal fantasies, thoughts, threats or attempts; circumstances at the time of the suicidal thought or behavior; concepts about suicide and death and previous experience with these; depression and other moods and feelings; acting-out behaviors; listening to music or reading books with morbid themes. Assessing lethality of plans is complicated by distorted concepts of death, immature ego functions, and lack of understanding of lethality.
Cultural Influences	Sensitivity to cultural influences is necessary to avoid inappropriate assessments. Eye contact, expression of feelings, and patterns of speech differ from culture to culture.

Cognitions must be evaluated in light of cultural beliefs. Folk medicine practices for the culture are also considered. |
| **Pervasive Developmental Disorders** | These disorders are characterized by severe and pervasive impairment of reciprocal social interaction and communication skills, usually accompanied by stereotyped behavior, interests, and activities. Mental retardation is often present. |
| **Autistic Disorder** | This is usually first observed before age 3 years. It is a behavioral syndrome resulting from abnormal left brain function (language, logic, reasoning).

Presenting symptoms of autism include the following:
1. Impairment in communication and imaginative activity: language delay or absence, immature grammatical structure, pronoun reversal, inability to name objects, stereotyped or repetitive use of language, high-pitched squealing or giggling, repetitive phrases, babbling, singsong speech, lack of spontaneous make-believe play, failure to imitate.
2. Impairment in social interactions: lack of responsiveness to and interest in others, lack of eye contact and facial response, indifference or aversion to affection and physical contact, lack of sharing interest or achievement with others, failure to develop cooperative play with peers, lack of friendships.
3. Markedly restricted, stereotyped patterns of behavior, interest, and activities: rigid adherence to routine and rituals with catastrophic reactions to minor changes; stereotyped and repetitive motor mannerisms; preoccupation with certain repetitive activities that is abnormal in intensity or focus. |
| **Asperger's Disorder** | This disorder is recognized later than autistic disorder. There are no significant delays in cognitive and language development or in self-help skills, but severe and sustained impairment in social interactions, development of restricted, repetitive patterns of behavior in interest and activities, and delayed motor milestones do occur. Social interaction problems are more noticeable when the child enters school, as are problems with empathy and modulating social relationships. |
| **Rett's Disorder** | This is seen only in females, with onset before age 4 years. Characteristics include persistent loss of manual skills, development of stereotyped hand movements (hand wringing), problems with coordination and gait, severe psychomotor retardation, severe problems with expressive and receptive language, and loss of interest in social interactions. |

Continued

Chapter 32   Disorders of Children and Adolescents

Childhood Disintegrative Disorder

Onset is between 2 and 10 years. Characteristics are marked regression in multiple areas of function after at least 2 years of normal development, loss of previously acquired skills in at least two areas (communication, social relationships, play, adaptive behavior, bowel and bladder control, motor skills), deficits in communication and social interactions, and stereotyped behaviors. Losses reach a plateau, then may show limited improvement.

Assessment Guidelines

Assess for developmental spurts, lags, uneven development, loss of previously acquired abilities.
1. Assess quality of relationship between child and caregiver for evidence of bonding, anxiety, tension, difficulty of fit of temperaments.
2. Be aware that children with behavioral and development problems are at risk for abuse.

Nursing Diagnosis

Delayed growth and development, impaired social interactions, impaired verbal communication are often useful.

Outcome Criteria

The Nursing Outcomes Classification (NOC) identifies a number of outcomes that are appropriate for a child with PDD. See Table 32-4.

Intervention

Interventions center around helping the child reach his or her full potential by fostering developmental competence and coping skills (e.g., increasing interest in reciprocal interactions, fostering social skill development, facilitating expression of appropriate emotional responses, fostering development of reciprocal communication, fostering cognitive skills, fostering development of self control, etc.).

Attention Deficit Hyperactivity Disorder and Disruptive Behavior Disorders

Attention Deficit Hyperactivity Disorder

Affected children show inappropriate inattention, impulsiveness, and hyperactivity. ADHD may be associated with oppositional defiant or conduct disorder or Tourette's disorder.

Presenting symptoms of ADHD include the following:
1. Inattention
2. Hyperactivity
3. Impulsivity

Oppositional Defiant Disorder

A recurrent pattern of negativistic, disobedient, hostile, defiant behavior toward authority figures without serious violations of the basic rights of others. Such children may exhibit the following characteristics: loses temper, argues with adults, actively defies, refuses to comply, deliberately annoys people, blames others for mistakes, is easily annoyed by others, is angry or resentful, spiteful or vindictive.

Conduct Disorder

This is characterized by a persistent pattern of behavior in which the rights of others and age-appropriate societal norms are violated. Rates for males range from 6% to 16% and for females 2% to 9%. Predisposing factors are ADHD, parental rejection, inconsistent parenting with harsh discipline, early institutional living, absence of father, alcoholic father, etc. Childhood-onset conduct disorder occurs prior to age 10 and is marked by physical aggression. The youth with adolescent-onset conduct disorder demonstrates less aggressive behaviors and more normal peer relationships, tending to act out misconduct with the peer group. Conduct disorders frequently progress to adult antisocial personality disorder.

Types of behavior noted: (1) aggressive conduct that causes harm to other people or animals, (2) destruction of property, (3) deceitfulness or theft, and (4) serious violation of rules.

Assessment Guidelines	For ADHD and disruptive behavioral disorders: 1. Assess quality of relationship between child and caregiver. 2. Assess caregiver's understanding of growth and development, parenting skills, and handling of problematic behaviors. 3. Assess cognitive, psychosocial, and moral development for lags or deficits. For attention deficit hyperactivity disorder: 1. Observe for level of physical activity, attention span, talkativeness, ability to follow directions, and impulse control. 2. Assess difficulty in making friends and performing in school. 3. Assess for problems with enuresis and encopresis. For oppositional defiant disorder: 1. Identify issues that result in power struggles, when they begin, and how they are handled. 2. Assess severity of defiant behavior and its impact on child's life at home, school, and with peers. For conduct disorder: 1. Assess seriousness of disruptive behavior, when it started, and attempts to manage it. 2. Assess levels of anxiety, aggression, anger and hostility toward others, and ability to control destructive impulses. 3. Assess moral development for ability to understand impact of hurtful behaviors on others, for empathy and feeling remorse.
Nursing Diagnosis	*Risk for self-directed violence, risk for other-directed violence, risk for injury, impaired social interaction, ineffective coping* are useful diagnoses. Table 32-3 lists other potential diagnoses.
Outcome Criteria	The Nursing Outcomes Classification (NOC) identifies a number of outcomes that are appropriate for a child with ADHD, oppositional defiant disorder, or conduct disorder. See Table 32-5.
Intervention	Behavior modification and pharmacological agents, such as methylphenidate (Ritalin), special education programs, play, psychotherapy. Nursing interventions for working with parents and caregivers: • Assess caregiver knowledge of disorder and give needed information. • Explore impact of behaviors on family life. • Assess caregiver's support system. • Discuss how to make home a safe environment. • Discuss realistic behavioral goals and how to set them. • Teach behavior modification techniques. • Give caregivers support. • Provide educational information about medications. • Refer caregiver to local chapter of self-help group. • Be child and parent advocate with the educational system.
Anxiety Disorders	Some anxiety is part of normal development. Anxiety becomes a problem when the individual cannot move beyond fears associated with the developmental stage or when anxiety interferes with normal functioning. Anxiety disorders affect as many as 10% of young people.
Separation Anxiety Disorder	In this disorder, the child becomes excessively anxious when separated or anticipating separation from home or parental figure. Other characteristics include excessive worry about being lost or kidnapped or that parental figures will be

Continued

155

harmed, fear of being home alone or in situations without significant adults present, refusal to sleep unless near a parental figure, refusal to attend school without a parental figure, and physical symptoms as a response to anxiety.

Posttraumatic Stress Disorder

Children of any age can develop PTSD. Younger children appear to react more with behaviors indicative of internalized anxiety, whereas older children and adolescents the anxiety is more often externalized.

Posttraumatic Stress Behaviors

Younger children do not relive the traumatic event, but rather develop nightmares featuring monsters, threats to self or others, and rescue of others. Repetitive playing out of the event may occur. The symptoms experienced by preschool children and those experienced by school-age children are listed in the text. Internalized anxiety is seen in the younger child, whereas the older child more often externalizes the anxiety.

Assessment Guidelines

The nurse will assess the quality of relationships, recent stressors, parent/caregiver's understanding of developmental norms; also assess developmental level and regression and assess for physical, behavioural, and cognitive symptoms of anxiety.

Nursing Diagnosis

Table 32-3 lists potential nursing diagnoses, in addition to *anxiety, ineffective coping,* and *delayed growth and development.*

Outcome Criteria

The NOC identifies a number of outcomes appropriate for the child with an anxiety disorder. See Table 32-6.

Intervention

- Protect from panic level anxiety and provide for biological and psychosocial needs.
- Accept regression, but give emotional support.
- Increase child's self-esteem and feelings of competence.
- Help child to accept and work through traumatic events or losses.

Mood Disorders

Symptoms of mood disorders in children and adolescents may be similar to adult symptoms. Symptoms of depression in children often include somatic complaints, irritability, and social withdrawal. Psychomotor retardation and hypersomnia are more evident in adolescent depression. Associated factors include, among other things, physical and sexual abuse, neglect, death, divorce, learning disabilities, conflicts with or rejection by family or peers. Complications include school failure, drug or alcohol abuse, promiscuity, running away, suicide, etc.

Tourette's Disorder

Tourette's disorder involves motor and vocal tics that cause marked distress and significant impairment in social and occupational function. Vulnerability is transmitted in an autosomal dominant pattern. Associated symptoms are obsessions, compulsions, hyperactivity, distractibility, and impulsivity. Low self-esteem is associated with tics.

Adjustment Disorder

Adjustment disorder is a residual category used for emotional responses to an identifiable stressor that do not meet other *DSM-IV-TR* axis I criteria for another disorder. The disorder is characterized by decreased performance at school and temporary changes in social relationships occurring within 3 months of the stress and lasting no longer than 6 months after the stress has ceased.

Feeding and Eating Disorders

These disorders include pica (persistent eating of nonnutritive substances), rumination disorder (the repeated regurgitation and rechewing of food), and feeding and eating disorders of infancy or early childhood (failure to eat adequate amounts of food though available).

CHAPTER OUTLINE	TEACHING STRATEGIES

Overall Interventions for Child and Adolescent Disorders

Family Therapy	To ensure optimal outcomes for children and adolescents, the family must be involved and educated. Both single-family therapy and multiple-family therapy are being used.
Group Therapy	For younger children, group therapy takes the form of play; for grade-school children, it combines play and talking. For older children and adolescents, group therapy takes the form of talking.
Milieu Therapy	Goals are to provide physical and psychological security, promote growth and mastery of developmental tasks, and ameliorate psychiatric disorders. Therapeutic factors include an environment with boundaries and limits, a reduction in stressors, opportunities for expression of feelings without fear of rejection or retaliation, available emotional support and comfort, assistance with reality testing and support for weak ego functions, interventions in impulsive or aggressive behavior, opportunities for learning and testing new adaptive behaviors, consistent constructive feedback, reinforcement of positive behaviors and development of self-esteem, corrective emotional experiences, role models for making healthy identifications, opportunities to be spontaneous and creative, and experiences leading to identity formation.
Behavioral Therapy	Desired behavior is rewarded; undesirable behavior is ignored or has limits set to prevent it. A point system awards points for age-appropriate desired behaviors and points are collected and used to obtain a specific reward. A level system has increasing levels of privileges that can be earned.
Modifying Disruptive Behavior	Disruptive behavior in the therapeutic milieu must be interrupted early to avoid causing chaos on the unit. Techniques include planned ignoring; use of signals or gestures to remind a child to use self-control; using closeness or touch to calm; redirecting child's attention toward an activity; giving additional affection; use of humor to help the child "save face"; direct appeals such as, "Please . . . not now"; extra assistance to avoid blowups due to frustration; clarifying the situation for the child; restructuring, such as shortening a story if the child becomes restless; and setting limits and giving permission to do what is expected. Interventions useful for modifying disruptive behaviors and preventing contagion include strategic removal, physical restraint, setting limits and giving permission, promises and rewards and threats, and punishment.
Removal and Restraint	These interventions may be used judiciously.
Seclusion	Use of seclusion is rare. Other methods are more effective, especially early intervention before loss of control occurs. The child or adolescent will always perceive seclusion as punishment and the experience of being overpowered by adults is terrifying to one who has been abused.
Quiet Room	An unlocked room used for removing a child from the situation to regain self-control with staff support is called the quiet room. The feelings room, which is carpeted and supplied with soft objects that can be punched or thrown, and the freedom room, which contains a large ball for throwing or kicking, are alternative approaches.
Time-Out	Time-out may require going to a designated room or sitting on the periphery of an activity until self-control is gained and the incident is reviewed with a staff member.
Therapeutic Holding	This limits self-destructive behavior by holding the child immobilized while talking to the child in a reassuring manner, providing comfort, and keeping the child's

Continued

157

self-esteem intact. Following the episode, the nurse reviews the event with the child to discuss alternative ways to cope. This fosters learning and self-control.

Cognitive-Behavioral Therapy

The goal of this therapy is to change cognitive and behavioral processes, thus reducing the frequency of maladaptive responses and replacing them with new competencies.

Play Therapy

Play is the child's way of learning to master impulses and adapt to the environment. Play therapy usually is a one-on-one session the therapist has with a child in a playroom. The guiding principles of play therapy include the following:

1. Accept the child as he or she is and follows the child's lead.
2. Establish a warm, friendly relationship that allows free expression of the child's feelings.
3. Recognize the child's feelings and reflect them back, to promote insight development.
4. Accept the child's ability to solve personal problems.
5. Set limits only to provide reality and security.

Dramatic Play

Psychodrama, often referred to as theater, uses dramatic techniques to act out emotional problems, develop new perspectives, and try out new behaviors. It is used with verbalizing children and adolescents.

Dramatic play is less formal than psychodrama. Hand puppets and puppet shows are a favorite way to act out problems and solutions. "Dress-up" with a box of clothes is another form of dramatic play.

Mutual storytelling is a technique for helping young children express themselves verbally. The child is asked to make up a story. At the end of the story the child is asked to give a lesson or the moral of the story. The nurse retells the story, selecting one or two of its important themes, and provides a healthy resolution.

Therapeutic Games

Playing a game with the child facilitates the development of a therapeutic alliance and provides an opportunity for conversation. Several therapeutic games exist that require the child to say something or tell a story about various objects in order to collect a chip. A more advanced game for older children requires talking, feeling, and doing activities.

Bibliotherapy

Bibliotherapy involves using children's literature to help the child express feelings in a supportive environment, gain insight, and learn new ways to cope with difficult situations. Books are chosen by the nurse to reflect the situations or feelings the child is experiencing.

Therapeutic Drawing

Drawing captures thoughts, feelings, and tensions a child may not be able to express verbally. Characteristics of human figures are general indicators of a child's emotions rather than indicators of psychopathology. A number of characteristics and their meanings are given in the text. The nurse may ask the child questions about the pictures and discuss emotions.

Psychopharmacology

Table 32-7 identifies child and adolescent disorders and medications used in the treatment of the disorders.

33 Adult Issues

THOUGHTS ABOUT TEACHING THE TOPIC

Many faculty will choose not to use lecture time for these topics, but may assign the chapter as required or recommended reading. Others may integrate the material in other contexts, including sleep disorders when sleep assessment is discussed, sexual disorders when sexual assessment is discussed. Adult onset ADHD can be discussed with development in children or can be made part of the introduction to adult type psychiatric disorder comorbidity disorders when teaching anxiety, mood disorders, psychotic disorders, or personality disorders. In some curricula, sleep disorders and sexual disorders are part of other courses and receive no attention in the psychiatric nursing module.

KEY TERMS AND CONCEPTS

dyspareunia, 679
dyssomnias, 662
exhibitionism, 681
fetishism, 681
frotteurism, 682
gender dysphoria, 678
gender identity, 678
gender identity disorder, 680
hypoactive sexual desire, 678
paraphilia, 681
parasomnias, 666
pedophilia, 681
polysomnography, 660
premature ejaculation, 679
primary insomnia, 662
sex, 677
sexual dysfunction, 679
sexual identity, 678
sleep deprivation, 659
sleep disorders, 662
sleep efficiency, 663
sleep fragmentation, 663
sleep latency, 663
transsexualism, 678
vaginismus, 679
voyeurism, 681

OBJECTIVES

After studying this chapter, the reader will be able to
1. Discuss the significance of sleep deprivation with regard to social problems, medical conditions, and psychiatric disorders.
2. Describe a normal sleep cycle.
3. Discuss the variation in normal sleep requirements, evaluate whether or not you are a short or a long sleeper, and analyze the impact of sleep deprivation on your daytime functioning.
4. Discuss the significance of primary insomnia.
5. Compare and contrast the use of polysomnography and the 2-week sleep diary in the assessment of sleep problems.
6. Discuss at least two interventions for primary insomnia.
7. Identify at least two sleep disorders that are life threatening.
8. Identify at least two factors that make diagnosis of adult attention deficit hyperactivity disorder (ADHD) difficult.
9. Discuss the importance of self-report questionnaires as well as family and spouse reports in the diagnosis of ADHD.
10. Describe the components of multimodal treatment for the adult with ADHD.
11. Discuss personal values and biases regarding sexuality and sexual behaviors.
12. Define at least three sexual disorders and describe their treatment.
13. Role-play with a classmate taking a sexual history and discuss how you feel and how your feelings influence your ability to perform this assessment.

CHAPTER OUTLINE	TEACHING STRATEGIES

SLEEP DISORDERS
The Problem

It is estimated that 47 million Americans suffer from sleep deprivation. Sleep deprivation is means that people are not getting an optimal amount of sleep every night, which can lead to chronic fatigue, memory problems, energy deficit, mood difficulties, and just feeling generally out of sorts. Many attribute this problem to the fact that we now have 24-hour-a-day access to supermarkets, airports, and

Continued

other services. Nurses, physicians, and other personnel work rotating shifts, and average only 5 hours of sleep nightly. During the last century, it is estimated that the average nightly sleeping time has been reduced by 2 hours.

Comorbidity

Social Issues

Sleep loss diminishes safety and results in loss of lives and property, especially when individuals are working in occupations where they are expected to work shifts around the clock.

Medical Conditions

Sleep apnea is associated with hypertension, heart failure, and diabetes. Sleep deprivation leads to the production of fewer infection-fighting antibodies, thereby increasing our vulnerability to infection.

Chronic sleep loss might lead to earlier onset and as well as an increase in severity of diabetes and obesity. Age-related diseases such as arthritis and Alzheimer's disease are affected by sleep as well.

Psychiatric Disorders

Prolonged sleep deprivation is linked to hallucinations and delusions. Current research indicates a relationship between sleep and dream disturbances and post-traumatic stress disorder. And there is also a correlation between sleep and relapse to alcoholism and drug addiction.

Normal Sleep Cycle

REM sleep is different from NREM sleep. NREM is a peaceful state compared to wakefulness, REM sleep is characterized by a high level of brain activity and physiological activity levels that are similar to the waking state. During a night's sleep, people begin usually begin with NREM sleep and proceed to the REM latency period. The cycling between NREM and REM sleep is regular, with REM sleep occurring every 90 to100 minutes. The first REM cycles each night usually last less than 10 minutes, whereas the following REM periods the rest of the night can last from 15 to 40 minutes each.

Sleep Patterns

Sleep patterns evolve over a person's lifetime—from newborns, where REM sleep comprises more than 50% of total sleep time, through a jdvancing age, where sleep becomes lighter and there is less REM sleep. Box 33-1 illustrates the distribution of time spent in each of the sleep states.

Evaluation of Sleep

Sleep cycles are evaluated through polysomnography, which monitors multiple processes during sleep including EEG activity, electrooculographic activity (eye movement), and electromyographic activity (muscle movement).

Regulation of Sleep

Researchers have identified anatomic areas that promote sleep, but regulation of sleep is not totally understood. It is thought that any change in neurotransmitters such as serotonin, norepinephrine, and acetylcholine can have an impact on the sleep cycle.

Functions of Sleep

It is believed that sleep serves to restore and maintain homeostasis.

Requirements of Sleep

Requirements for sleep are individual. Some people are considered short sleepers, whereas others are considered long sleepers. The body has a natural internal clock that follows a 25-hour cycle. Biological rhythms, including a woman's menstrual cycle, also influence sleep. The myth that a daytime nap compensates for lack of nighttime sleeping is untrue. This is important to note for those who work in occupations that require shift rotation.

Sleep Disorders

The *DSM-IV-TR* classifies sleep disorders into three major categories, including primary sleep disorders, sleep disorders related to other mental disorders, and other sleep disorders.

160

There are five major symptoms characteristic of most sleep disorders. These include: insomnia, hypersomnia, somnolence, parasomnia, and sleep-wake schedule disturbance. Box 32-2 describes these symptoms.

Primary Sleep Disorders
Dyssomnias

These are problems with initiation of or maintaining sleep. Box 33-3 lists and defines the dyssomnias.

Primary Insomnia

In primary insomnia, individuals have difficulty falling asleep and staying asleep. This type of sleep is also nonrestorative. This condition must last for 1 month and is not related to any known physical or medical condition.

In order to diagnose any sleep disorder there must be a thorough medical and psychiatric history. It is necessary to explore the entire 24-hour period with respect to sleep-wake behaviors.

The primary diagnostic tool for primary insomnia is the polysomnography. The treatment of primary insomnia includes several effective approaches, such as the use of medications, for example: alprazolam (Xanax), chlordiazepoxide (Librium, Novapam), triazolam (Halcion), and others. Increasingly, melatonin is being used by the elderly to deal with insomnia, and there are nonpharmacological interventions, including various relaxation therapies.

Sleep restriction therapy is another intervention that is useful in dealing with insomnia and is directed at reducing the amount of time spent awake in bed.

Parasomnias

Parasomnias are characterized by unusual or undesirable behaviors that intrude into sleep or occur at the threshold between waking and sleeping. They are listed and defined in Box 33-6.

Treatment for parasomnias includes reduction of stress, and other measures to protect the client such as use of a dental bite plate for sleep-related bruxism. Some medications can also be used for treatment of parasomnias.

Sleep Disorders Related
to Other Mental Disorders

There are two distinct sleep disorders associated with a major mental disorder: *insomnia related to another mental (axis I or axis II) disorder* and *hypersomnia related to another mental (axis I or axis II) disorder*. Both of these produce significant functional problems in social, occupational, and other important areas. Individuals can become so preoccupied with a sleep disorder that they ignore the symptoms of the related mental disorder, or even deny they have a mental disorder.

Clients with major depressive disorder frequently experience insomnia. Some clients with anxiety disorders have insomnias as well. Clients with schizophrenia frequently have prolonged sleep latencies and other sleep difficulties.

Hypersomnia related to another mental disorder is seen with many mental conditions including mood disorders. Daytime sleepiness is seen in clients with depression, bipolar I disorder, and uncomplicated grief. Personality disorders, dissociative disorders, somatoform disorders, and others can be associated with hypersomnia. Treatment is usually directed to the primary disorder.

Other Sleep Disorders

A client with *sleep disorder due to general medical condition* and *substance-induced sleep disorder* may report sleep disturbances such as insomnia, hypersomnia, parasomnia, or a combination.

Medical conditions such as those related to pain and discomfort such as arthritis and angina are frequently further complicated by the presence of insomnia.

Continued

161

A substance-induced sleep disorder can result from the use or recently discontinued use of a substance. These can include insomnia, hypersomnia, parasomnia or a combination.

Application of the Nursing Process

The application of the nursing process is focused on primary insomnia.

Assessment

The nurse can ask the client to keep a sleep diary in order for the client to begin to look at solutions to the sleep problems identified. There is also a set of important questions to ask the client who is having difficulty with a sleep disorder. These are listed in the text.

Nursing Diagnosis

There are two primary nursing diagnoses identified for primary insomnia: *sleep deprivation* related to insomnia with difficulty as sleep onset, and *disturbed sleep pattern* related to insomnia with difficulty maintaining sleep.

Outcome Criteria

The Nursing Outcomes Classification (NOC) identifies a number of appropriate outcomes for the client experiencing primary insomnia including: *Rest, Sleep, Mood Equilibrium,* and *Personal Well-Being.* See Table 33-2.

Planning

Most clients with sleep disorders are managed in the community unless the client has a primary psychiatric disorder or a medical condition that requires hospitalization. The role of the nurse is generally to conduct a full assessment, to provide support to the client and family while interventions are determined, and to teach the client and family strategies that may improve sleep.

Intervention
Basic Level Interventions
Counseling

This begins with the assessment of the sleep disorder and support and assurance that the sleep problems are amenable to treatment.

Health Teaching

There are many myths regarding sleep and what "good sleep" really is. The nurse's role as a health teacher cannot be overemphasized. See Box 33-5 for educational points for teaching how to obtain good sleep. The nurse can also teach the client relaxation techniques and effective use of medications.

Psychobiological Interventions

Many clients will use medication for sleep problems. The nurse can provide education about the benefits of a particular drug, side effects, untoward effects, and the fact that medications are usually prescribed for no more than 2 weeks because of the dangers of tolerance and withdrawal.

Box 33-7 lists interventions appropriate for sleep enhancement from the Nursing Interventions Classification (NIC).

Advanced Practice Interventions

The advanced practice nurse may be involved in establishing deconditioning techniques to improve sleep.

Evaluation

The evaluation is based on whether or not the client experiences improved sleep quality and can be accomplished through client report and through the maintenance of the sleep diary. The client's perception is also an important part of the evaluation process.

ADULT ATTENTION DEFICIT HYPERACTIVITY DISORDER

Adults with ADHD, especially those who are undiagnosed and untreated, struggle with life. Contrary to popular belief, there is no one ADHD personality profile.

Diagnosis

ADHD is usually first diagnosed in childhood. The *DSM-IV-TR* criteria for *attention-deficit hyperactivity disorder* and *attention-deficit hyperactivity disorder not otherwise specified* are shown in Boxes 33-8 and 33-9.

Many adults with ADHD may have been diagnosed with "hyperactivity" as children and received treatment until adolescence, when it probably stopped because professionals believed that the disorder resolved itself. But while the impulsive qualities tend to diminish, the inattentive and disorganized patterns of behavior remain constant.

It is believed that 10% to 20% of adults with histories of ADHD experience few problems moving into adult years. Approximately 60% continue to experience symptoms of ADHD that impact on the social, academic, and emotional arenas of their lives. Finally, 10% to 30% exhibit serious problems including antisocial behaviors coupled with their continued ADHD symptoms and other comorbid problems such as depression and anxiety.

Diagnosis of adult ADHD is largely subjective. The use of school records, self-report questionnaires, spousal reports and parent reports are all useful in the diagnosis. Most helpful is a record of behavior in childhood that indicates a history of ADHD. Before settling on the ADHD diagnoses, professionals need to rule out other co-occurrences of adult ADHD with psychiatric disorders such as borderline personality disorder, substance abuse disorders, as well as depression and anxiety.

Treatment

Treatment can consist of medication, cognitive therapy, and life coaching.

Medication

The psychostimulants including methylphenidate (Ritalin-SR, Concerta, and Metadate-CD), dexmethylphenidate (Focalin), and amphetamines (Adderall, Adderall XR, Dexedrine, Dexedrine Spansules, and Desoxyn), which constitute the cornerstone of treatment of both adult and childhood ADHD. Some tricyclic antidepressants are comparable to the psychostimulants; however, there are still individuals who respond either partially or not all to these medications.

Other medications often used for comorbid disorders or ADHD-related symptoms include the SSRIs and mood stabilizers. Table 33-3 provides dosage information on the most commonly prescribed medications used in ADHD.

Therapy

This is essential for treatment of ADHD and may be cognitive-behavioral, group, and/or family therapy, as well as vocational counseling.

Family or Marriage Counseling

Family or marriage counseling provides the opportunity for intimate partners and other family members to learn the dynamics of ADHD and to begin to reframe their own feelings because of behaviors that seemed willful, insensitive, and forgetful.

Vocational Counseling

Employment history of an individual with ADHD can be very erratic. With diagnosis and treatment, the individual can improve job skills and productivity.

Application of the Nursing Process
Assessment

It is not uncommon for ADHD to be diagnosed when a client presents with a complaint that is unrelated to adult ADHD. ADHD can present when the client is seeking treatment for a co-occurring disorder such as depression, anxiety, and/or substance abuse.

Also important to note is that it is not unusual that during an initial assessment process with a child that a parent begins to make connections between the child's present behaviors and the parent's lifelong difficulties. For many adults, this begins not only their children's journey toward management of ADHD but their own healing journey as well.

Continued

163

Self-Assessment

Before diagnosis and treatment of a client with ADHD, the nurse must examine personal experiences, feelings, and thoughts that might influence the care provided to a particular client. Behaviors of a client with ADHD, such as missed appointments, no follow through with treatment recommendations, etc., can lead a nurse to feeling irritated and frustrated. The guiding philosophy that all behavior has meaning can help the nurse avoid negative responses and encourage further exploration regarding the reasons behind the client's behavior.

Nursing Diagnosis

There are many appropriate NANDA diagnoses. Among potential diagnoses are *ineffective coping; readiness for enhanced coping;* and *chronic low self-esteem.*

Outcome Criteria

The Nursing Outcomes Classification (NOC) includes many outcomes including: *Coping, Anxiety Self-Control, Role Performance,* etc. See text for more details.

Planning

Nurses will provide care for clients with ADHD in many settings such as home, clinics, medical-surgical units, and outpatient settings, etc. Usually, when clients with ADHD are in an inpatient setting, it is for a co-occurring diagnosis. Adult ADHD is not a primary diagnosis warranting hospitalization. Therefore, planning for care usually involves selecting interventions that can be implemented in a community setting.

Intervention
Basic Level Interventions

Interventions for a basic level psychiatric mental health nurse include counseling, decision making, and self-esteem, psychobiological intervention focused on medication management and teaching. Identification of appropriate community resources is also an important function of the basic level psychiatric mental health nurse as is health teaching regarding strategies to deal with ADHD. See Box 33-10 for useful strategies.

Advanced Practice Interventions

The advanced practice nurse can provide cognitive-behavioral therapy, lead therapy groups, provide family and/or marital counseling, and offer individual "life coaching" for clients.

Evaluation

The client reports improvements in areas such as self-esteem, time-management and organizational skills, satisfaction with job performance, and improvement in family relationships.

GENDER IDENTITY AND SEXUAL DISORDERS

It is important that nurses assess the client's sexual practices, and be prepared to educate, dispel myths, assist with values clarification, refer to appropriate care providers when indicated, and share resources with clients concerning sexual disorders.

Definitions

Sex refers to a person's inherited biological sexual characteristics. Gender identity develops within the first 18 months of life and refers to the earliest sense of maleness or femaleness. Gender refers to the individual's psychological sense of being male or female. When sex differs from gender, the individual suffers from gender dysphoria. Transexualism is an example of the most extreme case of gender dysphoria.

Sexual Response Cycle

The *DSM-IV-TR* defines a four-phase response cycle: phase 1 is desire, phase 2 is excitement, phase 3 is orgasm, and phase 4 is resolution.

Desire Phase

In general, hypoactive sexual desire is a challenging disorder, associated with other psychiatric or medical conditions. Conversely, excessive sexual desire becomes a problem when this creates difficulties for the individual's partner or when such excessive desire drives that person to demand or force sexual compli-

164

ance from unwilling partners. Testosterone (present in both men and women) appears to be essential to sexual desire in both men and women.

Estrogen does not seem to have a direct effect on sexual desire in women.

In evaluating a client with a sexual desire disorder, the physical assessment, including laboratory studies, is performed before exploring psychological factors.

Excitement Phase

This is a period of time during which sexual tension continues to increase from preceding level of sexual desire.

Orgasm Phase

This is attained only at high levels of sexual tension in both women and men. It is produced by a combination of mental activity and erotic stimulation of erogenous areas.

Resolution Phase

During this phase, sexual tensions developed in prior phases subside to baseline levels, presuming that sexual stimulation has ceased.

Sexual Disorders

Sexual disorders are those things that cause the client discomfort, pain, or interference with a healthy adult sexual response.

Sexual Dysfunction

Sexual dysfunction includes sexual desire disorders, sexual arousal disorders, orgasm disorders, sexual pain disorders, sexual dysfunction due to a general medical condition, and substance-induced sexual dysfunction. See Box 33-12 for details.

Gender Identity Disorder

Gender identity disorder occurs when the individual's biological gender and psychological gender identity do not match. Childhood patterns of cross-gender interest are noted, with increasing intensity of gender dysphoria occurring in adolescence and adulthood. Individuals with gender identity disorder do not consider themselves homosexuals. Some seek sexual reassignment. This involves living in the cross-gender role, hormonal therapy, legal and social arrangements, and surgery.

Paraphilias

Paraphilias are recurrent and intense sexually arousing fantasies, urges, or behaviors generally involving inanimate objects, the suffering or humiliation of oneself or one's partner, the use of children or other nonconsenting persons. Paraphilias include the following:

Fetishism—requires a material object to be present in order to be sexually satisfied;

Pedophilia—sexual activity with a prepubescent child, which, within a family, is termed incest;

Exhibitionism—the intentional display of the genitals in a public place;

Voyeurism—viewing by stealth of other people in intimate situations;

Transvestism—obtaining sexual satisfaction via dressing in the clothing of the opposite sex;

Sadism and masochism—giving (sadism) and receiving (masochism) psychological or physical pain, or both, or domination to achieve sexual gratification;

Frotteurism—touching, rubbing against, or fondling another person to obtain sexual excitement.

The usual treatment for working with paraphilias is cognitive and behavioral therapy, psychodynamic techniques, or pharmacological agents when the practice is acutely or dangerously compulsive.

Continued

165

Sexual Problems Resulting from Head Trauma

Clients who have experienced head trauma with damage to the frontal lobe of the brain may display sexual problems.

Sexual Problems Resulting from Chromosomal Abnormalities

In Klinefelter's syndrome, the client has an extra X chromosome as his genetic makeup and frequently appears for treatment with immature genitalia and shows schizophrenic symptoms.

Sexual Problems Resulting from Psychosis

This is especially true for the client with schizophrenia who shows an inability to maintain stable relationships.

Application of the Nursing Process Assessment

The sexual assessment includes both subjective and objective data. Health history questions pertaining to the reproductive system may be limited to menstrual history, parity, history of sexually transmitted diseases, methods of contraception, and questions regarding "safer sex" practices.

Many nurses may experience discomfort exploring sexual issues with clients, because they are unsure of which questions to ask or why the questions should be asked. Clients may also feel uncomfortable during a sexual assessment and feel embarrassed.

Guidelines for Conducting a Sexual Assessment

The sexual assessment includes behavioral, emotional, and spiritual aspects of sexuality. It also includes religious beliefs in regard to sexual behavior and sexual knowledge base. With experience, the nurse is able to identify those clients that are at a greater risk for difficulties in sexual functioning. Key indicators might include clients with a history of medical problems such as diabetes, multiple sclerosis, history of myocardial infarction and other disease processes, as well as clients who are having difficulties because of medications, or those clients who are experiencing relationship difficulties.

Settings for a Sexual Assessment

The setting should be private and free from distractions. The interview is conducted in a nonjudgmental way that facilitates open discussion of sexual issues.

Conducting the Interview

The interview should begin with introductions, followed by an explanation of the purpose of the assessment. Questions proceed from least intrusive to more intrusive. Accepted medical terminology is used when discussing sexual issues, but the nurse must also have knowledge of commonly used slang expressions to understand what the client is saying. Table 33-4 presents some common slang expressions related to sexuality and their corresponding medical terms; Box 33-13 lists client cues that may indicate concerns about sexuality.

Self-Assessment

The nurse must always keep in mind that judgments regarding sexual behavior are inappropriate for the nurse. There may be reasons why the patient has demonstrated inappropriate behavior. The patient with schizophrenia may be responding to hallucinations, the alcoholic patient's behavior may be a reflection of diminished judgment, or a mentally retarded client may become involved with a child because of the lack of availability of adult partners and the lack of capacity to appreciate and understand fully the wrongful nature of his or her actions.

The nurse must also be sure to assess a client's temperament and traits of character. It is easy for a person who does not suffer the same illness as a client to say, "The client should just not do the behavior." But it is not only willpower that helps an individual to successfully resist desires, drives, or appetites such as hunger, thirst, pain, the need for sleep, or sex.

CHAPTER OUTLINE	TEACHING STRATEGIES
Nursing Diagnosis	Two important nursing diagnoses are *sexual dysfunction* related to martial problems evidenced in painful intercourse and inability to have orgasm, and *ineffective sexuality pattern* related to personal conflicts about sexual preferences evidenced by expressed desire to be the opposite gender.
Outcome Criteria	The Nursing Outcomes Classification (NOC) identifies a number of outcomes for clients with either sexual dysfunction or ineffective sexuality patterns. See Table 33-7 for selected intermediate and short-term indicators for *sexual identity* and *sexual functioning.*
Planning	Inpatient admissions are usually for primary diagnoses such as schizophrenia with sexual problems as secondary to the psychotic process. However, most clients will be encountered in outpatient and community settings.
Intervention **Basic Level Interventions**	In order to be a facilitator, the nurse must be nonjudgmental, have basic knowledge of sexual functioning, and the ability to conduct a basic sexual assessment. Sample interventions for the Nursing Interventions Classification (NIC) for sexual counseling can be found in Box 33-14.
Advanced Practice Interventions	Advanced practice nurses need to have specialized training to work with the client with sexual and gender identity disorders.
Evaluation	Evaluation of expected outcomes relate to the level of control and personal satisfaction that is achieved.

167

34 Psychosocial Needs of the Older Adult

THOUGHTS ABOUT TEACHING THE TOPIC

When time is limited, the instructor may choose to assign this chapter concurrently with Chapter 21, Cognitive Disorders. The material in Chapter 21 on dementia and delirium correlates well with material in this chapter, especially relating to disorders for which the elderly are at risk.

KEY TERMS AND CONCEPTS

adult day care, 700
advance directives, 706
ageism, 693
chemical restraints, 701
directive to physician, 706
durable power of attorney for health care, 707
living will, 706
Omnibus Budget Reconciliation Act (OBRA), 701
Patient Self-Determination Act (PSDA), 706
physical restraints, 701

OBJECTIVES

After studying this chapter, the reader will be able to
1. Discuss the facts and myths about aging.
2. Describe the impact of ageism in providing care to older adults.
3. Analyze how ageism affects your attitudes and willingness to care for the elderly.
4. Compare the different group interventions commonly used with elderly clients.
5. Explain the importance of a comprehensive geriatric assessment.
6. Describe the role of the nurse in different settings of care.
7. Identify the requirements for the use of physical and chemical restraints.
8. Discuss the importance of pain assessment and identify three tools used to assess pain in the elderly.
9. Identify the risk factors for elder suicide and the nurse's role in prevention of suicide.
10. Discuss institutional requirements related to the Patient Self-Determination Act (1990).
11. Discuss differences between a living will, a directive to physician, and durable power of attorney for health care.

CHAPTER OUTLINE	TEACHING STRATEGIES
The Older Population and the Health Care System	The growing number of elderly people and their percentage of the general population of the United States have had a significant impact on the country's economy and health and social services. As the population lives longer, chronic illness and disability have become major threats to the health of the elderly. At least 80% of people over age 65 have at least one chronic condition. Women outlive men. Husbands have their wives' assistance and support when their health starts to fail, whereas women often do not have that luxury.
	The elderly are divided into four groups: the young old (65 to 74), the middle old (75 to 84), the old-old (85 and older), and the elite old (95 and older). The older group is more vulnerable, frailer, at greater risk for falls and cognitive impairment, and are more adversely affected by the disorders of aging. The elderly are less likely to be accurately diagnosed or receive mental health treatment.
The Role of the Nurse	The author questions whether nurses are given enough information and sufficient exposure to the elderly during basic education to allow them to develop an interest in the elderly and to understand the aging process.
Ageism Among Health Care Workers	Ageism: A bias against older people because of their age. Reflected in dislike of the old by the young, and by the critical attitude of the elderly toward themselves. Ageism results in problems such as difficulty obtaining financial and political

support for programs for the elderly; health care personnel failing to share medical information, recommendations, and opportunities with the elderly; and failing to give mental health care to the elderly.

Health care workers' attitudes are often negative and based on stereotypes. To overcome misconceptions, the author suggests that educational programs provide students with information about the aging process, discussion of attitudes relating to care of the elderly, sensitization of participants to their clients' needs, and exploration of the dynamics of nurse and staff–client interactions. Facts and myths about aging are included in Table 34-2.

Unique Assessment Strategies

Figure 34-1 provides an example of a comprehensive geriatric assessment tool. Two particularly relevant rating tools, the Geriatric Depression Scale and the Michigan Alcohol Screening Test—Geriatric Version tool are also displayed in the text (Box 34-3 and Box 34-4).

Unique Intervention Strategies

Learners are reminded that the elderly who manifest mental problems are treatable and responsive. Techniques that work well with these clients are listening, crisis intervention, using empathetic understanding, encouraging ventilation of feelings, reestablishing emotional equilibrium when anxiety is moderate or higher, and explaining alternative solutions.

Inpatient Settings

Inpatient settings provide the acutely ill older adult with short-term or long-term care. Inpatient treatment is recommended for patients who are at high risk for self-harm or harm to others. Box 34-6 gives an example of a remotivation therapy that might be used in an inpatient setting.

Community-Based Programs

The hazards of institutionalization include increased mortality due to higher risk for nosocomial infections, injuries associated with disorientation to a new setting, learned helplessness, loss of interest in self-care activities, and decreased opportunities for socialization. Community-based programs provide an alternative whose purpose is to promote the elder's independent functioning. A multipurpose senior center provides a broad range of services: (1) health promotion and wellness programs; (2) health screening; (3) social, educational, and recreational activities; (4) meals; (5) information and referral services. Day care provides an alternative for seniors who are physically frail or cognitively impaired. Three types of day care programs exist: (1) Social day care affords clients recreation and social interaction. Nursing and rehabilitative care are usually not provided. (2) The adult day health or medical treatment model provides medical and psychiatric nursing rehabilitation for high-risk elderly clients and psychosocial interventions with the frail elderly. It requires physician referral. The goal is to prevent or slow mental, physical, or social deterioration and to maximize potential. (3) The maintenance day care model assists clients at high risk for institutionalization. Care is planned by an interdisciplinary team led by a psychiatrist. Clients include frail persons with dementia and those with severe and persistent psychiatric disorders. The goal is to maintain functional abilities as long as possible.

Issues That Affect the Mental Health of Some Elderly

Include use of restraints, pain management, death and dying, AIDS, suicide, alcoholism, and elder abuse (the latter is addressed in Chapter 25).

Use of Restraints
Physical Restraints

Physical restraints are any manual method or mechanical device, material, or equipment that inhibits free movement. Chemical restraints are drugs given for the specific purpose of inhibiting a specific behavior or movement.

Continued

Physical restraints can be humiliating and demoralizing. Physically restrained clients are more likely to sustain injury than those who are not restrained. Strangulation and asphyxiation are of greatest concern. Further, immobilization fosters constipation or impaction, disrupted vestibular function, reduced circulation, incontinence, skin abrasions or pressure sores, loss of bone mass, reduced metabolic rate, electrolyte losses, and muscle atrophy.

The Omnibus Budget Reconciliation Act (OBRA) mandates nursing homes may restrain only to ensure the physical safety of the resident or other residents and only upon the written order of a physician that specifies the duration and the circumstances under which restraints are to be used. It requires all physical restraints to be labeled with directions informing health care providers of the dangers. Furthermore, clients, or their representatives, must be informed of the contemplated action and its risks and benefits. Clients who are restrained must have ongoing observation and assessment. Surveys (inspections) evaluate the use of restraint and determine if less restrictive measures were attempted; if occupational and physical therapists were consulted; if the client and family received a complete explanation; if the device was used only for definite periods for therapeutic reasons; whether use of restraint was detrimental to the resident's physical, mental, or psychosocial well-being; and whether the client received ongoing observation, assessment, and care interventions.

Chemical Restraints

The Health Care Financing Administration (HCFA) will investigate to determine whether residents are free from unnecessary drugs, given antipsychotic drugs only to treat a specific condition, given gradual dose reductions, and drug holidays and behavioral programming, whenever possible, in lieu of medications.

Pain

Pain is common in the elderly and affects their well-being and quality of life. Up to 85% of the older population is thought to have problems, such as arthritis and diabetic neuropathy, which predispose them to pain. Pain decreases ability to perform ADLs, leads to delayed healing and decreased mobility, and interferes with sleep and appetite. It may cause psychological distress, including depression, low self-esteem, social isolation, and feelings of hopelessness. Nurses should perform a full pain assessment (i.e., of pain pattern, duration, location, character, exacerbating and relieving factors, and the probable cause of the pain).

Barriers to Accurate Pain Assessment

The elderly are often reluctant to label pain as pain, calling it, instead "discomfort," "hurting," or "aching." They may rank it as less important than other health problems. They may not wish to incur the cost of investigating the pain, or may be resigned to accepting serious disease as a natural part of aging. Sensory impairment, memory impairment, and depression are also barriers to assessment.

Assessment Tools

A number of pain assessment tools exist. The visual analogue scales, the Wong-Baker FACES Pain Rating Scale, and the present pain intensity rating scale have been found to be useful with the elderly.

Pain Management

Pharmacological pain management includes use of prescription and nonprescription medications. Nonpharmacological management includes a range of physical interventions and modalities such as exercise, positioning, acupuncture, heat or cold, massage, and transcutaneous electrical nerve stimulation (TENS). Cognitive strategies may emphasize relaxation, distraction, biofeedback, and hypnosis. Alternative medical approaches include homeopathy, naturopathy, and spiritual healing.

Decision Making
Patient Self-Determination Act

This act established that health care agencies receiving federal funds must provide, at the time of admission, written information to each client regarding his or her right to execute advance health care directives and to inquire if such directives already exist. Clients use such directives to indicate preferences for the types of medical care they want, or how much treatment they desire to have provided to them. Directives come into use if physical or mental incapacitation prevents clients from making health care decisions.

Living wills express wishes about future medical care, including restriction of medical intervention when technology or treatment can no longer advance a reasonable quality of life or chance of recovery. Only terminal illnesses are covered; it does not cover severe persistent illnesses such as Parkinson's or Alzheimer's disease. A living will can be rescinded orally.

Directive to a physician appoints a physician to serve as proxy and largely parallels a living will.

Durable power of attorney for health care (DPAHC) authorizes a person other than a physician to act as the client's agent. Individuals do not have to be terminally ill or incompetent for the person appointed to act on their behalf. The agent is the client's advocate in all medical matters and may even limit the institution from providing services to the client that the agent believes are not wanted.

Nursing Role in the
Decision-Making Process

Nurses are often involved in making decisions related to end-of-life care for clients who have not given clear instructions, since nurses have a broad understanding of the client based on the nurse-client relationship. Nurses are also responsible for orienting family members to death and dying and giving advance directives counseling to clients. Nurses are required to know the facility's policy on "coding" and to realize that affected clients should have orders in effect for implementation. (Nurses should never accept verbal no-code orders from physicians.) As client advocates, nurses must intervene on the client's behalf if advance directives are not being carried out.

Acquired Immunodeficiency
Syndrome

The elderly may well have contracted AIDS in the years prior to their current medical treatment. Nurses should use standard precautions. Transmission may occur among elderly sexually active individuals, making health teaching necessary even at advanced ages. Early AIDS dementia mimics Alzheimer's disease.

Suicide

The suicide rate for the elderly is higher than for any other group; elderly white males have the highest prevalence. Retirement; loss of status, influence, and community standing; feelings of uselessness; and financial need may contribute to suicide among the elderly. Suicide attempts among the elderly signify a desire to die rather than a cry for help.

Assessment of Suicide Risk
in the Elderly

Other high-risk factors for suicide in the elderly are depression, widowhood, illness and intractable pain, status change, and losses (of any sort). The elderly usually choose a reliable method of suicide (i.e., guns, jumping, hanging). The ratio of attempts to completed suicides for all ages is 10:1, but among the elderly it is 10:9. In the elderly, suicide is most closely associated with untreated depression. Early identification and treatment of depression are key measures in suicide prevention.

Right to Suicide

An ethical dilemma exists regarding the right to suicide. Society frowns on suicide; however, voluntary active euthanasia by an elderly person with a terminal illness may be viewed differently. Several nursing scholars support the perspective that affirms life by enhancing the individual's quality of life as opposed to assuring his or her of the right to die.

Continued

171

Depression Versus Dementia

Depression is often confused with dementia and may go unrecognized. Depression is treatable. Symptoms of depression in the elderly include change in sleep patterns and insomnia, change in eating pattern (loss of appetite), weight loss, excessive fatigue, increased concern with bodily functions, alterations in mood, expressions of apprehension and anxiety with reason, low self-esteem, and feelings of insignificance or pessimism. Depression can be caused by drugs or metabolic or endocrine diseases.

Antidepressant Therapy

Concern with antidepressants for the elderly is to provide a drug with a low side effect profile. SSRIs appear to be safer for use with the elderly, with sertraline being the drug of choice. In general, lower doses of medication are appropriate for the elderly.

Alcoholism and Substance Abuse

This is a hidden epidemic according to the American Medical Association. Identifying alcohol and substance abuse in the elderly is often difficult because personality and behavioral changes are not readily recognized and health care providers seldom assess the elderly for these problems.

Alcoholism

About 10% of the elderly have alcohol problems. Two patterns exist: the early-onset alcoholic, who has become an "aging alcoholic," and the late-onset or "geriatric problem drinker," who develops an alcohol abuse pattern in response to the stresses of aging.

Alcohol and Aging

Most elderly have an increased biological sensitivity to, or conversely, a decreased tolerance for, the effects of alcohol. This, combined with weakened muscles, poor balance, and low flexibility, increases the likelihood of falls, burns, and other accidents. In addition, alcohol elimination is slower in the elderly.

Alcohol and Medication

Alcohol potentiates the effects of many drugs and speeds the metabolism of others. Mixing alcohol with medication often creates problems.

Symptoms of Elder Dependence

Symptoms include contusions, malnutrition, self-neglect, depression, poor coordination, falls, signs of dementia, diarrhea, and urinary incontinence.

Treatment of the Elderly Alcoholic

The elderly are less likely to be referred for treatment due to reduced support systems or denial and hiding the symptoms from others. Screening can be done by the geriatric version of the Michigan Alcohol Screening Test (MAST-G). Treatment should emphasize social therapy. Although difficult to treat, the prognosis for late-onset alcoholism is excellent.

Drug Abuse
Illegal Drug Use

Currently use of illicit drugs among the elderly is low. However, there is a concern that this may change because the baby boomer generation is moving into the elderly population.

Prescription and Over-the-Counter Drug Use and Abuse

Because elderly clients use both prescription and over-the-counter drugs at a higher rate than the rest of the population, it is difficult to accurately estimate the extent to which they may be being abused.

35 Therapeutic Groups

THOUGHTS ABOUT TEACHING THE TOPIC

Although most nurses do not go into the field of psychiatric nursing, the importance of understanding group behavior cannot be ignored. Nurses work in groups. In the future it is highly likely that nurses will lead more educational groups as health promotion assumes greater value. Helping students realize that concepts such as group roles and group process are the same, whether used in medical-surgical settings or psychiatric settings, increases their value to the beginning student.

KEY TERMS AND CONCEPTS

OBJECTIVES

After studying this chapter, the reader will be able to
1. Identify basic concepts related to group work.
2. Describe the phases of group development.
3. Define task and maintenance roles group members may adopt within a group and give four examples.
4. Discuss the therapeutic factors that operate in all groups.
5. Name four facilitating techniques used by the group leader.
6. Describe a group intervention for a member who is silent or a member who is monopolizing the group.
7. Discuss four types of groups commonly led by basic level registered nurses.

CHAPTER OUTLINE	TEACHING STRATEGIES
Group Concepts	
Definition of Group	*Group* is defined as two or more people who develop a relationship that is interactive; these people share at least one issue or common goal. The specific characteristics of a group include the following: size, rules, boundaries, climate, defined purpose, apparent content and underlying process.
Phases of Group Development	During the initial phase, the leader's role is to set the atmosphere of confidentiality and respect while members are helped to relax and feel comfortable. The group task is for members to get to know one another and begin to take steps toward the working phase. In the working phase members are involved in working toward the group's goals, while the leader ties together common themes, encourages expression, and prevents hostile attacks. During the mature phase, the leader keeps the group focused on therapeutic goals of the individual members; members accept each other's differences. During the termination stage the group members prepare for separation and help each other prepare for the future.
Roles of Group Members	Growth-producing roles adopted by group members include opinion giver, opinion seeker, information giver, information seeker, initiator, elaborator, coordinator, orienter, evaluator, clarifier, recorder, and summarizer. A member may adopt more than one role.

Continued

173

CHAPTER OUTLINE	TEACHING STRATEGIES

Role of the Group Leader

A group leader has multiple responsibilities in starting, maintaining, and terminating a group. Cultural considerations must be taken into consideration as well. Table 35-2 describes communication techniques frequently utilized by the group leader, which include seeking clarification, encouraging description, presenting reality, focusing, reframing, providing feedback, and promoting the development of insight.

Therapeutic Factors Common to All Groups

Yalom's curative factors. They include imparting of information, instillation of hope, altruism, corrective recapitulation of the primary family group, development of socializing skills, imitative behavior, interpersonal learning, group cohesiveness, catharsis, existential factors, and universality.

Group Protocols

A protocol is a description of the actual nursing care involved in a group. It includes the objectives, methods or means to evaluate the success of the group; organization of such features as frequency of group meetings; qualifications of group leaders; and the description of the types of clients, their behaviors, and diagnoses that are most suited to a particular type of group.

Expected Outcomes

Measurable outcomes may be easier to accomplish with education and psychoeducation groups than with therapy groups. Key quality indicators should be identified. They can then be tracked over a period of time. Examples of quality indicators are listed in the text for a medication education group.

The Role of the Nurse in Therapeutic Groups
Basic Level Registered Nurse
Psychoeducational Groups

Psychiatric nurses, with their biopsychosocial and spiritual approach, are the ideal professionals to teach a variety of health subjects. These groups include a variety of specific somatic or psychological subjects, which also allow members to communicate about emotional concerns. Some of the psychoeducational groups include the following:

- Medication education groups are designed to teach clients about their medications, answer their questions, prepare them for discharge, and foster medication compliance after discharge. Clients should be taught the name of the medication, reasons for taking the medication, exact dose, time to take the medication, common side effects, ways to remember to take each dose, foods or OTC medications to avoid, what to do if the client wishes to change the regimen, and the importance of informing other health care providers of the medication being used (to prevent adverse medication interactions.)
- Sexuality education groups work with topics such as AIDS education, STD education, sexuality and psychotropic medication, effects of antidepressants on sexuality.
- Dual-diagnosis groups work with such topics as psychiatric illness and substance use. The RN may colead this group with a dual-diagnosis specialist (master's level clinician).
- Multifamily groups are usually found in the outpatient setting. The focus is on education about mental illness and strategies for the family to cope with long-term disability.
- Symptom management groups concentrate on a topic such as anger or psychosis. The focus is on sharing positive and negative experiences so that members learn coping skills from each other.
- Stress management groups teach members various relaxation techniques to reduce stress. They are usually time limited.

174

Therapeutic Milieu Groups

Goals: increase clients' self-esteem, decrease social isolation, encourage appropriate social behaviors, reeducate clients in basic living skills.

Leaders: occupational or recreational therapists with nurses as co-leaders.

Advanced Practice Registered Nurse

APRNs may lead any of the groups described and may also lead psychotherapy groups. Refer to Table 35-4 for an overview of theories for group therapy.

Self-Help Groups

Self-help groups are designed to serve people who have a common problem; they are led by a member rather than a professional. Strategies include promoting dialogue, self-disclosure, and encouragement. Concepts: psychoeducation, self-disclosure, mutual support. Characteristics: peer support, group teaching, counseling, using shared experiences. All self-help groups with the title _____ Anonymous use a 12-step method typical of the Alcoholics Anonymous program.

Challenging Client Behaviors
Person Who Monopolizes the Group

Compulsive speech by a client is an attempt to deal with anxiety. Intervention: Ask group why they have permitted the monopolizer to go on and on. This helps the group to recognize the role of their own passivity and to disclose their own feelings. Therapist helps group use "I" statements rather than "you" statements.

Person Who Complains but Continues to Reject Help (Yes. . .But)

This type of client takes pride in believing that his or her problem is insoluble. The group becomes concerned initially, then frustrated and angry with the client. Intervention: The therapist agrees with the content of the client's pessimism and maintains detached affect. With group cohesion a therapist can help client recognize the pattern of his or her relationships.

Person Who Demoralizes Others

Those who tend to challenge the group leader and demoralize the group are individuals who are self-centered, lack empathy, are depressive, angry, and refuse to take personal responsibility. Narcissistic individuals have problems in group therapy because they are defensive and have a grandiose sense of self-importance; may be initially charming, then demanding; may devalue the therapist, then feel elated; may monopolize the group. Intervention: The therapist must listen to the content that is being avoided and stay therapeutically objective. Only then can the therapist be empathetic in a matter-of-fact way.

Silent Person

This person may be silent for various reasons: because he or she is observing intently, trying to decide whether the group is safe; out of concern that he or she may not be as competent as the others; or hoping to avoid conflict. Intervention: The leader should exhibit patience, but encourage each member to offer comments to the group.

175

36 Family Therapy

THOUGHTS ABOUT TEACHING THE TOPIC

This chapter includes a wealth of information about families. There is good clarification of the differing roles of the basic level nurse and the advanced practice nurse. Although the basic level student needs to understand the complexity of family therapy, the focus of instruction should be on use of the nursing process in situations commonly seen at that level of practice: assessment of family structure and function, often-used nursing diagnoses, examples of outcome criteria, and strategies for intervention.

KEY TERMS AND CONCEPTS

behavioral family therapy, 736
boundaries, 731
clear boundaries, 731
diffuse or enmeshed boundaries, 731
double-bind theory, 735
family systems theory, 736
family triangle, 738
flexibility, 736
genogram, 740
insight-oriented family therapy, 736
multigenerational issues, 740
nuclear family, 739
psychoeducational family therapy, 745
rigid or disengaged boundaries, 731
sociocultural context, 739

OBJECTIVES

After studying this chapter, the reader will be able to
1. Discuss the characteristics of a healthy family using clinical examples.
2. Differentiate between functional and dysfunctional family patterns of behavior as they relate to the five family functions.
3. Compare and contrast insight-oriented family therapy and behavioral family therapy.
4. Identify five family theorists and their contributions to the family therapy movement.
5. Analyze the meaning and value of the family's sociocultural context when assessing and planning intervention strategies.
6. Construct a genogram using a three-generation approach.
7. Formulate seven outcome criteria that a counselor and family might develop together.
8. Identify some strategies for family intervention.
9. Distinguish between the nursing intervention strategies of a basic level nurse and those of an advanced practice nurse with regard to counseling and psychotherapy and psychobiological issues.

CHAPTER OUTLINE	TEACHING STRATEGIES
	According to Wynne, family therapy is a psychotherapeutic approach that focuses on altering interactions between a couple, within a nuclear or extended family, or between a family and other interpersonal systems, with the goal of alleviating problems initially presented by individual family members, family subsystems, the family as a whole, or other referral sources. Family therapy is essentially about changing relationships through changing the interactions between the people who make up the family. The definition of family has become more complicated over the past 2 decades.
Theoretical Premises **Family Functions**	Healthy families provide individuals with the tools that guide how they will function in intimate relationships, the workplace, within their culture, and in society. These tools are acquired through activities associated with family life and are divided into five functions: management, boundary, communication, emotional-supportive, and socialization.

CHAPTER OUTLINE	TEACHING STRATEGIES
Management Function	This includes the use of power for all family members, clear rule making, adequate fiscal support, successful negotiation with extrafamilial systems, and plans for the future. It is usually the adults in the family who agree on how these functions are to be performed.
Boundary Function	Boundaries maintain a distinction between individuals in the family. Ideally, there will be clear individual boundaries, clear generational boundaries, and clear family boundaries. Diffused or enmeshed boundaries refer to a blending together of the roles, thoughts, and feelings of the individuals so that clear distinctions fail to emerge. Families with diffused boundaries are more prone to psychological or psychosomatic symptoms.
	Rigid or disengaged boundaries are those in which the rules and roles are adhered to no matter what. This prevents trying new roles or taking on different functions. Isolation may be marked.
Communication Function	Healthy communication uses clear, direct messages, asking for what one wants, no manipulation, and expression of positive and negative feelings allowed.
Emotional-Supportive Function	Affection is uppermost and anger and conflict do not dominate interactions. Healthy families give mutual positive regard, resolve conflicts, use resources for all family members, and promote growth in all family members.
Socialization Function	The healthy family develops in a healthy pattern, using mutual negotiation of roles by age and ability. Parents feel good about parenting, and spouses are happy with each other's role behavior.
Family Life Cycle	A family is a system moving through time, with each stage having tasks. Family stress is often greatest at transition points from one stage to another. Symptoms are likely to appear when there is an interruption in the unfolding of the family life cycle (illness, death, divorce). Six main stages exist in the changing family life cycle: 1. Launching the single young adult 2. Joining families: the couple forms 3. Becoming parents—families with young children 4. Families with adolescents 5. Launching children and moving on 6. The family in later life
Theories, Theorists, and Approaches to Family Therapy	Family systems perspective is rooted in observing the client in terms of social systems and has an interactive, interpersonal context rather than an intrapsychic focus.
	Jay Haley describes double-bind theory, a situation in which two conflicting messages are given simultaneously on two levels, verbal and nonverbal. The individual is placed in a position in which no acceptable response exists.
	Virginia Satir became interested in client's position and relationships within family. She saw poor self-esteem and symptoms as expressions of family pain.
	Milan group used paradox to challenge the family about present situations as a way of delivering therapy.
	Minuchin looked at organizational patterns and boundaries.
	Murray Bowen used family systems model.

Continued

177

Frameworks for family therapy include the strategic model, which assumes that changing any element in the family system brings change to the entire system, and the structural model, which emphasizes the boundaries between family subsystems and the establishment, and maintenance of a clear hierarchy based on parental competence. Further, two basic forms of marital family therapy exist: (1) insight-oriented marital and family therapy and (2) behavioral marital and family therapy.

Basic Concepts in Family Therapy

Many concepts are used in working with families. The concepts of the identified patient, the family triangle, and the nuclear family emotional system are discussed. Other concepts are explained in Box 36–2.

The Family as a System

All families can be viewed as unique systems, each with its own structure, rules, and history of handling problems and crises. In marital and family therapy the focus is not on the individual but on family patterns and interactions.

The Identified Client

The identified patient is the individual regarded by others as having the problem. He or she is usually responding to problems within the family system. The presenting problem should be assessed by looking at circular causality (i.e., viewing it from many different perspectives).

Family Triangles

Interlocking triangles occur within families. When major tension is experienced between two people, the tension is relieved by bringing in a third person to help lower the tension. In triangles there is a close side, a distant side, and a side where tension exists. Differentiation refers to the ability of the individual to establish a unique identity while still remaining emotionally connected to the family of origin: the lower the differentiation, the higher the tension and the greater the need for triangles. Triangles become active in the event of any change. A nurse's task is to calm down the system and help the family explore alternative ways of dealing with change while avoiding being "triangled in."

The Nuclear Family Emotional System

Nuclear family refers to parent(s) and children under the parents' care. A nuclear family emotional system is the flow of emotional processes within the nuclear family; symptoms belong to the family rather than to the identified patient.

Application of the Nursing Process Assessment

Assessment is typically intermixed with treatment and has multiple foci, including the family system, the subsystems, the individuals. Nichols suggests three areas of consideration: stage of the family life cycle, multigenerational issues, and sociocultural context.

Sociocultural Context

This context considers issues of gender, race, ethnicity, class, sexual orientation, and religion as each affects values, norms, traditions, roles, and rules. The nurse will seek to understand how the family's beliefs affect the presenting problem and impact the family's options.

Multigenerational Issues

Three to four previous generations influence a family. Patterns are handed down over generations. The nurse will seek to understand how the messages and legacies relate to the presenting problem

Constructing a Genogram

A genogram is one format for summarizing information and relationships across three or more generations. It incorporates the stage of the family life cycle, multigenerational issues, and sociocultural context. The genogram provides a graphic display of complex patterns and becomes a source of hypotheses that indicate how the presenting problem connects to the family over time.

178

CHAPTER OUTLINE	TEACHING STRATEGIES
Self-Assessment	Self-assessment is necessary when working with families due to the potential for multiple transferences and triangulations. Nurses must become aware of their own potential for forming triangles when anxious, to become defensive when personal family anxieties are aroused, and to experience role blurring when sensitive personal issues and conflicts are triggered.
Other Assessment Tools	Focused interviews and family assessment devices can be of help to the nurse.
Nursing Diagnosis	Box 36-3 identifies a number of nursing diagnoses that may be useful when working with families: *impaired parenting; sexual dysfunction; interrupted family processes; caregiver role strain; risk for caregiver role strain; parental role conflict; spiritual distress; impaired adjustment; ineffective denial; compromised family coping; ineffective family therapeutic regimen management; deficient knowledge; impaired verbal communication; defensive coping.*
	In addition, the *DSM-IV-TR* heading "Other Conditions That May Be a Focus of Clinical Attention" contains the following categories: Relational problems, Problems related to abuse or neglect, and Bereavement.
Outcome Criteria	Useful goals include reducing dysfunctional behavior of individual family members; reducing intrafamily relationship conflicts; mobilizing family resources and encouraging adaptive family problem solving; improving family communication skills; increasing awareness and sensitivity of other family members' emotional needs; helping family members meet needs of their members; strengthening family's ability to cope with major life stressors and traumatic events; and improving integration of family system into societal system. Other goals related to psychoeducational interventions, self-help groups, or professional counseling are learning to accept illness of a family member; learning to deal effectively with ill member's symptoms; understanding what medications can and cannot do, when to seek medical advice; and assisting in locating community resources.
Planning	Careful analysis of a sound assessment helps identify the most appropriate interventions. Factors to be considered include immediate and long-term needs of the family, crisis at a family developmental stage, coping mechanisms being used, and identification of new skills family members need such as conflict management, parenting, limit setting, or need for psychoeducational family interventions.
Intervention	Outcome research has shown that family therapy is effective for the following situations: • The child is the patient and the disorder is one of conduct. • The wife of the couple is depressive. • A substance-abusing person enters treatment and then is maintained after treatment. • A schizophrenic individual is the client and family therapy is used to reduce relapse.
Communication Guidelines	1. A nonblaming manner promotes open and flexible communication among all professionals and family members in the caregiving system. 2. Imparting information should be clear and understandable to all family members and allow them to choose and decide what to do with the information. 3. The perspective of each family member must be elicited and heard.
Family Interventions	Family therapy is appropriate for most situations. Exceptions are (1) when there is an unsafe environment in which someone will be harmed by information, uncontrolled anxiety, or hostility; (2) when there is lack of willingness to be honest; (3) when there is unwillingness to maintain confidentiality.

Continued

179

CHAPTER OUTLINE	TEACHING STRATEGIES
Traditional Family Therapy	Some therapists focus on here-and-now interactions, others on family history and what happened between sessions; still others are eclectic in choice of techniques. Multiple-family therapy may be useful for families with a hospitalized member to help gain insight and offer support.
Psychoeducational Family Therapy	The goal, through sharing of mental health care information, is to help members understand their family member's illness, prodromal symptoms, medication needed to reduce symptoms, etc. Painful issues and feelings can be shared and put in perspective.
Self-Help Groups	There are two types: one for people suffering from a personal problem or social deprivation (e.g., AA); the other for families with a member with a specific problem or condition (e.g., Al-Anon).
Case Management	Case management involves teaching, giving appropriate referrals, offering emotional support, and making ongoing assessments of family strengths and weaknesses.
Psychopharmacological Issues	Nurses explain to the family the purpose for a prescribed medication, the desired effects, and the possible side effects and adverse reactions.
Evaluation	The nursing process is not concluded until members of the family are demonstrating changes in behaviors, communication and coping skills, conflict resolution, and the family being more integrated into the societal system.

37 Integrative Care

THOUGHTS ABOUT TEACHING THE TOPIC

Instructors may wish to avoid this topic, since so little research-based evidence of effectiveness is available. However, since so may consumers are choosing to use or, at least, investigate complementary and alternative medicine, students should be made as knowledgeable as possible, since their clients will be using them as sources of information. In lieu of a separate lecture on the topic of CAM, the information about herbal supplements might be included as a topic when psychopharmacology is taught, and the other modalities might be integrated when traditional treatments are discussed.

This topic could also be a topic for discussion in a website or as part of a clinical post-conference. If the instructor knows that there is an advanced nurse practitioner available, he or she may wish to be a guest at a particular post-conference to share some expert knowledge about CAM and how it is used in practice.

KEY TERMS AND CONCEPTS

acupuncture, 760
aromatherapy, 761
chiropractic, 754
complementary and alternative medicine (CAM), 749
conventional health care system, 750
herbal therapies, 761
homeopathy, 753
integrative care, 749
naturopathy, 753
prayer, 763
therapeutic touch, 760

OBJECTIVES

After studying this chapter, the reader will be able to
1. Describe integrative care.
2. Explore the philosophies behind various complementary and alternative therapies, including acupressure and acupuncture, aromatherapy, chiropractic medicine, herbal medicine, homeopathy, and massage.
3. Discuss the techniques used in major complementary therapies and the nurse's role.
4. Discuss how the public can be misled through quackery and fraud related to the use of alternative and complementary therapies.
5. Explore information resources available through literature and on-line sources.

CHAPTER OUTLINE	TEACHING STRATEGIES

Movement Toward Integrative Care
Overview of Complementary and Alternative Medicine
Complementary and Alternative Medicine Defined

Complementary and alternative medicine (CAM) is being sought by individuals to help manage or sometimes prevent the onset of chronic illness, increase longevity, improve cognitive function, or increase feelings of well-being. Caution is advised since sources of information about CAM, often friends or the Internet, may not be entirely reliable. The dominant health care system of biomedicine in the United States (allopathy) is research-based, whereas CAM is based on cultural or historical beliefs that do not necessarily have scientific underpinnings. Conventional medicine often focuses on treating a disease, whereas CAN focuses on healing the whole person.

Complementary and alternative medicine covers a broad range of healing philosophies that are not widely taught in medical schools, not generally used in hospitals, and usually not reimbursed by insurance companies. Such therapies used alone are called alternative therapies, whereas those used with conventional treatments are called complementary.

Continued

181

Consumers of traditional health care practices are requesting information about complementary and alternative medical treatments from their health care practitioners. Some question traditional medical practices, whereas others who are actually using medicinal herbs are seeking advice regarding their use. It is estimated that one third of Americans use herbs for health purposes. Traditional practitioners must expand their understandings of CAM. Internet sites developed by individual organizations may present biased information; therefore, practitioners are referred to NIH center sites for unbiased information.

Consumers and Health Care

Reasons consumers are attracted to CAM include a desire to: be an active participant in his or her health care and engage in holistic practices; find lower-risk therapeutic approaches; find health care less expensive than conventional health care. Additional reasons include dissatisfaction with the practice style of conventional medicine and positive experiences with CAM practitioners.

Cost of Alternative Therapies

The growth in the use of CAM therapies is linked to the rising cost of conventional health care. Though the CAM therapies are less expensive, before we can adopt them, health care workers must be sure that the alternatives are safe, reliable and effective.

Categories of Complementary and Alternative Medicine

There are five major domains: (1) alternative medical systems, (2) mind-body interventions, (3) biologically based treatments, (4) manipulative and body-based methods, and (5) energy therapies.

Alternative Medical Systems

What we consider alternative medical systems are often traditional systems of medicine in other cultures (e.g., traditional oriental medicine, which emphasizes the proper balance or disturbances of qi, or vital energy). Therapeutic techniques include acupuncture, herbal medicine, and oriental massage. Other examples of alternative medical systems are homeopathy, which uses small doses of specially prepared plant extracts and minerals to stimulate the body's defenses, and naturopathy, which emphasizes health restoration rather than disease treatment. Naturopathy uses diet, homeopathy, acupuncture, herbal medicine, hydrotherapy, spinal and soft tissue manipulation, physical therapies, and counseling.

Mind-Body Interventions

Mind-body interventions include meditation, spiritual healing and some therapies classified as alternative and complementary are hypnosis, dance, and music and art therapy, as well as prayer.

Biologically Based Therapies

Biologically based therapies may overlap with conventional medicine's use of dietary supplements such as vitamins, minerals, etc.

Manipulative and Body-Based Methods

Chiropractors focus on the relationship between structure and function by using manipulative therapy. Massage therapists manipulate soft tissues to normalize these tissues.

Energy Therapies

Energy therapies focus on energy fields. Reiki is an example of energy therapy.

Review of Selected Therapies
Diet and Nutrition

Dietary supplements are sold without premarketing safety evaluations. Nutritional therapies used for addictions have not been subjected to research, but if standardized through research programs may result in having a significant impact on the treatment of addiction. Individuals who experienced major depression were found to be twice as likely to be taking nonprescription dietary supplements as were individuals without depression, suggesting that such individuals may seek self-medication for depression rather than seek traditional treatment. Of additional concern to health care providers is the fact that many nutritional supple-

182

Chapter 37   Integrative Care

	ments may have problematic interactions with medications. Clients should be encouraged to discuss intake of supplements with health care practitioners.
Acupressure and Acupuncture	Acupuncture consists of placement of needles into the skin at certain points to modulate the flow of energy (qi) through pathways called meridians. Acupressure consists of the use of pressure instead of needles. There is interest in acupuncture to treat alcoholism and other substance abuse. NIH in 1997 identified acupuncture as an acceptable adjunct treatment in a comprehensive management program. Research is presently being conducted into the effectiveness of acupuncture in emotional disorders.
Therapeutic Touch	In therapeutic touch healing is promoted when the body's energies are in balance; the therapist pass their hands over the client, and the healer can feel the body's imbalances. Practitioners center themselves before they begin a treatment session so that they can focus on helping the client without any preoccupation. After a session, many clients express a sense of deep relaxation.
Aromatherapy	Aromatherapy employs the use of essential oils for inhalation or skin application to reduce stress, regulate emotions, relieve anxiety, and reduce insomnia by stimulating the olfactory nerve to send messages to the limbic area.
Chiropractic Medicine	Chiropractic is the most widely used complementary or alternative therapy. It is practiced for relief of musculoskeletal pain and involves manipulation of the spinal column, called adjustments.
Herbal Medicine	There is a need for standardization and regulation of herbal products, for these psychoactive substances are neither benign nor without potential for drug-drug interactions. St. John's wort is used for depression and ginkgo biloba for dementia. Serotonin syndrome has been noted in the elderly who combine use of St. John's wort and other antidepressants. Warnings have been published about interactions with drugs used to treat HIV infections and with immunosuppressant drugs. Side effects of St John's wort include dry mouth, dizziness, fatigue, constipation, nausea, and photosensitivity.
	Gingko biloba has been used for cerebral insufficiency. One research study suggests mild to severely demented individuals may see improvement with 4 to 6 weeks of therapy. Of concern is the fact that gingko interacts with anticoagulants and antiplatelet agents to cause spontaneous bleeding. Gingko must also be used with caution by clients who consume alcohol or who have other risk factors for hemorrhagic stroke.
	Other herbs: Black cohosh is said to have a calming effect but is toxic in high doses and should be avoided by clients with hypertension or heart disease. Kava kava is used for analgesic antianxiety effect, but may potentiate the action of other tranquilizing agents, especially benzodiazepines, and alcohol. Valerian is used as a treatment for insomnia. It may potentiate the effects of other CNS depressants, and may cause headache and upset stomach. Herbal teas are said to have a sedative-hypnotic effect. The most studied is chamomile, which has been found to bind with GABA receptors.
Homeopathy	Homeopathy is based on the concept that like cures like (law of similars). Small doses of diluted preparations that mimic an illness are used to heal. Treatments are individualized according to the client's symptoms, so generalization is impossible.
Prayer	Historically, spiritual care was very much a part of the psychiatric care that clients received. Today, there is an increasing interest in the importance of spiritual in-

Continued

183

terventions for some psychiatric clients. The challenge in meeting these spiritual needs of the client occurs with respecting boundary issues. There is abundant research demonstrating the positive relationship between religion and measures of well-being. Therefore asking clients about issues such as prayer, sources of hope and strength, and the client's preferred spiritual practices allows us to know how we can provide spiritual support for the client.

Quackery and Fraud

Consumers waste billions of dollars on unproven, fraudulently marketed, sometimes useless, and sometimes harmful health care products and treatments. Claims that should warn of fraud: the product is a quick and effective cure-all for a wide range of ailments; the substance contains a secret ingredient or ancient remedy; undocumented case histories claiming amazing results; the product is available from only one source and advance payment is required.

Credibility of CAM: Research, Reimbursement, and Credentialing

The National Center for Complementary and Alternative Medicine (NCCAM), part of the NIH, supports fair and scientific evaluation of complementary and alternative modalities.

Information Resources

NCCAM disseminates information on complementary and alternative medicine through the NCCAM Clearinghouse. NCCAM has a website or can be contacted by mail or fax. The National Library of Medicine MEDLINE may be used to search a particular condition.

Chapter 37   Integrative Care

Test Bank

CHAPTER 1

1. A nurse explaining the multiaxial *DSM-IV-TR* a psychiatric technician can accurately say that it
   1. focuses on plans for treatment.
   2. includes nursing and medical diagnoses.
   3. includes assessments of several aspects of functioning.
   4. uses the framework of a specific biopyschosocial theory.

   Answer: 3
   Rationale: The use of five axes requires assessment beyond diagnosis of a mental disorder and includes relevant medical conditions, psychosocial and environmental problems, and global assessment of functioning. Option 1: The *DSM-IV-TR* does not include a treatment plan. Option 2: Nursing diagnoses are not included. Option 4: The *DSM-IV-TR* does not use a specific biopsychosocial theory.
   Cognitive level: Application
   Nursing process: Implementation
   NCLEX: Safe and Effective Care Environment
   See text page: 9

2. A 23-year-old college student wrote about herself, "Most of the time I'm happy and feel pretty good about myself. I've learned that what I get out of something is often proportional to the effort I put into it. My grades are OK." Based on this information, what number on the mental health continuum should the nurse select as best reflecting the individual's state of mental health/illness?

Mental	Illness	Mental	Health
1	2	3	4

   1. 1
   2. 2
   3. 3
   4. 4

   Answer: 4
   Rationale: The student states she's happy. Her self-concept is adequate. She is reality oriented, effective in her work, and has control over her behavior. Option 1 would be appropriate for an individual with severe impairment of functioning. Option 2 would be appropriate for an individual with moderate impairment of functioning. Option 3 would be appropriate for an individual with mild impairment of functioning.
   Cognitive level: Analysis
   Nursing process: Assessment
   NCLEX: Psychosocial Integrity
   See text pages: 5, 7

3. A client has been admitted to the psychiatric hospital for assessment and evaluation. What behavior might indicate that the client has a mental disorder? The client
   1. is able to see the difference between the "as if" and the "for real."
   2. describes her mood as consistently sad, discouraged, down in the dumps, and hopeless.
   3. responds to the rules, routines, and customs of any group to which she belongs.
   4. can perform tasks she attempts within the limits set by her abilities.

   Answer: 2
   Rationale: Option 2 describes a mood alteration. Options 1, 3, and 4 describe mentally healthy behaviors.
   Cognitive level: Application
   Nursing process: Assessment
   NCLEX: Psychosocial Integrity
   See text page: 5

4. An outcome for a client is that he will demonstrate mentally healthy behavior. The behavior that indicates the outcome is being met is that the client
   1. behaves without considering the consequences of his actions.
   2. sees himself as approaching his ideals and as capable of meeting demands.
   3. passively allows others to assume responsibility for major areas of his life.
   4. is aggressive in meeting his own needs without considering the rights of others.

   Answer: 2
   Rationale: Option 2 describes an adaptive, healthy behavior. Options 1, 3, and 4 are considered maladaptive behaviors.
   Cognitive level: Analysis
   Nursing process: Evaluation
   NCLEX: Psychosocial Integrity
   See text page: 5

185

5. A float nurse working at a behavioral health clinic notes a diagnosis of a psychiatric disorder with which he is unfamiliar on a client's insurance form. To discern the criteria used to establish this diagnosis, the nurse should consult the
1. *DSM-IV-TR*.
2. *Nursing Diagnosis Manual*.
3. a psychiatric nursing textbook.
4. a behavioral health reference manual.

Answer: 1
Rationale: The *DSM-IV-TR* gives the criteria used to diagnose each mental disorder. Option 2 focuses on nursing diagnoses. Options 3 and 4 may not contain diagnostic criteria.
Cognitive level: Application
Nursing process: Assessment
NCLEX: Safe and Effective Care Environment
See text page: 8

6. The nurse must assess the mental health/mental illness of several new clients at the mental health clinic. Conclusions about current functioning should be made on the basis of
1. the degree of conformity of the individual to society's norms.
2. the degree to which an individual is logical and rational.
3. the rate of intellectual and emotional growth.
4. a continuum from healthy to psychotic.

Answer: 4
Rationale: Because mental health and mental illness are relative concepts, assessment of functioning is made by using a continuum. Option 1: Mental health is not based on conformity. Some mentally healthy individuals do not conform to society's norms. Option 2: Most individuals occasionally display illogical or irrational thinking. Option 3: The rate of intellectual and emotional growth is not the most useful criteria to assess mental health or mental illness.
Cognitive level: Application
Nursing process: Assessment
NCLEX: Psychosocial Integrity
See text pages: 3, 4

7. A 22-year-old college student is highly confident of his own intellectual abilities and strives to excel to the point of always wanting to be first or better than others in academic standing, sports, and other endeavors. Peers find him aggressive, but he ignores this opinion, stating "Too bad. I'm happy when I'm getting ahead. I get my work done and don't break any laws." The nurse assessing this individual would be most concerned about the aspect of mental health known as

1. control over behavior.
2. appraisal of reality.
3. effectiveness in work.
4. healthy self-concept.

Answer: 1
Rationale: The individual accurately appraises reality, is effective in his work, and is self-confident. The trait of control over behavior is of greatest concern because he is not sensitive to the rules, routines, and customs of his peer group, and he violates the rights of others.
Cognitive level: Application
Nursing process: Assessment
NCLEX: Psychosocial Integrity
See text page: 5

8. A 40-year-old woman who lives with her parents and works at a highly routine clerical job states "I'm as happy as the next person even though I don't socialize much outside of work. My work is routine, but when new things come up my boss explains things a few times to make sure I catch on. At home, my parents make all the decisions for me and I go along with their ideas." The nurse should identify interventions to increase this client's
1. self-concept.
2. overall happiness.
3. appraisal of reality.
4. control over behavior.

Answer: 1
Rationale: The client sees herself as needing multiple explanations of new tasks at work and allows her parents to make decisions for her even though she is 40 years old. These behaviors indicate a poorly developed self-concept.
Cognitive level: Application
Nursing process: Planning
NCLEX: Psychosocial Integrity
See text page: 5

9. A client tells the nurse, "I'm a real freak. I'm a psychiatric patient, in and out of hospitals all the time. None of my friends or relatives is crazy like this." The reply that would help the client understand the prevalence of mental illness is
1. "Comparing yourself with others has no real advantages."
2. "Mental illness affects 50% of the adult population in any given year."
3. "Nearly 50% of all people aged 15 to 55 years have had a psychiatric disorder at some time in their lives."
4. "You are not to blame for having a psychiatric illness. The important thing is to recognize your need for treatment."

Answer: 3

Rationale: The question calls for an answer relating to the prevalence of mental illness. Only options 2 and 3 address this, and option 2 is untrue.

Cognitive level: Application
Nursing process: Implementation
NCLEX: Psychosocial Integrity
See text page: 8

10. The best response for the nurse who receives a query from another mental health professional seeking to understand the difference between a *DSM-IV-TR* diagnosis and a nursing diagnosis would be
    1. "There is no functional difference between the two; both serve to identify a human deviance."
    2. "The *DSM-IV-TR* diagnosis disregards culture, whereas the nursing diagnosis takes culture into account."
    3. "The *DSM-IV-TR* diagnosis is associated with present distress or disability, whereas a nursing diagnosis considers past and present responses to actual mental health problems."
    4. "The *DSM-IV-TR* diagnosis affects the choice of medical treatment, whereas the nursing diagnosis offers a framework for identifying interventions for phenomena a client is experiencing."

Rationale: 4

Rationale: The medical diagnosis is concerned with the client's disease state, causes, and cures, whereas the nursing diagnosis focuses on the client's response to stress and possible caring interventions. Options 1 and 2 are not true statements. Both consider culture. Option 3: The *DSM-IV-TR* is multiaxial. Nursing diagnoses also consider potential problems.

Cognitive level: Analysis
Nursing process: Implementation
NCLEX: Safe and Effective Care Environment
See text pages: 11, 12

11. A client mentions to a nursing student, "I'd never want to be a nurse working with psychiatric clients because none of us ever gets well." The reply by the nursing student that best addresses the stated bias is
    1. "People with mental disorders should not be stereotyped as hopeless cases."
    2. "The media tend to focus on the sensational, so the public hears only about the poorest outcomes."
    3. "Treatment of bipolar disorder has an 80% success rate, whereas angioplasty is successful 41% of the time."
    4. "Some mental disorders such as panic disorder are highly treatable, whereas other disorders result in progressive deterioration."

Answer: 3

Rationale: Providing information about treatment efficacy is a concrete way to refute the myth that clients with mental disorders are untreatable. Option 1 does not provide information to refute the myth. Option 2 gives general information, whereas option 3 is more specific. Option 4 provides general information, some of which is discouraging.

Cognitive level: Application
Nursing process: Implementation
NCLEX: Psychosocial Integrity
See text pages: 3, 4

12. The nurse caring for a client finds the client uncommunicative about recent life events. The nurse suspects marital and perhaps economic problems exist. The social worker's intake note has been dictated, but not typed, and is placed in the medical record. The most effective action the nurse could take is to
    1. focus questions on these two topics.
    2. ask the client who shares a room with this client.
    3. try to work around the lack of pertinent information.
    4. look at axis IV of the *DSM-IV-TR* in the medical record.

Answer: 4

Rationale: The intake physician would use axis IV to note psychosocial and environmental problems pertinent to the client's situation, providing another source of information for the nurse. Option 1: Persistent questioning will likely result in client withdrawal. Option 2 violates client privacy rights. Option 3 is not an effective solution.

Cognitive level: Application
Nursing process: Assessment
NCLEX: Safe and Effective Care Environment
See text pages: 9-11

13. The nurse making an admission assessment notes the client is profoundly depressed to the point of being mute and motionless. The client has refused to bathe and eat for a week, according to her parents. The nurse should code the client's global assessment of functioning as
    1. 100
    2. 50
    3. 25
    4. 10

Answer: 4

Rationale: The client is unable to maintain personal hygiene, oral intake, or verbal communication. She is a persistent danger to herself because she refuses to eat. Option 1 indicates high-level functioning. Options 2 and 3 suggest higher functional abilities than the client presently displays.

Chapter 1   Mental Health and Mental Illness

Cognitive level: Analysis
Nursing process: Assessment
NCLEX: Safe and Effective Care Environment
See text page: 10

14. The nurse tells a peer, "I'm assigned to an interdisciplinary team working with a group of depressed clients, half of whom are receiving supportive interventions and antidepressant medication. The others are receiving only antidepressants. We are concerned with treatment outcomes for each group." The peer should identify the work described as
   1. analytical epidemiology.
   2. clinical epidemiology.
   3. descriptive epidemiology.
   4. experimental epidemiology.

Answer: 2
Rationale: Clinical epidemiology is a broad field that addresses what happens to people with illnesses who are seen by providers of clinical care. This study is concerned with the effectiveness of various interventions. Option 1 explores the rates of variation in illness among different groups, seeking to identify risk factors contributing to development of the disorder. Option 3 provides estimates of the rates of disorders in a general population and its subgroups. Option 4 tests presumed assumptions between a risk factor and a disorder.
Cognitive level: Comprehension
Nursing process: NA
NCLEX: Safe and Effective Care Environment
See text pages: 4, 5

15. The husband of a client with schizophrenia tells the nurse, "I simply don't understand why how my wife was nurtured or toilet trained has anything to do with the incredibly disabling illness she has!" The response by the nurse that will help the husband better understand his wife's condition is
   1. "It must be frustrating for you that your wife is sick so much of the time."
   2. "You can count on the fact that her illness is the result of genetic factors."
   3. "Although it seems impossible, psychological stress really is at the root of most mental disorders."
   4. "New findings tell us that your wife's condition is more likely biological than psychological in origin."

Answer: 4
Rationale: Many of the most prevalent and disabling mental disorders have been found to have strong biological influences. Option 1 is empathetic but does not address increasing the husband's level of knowledge about the cause of his wife's condition. Option 2 is not an established fact. Option 3 is not true.
Cognitive level: Application
Nursing process: Implementation
NCLEX: Psychosocial Integrity
See text page: 6

16. A client asks the nurse, "The pamphlet I read about depression mentions that psychosocial factors influence depression. What does that mean?" Examples a nurse could cite to support the premise that a client's depression can be influenced by psychosocial factors include (more than one answer may be correct)
   1. having a hostile and overinvolved family.
   2. having two first-degree relatives with bipolar disorder.
   3. feeling strong guilt over having an abortion when one's religion forbids it.
   4. experiencing the death of a parent a month before the onset of depression.
   5. experiencing symptom remission when treated with antidepressant medication.

Answers: 1, 3, and 4
Rationale: Option 1: Family influence is considered a psychosocial factor affecting a client's mental health. A hostile, overinvolved family is critical of the client and contributes to low self-esteem. Option 2: This example would be considered a genetic factor that influences the individual's risk for mental disorder, not a psychosocial factor. Option 3: Religious influences are considered psychosocial in nature. Option 4: Life experiences, especially crises and losses, are considered psychosocial influences on mental health. Option 5: Treatment with a biological agent such as antidepressant medication is an example of a biological influence.
Cognitive level: Analysis
Nursing process: Implementation
NCLEX: Psychosocial Integrity
See text page: 8

17. The understanding on the part of the nurse that should result in the nurse providing the highest degree of client advocacy during a multidisciplinary client care planning session is
   1. all mental illnesses are culturally determined.
   2. schizophrenia and bipolar disorder are cross-cultural disorders.
   3. symptoms of mental disorders are unchanged from culture to culture.
   4. symptoms of mental disorders reflect a person's cultural patterns.

Answer: 4

Rationale: A nurse who understands that a client's symptoms are influenced by culture will be able to advocate for the client to a greater degree than a nurse who believes that culture is of little relevance. Option 1 is an untrue statement. Option 2 is a true statement but has little relevance to client advocacy. Option 3 is an untrue statement.

Cognitive level: Analysis

Nursing process: Implementation

NCLEX: Safe and Effective Care Environment

See text pages: 11, 12

18. A client comes to the emergency department with the chief symptom of "I'm hearing voices telling me that someone is stalking me. They want to kill me because I have developed a cure for cancer." The client tells the nurse that he carries a knife and will stab anyone he thinks is a threat to him. Which aspects of mental health should be of greatest immediate concern to the nurse? (More than one answer may be correct.)
   1. Happiness
   2. Appraisal of reality
   3. Control over behavior
   4. Effectiveness in work
   5. Healthy self-concept

Answers: 2, 3, 5

Rationale: The aspects of mental health of greatest concern are the client's appraisal of and his control over behavior. His appraisal of reality is inaccurate. He has auditory hallucinations, delusions of persecution, and delusions of grandeur. In addition, the client's control over behavior is tenuous, as evidenced by his plan to stab anyone who seems threatening. A healthy self-concept is lacking, as evidenced by the delusion of grandeur. Data are not present to suggest that the other aspects of mental health (happiness [option 1] and effectiveness in work [option 4]) are of immediate concern.

Cognitive level: Analysis

Nursing process: Assessment

NCLEX: Safe and Effective Care Environment

See text page: 5

19. A nurse visiting a U.S. senator's office to lobby for greater insurance parity for psychobiological disorders can establish need for parity by accurately stating that approximately 1 in _____ adults per year in the United States has a diagnosable mental disorder.

Answer: 5

Rationale: An estimated 21.1% of Americans aged 18 years and older have a diagnosable mental disorder each year. This statistic is roughly equivalent to 1 in 5 adults.

Cognitive level: Knowledge

Nursing process: Implementation

NCLEX: Safe and Effective Care Environment

See text pages: 4-6

20. The nurse reading a client's medical record determines that the client's relationships with both men and women tend to be intense and unstable, with the client initially idealizing the significant other and then devaluing him or her when the individual does not meet the client's needs. Furthermore, the client experiences feelings of emptiness and resorts to self-mutilation. The aspect of mental health the nurse can assess as lacking is
   1. effectiveness in work.
   2. communication skills.
   3. productive activities.
   4. fulfilling relationships.

Answer: 4

Rationale: The information given centers on relationships with others, which are described as intense and unstable. The relationships of mentally healthy individuals are stable, satisfying, and socially integrated. Data are not present to describe work effectiveness, communication skills, or activities (options 1, 2, and 3).

Cognitive level: Analysis

Nursing process: Assessment

NCLEX: Psychosocial Integrity

See text page: 5

21. In the majority culture of the United States, the individual at greatest risk for being labeled mentally ill is
   1. one who is wealthy and goes around the city giving away $20 bills to needy individuals.
   2. one who attends a charismatic church and describes hearing God's voice speaking to her.
   3. one who always has an optimistic viewpoint about her life situation and the possibility of having her needs met.
   4. one who is usually pessimistic about possible outcomes but strives to meet personal goals.

Answer: 2

Rationale: Hearing voices is generally associated with mental illness; however, in charismatic religious groups, hearing the voice of God or a prophet is a desirable event.

In this situation cultural norms vary, making it more difficult to make an accurate *DSM-IV-TR* diagnosis. The individuals described in the other options are less likely to be labeled as mentally ill.

Cognitive level: Analysis

Nursing process: Assessment

NCLEX: Psychosocial Integrity

See text page: 12

22. To effectively use the *DSM-IV-TR* the nurse must be cognizant of the fact that this tool classifies
  1. deviant behavior.
  2. people with mental disorders.
  3. disorders that people have.
  4. present disability or distress.

Answer: 3

Rationale: The *DSM-IV-TR* classifies disorders that people have rather than people themselves. The terminology of the tool reflects this distinction by referring to individuals with a disorder rather than as a "schizophrenic" or "alcoholic," for example. Option 1: Deviant behavior is generally not considered a mental disorder. Option 4: Present disability or distress is associated with having a mental disorder.

Cognitive level: Comprehension
Nursing process: Implementation
NCLEX: Safe and Effective Care Environment
See text page: 8

23. The psychiatric nurse addresses axis I of the *DSM-IV-TR* as the focus of treatment but must also consider the presence of a long-term disorder that affects treatment. This information is accessed by noting axis
  1. II.
  2. III.
  3. IV.
  4. V.

Answer: 1

Rationale: Axis II refers to personality disorders and mental retardation. Together they constitute the classification of abnormal behavior diagnosed in the individual. Option 2: Axis III indicates any relevant general medical conditions. Option 3: Axis IV reports psychosocial and environmental problems that may affect the diagnosis, treatment, and prognosis. Option 4: Axis V is the global assessment of functioning.

Cognitive level: Comprehension
Nursing process: Assessment
NCLEX: Psychosocial Integrity
See text pages: 9, 10

24. For the psychiatric nurse whose client care focus is holistic, awareness of which *DSM-IV-TR* axes is most important?
  1. I and II
  2. III and IV
  3. V
  4. I through V

Answer: 4

Rationale: A holistic focus requires the nurse to be aware of the entire client, thus allowing more comprehensive and appropriate interventions.

Cognitive level: Application
Nursing process: Assessment
NCLEX: Psychosocial Integrity
See text page: 13

25. When the nurse providing psychoeducation about mental disorders is asked "What is the most prevalent mental disorder in the United States?" the response should be
  1. "why do you ask?"
  2. schizophrenia.
  3. affective disorders.
  4. substance abuse.

Answer: 4

Answer: The prevalence for schizophrenia is 1.1% per year. The prevalence of all affective disorders (depression, dysthymia, bipolar) is 9.5%, and the prevalence of substance abuse is 11.3%. Option 1 does not provide an answer.

Cognitive level: Knowledge
Nursing process: Implementation
NCLEX: Health Promotion and Maintenance
See text page: 7

CHAPTER 2

1. At the well-child clinic the nurse notices that a 26-month-old boy is displaying negative behavior. His mother relates that he refuses to have anything to do with toilet training and often shouts "no!" when given direction. His mother asks what might be the matter with her son. On the basis of knowledge of growth and development, the nurse should reply
  1. "He is behaving normally for his age. He is striving for independence."
  2. "He needs firmer control. He should be scolded when he tells you 'no' and is defiant."
  3. "I suspect he has a serious developmental problem because most children are toilet trained by the age of 2 years."
  4. "He seems to be developing some undesirable attitudes. A child psychologist might be able to help you develop a remedial plan."

Answer: 1

Rationale: Options 2, 3, and 4 all indicate the child's behavior is abnormal when, in fact, this behavior is typical of a child around the age of 2 years whose developmental task is to develop autonomy.

Cognitive level: Application
Nursing process: Implementation
NCLEX: Health Promotion and Maintenance
See text page: 19

2. A 26-month-old child often displays negative behavior, refuses to have anything to do with toilet training, and often shouts "no!" when given direction. By using Freud's stages of psychosexual development, the nurse would assess the child's behavior as being consistent with the stage of development termed
1. oral.
2. anal.
3. phallic.
4. genital.

Answer: 2

Rationale: The anal stage occurs from age 1 to 3 years and has as its focus toilet training and learning to delay immediate gratification. Option 2: The oral stage occurs between birth and 1 year. Options 3 and 4: The phallic stage occurs between 3 and 5 years, and the genital stage occurs between age 13 and 20 years.

Cognitive level: Application
Nursing process: Assessment
NCLEX: Health Promotion and Maintenance
See text page: 8

3. A 26-month-old child often displays negative behavior, refuses to have anything to do with toilet training, and often shouts "no!" when given direction. His mother asks the nurse what might be the matter with the child. The counseling the nurse gives the mother should be based on the premise that the child is engaged in the psychosocial crisis of
1. trust versus mistrust.
2. initiative versus guilt.
3. industry versus inferiority.
4. autonomy versus shame and doubt.

Answer: 4

Rationale: The crisis of autonomy versus shame and doubt is related to the developmental task of gaining control of self and environment, as exemplified by toilet training. This psychosocial crisis occurs during the period of early childhood. Option 1: Trust versus mistrust is the crisis of the infant. Option 2: Initiative versus guilt is the crisis of the preschool and early school-aged child. Option 3: Industry versus inferiority is the crisis of the 6- to 12-year-old child.

Cognitive level: Application
Nursing process: Assessment
NCLEX: Health Promotion and Maintenance
See text page: 19

4. A 4-year-old child seen at the well-child clinic is noted to grab toys from his sibling, saying, "I want that toy, now!" The sibling usually cries, and the child's mother becomes upset with the behavior. By using Freudian theory the nurse can interpret this behavior to the mother as being as a product of impulses originating in the
1. id.
2. ego.
3. superego.
4. preconscious.

Answer: 1

Rationale: The id operates on the pleasure principle, seeking immediate gratification of impulses. Option 2: The ego acts as a mediator of behavior and would weigh the consequences of the action, perhaps determining that taking the toy is not worth the mother's wrath. Option 3: The superego would oppose the impulsive behavior as "not nice." Option 4: The preconscious is a level of awareness.

Cognitive level: Application
Nursing process: Assessment
NCLEX: Health Promotion and Maintenance
See text pages: 16, 17

5. The mother of a 4-year-old child rewards and praises the child for helping his younger brother and for being polite and using good manners. The nurse supports the use of praise because the qualities of politeness and helpfulness will likely be internalized and become part of the child's
1. id.
2. ego.
3. superego.
4. preconscious.

Answer: 3

Rationale: The superego contains the "thou shalts," or moral standards internalized from interactions with significant others. Praise fosters internalization of desirable behaviors. Option 1: The id is the center of basic instinctual drives, and the ego is the mediator. Option 2: The ego is the problem-solving and reality-testing portion of the personality that negotiates solutions with the outside world. Option 4: The preconscious is a level of awareness from which material can be retrieved rather easily with conscious effort.

Cognitive level: Application
Nursing process: Implementation
NCLEX: Health Promotion and Maintenance
See text pages: 16, 17

6. The nurse who supports parental praise of a child who is behaving in a helpful way can hypothesize that in adulthood, when the individual behaves with politeness and helpfulness, she will feel

1. guilt.
2. anxiety.
3. unsatisfied.
4. positive self-esteem.

Answer: 4

Rationale: The individual will be living up to her ego ideal, which will result in positive feelings about herself. The other options are incorrect because each represents a negative feeling.

Cognitive level: Application
Nursing process: Implementation
NCLEX: Health Promotion and Maintenance
See text pages: 16, 17

7. A client says, "I never know the answers" or "My opinion doesn't count for much." The nurse can correctly assess that, according to Erikson, the client has had difficulty resolving the crisis of
   1. initiative versus guilt.
   2. trust versus mistrust.
   3. autonomy versus shame and doubt.
   4. generativity versus self-absorption.

Answer: 3

Rationale: These statements show severe self-doubt, indicating that the crisis of gaining control over the environment was not successfully met. Option 1: Unsuccessful resolution of the crisis of initiative versus guilt would result in feelings of guilt. Option 2: Unsuccessful resolution of the crisis of trust versus mistrust results in poor interpersonal relationships and suspicion of others. Option 4: Unsuccessful resolution of the crisis of generativity versus self-absorption results in self-absorption that limits the ability to grow as a person.

Cognitive level: Application
Nursing process: Assessment
NCLEX: Psychosocial Integrity
See text page: 19

8. Which client statement would lead the nurse to suspect that the developmental task of infancy was not successfully completed by the client?
   1. "Andy and I are very warm and close friends."
   2. "I'm afraid to allow anyone to really get to know me."
   3. "I'm always absolutely right, so don't bother saying more."
   4. "I'm so ashamed because I didn't do it correctly in the first place."

Answer: 2

Rationale: According to Erikson the developmental task of infancy is the development of trust. Option 2 is the only statement clearly showing lack of ability to trust others. Option 1 suggests the developmental task of infancy was successfully completed. Option 3 suggests rigidity rather than mistrust. Option 4 suggests failure to resolve the crisis of initiative versus guilt.

Cognitive level: Analysis
Nursing process: Assessment
NCLEX: Health Promotion and Maintenance
See text page: 19

9. The nurse caring for a client makes the assessment that the client is suspicious of others and frequently engages in manipulation of others. To plan care, the nurse should consider these traits as being related to Freud's
   1. oral stage.
   2. anal stage.
   3. phallic stage.
   4. genital stage.

Answer: 1

Rationale: Each of the behaviors mentioned develops as the result of attitudes formed during the oral stage, when an infant first learns to relate to the environment. Option 2: Anal stage traits include stinginess, stubbornness, orderliness, or their opposites. Option 3: Phallic stage traits include flirtatiousness, pride, vanity, difficulty with authority figures, and difficulties with sexual identity. Option 4: Genital stage traits include the ability to form satisfying sexual and emotional relationships with members of the opposite sex, emancipation from parents, a strong sense of personal identity, or the opposites of these traits.

Cognitive level: Application
Nursing process: Planning
NCLEX: Psychosocial Integrity
See text page: 18

10. The nurse notes that an assigned client expresses the wish to be taken care of and that the client often behaves in a helpless fashion. The client can be assessed as having needs related to the stage of psychosexual development termed the
    1. latency stage.
    2. phallic stage.
    3. anal stage.
    4. oral stage.

Answer: 4

Rationale: Fixation at the oral stage sometimes produces dependent infantile behaviors in adults. Option 1: Latency fixations often result in difficulty identifying with others and developing social skills, resulting in a sense of inadequacy and inferiority. Option 2:

Phallic fixations result in having difficulty with authority figures and poor sexual identity. Option 3: Anal fixation sometimes results in retentiveness, rigidity, messiness, destructiveness, and cruelty.

Cognitive level: Application
Nursing process: Assessment
NCLEX: Health Promotion and Maintenance
See text page: 18

11. A is a 55-year-old retiree who volunteers 5 days a week helping with Meals on Wheels, coaching teen sports, and doing church visitation. B is a 58-year-old retiree who laughs at A and says, "I'm too busy taking care of myself to volunteer. I don't care much about doing good for others." These behaviors can be assessed as showing the difference between
    1. trust and mistrust.
    2. industry and inferiority.
    3. intimacy and isolation.
    4. generativity and self-absorption.

Answer: 4
Rationale: Both men are in middle adulthood, when the developmental crisis to be resolved is generativity versus self-absorption. A exemplifies generativity; B embodies self-absorption. Option 1: This developmental crisis would show a contrast between relating to others in a trusting fashion or being suspicious and lacking trust. Option 2: Failure to negotiate this developmental crisis would result in a sense of inferiority or difficulty learning and working as opposed to the ability to work competently. Option 3: Behaviors that would be contrasted would be emotional isolation and the ability to love and commit oneself.

Cognitive level: Application
Nursing process: Assessment
NCLEX: Health Promotion and Maintenance
See text page: 19

12. The student nurse notes that a client uses a number of behaviors designed to relieve anxiety. The student asks the coassigned staff nurse if ego defense mechanisms and security operations are identical. The nurse should explain that, although both are unconsciously determined and designed to relieve anxiety, the major difference is that
    1. defense mechanisms are always intrapsychic and not observable.
    2. defense mechanisms always lead to arrested personal development.
    3. security operations are interpersonal relationship activities.
    4. security operations are masterminded by the id and superego.

Answer: 3
Rationale: Sullivan's theory explains that security operations are interpersonal relationship activities designed to relieve anxiety. Because they are interpersonal in nature they can be observed. Option 1: Defense mechanisms are unconscious and automatic. Repression is entirely intrapsychic, but other mechanisms result in observable behaviors. Option 2: Frequent, continued use of many defense mechanisms often results in reality distortion and interference with healthy adjustment and emotional development. Occasional use of defense mechanisms is considered normal and does not markedly interfere with development. Option 4: Security operations are ego centered.

Cognitive level: Application
Nursing process: Implementation
NCLEX: Health Promotion and Maintenance
See text pages: 17, 18

13. A student nurse tells the clinical instructor, "I've found that I do not need to interact with my assigned clients. I learn what I need to know simply by observing them." The instructor can best interpret the nursing implications of Sullivan's theory to the student by responding
    1. "Nurses cannot be isolated from the therapeutic situation. We need to interact with clients to provide opportunities for them to practice interpersonal skills."
    2. "Observing client interactions can provide sufficient data to formulate priority nursing diagnoses and appropriate interventions."
    3. "I wonder how accurate your assessment of the client's needs hierarchy can be if you do not interact with the client."
    4. "It is important to note client behavioral changes because these signify changes in personality."

Answer: 1
Rationale: Sullivan believed that the nurse's role includes educating clients and assisting them in developing effective interpersonal relationships. Mutuality, respect for the client, unconditional acceptance, and empathy are cornerstones of Sullivan's theory. These cornerstones cannot be demonstrated by the nurse who does not interact with the client. Option 2: Observations provide only objective data. Priority nursing diagnoses usually cannot be accurately established without subjective data from the client. Option 3: This response pertains to Maslow's theory. Option 4: This response pertains to behavioral theory.

Cognitive level: Application
Nursing process: Implementation
NCLEX: Safe and Effective Care Environment
See text pages: 18, 19

14. A psychiatric technician mentions that little of what takes place on the behavioral health unit seems to be theory based. The nurse can enlighten the technician by citing the fact that many of Sullivan's theoretic constructs are used in
   1. the ongoing use of restraint and seclusion as behavior management tools.
   2. the structure of the therapeutic milieu of most behavioral health units.
   3. assessment tools based on age-appropriate versus arrested behaviors.
   4. the method nurses use to determine the best sequence for nursing actions.

Answer: 2

Rationale: The structure of the therapeutic environment has as foci an accepting atmosphere and provision of opportunities for practicing interpersonal skills. Both constructs are directly attributable to Sullivan's theory of interpersonal relationships. Option 1: Sullivan's interpersonal theory did not specifically consider use of restraint or seclusion. Option 3: Assessment based on developmental level is more the result of Erikson's theories. Option 4: Sequencing nursing actions based on client priority needs is related to Maslow's need hierarchy.

Cognitive level: Application
Nursing process: Implementation
NCLEX: Safe and Effective Care Environment
See text pages: 18, 19

15. When the nurse uses Maslow's needs hierarchy to plan care for a client who is psychotic, which client problem below will receive priority?
   1. Refusal to eat
   2. Feelings of alienation from family
   3. Reluctance to participate in unit social activities
   4. Need to be taught about medication action and side effects

Answer: 1

Rationale: The need for food is a physiological need; therefore it takes priority over psychological or meta-needs in care planning.

Cognitive level: Analysis
Nursing process: Planning
NCLEX: Safe and Effective Care Environment
See text pages: 20, 21

16. Operant conditioning will be used to encourage speech in a child who is nearly mute. Which technique would the nurse include in the treatment plan?
   1. Spanking the child for silence
   2. Having the child observe others talking
   3. Giving the child a small candy for speaking

4. Teaching the child relaxation techniques, then coaxing speech

Answer: 3

Rationale: Operant conditioning involves giving positive reinforcement for a desired behavior. Presuming the child likes candy, candy will reinforce speech. Option 1 describes an aversive therapy technique. Option 2 describes modeling. Option 4 is an example of systematic desensitization.

Cognitive level: Application
Nursing process: Planning
NCLEX: Safe and Effective Care Environment
See text page: 22

17. The mother of a young adult client who has schizophrenia tearfully asks the nurse what she could have done differently to prevent her child's illness. The most reassuring response for the nurse would be
   1. "Although schizophrenia is caused by impaired interpersonal relationships between parents and the child, try not to feel guilty. No one can predict how a child will respond to parental guidance."
   2. "Most of the damage is done, but there is still hope. By changing your parenting style, you can help your child learn to cope more effectively with the environment."
   3. "Schizophrenia is a biological illness not unlike diabetes and heart disease. You are not to blame for your child's illness."
   4. "Most mental illnesses result from genetic inheritance. Your genes are more at fault than your parenting."

Answer: 3

Rationale: Clients and families need reassurance that the major mental disorders are biological in origin and are not the "fault" of parents. Knowing the biological nature of the disorder relieves feelings of guilt over being responsible for the illness. Option 1 is neither wholly accurate nor reassuring. Option 2 falls short of being reassuring. Option 4 places the burden of having faulty genes on the shoulders of the parents.

Cognitive level: Application
Nursing process: Implementation
NCLEX: Health Promotion and Maintenance
See text pages: 22-24

18. A nurse using Peplau's interpersonal therapy while working with an anxious, withdrawn client will plan interventions focusing on
   1. changing the client's cognitions about self.
   2. improving the client's interactional skills.
   3. reinforcing specific behaviors.
   4. liberally using medications to relieve anxiety.

Answer: 2

Rationale: The nurse-client relationship is structured to provide a model for adaptive interpersonal relationships that can be generalized to others. Option 1 would be appropriate for cognitive therapy. Option 3 would be used in behavioral therapy. Option 4 would be the focus of biological therapy.

Cognitive level: Application
Nursing process: Planning
NCLEX: Psychosocial Integrity
See text page: 24

19. Desired outcomes of a nurse assuming the role of participant observer during an interaction with a client would include (more than one answer may be correct)
    1. client anxiety level decreases
    2. nurse self-awareness is enhanced
    3. the nurse views the client as a unique individual
    4. the focus of the interaction remains client centered

Answers: 2, 3, 4

Rationale: Option 2 is a desirable outcome. Being a participant observer involves participating in an interaction with a client and simultaneously being aware of both the client's reactions and one's own reactions. Self-awareness promotes true mutuality. Option 3: Participant observation promotes viewing the client as a person with unique attributes. Seeing the client as a unique individual diminishes distortions and stereotyping. Option 4: Participant observation promotes self-awareness. The nurse who has self-awareness is able to separate his or her own needs from those of the client and remain client focused. Option 1: Although anxiety reduction would be a desirable outcome, it cannot be seen as resulting from the nurse acting as a participant observer. Other interventions would probably be necessary.

Cognitive level: Analysis
Nursing process: Planning (Outcome Identification)
NCLEX: Psychosocial Integrity
See text page: 24

20. A client tells the nurse she had psychotherapy weekly for 3 years. The client states the therapist used the techniques of free association, dream analysis, and facilitation of awareness of transference feelings to help her understand unconscious processes and foster personality change. The nurse can determine that the client was treated with
    1. short-term dynamic psychotherapy.
    2. transactional analysis.
    3. cognitive therapy.
    4. psychoanalysis.

Answer: 4

Rationale: The client described traditional psychoanalysis. Option 1: Short-term dynamic psychotherapy would last less than a year. Options 2 and 3: Neither transactional analysis nor cognitive therapy makes use of the techniques described.

Cognitive level: Application
Nursing process: Assessment
NCLEX: Psychosocial Integrity
See text page: 25

21. The nurse states "The patient is a lesbian and is experiencing severe anxiety and depression as she anticipates a problem with acceptance by her family when she reveals her sexual orientation." The nurse has formulated the client's problem from the vantage point of a therapist who uses
    1. cognitive therapy.
    2. behavioral therapy.
    3. interpersonal psychotherapy.
    4. psychodynamic psychotherapy.

Answer: 3

Rationale: By using the interpersonal model, the therapist sees the anxiety and depression as resulting from unmet interpersonal security needs. Option 1: A cognitive theory formulation would focus on faulty cognitions of the client. Option 2: A behavioral formulation would focus on changing specific behaviors of the client. Option 4: A psychodynamic formulation would focus on uncovering unconscious material that relates to the client problem.

Cognitive level: Application
Nursing process: Assessment
NCLEX: Psychosocial Integrity
See text pages: 25-28

22. The nurse psychotherapist is working with an anxious, dependent client. The therapeutic strategy most consistent with the framework of psychodynamic or psychoanalytic psychotherapy would be
    1. emphasizing medication compliance.
    2. identifying client strengths and assets.
    3. using psychoeducational materials.
    4. focusing on feelings developed by the client toward the nurse.

Answer: 4

Rationale: Positive or negative feelings of the client toward the nurse or the therapist are called transference. Transference is a psychoanalytic concept. Transference can be used to explore previously unresolved conflicts. Option 1 would be more related to biological therapy. Option 2 would be consistent with supportive psychotherapy. Option 3: Use of

195

psychoeducational materials is a common "homework" assignment used in cognitive therapy.
Cognitive level: Application
Nursing process: Implementation
NCLEX: Psychosocial Integrity
See text pages: 26, 27

23. A client tells the nurse, "I was the lone survivor in a small plane crash in which three of my business associates were killed. I got anxious and depressed and saw a counselor three times a week for 4 weeks. The therapist and I talked about my feelings about being a survivor. I'm OK now, back to being my old self." The nurse can correctly conclude that the type of therapy the client underwent was
    1. milieu therapy.
    2. psychoanalysis.
    3. behavior modification.
    4. interpersonal psychotherapy.

Answer: 4
Rationale: Interpersonal psychotherapy returned the client to his former level of functioning by helping him come to terms with the loss of friends and guilt over being a survivor. Option 1: Milieu therapy refers to environmental therapy. Option 2: Psychoanalysis would call for a long period of exploration of unconscious material. Option 3: Behavior modification would focus on changing a behavior rather than helping the client understand what is going on in his life.
Cognitive level: Application
Nursing process: Assessment
NCLEX: Psychosocial Integrity
See text page: 26

24. A cognitive strategy the nurse could use to help an excessively dependent client would be to have the client
    1. reveal his or her dreams.
    2. take prescribed medications.
    3. examine his or her thoughts about being independent.
    4. choose an applicable diagnostic label from the *DSM-IV-TR*.

Answer: 3
Rationale: Cognitive theory suggests that one's thought processes are the basis of emotions and behavior. Changing faulty learning makes development of new adaptive behaviors possible. Option 1 would be used in psychoanalytically oriented therapy. Option 2 is an intervention associated with biological therapy. Option 4 is not an appropriate intervention. Medical diagnosis is the prerogative of the medical practitioner or advanced practice registered nurse.
Cognitive level: Application

Nursing process: Implementation
NCLEX: Psychosocial Integrity
See text pages: 26, 27

25. A 39-year-old businesswoman and single parent of three is experiencing many feelings of inadequacy in her job and family situation since her 16-year-old daughter ran away several weeks ago. She seeks the help of a therapist specializing in cognitive therapy. The nurse psychotherapist who uses cognitive therapy will treat the client by
    1. focusing on unconscious mental processes.
    2. negatively reinforcing an undesirable behavior.
    3. discussing ego states.
    4. helping her identify and change faulty thinking.

Answer: 4
Rationale: Cognitive therapy emphasizes the importance of changing erroneous ways people think about themselves. Once faulty thinking is changed, the individual's behavior changes. Option 1 describes a psychoanalytic approach. Option 2 describes behavior modification, and option 3 relates to transactional analysis.
Cognitive level: Application
Nursing process: Implementation
NCLEX: Psychosocial Integrity
See text pages: 26, 27

26. A client states "I'm going to be engaging in cognitive therapy. What can I expect from the sessions?" Which responses by the nurse would be appropriate? (More than one answer may be correct.)
    1. "The therapist will be active and questioning."
    2. "You may be given homework assignments."
    3. "The therapist will help you look at ideas and beliefs you have about yourself."
    4. "The goal is to increase your subjectivity about the thoughts that govern your behavior."

Answers: 1, 2, 3
Rationale: Option 1: Cognitive therapists are active rather than passive during therapy sessions because they help clients reality test their thinking. Option 2: Homework assignments are given and are completed outside the therapy sessions. Homework is usually discussed at the next therapy session. Option 3: The goal of cognitive therapy is to assist the client in identifying inaccurate cognitions and in reality testing and formulating new, accurate cognitions. Option 4: The desired outcome of cognitive therapy is to assist the client in increasing his or her objectivity, not subjectivity, about the cognitions that influence behavior.
Cognitive level: Application
Nursing process: Implementation
NCLEX: Psychosocial Integrity
See text pages: 26, 27

196

27. A college student has been invited to be the best man at the wedding of a college friend who lives across the country. The wedding is in 6 weeks. He must travel by plane but is afraid of flying. A nurse suggests seeing a therapist. What type of therapy would the nurse be most likely to recommend?
   1. Psychoanalysis
   2. Milieu therapy
   3. Systematic desensitization
   4. Short-term dynamic therapy

Answer: 3

Rationale: Systematic desensitization is a type of therapy aimed at extinguishing a specific behavior, such as the fear of flying. Options 1 and 4: Psychoanalysis and short-term dynamic therapy are aimed at uncovering conflicts. Option 2: Milieu therapy involves environmental factors. None of these would be likely to cause behavioral change in 6 weeks.

Cognitive level: Analysis
Nursing process: Planning
NCLEX: Psychosocial Integrity
See text page: 29

28. The advanced practice nurse concludes a client would profit from the type of therapy in which peers and interdisciplinary staff all have a voice in determining the level of client privileges. The nurse would arrange for
   1. milieu therapy.
   2. cognitive therapy.
   3. short-term dynamic therapy.
   4. systematic desensitization.

Answer: 1

Rationale: Milieu therapy is based on the idea that all members of the environment contribute to the planning and functioning of the setting. The other therapies are all individual therapies that do not fit the description given.

Cognitive level: Application
Nursing process: Planning
NCLEX: Safe and Effective Care Environment
See text pages: 30, 31

29. A client expresses suicidal ideation and admits to having a plan for committing suicide.
   The advanced practice nurse assesses the client as being at risk for suicide. In arranging for the client's admission to the inpatient unit, the nurse has used principles of
   1. a practice beyond the scope of nursing licensure.
   2. interpersonal relationship therapy.
   3. short-term dynamic therapy.
   4. milieu therapy.

Answer: 4

Rationale: One aspect of milieu therapy involves providing safe and effective care environments for clients. Option 1: The nurse's action is within the scope of nursing practice. Option 2: The information provided is not sufficient to determine if principles of interpersonal relationship therapy were used. Option 3: The information given does not describe short-term dynamic therapy.

Cognitive level: Application
Nursing process: Implementation
NCLEX: Safe and Effective Care Environment
See text pages: 30, 31

30. A nurse sees the nursing theory of Dorothea Orem as providing a suitable framework for practice. This nurse would plan care to
   1. acknowledge the client's suffering related to illness.
   2. support client coping strategies to enhance adaptation.
   3. assist the client to discover and use stress reduction strategies.
   4. promote self-care activities of the seriously and persistently mentally ill client.

Answer: 4

Rationale: The focus of Orem's theory suggests that the goal of care for clients should be to maximize client self-care activities and abilities. Option 1 is associated with Benner's caring theory. Option 2 is emphasized in the adaptation theory of Sister Calista Roy. Option 3: Betty Neuman's theory focuses on the impact of internal and external stressors of the equilibrium of the client.

Cognitive level: Analysis
Nursing process: Planning
NCLEX: Psychosocial Integrity
See text page: 25

31. The nurse providing cognitive therapy for a client who believes she is stupid would evaluate cognitive intervention as effective when the client states
   1. "I'm disappointed in my lack of ability."
   2. "Sometimes I do stupid things."
   3. "Things always go wrong for me."
   4. "I always fail when I try new things."

Answer: 2

Rationale: "I'm stupid" is an irrational thought. A more rational thought is "Sometimes I do stupid things." The latter thinking promotes emotional self-control. Options 1, 3, and 4 reflect irrational thinking.

Cognitive level: Evaluation
Nursing process: Evaluation
NCLEX: Psychosocial Integrity
See text page: 27

1. A client asks the nurse, "What are neurotransmitters? My doctor says they are at the root of my problem." The best reply would be
   1. "You must feel relieved to know that your problem has a physical basis."
   2. "It is a rather high-level concept to explain. Perhaps you should ask the doctor to tell you more."
   3. "Neurotransmitters are substances we eat daily that influence the brain functions of memory and mood."
   4. "Neurotransmitters are chemicals manufactured in the brain that are responsible for passing messages between brain cells."

Answer: 4
Rationale: Option 4 gives the most accurate information. Neurotransmitters are chemical substances that function as neuromessengers. They are released from the axon terminal and diffuse across the synapse and attach to specialized receptors on the postsynaptic neuron. Option 1 does not answer the client's question. Option 2 does not answer the client's question and is somewhat demeaning. Option 3 provides untrue, misleading information.
Cognitive level: Application
Nursing process: Implementation
NCLEX: Psychosocial Integrity
See text pages: 38-40

2. The mother of an adolescent client with obsessive-compulsive disorder tells the nurse, "My daughter's doctor wants her to be in a research study and to have a PET [positron emission tomography] scan. I do not want her to have to go through any tests that are painful. What should I do?" The best reply for the nurse would be
   1. "The doctor has made the diagnosis, but having a PET scan would confirm it."
   2. "You might want to ask who will pay for the PET scan because they are very expensive."
   3. "PET scans involve an injection and lying still while a machine visualizes brain activity."
   4. "PET scans involve passing an electrical current through the brain and can be uncomfortable."

Answer: 3
Rationale: The mother is seeking information about PET scans. Option 3 is the only option that provides factual information on which the mother can base a decision.
Cognitive level: Application
Nursing process: Implementation
NCLEX: Psychosocial Integrity
See text pages: 44-46

3. The physician mentions that a client's dementia may be associated with either Alzheimer's disease or multiple infarcts. For the physician to make a differential diagnosis with the least expensive test, the nurse should expect to prepare the client for a
   1. computed tomography (CT) scan.
   2. magnetic resonance imaging (MRI) scan.
   3. PET scan.
   4. single-photon emission computed tomography (SPECT) scan.

Answer: 1
Rationale: The CT scan could be expected to show the presence or absence of cortical atrophy, ventricular enlargement, and areas of infarct, information that would be helpful to the physician. The CT scan is the least expensive of the imaging techniques listed.
Cognitive level: Application
Nursing process: Planning
NCLEX: Physiological Integrity
See text page: 44

4. A client has delusions and hallucinations. Before beginning treatment with psychotropic drugs, the physician wishes to rule out the presence of a brain tumor. For which test will the nurse need to prepare the client?
   1. CT or MRI scan
   2. PET or SPECT scan
   3. Cerebral arteriogram
   4. Neuronal depolarization

Answer: 1
Rationale: CT and MRI scans visualize neoplasms and other structural abnormalities. Options 2 and 3: A scan giving information about brain function is not called for, and an arteriogram would not be appropriate. Option 4: Neuronal depolarization is not a diagnostic test.
Cognitive level: Application
Nursing process: Planning
NCLEX: Physiological Integrity
See text page: 44

5. A client who is being admitted for depression should be assessed for disturbances in circadian rhythms. The question that best implements this assessment is
   1. "What time of day do you feel worst and when do you feel best?"
   2. "Do you ever see or hear things that others do not?"
   3. "How would you describe your thinking?"
   4. "Would you say your memory is failing?"

Answer: 1

Rationale: Mood changes throughout the day are related to circadian rhythms. Questions about sleep pattern would also be relevant to circadian rhythms. Option 2 is relevant to the assessment for illusions and hallucinations. Option 3 is relevant to the assessment of thought processes. Option 4 is relevant to the assessment of memory.

Cognitive level: Application
Nursing process: Assessment
NCLEX: Psychosocial Integrity
See text pages: 37, 38

6. When the wife of a client with schizophrenia asks which neurotransmitter is implicated in the development of schizophrenia, the nurse should state "The current thinking is that the thought disturbances are related to
   1. excess dopamine."
   2. serotonin deficiency."
   3. histamine decrease."
   4. increased γ-aminobutyric acid [GABA]."

Answer: 1

Rationale: Dopamine plays a role in integration of thoughts and emotions, and excess dopamine is implicated in the thought disturbances of schizophrenia. Option 2: Serotonin deficiency is implicated in some forms of depression. Option 3: Histamine decrease is associated with depression. Option 4: Increased GABA is associated with anxiety reduction.

Cognitive level: Application
Nursing process: Implementation
NCLEX: Physiological Integrity
See text page: 40

7. Ongoing assessment and outcome planning for a client with schizophrenia are facilitated if the nurse understands that the medication prescribed to reduce the client's symptoms targets the neurotransmitter
   1. dopamine.
   2. serotonin.
   3. norepinephrine.
   4. acetylcholine.

Answer: 1

Rationale: Dopamine is a neurotransmitter found in areas of the brain responsible for decision making and integrating thoughts and emotions. Knowing this, the nurse can formulate related outcomes. Because dopamine is a neurotransmitter found in the extrapyramidal system, the nurse can also provide ongoing assessment for movement disorders. Option 2: Serotonin is the target of selective serotonin reuptake inhibitors (SSRIs). Option 3: Norepinephrine is targeted by selected anti-depressant medications. Option 4: Acetylcholine is affected by drugs with cholinergic effects.

Cognitive level: Application
Nursing process: Planning
NCLEX: Physiological Integrity
See text page: 50

8. The nurse should provide ongoing assessment for a client receiving medication that potentiates the action of GABA relative to
   1. reduced anxiety.
   2. improved memory.
   3. more organized thinking.
   4. fewer sensory perceptual alterations.

Answer: 1

Rationale: Increased levels of GABA reduce anxiety; thus any potentiation of GABA action should result in anxiety reduction. Option 2: Acetylcholine and substance P, rather than GABA, are associated with memory enhancement. Option 3: Thought disorganization is associated with dopamine rather than GABA. Option 4: GABA is not associated with sensory perceptual alterations.

Cognitive level: Application
Nursing process: Planning
NCLEX: Physiological Integrity
See text page: 40

9. On the basis of current knowledge of neurotransmitter effects, the nurse could anticipate that the treatment plan for a client with memory difficulties might include orders to administer medication designed to
   1. inhibit GABA.
   2. increase dopamine at receptor sites.
   3. decrease dopamine at receptor sites.
   4. prevent destruction of acetylcholine.

Answer: 4

Rationale: Increased acetylcholine plays a role in learning and memory. Preventing destruction of acetylcholine by acetylcholinesterase would result in higher levels of acetylcholine, with the potential for improved memory. Option 1: GABA is known to affect anxiety level rather than memory. Option 2: Increased dopamine would cause symptoms associated with schizophrenia or mania rather than improve memory. Option 3: Decreasing dopamine at receptor sites is associated with Parkinson's disease rather than improving memory.

Cognitive level: Application
Nursing process: Planning
NCLEX: Physiological Integrity
See text page: 40

199

10. A client demonstrates disorganized and delusional thinking. The tentative diagnosis is schizophrenia. The nurse can anticipate that a PET scan would be most likely to show dysfunction in the part of the brain called the
 1. temporal lobe.
 2. cerebellum.
 3. brainstem.
 4. frontal lobe.

Answer: 4

Rationale: The frontal lobe is responsible for intellectual functioning. Option 1: The temporal lobe is responsible for the sensation of hearing. Option 2: The cerebellum regulates skeletal muscle coordination and equilibrium. Option 3: The brainstem regulates internal organs.

Cognitive level: Analysis
Nursing process: Assessment
NCLEX: Physiological Integrity
See text pages: 43-47

11. The nurse should assess clients taking a drug known to have anticholinergic properties for symptoms of inhibition of function of the
 1. parasympathetic nervous system.
 2. sympathetic nervous system.
 3. reticular activating system.
 4. medulla oblongata.

Answer: 1

Rationale: Acetylcholine is the neurotransmitter found in high concentration in the parasympathetic nervous system. When acetylcholine action is inhibited by anticholinergic drugs, parasympathetic symptoms such as blurred vision, dry mouth, constipation, and urinary retention appear. Options 2, 3, and 4: The functions of these parts of the nervous system are not affected by anticholinergics.

Cognitive level: Application
Nursing process: Assessment
NCLEX: Physiological Integrity
See text page: 51

12. The nurse can explain the therapeutic action of monoamine oxidase (MAO) inhibitors as blocking neurotransmitter reuptake, causing
 1. increased concentration of neurotransmitter in the synaptic gap.
 2. decreased concentration of neurotransmitter in the synaptic gap.
 3. destruction of receptor sites.
 4. limbic system stimulation.

Answer: 1

Rationale: If the reuptake of a substance is inhibited, it accumulates in the synaptic gap and its concentration increases, permitting ease of transmission of impulses across the synaptic gap. Normal transmission of impulses across synaptic gaps is consistent with normal rather than depressed mood. The other options are not associated with blocking neurotransmitter reuptake.

Cognitive level: Comprehension
Nursing process: Implementation
NCLEX: Physiological Integrity
See text page: 41

13. A client taking medication for his mental illness develops a profound sense of restlessness and an uncontrollable need to be in motion. The nurse can correctly hypothesize that these symptoms are related to the drug's
 1. dopamine-blocking effects.
 2. anticholinergic effects.
 3. endocrine-stimulating effects.
 4. ability to stimulate spinal nerves.

Answer: 1

Rationale: Medication that blocks dopamine is often seen to produce disturbances of movement such as akathisia because dopamine affects neurons involved in both thought processes and movement regulation. Option 2: Anticholinergic effects include dry mouth, blurred vision, urinary retention, and constipation. Options 3 and 4: Akathisia is not caused by endocrine stimulation or spinal nerve stimulation.

Cognitive level: Application
Nursing process: Assessment
NCLEX: Physiological Integrity
See text pages: 50, 51

14. A nurse makes the assessment that the client demonstrates anxiety and a number of responses consistent with sympathetic nervous system stimulation. The nurse would suspect the presence of a high concentration of brain
 1. GABA.
 2. histamine.
 3. acetylcholine.
 4. norepinephrine.

Answer: 4

Rationale: Norepinephrine is the neurotransmitter associated with sympathetic nervous system stimulation, preparing the individual for "fight or flight." Option 1: GABA is a mediator of anxiety level. Option 2: A high concentration of histamine is associated with an inflammatory response. Option 3: A high concentration of acetylcholine is associated with parasympathetic nervous system stimulation.

Cognitive level: Application
Nursing process: Assessment
NCLEX: Physiological Integrity
See text page: 40

15. A client's laboratory reports show marked deficiencies of both serum sodium and potassium. On the basis of this finding, the nurse should assess the client for symptoms of electrical conduction problems
   1. throughout the body.
   2. in skeletal muscle function only.
   3. in the central nervous system only.
   4. in the cardiac conduction system only.

Answer: 1
Rationale: The brain is involved in mental activity, maintenance of homeostasis, and control of all physiological functions. Brain neuronal activity involves conducting electrical impulses from one end of the cell to the other, involving inward movement of sodium followed by outward movement of potassium. Without sufficient sodium and potassium, electrical conduction of impulses is impaired. Physical and mental symptoms result.

Cognitive level: Application
Nursing process: Assessment
NCLEX: Physiological Integrity
See text page: 38

16. A client is seen in the emergency department for symptoms of acute anxiety related to the death of her mother in an automobile accident 2 hours ago. To prepare a care plan, the nurse must correctly hypothesize that the client will need teaching about a drug from the group called
   1. tricyclic antidepressants.
   2. antimanic drugs.
   3. benzodiazepines.
   4. neuroleptic drugs.

Answer: 3
Rationale: Benzodiazepines provide anxiety relief. Option 1: Tricyclic antidepressants are used to treat symptoms of depression. Option 2: Antimania drugs are used to treat bipolar disorder. Option 4: Neuroleptic drugs are major tranquilizers and are used to treat psychosis.

Cognitive level: Application
Nursing process: Planning
NCLEX: Physiological Integrity
See text pages: 57, 58

17. A client is hospitalized for severe depression. Of the medications listed below, the nurse can expect to provide the client with teaching about
   1. clozapine (Clozaril).
   2. chlordiazepoxide (Librium).
   3. tacrine (Cognex).
   4. fluoxetine (Prozac).

Answer: 4
Rationale: Fluoxetine is an SSRI. It is an antidepressant that blocks the reuptake of serotonin with few anticholinergic and sedating side effects. Option 1: Clozapine is an antipsychotic. Option 2: Chlordiazepoxide is an anxiolytic. Option 3: Tacrine is used to treat Alzheimer's disease.

Cognitive level: Application
Nursing process: Planning
NCLEX: Physiological Integrity
See text page: 55

18. A client hospitalized with a mood disorder displays an elevated, unstable mood, aggressiveness, agitation, talkativeness, and irritability. The nurse can begin care planning based on the expectation that the psychiatrist is most likely to prescribe a medication classified as a(n)
   1. anticholinergic.
   2. mood stabilizer.
   3. psychostimulant.
   4. antidepressant.

Answer: 2
Rationale: The symptoms describe a manic attack. Mania is effectively treated by the antimania drug lithium and selected anticonvulsants such as carbamazepine, valproic acid, and lamotrigine. No drugs from the other classifications listed are effective in the treatment of mania.

Cognitive level: Application
Nursing process: Planning
NCLEX: Physiological Integrity
See text page: 53

19. The *Physician's Desk Reference* gives the nurse information that a certain drug causes muscarinic receptor blockade. This alerts the nurse to assess the client for
   1. gynecomastia.
   2. pseudoparkinsonism.
   3. orthostatic hypotension.
   4. dry mouth.

Answer: 4
Rationale: Muscarinic receptor blockade includes atropinelike side effects such as dry mouth, blurred vision, and constipation. Option 1: Gynecomastia is

201

associated with decreased prolactin levels. Option 2: Movement defects are associated with dopamine blockade. Option 3: Orthostatic hypotension is associated with α_1 antagonism.

Cognitive level: Application
Nursing process: Assessment
NCLEX: Physiological Integrity
See text page: 51

20. When the nurse understands that clozapine preferentially blocks dopamine receptors in the limbic system rather than in the basal ganglia, the nurse will plan to assess the client for
   1. seizures.
   2. marked motor disturbances.
   3. strong suicidal tendencies.
   4. greatly increased appetite.

Answer: 1
Rationale: Clozapine has the potential for inducing convulsions in approximately 3% of clients. All clients receiving this drug should be monitored for seizure activity. Option 2: The blockade of dopamine receptors in the basal ganglia is responsible for movement disorders associated with administration of standard antipsychotics. Clozapine selectively targets the limbic system, which is not involved in movement. Option 3: Clozapine therapy is not associated with producing suicidal ideation. Option 4: Clozapine therapy is not associated with increased appetite.

Cognitive level: Application
Nursing process: Assessment
NCLEX: Physiological Integrity
See text page: 52

21. A client has begun phenothiazine therapy. What teaching should the nurse provide related to the drug's strong dopaminergic effect?
   1. Chew sugarless gum
   2. Eat plenty of roughage
   3. Arise slowly from bed
   4. Report muscle stiffness

Answer: 4
Rationale: Phenothiazines block dopamine receptors in both the limbic system and basal ganglia. The movement disorder dystonia is likely to occur early in the course of treatment and is often heralded by sensations of muscle stiffness. Early intervention with anti-Parkinson medication can increase the client's comfort and prevent dystonic reactions.

Cognitive level: Application
Nursing process: Implementation
NCLEX: Physiological Integrity
See text pages: 50, 51

22. During the administration of the abnormal involuntary movement scale, the nurse should
   1. have the client sit with hands over the head.
   2. ask the client to protrude the tongue.
   3. have the client lie prone on the floor.
   4. direct the client to touch the nose with the tip of each finger.

Answer: 2
Rationale: The client is asked to protrude the tongue for several seconds to enable the nurse to assess for fine movements of the tongue, a possible indicator of tardive dyskinesia related to long-term phenothiazine therapy. Administration of the abnormal involuntary movement scale does not call for any of the other client actions.

Cognitive level: Application
Nursing process: Implementation
NCLEX: Health Promotion and Maintenance
See text page: 50

23. The client tells the nurse "My doctor prescribed Prozac [fluoxetine]. I suppose I'll have to get used to the side effects like the ones I experienced when I was taking Tofranil [imipramine]." The nurse's reply should be based on the knowledge that fluoxetine is a(n)
   1. tricyclic antidepressant.
   2. MAO inhibitor.
   3. SSRI.
   4. selective norepinephrine reuptake inhibitor.

Answer: 3
Rationale: Fluoxetine is an SSRI and will not produce the same side effects as imipramine, a tricyclic antidepressant. The client will probably not experience dry mouth, constipation, or orthostatic hypotension.

Cognitive level: Application
Nursing process: Implementation
NCLEX: Physiological Integrity
See text page: 55

24. A nurse can anticipate that anticholinergic side effects may occur when a client is taking
   1. lithium.
   2. risperidone.
   3. buspirone.
   4. fluphenazine.

Answer: 4
Rationale: Fluphenazine, a first-generation antipsychotic, exerts muscarinic blockade, resulting in dry mouth, blurred vision, constipation, and urinary retention. Option 1: Lithium therapy is more often associated with fluid balance problems, including polydipsia,

202

polyuria, and edema. Option 2: Risperidone therapy is more often associated with movement disorders, orthostatic hypotension, and sedation. Option 3: Buspirone is associated with anxiety reduction without major side effects.

Cognitive level: Application
Nursing process: Planning
NCLEX: Physiological Integrity
See text pages: 50, 51

25. The teaching plan for a client taking clozapine should include the following instruction:
    1. Report sore throat and fever immediately.
    2. Avoid foods high in polyunsaturated fats.
    3. Practice unprotected sex.
    4. Use over-the-counter preparations for rashes.

Answer: 1
Rationale: Clozapine therapy may produce agranulocytosis; therefore signs of infection should be immediately reported to the physician. In addition, the client should have white blood cell levels measured weekly. The other options are not relevant to clozapine administration.
Cognitive level: Application
Nursing process: Planning
NCLEX: Health Promotion and Maintenance
See text page: 52

26. The nurse is caring for clients taking various medications, including buspirone (Buspar), haloperidol (Haldol), carbamazepine (Tegretol), trazodone (Desyrel), phenelzine (Nardil), and risperidone (Risperdal). The nurse must check to ensure that a special diet has been ordered for each client receiving
    1. buspirone and haloperidol.
    2. trazodone and carbamazepine.
    3. phenelzine.
    4. risperidone.

Answer: 3
Rationale: Clients taking phenelzine, an MAO inhibitor, must be on a tyramine-free diet to prevent hypertensive crisis.
Cognitive level: Application
Nursing process: Planning
NCLEX: Safe and Effective Care Environment
See text pages: 55, 56

27. The nurse must tell a client taking a drug that acts by inhibiting MAO to avoid certain foods and drugs or risk
    1. hypotensive shock.
    2. hypertensive crisis.
    3. cardiac dysrhythmia.
    4. cardiogenic shock.

Answer: 2
Rationale: Clients taking MAO inhibiting drugs must be on a tyramine-free diet to prevent hypertensive crisis. In the presence of MAO inhibitors, tyramine is not destroyed by the liver and in high levels produces intense vasoconstriction, resulting in elevated blood pressure.
Cognitive level: Application
Nursing process: Planning
NCLEX: Health Promotion and Maintenance/Safe and Effective Care Environment
See text pages: 55, 56

28. The nurse caring for a client taking SSRIs will develop evaluation parameters and outcome criteria related to
    1. mood improvement.
    2. logical thought processes.
    3. reduced levels of motor activity.
    4. increased extrapyramidal symptoms.

Answer: 1
Rationale: SSRIs affect mood, relieving depression in many cases. Option 2: SSRIs do not act to reduce thought disorders. Option 3: SSRIs reduce depression but have little effect on motor hyperactivity. Option 4: SSRIs do not produce extrapyramidal symptoms.
Cognitive level: Evaluation
Nursing process: Evaluation
NCLEX: Physiological Integrity
See text page: 50

29. A client's husband is a chemist. He asks the nurse the action by which SSRIs lift depression. The nurse should explain that SSRIs
    1. make more serotonin available at the synaptic gap.
    2. destroy increased amounts of neurotransmitter.
    3. increase production of acetylcholine and dopamine.
    4. block muscarinic and α_1 norepinephrine receptors.

Answer: 1
Rationale: Depression is thought to be related to lowered availability of the neurotransmitter serotonin. SSRIs act by blocking reuptake of serotonin, leave a higher concentration available at the synaptic cleft. Option 2: SSRIs actually prevent destruction of serotonin. Option 3: SSRIs have no effect on acetylcholine and dopamine production. Option 4: SSRIs do not produce muscarinic or α_1 norepinephrine blockade.
Cognitive level: Application
Nursing process: Implementation
NCLEX: Health Promotion and Maintenance
See text page: 55

203

30. A client has taken a number of conventional and standard antipsychotic drugs over the years. The physician, concerned about the client's lack of response to these drugs and the development of tardive dyskinesia, has prescribed risperidone. The nurse planning care for the client must consider that atypical antipsychotics
1. are more readily available.
2. are of higher potency.
3. are less costly.
4. produce fewer motor side effects.

Answer: 4

Rationale: Atypical antipsychotic drugs often exert their action on the limbic system rather than the basal ganglia. The limbic system is not involved in motor disturbances. Option 1: These drugs are not more readily available. Option 2: These drugs are not considered to be of higher potency; rather, they have different modes of action. Option 3: The atypical antipsychotic drugs tend to be more expensive.

Cognitive level: Application
Nursing process: Planning
NCLEX: Physiological Integrity
See text page: 51

31. The laboratory reports for a client who is taking clozapine show a white blood cell count of 3000 mm^3 and a granulocyte count of 1500 mm^3. The nurse should
1. give the next dose as ordered.
2. report the laboratory results to the physician.
3. repeat the laboratory tests.
4. give aspirin and force fluids.

Answer: 2

Rationale: These laboratory values indicate the possibility of agranulocytosis, a serious side effect of clozapine therapy. These results must be immediately reported to the physician. Option 1: The drug should be withheld because the physician will discontinue it. Option 3: The physician may repeat the test, but in the meantime the drug should be withheld. Option 4: These measures are less important than stopping administration of the drug.

Cognitive level: Application
Nursing process: Implementation
NCLEX: Safe and Effective Care Environment
See text page: 52

32. The nurse administering psychotropic medications should be prepared to intervene when giving a drug that blocks the attachment of norepinephrine to α_1 receptors because the client may experience

1. an increase in psychotic symptoms.
2. hypertensive crisis.
3. orthostatic hypotension.
4. severe appetite disturbance.

Answer: 3

Rationale: Sympathetic mediated vasoconstriction is essential for maintaining normal blood pressure in the upright position. Blockage of α_1 receptors leads to vasodilation and orthostatic hypotension. Orthostatic hypotension may cause fainting and falls. Clients should be taught ways of minimizing this phenomenon.

Cognitive level: Application
Nursing process: Implementation
NCLEX: Physiological Integrity
See text page: 50

33. A nurse is caring for four clients who are receiving clozapine, lithium, fluoxetine, and venlafaxine, respectively. In which client should the nurse be most alert for alterations in cardiac or cerebral electrical conductivity and fluid and electrolyte imbalance?
1. The client receiving lithium (Lithobid)
2. The client receiving clozapine (Clozaril)
3. The client receiving fluoxetine (Prozac)
4. The client receiving venlafaxine (Effexor)

Answer: 1

Rationale: Lithium is known to alter electrical conductivity, producing cardiac dysrhythmias, tremor, convulsions, polyuria, edema, and other symptoms of fluid and electrolyte imbalance. Option 2: Clients receiving clozapine should be monitored for agranulocytosis. Option 3: Clients receiving fluoxetine should be monitored for acetylcholine block. Option 4: Clients receiving venlafaxine should be monitored for heightened feelings of anxiety.

Cognitive level: Application
Nursing process: Assessment
NCLEX: Physiological Integrity
See text page: 53

34. To evaluate the efficacy of tacrine (Cognex), the nurse would consider outcome criteria related to
1. improvement in mood.
2. memory improvement.
3. reduction of hyperactivity.
4. absence of auditory hallucinations.

Answer: 2

Rationale: Tacrine is an anticholinesterase drug that works by increasing the concentration of acetylcholine at the synapse. It is used to treat Alzheimer's disease. The other options do not reflect expected outcomes of tacrine therapy.

Cognitive level: Application
Nursing process: Planning (Outcome Identification)
NCLEX: Physiological Integrity
See text page: 59

35. During a care planning meeting for an obese client who has been diagnosed with schizophrenia, the nurse suggests to the physician that it would be appropriate to select a medication that does not block the receptors for
   1. H_1.
   2. GABA.
   3. Acetylcholine.
   4. 5 HT_2.

Answer: 1
Rationale: H_1 receptor blockade results in weight gain, which is undesirable for an obese client. Blocking of the other receptors would have little or no effect on the client's weight.
Cognitive level: Application
Nursing process: Planning
NCLEX: Physiological Integrity
See text pages: 50, 51

36. A client who has had excellent symptom reduction as a result of taking a conventional/standard antipsychotic tells the nurse that his medication makes him so sleepy that he is concerned his supervisor may terminate his employment. A solution the nurse should discuss with the physician is
   1. reducing the dose by half.
   2. discontinuing the medication.
   3. having the client take the medication at bedtime.
   4. switching from the conventional antipsychotic to risperidone (Risperdal).

Answer: 3
Rationale: Taking the medication at bedtime when the sedation would not be problematic may also reduce daytime sleepiness. Option 1 might prompt symptom exacerbation. Option 2 is undesirable because it may prompt relapse. Option 4 would not resolve the problem because risperidone also produces sedation.
Cognitive level: Application
Nursing process: Planning
NCLEX: Physiological Integrity
See text page: 51

37. During a medication information group, the nurse responds to a question about the basis on which the antiepileptic drugs carbamazepine (Tegretol), valproic acid (Depakene), and lamotrigine (Lamictal) act to relieve symptoms of mania by saying that these drugs
   1. preferentially block the reuptake and destruction of serotonin.

2. reduce the firing rate of high-frequency brain neurons.
3. exert a powerful and rapid sleep-inducing effect.
4. produce paradoxical psychostimulation.

Answer: 2
Rationale: The anticonvulsants mentioned alter electrical conductivity in membranes, slowing the firing rate of brain neurons. This membrane-stabilizing effect probably accounts for the reduction in mood swings seen in bipolar clients. Option 1 is the action of SSRIs. Option 3 is the action of soporific benzodiazepines such as flurazepam (Dalmane). Option 4: Psychostimulation is produced by drugs such as methylphenidate (Ritalin), which are used to treat attention deficit hyperactivity disorder.
Cognitive level: Application
Nursing process: Implementation
NCLEX: Health Promotion and Maintenance
See text pages: 53, 54

38. Questions that would be nonjudgmental approaches to obtaining information about client use of herbal remedies include (more than one answer may be correct)
   1. "You don't regularly take herbal remedies, do you?"
   2. "What herbal medicines have you used to relieve your symptoms?"
   3. "Have you ever experienced toxic effects from mixing herbals and prescription drugs?"
   4. "What over-the-counter medicines and nutritional supplements do you use?"

Answers: 2, 3, 4
Rationale: These queries are neutral in tone and do not express bias for or against the use of herbal medicines. Option 1 is worded in a negative way that makes the nurse's bias plain.
Cognitive level: Application
Nursing process: Assessment
NCLEX: Psychosocial Integrity
See text pages: 59, 60

CHAPTER 4

1. The managed behavioral health care organization nurse speaking to a group of employers concerned about health care costs should explain that new strategies designed to decrease the high cost of inpatient treatment include (more than one answer may be correct)
   1. milieu therapy.
   2. shortened in-patient stays.
   3. introduction of nurse practitioners.
   4. development of new levels of outpatient care.

205

Answers: 2, 3, 4

Rationale: Hospital stays have been shortened or denied on the basis of external oversight and written criteria to approve or deny requests for treatment. New levels of outpatient care such as partial hospitalization programs, intensive outpatient treatment, home care, and school-based services have been introduced. The use of nurse practitioners with admitting privileges, prescriptive privileges, and consultative skills has also been instrumental in moderating health care costs. Option 1: Milieu therapy, although useful, is not a new strategy developed to reduce cost.

Cognitive level: Comprehension
Nursing process: Implementation
NCLEX: Safe and Effective Care Environment
See text pages: 66, 67

2. An advanced practice psychiatric mental health nurse practitioner has taken a new position at a managed behavioral health agency. The nursing activity that would best use the advanced practice nurse's unique qualifications is
   1. milieu management.
   2. assisting clients with self-care.
   3. monitoring biological treatments.
   4. consultation-liaison activities.

Answer: 4

Rationale: Consultation-liaison activities are reserved for the advanced practice nurse. The other nursing activities may be performed by basic level psychiatric mental health nurses.

Cognitive level: Application
Nursing process: Implementation
NCLEX: Safe and Effective Care Environment
See text page: 66

3. A nurse who has a bachelor's of science in nursing degree and certification in psychiatric mental health nursing would be considered competent to
   1. provide psychotherapy.
   2. provide crisis intervention.
   3. prescribe psychopharmacologic agents.
   4. provide consultation regarding client treatment.

Answer: 2

Rationale: The certified psychiatric mental health nurse at the basic level can provide crisis intervention services. The other activities are reserved for advanced practice psychiatric mental health nurses.

Cognitive level: Application
Nursing process: Implementation
NCLEX: Safe and Effective Care Environment
See text page: 66

4. A client has had the following problems identified: ineffective coping related to mastectomy for breast cancer, deficient knowledge of cancer treatment options, dysfunctional grieving related to perception of loss, and disturbed body image related to mastectomy. A psychiatric mental health liaison nurse has been called. The problem that the liaison nurse should suggest an oncology nurse address is
   1. ineffective coping.
   2. deficient knowledge.
   3. dysfunctional grieving.
   4. disturbed body image.

Answer: 2

Rationale: The psychiatric mental health liaison nurse will intervene in the phenomena of emotional stress components of illness, self-concept changes, and grief. The knowledge deficit will be important to address but is the domain of an oncology nurse.

Cognitive level: Application
Nursing process: Planning
NCLEX: Physiological Integrity
See text page: 66

5. A community mental health nurse visits a client who lives in a community residence. On two sequential visits, the client makes veiled references to receiving verbally abusive treatment at the hands of one of the residence aides. The action the nurse should take is to
   1. understand that psychiatric clients often feel abused.
   2. listen and wait to see if the client continues to report the abuse.
   3. confront the residence aide with the client's allegations.
   4. report the client's comments to the protection and advocacy agency.

Answer: 4

Rationale: Nurses must advocate for the client's right to nonabusive treatment. Reporting to a protection and advocacy agency is the ethical duty of the nurse. Options 1 and 2 do nothing to investigate and resolve the situation. Option 3: The investigation is best conducted by skilled professionals trained to investigate such allegations.

Cognitive level: Application
Nursing process: Implementation
NCLEX: Safe and Effective Care Environment
See text page: 67-69

6. Regarding client use of psychotropic medication, the activities in which the basic level psychiatric mental health nurse can engage in include (more than one answer may be correct)

206

1. listening to the client's concerns about medication dose.
2. noting and addressing medication side effects.
3. adjusting medication dosage as symptoms change.
4. providing understandable medication teaching.

Answers: 1, 2, 4

Rationale: A basic level psychiatric mental health nurse does not have prescriptive privileges to adjust medication dosages. All other activities are within the realm of the basic level psychiatric mental health nurse and are important in promoting medication compliance.

Cognitive level: Application
Nursing process: Implementation
NCLEX: Safe and Effective Care Environment
See text page: 66

7. The nurse using the Forchuck model of case management will see the essential component of case management as
   1. the one-on-one therapeutic relationship between nurse and client.
   2. monitoring the cost-effect ratio of care provided by a managed care organization.
   3. a melding of nursing roles to meet all manifest needs of a particular client.
   4. advocacy for the client in the community in which he or she lives and works.

Answer: 1

Rationale: Forchuck incorporates Peplau's model as a basis for explaining case management activities and responsibilities and suggests that the most important component is the supportive interpersonal relationship of the nurse and patient. The other options are not central to case management as Forchuck sees it.

Cognitive level: Application
Nursing process: Planning
NCLEX: Safe and Effective Care Environment
See text page: 68

8. A client states "I'm pretty fed up with my wife. I'm thinking I should just get a divorce, but I worry about how that will affect my kids. What do you think I should do?" The psychiatric mental health nurse responds "Tell me what is happening between you and your wife." Which basic nursing intervention does this interchange characterize?
   1. Advocacy
   2. Counseling
   3. Health teaching
   4. Milieu management

Answer: 2

Rationale: The nurse is intervening to assist the client to clarify his thoughts and feelings, which is an activity related to counseling. Option 1: Advocacy is taking the client's side. Option 2: Health teaching involves imparting information to the client. Option 4: Milieu therapy involves using the environment to influence behavior.

Cognitive level: Application
Nursing process: Implementation
NCLEX: Physiological Integrity
See text page: 66

9. Approximately 45 minutes ago, the nurse administered a prn anxiolytic to a client who was feeling acutely anxious. The nurse, who has been sitting with the client, asks "On a scale of 1 to 10, how would you rate your anxiety at the moment?" Which basic nursing intervention does this interaction characterize?
   1. Counseling
   2. Milieu management
   3. Culturally relevant health promotion
   4. Administering and monitoring psychobiological interventions

Answer: 4

Rationale: Administering psychopharmacological drugs and monitoring the client's response to them is the basic level intervention described. Option 1: Counseling would involve activities such as interviewing, problem solving, and conflict resolution. Option 2: Milieu management would involve use of the environment to influence behavior. Option 3: Health promotion would involve activities to enhance mental health.

Cognitive level: Application
Nursing process: Implementation
NCLEX: Physiological Integrity
See text page: 66

10. The nurse meets with a client and his wife and explains the biological basis of the client's illness and the importance of taking neuroleptic medication daily to reduce symptoms. The nurse asks if either of them can foresee any reasons this might be difficult to do. Which basic intervention does this interaction characterize?
    1. Counseling
    2. Milieu therapy
    3. Health teaching
    4. Health promotion

Answer: 3

Rationale: A basic intervention of psychiatric mental health nurses is health teaching. This example of

207

giving information and assessing potential problems in compliance is part of health teaching, which is also called psychoeducation. Option 1: Counseling is described as interviewing, problem-solving, crisis intervention, conflict resolution, and support groups. Option 2: Milieu therapy involves use of the environment to influence behavior. Option 4: Health promotion includes activities designed to prevent mental illness.

Cognitive level: Application
Nursing process: Implementation
NCLEX: Health Promotion and Maintenance
See text page: 66

11. The nurse has instructed the client of the need to come to the mental health clinic each Tuesday at 10 AM. The client tells the nurse "I have no transportation." The nurse calls and arranges to have a car from the medical transportation volunteer pool pick him up at 9:30 AM. This basic intervention is part of
    1. advocacy.
    2. health promotion.
    3. case management.
    4. assisting clients with self-care.

Answer: 3
Rationale: Facilitating clinic appointments can be considered part of case management duties. Option 1: Advocacy is seen as taking the part of the client. Option 2: Health promotion includes activities designed to prevent mental illness. Option 4: Self-care activities refer to activities of daily living necessary for independence (grooming, eating, etc.).

Cognitive level: Application
Nursing process: Implementation
NCLEX: Physiological Integrity
See text page: 66

12. The clinical nurse specialist meets with a client receiving lithium. The nurse tells the client that her lithium level is 0.6 mEq/L, a finding in the desirable range. The nurse reinforces the importance of continuing to take the lithium as directed and the need to drink adequate amounts of fluids. This action is part of the advanced practice intervention of
    1. psychotherapy.
    2. consultation.
    3. prescriptive authority.
    4. complementary interventions.

Answer: 3
Rationale: Monitoring laboratory tests for serum lithium level and interpreting results for the client is an advanced practice level nursing intervention associated with prescriptive authority and treatment. Option 1: Psychotherapy refers to individual, group, or family therapy. Option 2: Consultation refers to providing clinical feedback to nurses or other disciplines to enhance the treatment of clients or systems issues. Option 4: Complementary interventions refer to the use of alternative therapies.

Cognitive level: Application
Nursing process: Implementation
NCLEX: Health Promotion and Maintenance
See text page: 66

13. The clinical nurse specialist meets with the interdisciplinary staff members planning care for a client with borderline personality disorder hospitalized on a surgical unit after a suicide attempt. The staff members are seeking ways to prevent the client from manipulating and splitting staff. The clinical specialist offers several suggestions for interventions. The clinical specialist is intervening by providing
    1. basic-level client interventions.
    2. complementary interventions.
    3. liaison consultation.
    4. expanded advocacy.

Answer: 3
Rationale: This interaction with the surgical team is an example of liaison consultation activity on the part of the clinical specialist. Option 1: This intervention is beyond the basic-level interventions oriented to the individual client, such as counseling, milieu therapy, and promotion of self-care activities. Option 2: Complementary interventions refer to alternative and complementary therapies such as massage and the use of herbal preparations. Option 4: No recognized intervention category of expanded advocacy exists.

Cognitive level: Application
Nursing process: Implementation
NCLEX: Safe and Effective Care Environment
See text page: 66

14. The psychiatric mental health nurse in the mental health clinic sees a client whose auditory hallucinations have worsened since his landlord told him he was being evicted. The nurse explores possible alternative living arrangements with the client and offers a 36-hour hospitalization while arrangements are being made. The phenomena in which the nurse is intervening is
    1. self-concept change.
    2. difficulty relating to others.
    3. problems related to loneliness.
    4. environmental events affecting client well-being.

Answer: 4

Rationale: Being evicted is an example of a situational crisis. The nurse is performing crisis intervention in response to an environmental circumstance that affects the emotional well-being of the client. Option 1: The scenario does not describe self-concept change on the part of the client. Option 2: The scenario does not specifically refer to client difficulty relating to others. Option 3: The scenario does not describe the client problem of loneliness or other emotions.

Cognitive level: Application
Nursing process: Implementation
NCLEX: Safe and Effective Care Environment
See text page: 64

15. Which task can the clinical nurse leader who is creating the work assignment give to either a basic level or an advanced level psychiatric mental health nurse?
    1. Responding to "telehealth" calls
    2. Providing psychotherapy for a new client
    3. Performing clinical supervisory activities with a new nurse
    4. Meeting with community leaders to expand advocacy for residents of a group home for persistently mentally ill clients

Answer: 1

Rationale: Telehealth is as a basic-level intervention suitable for basic level or advanced practice psychiatric mental health nurses. The other options are reserved for advanced practice nurses.

Cognitive level: Application
Nursing process: Implementation
NCLEX: Safe and Effective Care Environment
See text page: 66

16. The psychiatric mental health nurse engages in daily sessions with a client with bipolar disorder to teach about the desired effects of prescribed medications, their side effects, and ways to manage the side effects. The problem for which the nurse is intervening is
    1. self-care limitation.
    2. difficulties relating to others.
    3. symptom management.
    4. problems related to emotions.

Answer: 3

Rationale: Each of the options listed is a phenomenon of concern to psychiatric mental health nurses. The problem described is symptom management associated with psychopharmacological intervention. It includes consideration of side effects and toxic effects of medication. No mention is made in the scenario of the problems listed in the other options.

Cognitive level: Analysis
Nursing process: Implementation
NCLEX: Physiological Integrity
See text page: 64

17. The phenomenon of highest priority to a psychiatric nurse caring for a client with the following nursing diagnoses would be
    1. risk for suicide.
    2. disturbed thought processes.
    3. situational low self-esteem.
    4. self-care deficit: grooming.

Answer: 1

Rationale: Risk for suicide is the nursing diagnosis of highest priority. Safety needs transcend psychological needs. Options 2, 3, and 4 do not provide an immediate threat to the client, whereas option 1 does.

Cognitive level: Analysis
Nursing process: Diagnosis
NCLEX: Safe and Effective Care Environment
See text page: 64

18. A new nurse is concerned with identifying outcomes pertaining to client social interactions and client self-control. The nurse's mentor should suggest
    1. using the *DSM-IV-TR*.
    2. daily discussions with the mentor.
    3. referring to the Nursing Outcomes Classification reference.
    4. searching the Internet for hints.

Answer: 3

Rationale: The Nursing Outcomes Classification is a comprehensive list of standardized outcomes, definitions, and measures to describe client outcomes influenced by nursing practice. Two categories found in the classification include social interaction and self-control. Option 1: The *DSM-IV-TR* contains diagnostic information. Option 2: Daily discussions with the mentor might be helpful but would not yield the quantity of information found in the Nursing Outcomes Classification. Option 4: This option would not provide the focused information found in the Nursing Outcomes Classification.

Cognitive level: Comprehension
Nursing process: Implementation
NCLEX: Safe and Effective Care Environment
See text pages: 64, 65

19. The nurse planning care for a client should strive to select valid nursing interventions. The best way of achieving this outcome is to select relevant interventions
    1. suggested by experienced unit nurses.
    2. clients have reported to be helpful.

209

3. that are research derived.
4. that seem logical.

Answer: 3

Rationale: Research-derived interventions are evidence-based interventions. The nurse can rely on their proven effectiveness. Option 1: Interventions suggested by unit nurses may be largely unproven and subjectively derived. Option 2: Client-reported preferences can be skewed. Option 4: This criteria is quite subjective because what one nurse sees as logical might be perceived differently by another.

Cognitive level: Analysis
Nursing process: Planning
NCLEX: Safe and Effective Care Environment
See text pages: 64, 65

20. Which of the following trends should the psychiatric nurse consider when engaged in planning for future managed behavioral health organization services? (More than one answer may be correct.)
    1. Cost constraints will continue.
    2. Community-based care will evolve.
    3. Case management is a necessary skill.
    4. The prevalence of dementia is falling.
    5. Cultural diversity in the United States is decreasing.

Answers: 1, 2, 3

Rationale: Cost constraints will continue. More people will need mental health services, making scarce services even more scarce. Costs will rise because of the sheer numbers of individuals requiring care. Community-based care will continue to increase in an attempt to keep costs as low as possible. New services will evolve as innovative responses to need. Case management is necessary because it ensures that care is provided as efficiently and effectively as possible, thus saving scarce dollars. Option 4 is incorrect. The prevalence of dementia is expected to rise as the population ages. Increased need for institutions to care for clients with dementia is expected. Option 5 is incorrect. Cultural diversity in the United States is increasing. Nursing cultural competence is necessary.

Cognitive level: Analysis
Nursing process: Planning
NCLEX: Safe and Effective Care Environment
See text pages: 66, 67, 69

21. Which of the statements made by a nurse applying for a position as a case manager suggests the nurse does not have the requisite attitude or skill and should not be given the position?
    1. "I most enjoy taking care of clients who are dependent."

2. "I am rewarded when I see a client functioning in the community."
    3. "I am able to identify a client's changing needs and shift roles accordingly."
    4. "My interpersonal skills are excellent and I know the resources of the community."

Answer: 1

Rationale: A case manager must provide a consistent, supportive, one-to-one, long-term relationship that helps clients develop their strengths and increase and maintain an optimal level of independence. The nurse who prefers to work with dependent clients may unconsciously sabotage client movement toward independence. The other statements refer to attitudes and skills consistent with Forchuck's case management model.

Cognitive level: Analysis
Nursing process: Assessment
NCLEX: Safe and Effective Care Environment
See text page: 68

22. The most important issue a nurse who wishes to become involved in political action on behalf of clients and families affected by mental illness could choose is
    1. the need to do away with utilization review.
    2. passing a national mental health parity law.
    3. stopping computerization of medical records.
    4. the need for accurate mental health information on the Internet.

Answer: 2

Rationale: A national mental health parity law would provide better insurance benefits for insured clients with mental health problems. Insurance equality would be achieved for clients with physical and mental illness. Option 1: Utilization review is an important cost-containment tool. The nurse would not want to speak against this. Option 3: The nurse should not adopt this cause. Communication technology should be used to benefit clients and staff. Although confidentiality is currently an issue, it is not insurmountable. Option 4: This is not a cause for political action.

Cognitive level: Analysis
Nursing process: NA
NCLEX: Safe and Effective Care Environment
See text pages: 67-69

23. A mentoring nurse tells a new nurse that "Documentation is a critically important skill for you to develop." The rationale for this advice is that documentation (more than one answer may be correct)

Chapter 4   Psychiatric Mental Health Nursing
and Managed Care Issues

1. ensures that clients receive necessary care.
2. justifies payment for the client's care.
3. keeps evaluators from giving deficiencies.
4. makes risk management more effective.

Answers: 1, 2

Rationale: Progress notes written on a daily basis document behavior, behavioral outcomes, and daily interventions. Client change necessitates revised planning. Only when documentation is relevant, accurate, and timely will the client receive optimal care. Payors are unwilling to pay for care that is not justified or not received; thus documentation is the foundation on which payment is based. The other options bear no relevance to the importance of documentation.

Cognitive level: Application
Nursing process: Implementation
NCLEX: Safe and Effective Care Environment
See text pages: 66, 67

24. Trends that have significant bearing on the skill set needed by psychiatric nurses over the next 5 years include (more than one answer may be correct)
    1. increasing cultural diversity.
    2. the decreasing age of the population.
    3. community-based care case management.
    4. increased funding prospects for psychiatric care.

Answers: 1, 3

Rationale: Increasing cultural diversity calls for the nurse to be more culturally competent. By 2050 the majority of the U.S. population will be people of color. Demand for community-based care case management is expected to increase in keeping with continuing need to hold costs down. Option 2: The population is expected to age, requiring more psychiatric home care for the aged and long-term treatment for those with mental disorders. Option 4: Funding prospects for psychiatric care are not expected to increase.

Cognitive level: Application
Nursing process: NA
NCLEX: Safe and Effective Care Environment
See text pages: 67-69

25. The situation in which the nurse's primary role can be assessed as advocacy is
    1. treating the self-inflicted injuries of psychiatric clients.
    2. providing preventive counseling regarding violence.
    3. providing care to the family of a suicide victim.
    4. participating in consumer mental health groups to destigmatize mental illness.

Answer: 4

Rationale: Destigmatization efforts are a form of advocacy. The other options are examples of the care provider role. Option 1 provides secondary prevention. Option 2 offers primary prevention. Option 3 offers tertiary prevention.

Cognitive level: Application
Nursing process: Implementation
NCLEX: Safe and Effective Care Environment
See text pages: 67-69

CHAPTER 5

1. A group of nurses at the managed behavioral health organization have the task of revising the current admission criteria:
   1. Clear risk of client danger to self or others
   2. Dangerous decompensation of a client under long-term treatment
   3. Failure of community-based treatment demonstrating clear need for intensive, structured treatment
   4. Medical need unassociated with psychiatric treatment or associated with treatment
   5. Provision of respite for caregivers

   Which, if any, of the criteria should be deleted?
   1. none
   2. 1
   3. 2
   4. 3
   5. 4
   6. 5

Answer: 6

Rationale: The goal of caregiver respite can be accomplished without hospitalizing the client. The other options are acceptable, evidence-based criteria for admission of a client to a managed behavioral health organization.

Cognitive level: Application
Nursing process: Implementation
NCLEX: Safe and Effective Care Environment
See text pages: 74, 75

2. The nurse manager has the task of introducing staff to the use of clinical pathways. The nurse manager will need to explain that clinical pathways are used in managed care settings to
   1. identify obstacles to effective care.
   2. stabilize aggressive clients.
   3. relieve nurses of planning responsibilities.
   4. streamline the care process and save money.

Answer: 4

Rationale: Clinical pathways provide guidelines for assessments, interventions, treatments, and outcomes as well as a designated timeline for accomplishment. Deviations from the timeline must be reported and investigated. Clinical pathways streamline the care process and save money. Option 1: Care pathways do not identify obstacles; staff do this. Option 2: Care pathways do not stabilize aggressive clients; staff are responsible for the necessary interventions. Option 3: Care pathways do not relieve nurses of the responsibility of planning; pathways may, however, make the task easier.

Cognitive level: Application
Nursing process: Implementation
NCLEX: Safe and Effective Care Environment
See text pages: 76, 77

3. Planning for clients with mental illness is facilitated by understanding that under behavioral health managed care, inpatient hospitalization is generally reserved for clients who
   1. are noncompliant with medication at home.
   2. present a clear danger to self or others.
   3. develop new symptoms during the course of the illness.
   4. have no support systems in the community.

Answer: 2

Rationale: Hospitalization is justified when the client is a danger to self or others, has dangerously decompensated, or needs intensive medical treatment. Options 1, 3, and 4 do not necessarily describe clients who would require inhospital treatment.

Cognitive level: Application
Nursing process: Assessment
NCLEX: Safe and Effective Care Environment
See text pages: 74, 75

4. An intervention strategy in which all psychiatric mental health nurses need to be competent and that is useful in reducing the number of clients who are admitted to psychiatric units is
   1. milieu therapy.
   2. utilization review.
   3. use of clinical pathways.
   4. community-based crisis intervention.

Answer: 4

Rationale: Community-based crisis intervention, by a case manager or at a crisis clinic, often resolves or manages client problems so hospitalization may be averted. Options 1, 2, and 3 refer to interventions and processes that take place after admission.

Cognitive level: Comprehension

Nursing process: Implementation
NCLEX: Safe and Effective Care Environment
See text pages: 74, 75

5. A client who is a member of a health maintenance organization was hospitalized after a severe reaction to a psychotropic medication. He was treated for the reaction, a new medication was ordered, and he was closely observed for side effects for 24 hours. The case manager visited before the client's discharge to give him an appointment for an outpatient visit in 2 days and learned that the client had neglected to mention that he received notice of eviction from his apartment on the day he was admitted. The most appropriate intervention for the case manager is to
   1. cancel the client's discharge from the hospital.
   2. file a restraining order against the landlord who evicted the client.
   3. arrange a place for the client to stay until a new apartment can be found.
   4. call the health maintenance organization and obtain permission to transfer the client to a medical unit in the hospital.

Answer: 3

Rationale: The case manager should intervene by arranging temporary shelter for the client until an apartment can be found. This is part of the coordination and delivery of services that falls under the case manager role. None of the other options is a viable alternative.

Cognitive level: Application
Nursing process: Implementation
NCLEX: Safe and Effective Care Environment
See text page: 77

6. Under managed care, how are the client and family likely to view the experience of hospitalization?
   1. As an unpleasant interruption of daily life
   2. Too short to produce complete wellness
   3. Too restrictive to help with adjustment to the community
   4. A pleasant vacation from the pressures of life in the community

Answer: 2

Rationale: Managed care has resulted in very short hospital stays, much shorter than clients experienced in the past when discharge occurred only when the client was reasonably well suited to resume community responsibilities. Option 1: Crisis situations often precede admission. Generally, both client and family are relieved. Option 3: Hospitalization is currently no more restrictive or unpleasant than before the advent of managed care. Option 4:

Hospitalization can be guaranteed not to be long enough to be considered a vacation.

Cognitive level: Application
Nursing process: Assessment
NCLEX: Safe and Effective Care Environment
See text pages: 74, 75

7. A teenage client is hospitalized after a serious suicide attempt related to feelings of hopelessness. The client comes from an upper-middle-class home in the suburbs and has never had psychiatric care before. Two hours after admission, when the nurse asks about the client's reaction to hospitalization, the client is most likely to label the experience as
   1. necessary.
   2. exciting.
   3. enjoyable.
   4. frightening.

Answer: 4
Rationale: Because only the most acutely ill clients are hospitalized, the client is in a milieu in which many behavioral manifestations of mental illness are apparent. The client is most likely frightened. Option 1: Insight into the necessity for hospitalization only hours after making a suicide attempt is unlikely. Options 2 and 3: Finding hospitalization enjoyable or exciting is also unlikely.

Cognitive level: Application
Nursing process: Assessment
NCLEX: Psychosocial Integrity
See text pages: 80, 81

8. The interdisciplinary health care team meets 12 hours after a teenage client was admitted after a suicide attempt. Members of the team report assessments. What other outcome can be expected from this meeting?
   1. A clinical pathway will be selected.
   2. The nurse will assume the surrogate mother role.
   3. The team will request a court-appointed advocate for the client.
   4. Assessment of client need for placement outside the home will be undertaken.

Answer: 1
Rationale: Clinical pathways are selected early in the course of treatment to streamline the treatment process and reduce costs. Option 2 would be inappropriate. Option 3 would rarely be required. Option 4: It would be too early to determine the need for alternative postdischarge living arrangements.

Cognitive level: Application
Nursing process: Planning (Outcome Identification)
NCLEX: Safe and Effective Care Environment
See text pages: 76, 77

9. A client with a thought disorder is to be discharged home today, 4 days after having severe decompensation related to medication noncompliance. The client's medication was restarted, and the client's thought processes are now noted to be more logical and less interrupted by hallucinations. When the client's husband comes to pick her up, he becomes upset and tells the nurse "She shouldn't come home so soon. She's still sick. You must keep her at least a month." The nurse should
   1. call the psychiatrist to come to the unit to explain discharge rationale.
   2. explain that health insurance won't pay for a longer stay for the client.
   3. explain that the client will continue to improve if she takes medication regularly.
   4. call security to handle the disturbance and escort the husband off the unit.

Answer: 3
Rationale: Under managed care clients no longer stay in the hospital until every vestige of a symptom disappears. The nurse must assume responsibility to advocate for the client's right to the least restrictive setting as soon as the symptoms are under control and for the right of citizens to control health care costs. Option 1 will ultimately produce the same result because the physician will use the same rationale. Option 2 simply shifts blame but will not change the discharge. Option 4 is unnecessary; the nurse can handle the matter.

Cognitive level: Application
Nursing process: Implementation
NCLEX: Psychosocial Integrity
See text page: 82

10. The nurse receives three telephone calls regarding a newly admitted client. The psychiatrist wishes to see the client for an assessment interview, the medical doctor wants to perform a physical examination, and the client's lawyer wishes to set up an appointment to see the client. The nurse schedules the three activities for the client. This exemplifies the role of the nurse known as
    1. advocate.
    2. milieu manager.
    3. care manager.
    4. provider of care.

Answer: 3
Rationale: Nurses on psychiatric units routinely coordinate client services as described in this scenario. Option 1: The role of advocate would require the nurse to speak out on the client's behalf. Option 2: The role of milieu manager refers to maintaining a

Chapter 5   Mental Health Nursing in Acute Care Settings

therapeutic environment. Option 4: Provider of care refers to giving direct care to the client.

Cognitive level: Application
Nursing process: Planning
NCLEX: Safe and Effective Care Environment
See text page: 78

11. The nurse moves about the psychiatric unit, noting that exits are free from obstruction, no one is smoking in any area other than the smoking room, the janitor's closet is locked, and all sharp objects are being used under supervision of staff. These observations relate to
   1. management of milieu safety.
   2. coordinating care of clients.
   3. management of the interpersonal climate.
   4. use of therapeutic intervention strategies.

Answer: 1
Rationale: Nursing staff are responsible for all aspects of milieu management. The observations mentioned in this question directly relate to the safety of the unit. The other options, although part of the nurse's concerns, are unrelated to the observations cited.

Cognitive level: Application
Nursing process: Implementation
NCLEX: Safe and Effective Care Environment
See text page: 80

12. Which aspect of direct care is the hospital psychiatric nurse most likely to provide for a client?
   1. Hygiene assistance
   2. Assertiveness training
   3. Diversional activity
   4. Assistance with job hunting

Answer: 2
Rationale: Assertiveness training relies on the counseling and psychoeducational skills of the nurse. The other tasks are usually performed by the lowest cost staff member who can effectively perform the task. Option 1: Assistance with personal hygiene would usually be accomplished by a psychiatric technician or nursing assistant. Option 3: Diversional activities are usually the province of activities therapists. Option 4: The client would probably be assisted in job hunting by the social worker.

Cognitive level: Application
Nursing process: Implementation
NCLEX: Health Promotion and Maintenance
See text pages: 76, 77

13. The nurse writes in the client's progress notes: "3/5/year 10 AM. Client brought to unit by ER nurse. Client's clothing and body are dirty. In interview room, client sat with hands over face, sobbing softly. Did not acknowledge nurse and did not reply to questions. After several minutes abruptly arose and ran to window and pounded window screen, shouting, 'Let me out of here!' repeatedly. Verbal intervention unsuccessful. Order for stat dose 2 mg haloperidol po obtained. Medication administered with result that client stopped shouting and returned to sit wordlessly in chair. Client placed on one-to-one observation until seen by psychiatrist." How should this documentation be evaluated?
   1. Meets agency standards
   2. Contains subjective material
   3. Too brief to be of value
   4. Excessively wordy

Answer: 1
Rationale: This narrative note describes client appearance, behavior, and conversation. It mentions that less-restrictive measures were attempted before administering medication and documents client response to medication. This note would probably meet agency standards. A complete nursing assessment would be in order as soon as the client is able to participate. Option 2: Subjective material is absent from the note. Options 3 and 4 are inaccurate evaluations based on the explanation for option 1.

Cognitive level: Evaluation
Nursing process: Assessment
NCLEX: Safe and Effective Care Environment
See text page: 80

14. For the nurse managing the therapeutic milieu, the most heavily weighted factor in determining whether a client should receive a prn dose of neuroleptic medication is whether
   1. the client is willing to accept the medication.
   2. less-restrictive alternatives have been tried without success.
   3. the client's behavior indicates possible danger to self, others, or the environment.
   4. administration of the medication will make the work of the staff easier or safer.

Answer: 3
Rationale: Although options 1 and 2 are factors to be considered, the client's behavior is the factor of greatest importance. Option 4 is irrelevant.

Cognitive level: Application
Nursing process: Assessment
NCLEX: Safe and Effective Care Environment
See text pages: 80, 81

15. A client was admitted after police brought him to the hospital after a fight with his roommate at a com-

munity residence. The client tells the nurse that he had been suspicious for several days, then noted his roommate was casting a spell on him by looking at him intently, so he hit the roommate with his fists. The client admits he stopped taking his antipsychotic medication a week ago when the prescription needed to be refilled. Which outcome should the nurse working in a managed behavioral health inpatient unit select for this client?
1. Symptoms will be stabilized with medication within 48 hours.
2. A trusting relationship with the nurse will be developed within 5 days.
3. A high level of ease with other clients will be reported within 1 week.
4. The client will agree to placement in a new residence within 3 weeks.

Answer: 1

Rationale: Managed care requires the shortest possible hospital stay. Stabilization of symptoms can occur rapidly when medication is restarted. Discharge can occur shortly after stabilization. Options 2, 3, and 4: These outcomes are inappropriate because they presume a long hospitalization.
Cognitive level: Application
Nursing process: Planning (Outcome Identification)
NCLEX: Physiological Integrity
See text page: 82

16. The following clients are seen in the emergency department. The psychiatric unit has one bed. The advanced practice nurse acting as admitting officer should recommend for admission to the hospital the client who
1. is experiencing dry mouth and tremor related to haloperidol and wants his dose of haloperidol reduced.
2. is experiencing anxiety and a saddened mood after separation from her husband of 10 years.
3. argued with her boyfriend and inflicted a superficial cut on her forearm with a knife.
4. is a single parent and hears voices telling her to smother her infant son.

Answer: 4

Rationale: Admission to the hospital would be justified by the risk of client danger to self or others. The other clients have issues that can be handled without hospitalization.
Cognitive level: Analysis
Nursing process: Assessment
NCLEX: Safe and Effective Care Environment
See text pages: 74, 75

17. Which document pertaining to client care would a student beginning clinical experience on a psychiatric inpatient unit be justified in reading last?
1. Clients' Bill of Rights
2. Unit Policy on Suicide Precautions
3. Unit Seclusion and Restraint Policies
4. Employee Directive on Overtime Refusal

Answer: 4

Rationale: Because the student is not an employee, information about overtime refusal is of less relevance. Options 1, 2, and 3: The student will be directly involved with client rights, implementing suicide precautions, and seclusion and restraint policies.
Cognitive level: Analysis
Nursing process: NA
NCLEX: Safe and Effective Care Environment
See text pages: 76, 80

18. A student nurse is assigned to administer oral medications to her assigned client. The client refuses to take the medication. The student nurse should
1. tell the client that she will receive a poor grade if she doesn't administer the medication.
2. tell the client that refusal is not permitted and staff will require him to take the medication.
3. document the client's refusal on the medication administration record without comment.
4. ask the client's reason for refusing and report to the coassigned nurse.

Answer: 4

Rationale: The client has the right to refuse medication unless a court order to medicate has been obtained. The client's reason for refusing should be ascertained, and the refusal should be reported to a unit nurse. Sometimes refusals are based on unpleasant side effects that can be ameliorated. Options 1 and 2: Threats and manipulation are inappropriate. Option 3: Medication refusal should be reported to permit appropriate intervention.
Cognitive level: Application
Nursing process: Implementation
NCLEX: Psychosocial Integrity
See text pages: 80, 81

19. Which nursing intervention is most likely to be listed in the clinical pathway as part of a basic level psychiatric nurse's duties to a psychiatric client on day 1 of hospitalization?
1. Provide a safe environment.
2. Assign therapeutic activities.
3. Order admission laboratory studies.
4. Educate client and family about illness and medications.

Chapter 5   Mental Health Nursing in Acute Care Settings

Answer: 1

Rationale: The nurse is responsible for options 1 and 4, but client education about illness and medications usually begins on day 2 after assessments are completed. Providing a safe environment begins at the time of admission. Option 2 is usually the responsibility of activities therapists. Option 3 would be the responsibility of a physician, physician assistant, or nurse practitioner.

Cognitive level: Application
Nursing process: Implementation
NCLEX: Safe and Effective Care Environment
See text page: 80

20. The unit secretary is away from the unit desk, the phone rings, and the student nurse answers. The caller is the health insurer for one of the inpatients, seeking information about the client's projected length of stay. How should the student nurse handle the request?
   1. Obtain the information from the client's medical record and relay it to the caller.
   2. Inform the caller that information about clients is confidential.
   3. Refer the request for information to the client's case manager.
   4. Refer the request to the unit psychiatrist.

Answer: 3

Rationale: The case manager usually confers with insurers and provides the treatment team with information about available resources. The student nurse should be mindful of client confidentiality and should neither confirm that the client is an inpatient nor disclose other information.

Cognitive level: Application
Nursing process: Implementation
NCLEX: Safe and Effective Care Environment
See text page: 77

21. The nurse is surveying medical records to look for violations of client rights. The finding that would signal a violation of client rights is
   1. no treatment plan present in record.
   2. client belongings searched at admission.
   3. physical restraint used to prevent harm to self.
   4. client was placed on one-to-one continuous observation.

Answer: 1

Rationale: The client has the right to have a treatment plan. Option 2: Inspecting client belongings is performed as a safety measure. Clients have the right to a safe environment. Options 3 and 4: Clients have the right to be protected against the possible impulse to harm oneself that occurs as a result of a mental disorder.

Cognitive level: Analysis
Nursing process: Evaluation
NCLEX: Safe and Effective Care Environment
See text page: 76

22. When responding to a client who exhibits agitated, hostile behavior during a community meeting, the initial action the nurse should take is to
   1. offer prn medication.
   2. follow the treatment plan.
   3. place the client in seclusion.
   4. permit the angry outburst if no harmful behavior is threatened.

Answer: 2

Rationale: Consistency in response is vital to positive outcomes; hence, following the treatment plan is the correct answer. The response of staff might take different forms depending on the treatment plan.

Cognitive level: Application
Nursing process: Implementation
NCLEX: Safe and Effective Care Environment
See text page: 81

23. A student nurse tells the instructor "I don't feel as though I'm helping my assigned client. I don't have the opportunity to engage him in formal counseling sessions. I only spend time with him as he has time between appointments." The best reply for the instructor would be
   1. "It is appropriate for beginners to progress slowly and develop skills."
   2. "It's all new to you. By the end of your second week on the unit you will find you feel more helpful."
   3. "I'm sorry you're feeling disappointed. Have you considered whether your goals for the experience were realistic?"
   4. "In informal contacts your psychosocial communication skills help him feel listened to and supported. You provide feedback and encourage use of adaptive coping skills."

Answer: 4

Rationale: Nurses should be aware that informal contacts are often as significant as formal contacts because they occur during natural activities of daily and social living and are therefore based on reality.

Cognitive level: Application
Nursing process: Implementation
NCLEX: Psychosocial Integrity
See text page: 79

24. The psychiatric nurse should plan interventions based on the knowledge that clients may be intolerant of, or resistant to, common procedures such as

vital signs, blood glucose monitoring, or insulin administration. Common reasons for resistance include (more than one answer may be correct)
1. anxiety.
2. obstinacy.
3. lack of trust.
4. thought impairment.

Answers: 1, 3, 4
Rationale: Resistance to routine procedures is rarely related to the psychiatric client being perverse or having an uncooperative personality trait. More often resistance is related to anxiety, fear, suspicion, cognitive impairment, or lack of knowledge.
Cognitive level: Analysis
Nursing process: Planning
NCLEX: Psychosocial Integrity
See text pages: 80, 81

25. Which of the following would the psychiatric nurse assess as a behavioral crisis? A client is
1. found crying hysterically after receiving a phone call from her boyfriend.
2. noted curled up in a corner of the bathroom with a towel wrapped around her head.
3. performing push-ups in the middle of the hall, forcing everyone to walk around him.
4. waving his fists and shouting threats at a nurse who offered him prn medication.

Answer: 4
Rationale: This behavior constitutes a behavioral crisis because the client is threatening harm to another individual. Intervention is called for to defuse the situation. The other options speak of behaviors that may require intervention of a less urgent nature because the clients in question are not threatening harm to self or others.
Cognitive level: Analysis
Nursing process: Assessment
NCLEX: Safe and Effective Care Environment
See text page: 81

26. Which principle should be followed by psychiatric inpatient staff when addressing a behavioral crisis?
1. Resolve it with the least restrictive intervention possible.
2. Individual client rights are superseded by the rights of the majority.
3. Swift intervention is preferable to planned, structured intervention in nearly all instances of dyscontrol.
4. Allow the client the opportunity to regain control without intervention when safety of other clients is not compromised.

Answer: 1
Rationale: The rule of using the least restrictive treatment or intervention possible to achieve the desired outcome is the client's legal right. Option 2: This is not strictly true. Option 3: Planned interventions are nearly always preferable. Option 4: Intervention may be necessary when the client is threatening harm to self.
Cognitive level: Analysis
Nursing process: Implementation
NCLEX: Safe and Effective Care Environment
See text page: 81

27. A nurse performed the following actions and interventions in the course of a day while caring for a client with psychosis:
1. Removed embroidery scissors from client's possession
2. Arranged for client to make an appointment with a lawyer
3. In client's presence, opened a package mailed to client
4. Remained within arm's length of client during the shift
5. Permitted client to refuse oral psychotropic medication

Which intervention, if any, violated a right of the client?
1. none
2. 1
3. 2
4. 3
5. 4
6. 5

Answer: 1
Rationale: Options 1 and 4 preserve the client's right to be protected against the possible impulse to harm self or others. Option 2 preserved the client's right to legal counsel. Option 3 preserved the client's rights to send and receive mail and be present during package inspection. Option 5 preserved the client's right to refuse treatment.
Cognitive level: Analysis
Nursing process: Implementation
NCLEX: Safe and Effective Care Environment
See text page: 76

28. When the clinical nurse leader is asked to defend the use of clinical pathways to a hospitalwide committee, which should be stated as an advantage? Clinical pathways
1. obscure resource management.
2. deter collaborative practice.
3. are generic rather than individualized.
4. make it easy to monitor treatment progression.

217

Answer: 4

Rationale: When treatment and outcomes are projected on a day-to-day basis, monitoring and outcome evaluation are simplified. Exceptions are quickly noted. This is of considerable advantage to the treatment team. Option 1: Pathways actually facilitate resource management, particularly in the area of staffing. Option 2: Pathways support collaborative practice. Option 3: Generic treatment plans are useful because they are evidence based and complete plans for a client with a specific disorder. They can easily be modified to meet individual needs.

Cognitive level: Application
Nursing process: NA
NCLEX: Safe and Effective Care Environment
See text pages: 76, 77

29. A new client asks the nurse "So what goes on at this community meeting scheduled this afternoon?" The best reply by the nurse would be
    1. "You and your therapist will discuss problems and goals for problem resolution."
    2. "You and a small group of other clients will meet to discuss common issues."
    3. "You, the staff, and the other clients will meet to discuss problems occurring on the unit."
    4. "We never know what will go on at a community meeting because clients determine the agenda."

Answer: 3

Rationale: Community meetings involve staff and clients. Items pertinent to the functioning of the community are topics for exploration. Ideas for activities, community problems, clarifications of unit rules, greeting new clients, and saying goodbye to clients being discharged might be included. Option 1 describes individual therapy. Option 2 describes group therapy. Option 4 is evasive.

Cognitive level: Application
Nursing process: Implementation
NCLEX: Safe and Effective Care Environment
See text page: 79

30. The nurse observes a client's anger escalating. He begins to pace the hall and shouts "You all had better watch out. I'm going to hurt anybody who gets in my way." Assuming each of the following interventions is appropriate, put them in the order in which they should occur. (Type answer in order from first to last without using commas.)
    1. Take the client to a seclusion room and administer medication.
    2. Have a nurse prepare prn medication.
    3. Calmly tell the client that "staff will help you control your impulse to hurt someone."

4. Gather a show of force.
5. Remove clients from the area.

Answer: 5, 3, 2, 4, 1

Rationale: The ideal sequence provides a rapid, organized response that provides safety for the other clients and progresses from verbal limit setting to immobilization and concurrent use of medication.

Cognitive level: Analysis
Nursing process: Implementation
NCLEX: Safe and Effective Care Environment
See text page: 81

CHAPTER 6

1. Nurse A works in an inpatient unit in the community mental health center. Nurse B is a community mental health nurse. To provide comprehensive care to clients, which skill must nurse B use that nurse A does not currently use?
    1. A calm external manner
    2. Problem-solving skills
    3. Ability to cross service systems
    4. Knowledge of psychopharmacology

Answer: 3

Rationale: A community mental health nurse must be able to work with schools, corrections facilities, shelters, health care providers, and employers. The mental health nurse working in an inpatient unit needs only to be able to work within the single setting. Option 1: This manner would be needed by nurses in both settings. Option 2: Problem-solving skills are needed by all nurses. Option 4: Nurses in both settings must have knowledge of psychopharmacology.

Cognitive level: Analysis
Nursing process: Implementation
NCLEX: Safe and Effective Care Environment
See text pages: 89, 90

2. The community mental health nurse calls on a highly suspicious psychiatric client, saying "I'm a nurse from the mental health center. I'd like to come in and find out how you're doing." The client refuses to allow the nurse access to her apartment, saying "My neighbor talks to me every day. I don't know you. You could be from the IRS or the CIA. The less you know about me, the better." The best initial intervention for the nurse to take to try to gain access would be to
    1. ask the client's neighbor to go with her.
    2. have the police accompany her.
    3. deny a relationship with the IRS or CIA.
    4. mention the client will have to go to the hospital unless she sees the nurse.

218

Answer: 1

Rationale: Having a person the client trusts intercede on the nurse's behalf may smooth the way for the nurse and client to develop a trusting relationship. Option 2: This measure would be a last resort. Option 3: This would be ineffective because of the client's high level of suspicion. Option 4: This is a threat that could be construed as an assault.

Cognitive level: Application
Nursing process: Implementation
NCLEX: Safe and Effective Care Environment
See text pages: 86, 87

3. A desirable treatment outcome for a seriously mentally ill client in an inpatient setting might be that "The client will show stabilization of symptoms and return to the community." In contrast, an identified outcome for a seriously mentally ill client being treated in a community setting should be that "The client will demonstrate
   1. the ability to maintain stability in the community."
   2. an absence of symptoms and improved level of functioning."
   3. functioning at a moderate to high level of social integration."
   4. socially acceptable interactions within the community, good self-care, and adequate nutrition."

Answer: 1

Rationale: Symptoms often worsen when the client is discharged from the hospital and no longer has the support and structure of the hospital setting. The client can remain in the community if he or she can cope with the symptoms and situational demands (i.e., maintain stability). The goals listed in the other options are unrealistically high.

Cognitive level: Application
Nursing process: Planning (Outcome Identification)
NCLEX: Psychosocial Integrity
See text page: 88

4. Which intervention strategy would the community psychiatric nurse include when planning care for a mentally ill client being cared for in the community?
   1. Enforce boundaries by way of seclusion
   2. Develop a long-term relationship
   3. Administer prescribed medication three times daily
   4. Provide three nutritious meals with snacks between meals

Answer: 2

Rationale: A long-term relationship is necessary to care for clients in the community because the time span of care is lengthy. Because hospitalizations are cur-

rently so brief, establishing a short-term relationship is all that can be expected. Options 1, 3, and 4 are interventions that would occur in the hospital rather than in the community.

Cognitive level: Application
Nursing process: Planning
NCLEX: Psychosocial Integrity
See text page: 88

5. A client states "I don't understand all these levels of nurses." Which reply provides the client with accurate information? "In contrast to the role of the psychiatric nurse prepared to provide basic and direct nursing care, the advanced practice psychiatric mental health nurse is exclusively able to
   1. provide mental health care if under the direct supervision of a physician."
   2. contract to provide mental health services for individuals or groups."
   3. participate in research projects if protocols have been approved by senior researchers."
   4. assist with medication management but not actually prescribe it."

Answer: 2

Rationale: The only exclusive role of the advanced practice nurse mentioned in the options is contracting to provide mental services to individuals or groups. Options 1, 3, and 4 are functions the nurse with basic preparation can perform.

Cognitive level: Application
Nursing process: Implementation
NCLEX: Safe and Effective Care Environment
See text page: 88

6. The community psychiatric nurse learns that a suspicious and socially isolated client who lives alone chooses to eat one meal a day at a nearby soup kitchen and spend the remainder of his daily food allowance on cigarettes. The nurse's initial action should be to
   1. tell the client he must stop smoking to save money.
   2. assess weight and determine foods and amounts eaten.
   3. report the situation to the manager of the soup kitchen.
   4. seek rehospitalization for the client while a new plan is put into place.

Answer: 2

Rationale: Assessment of biopsychosocial needs and general ability to live in the community is called for before any action is taken. Both nutritional status and income adequacy are critical assessment parameters. Option 1: This demand would probably be ignored.

Chapter 6   Mental Health Nursing in Community Settings

Remember, a client may be able to maintain adequate nutrition while eating only one meal a day. Option 3: The rule is to assess before taking action. Option 4: Hospitalization may not be necessary.

Cognitive level: Application
Nursing process: Assessment
NCLEX: Physiological Integrity
See text pages: 87, 88

7. The community psychiatric nurse notes that a client with schizophrenia has remained stable in the community for 6 weeks after discharge from the hospital. Two weeks after making this notation in the medical record, the nurse is called by the client's husband to say that the client is delusional and explosive. During the home visit the nurse learns that the client is willing to take medication, but when her 90-day supply ran out she had none to take. The nurse arranges for a prescription refill. To avoid recurrence of this situation
   1. the nurse will obtain the prescription refill every 90 days and deliver it to the client.
   2. the client's husband will mark dates to obtain prescription refills on the calendar.
   3. the client will report to the hospital for medication follow-up every week.
   4. the client will call the nurse weekly to discuss medication-related issues.

Answer: 2
Rationale: The nurse will attempt to use the client's support system to meet client needs whenever possible. Option 1 should be unnecessary for the nurse to do if client or a significant other can be responsible. Option 3: The client may not need more intensive follow-up as long as she continues to take medication as prescribed. Option 4: This is probably unnecessary because no client issues except failure to obtain medication refill were identified.

Cognitive level: Application
Nursing process: Planning
NCLEX: Safe and Effective Care Environment
See text page: 88

8. The nurse assigned to an assertive community treatment program should explain the program's treatment goals as
   1. assisting clients to maintain abstinence from alcohol and other substances of abuse.
   2. maintaining medications and stable psychiatric status for incarcerated inmates who have a history of mental illness.
   3. providing assessment and intervention for mentally ill individuals who would otherwise have no access to care.

4. providing structure and a therapeutic milieu for mentally ill clients whose symptoms require stabilization.

Answer: 3
Rationale: A mobile health care unit cares for individuals who would not come to a treatment facility or an established site. Assessment and intervention are the primary aspects of the nursing process used. Little time for extensive planning and little opportunity for evaluation of outcomes exist. Option 1 is a goal relevant to a substance abuse treatment program. Option 2 is a goal relevant to a forensic setting. Option 4 is a goal of an inpatient unit.

Cognitive level: Application
Nursing process: Planning
NCLEX: Safe and Effective Care Environment
See text pages: 92-94

9. The nurse assigned to the assertive community treatment program is responsible for determining the location of a new inner city site for a 3-hour block of time each Tuesday. The nurse has learned the following facts: A conference room is available on the sixth floor of city hall as well as a large lobby area on the first floor, either of which could each be used as a site between 9 AM and noon. City police have been successful in clearing homeless individuals from a two-block area around city hall. A firehouse near city hall has offered a room that could be used on alternate Tuesdays from 2 to 5 PM. A fast-food restaurant located approximately four blocks from city hall is willing to allow use of its "party room" from 7 to 10 AM. The most preferable site would be the
   1. city hall conference room.
   2. city hall lobby.
   3. firehouse room.
   4. restaurant "party room."

Answer: 4
Rationale: The room in the fast-food restaurant is preferable because it could be used consistently each week and because inner city residents, including those from the homeless shelter, could go there without interference.

Cognitive level: Analysis
Nursing process: Planning
NCLEX: Safe and Effective Care Environment
See text pages: 92-94

10. A nurse can best address factors of critical importance to successful community treatment during a new client interview by including assessments relative to (more than one answer may be correct)
    1. housing adequacy and stability.
    2. income adequacy and stability.

220

3. family and other support systems.
4. early psychosocial development.
5. substance abuse history and current use.

Answers: 1, 2, 3, 5

Rationale: Early psychosocial developmental history is less relevant to successful outcomes in the community than the assessments listed in the other options. If a client is homeless or fears homelessness, focusing on other treatment issues is impossible. Option 2: Sufficient income for basic needs and medication is necessary. Option 3: Adequate support is a requisite to community placement. Option 4: This information has less bearing on the success of community treatment than the issues related to daily living arrangements. Option 5: Substance abuse undermines medication effectiveness and interferes with community adjustment.

Cognitive level: Application
Nursing process: Assessment
NCLEX: Psychosocial Integrity
See text pages: 87, 88

11. A community mental health nurse has been working for 6 months to establish a trusting relationship with a delusional and suspicious client. The client recently lost his job, stopped taking medication because he had no money, and then decompensated. The client states "only a traitor would make me go to the hospital." The nurse must decide whether to arrange for hospitalization or try to provide medication so he can remain at home. The solution most in keeping with current practices in health care calls for
1. hospitalization for up to a week.
2. negotiating a way to provide medication.
3. hospitalization until he is asymptomatic.
4. arranging for a bed in a homeless shelter.

Answer: 2

Rationale: Although no absolutely "right" answer exists, hospitalization will damage the nurse-client relationship even if it provides an opportunity for rapid stabilization. If medication can be obtained and restarted, the client can possibly be stabilized in the home setting, even if it takes a little longer. Option 4: A homeless shelter is inappropriate and unnecessary.

Cognitive level: Analysis
Nursing process: Planning
NCLEX: Safe and Effective Care Environment
See text page: 86

12. An activity a nurse engaged exclusively in community-based primary prevention would implement is
1. substance abuse counseling.
2. teaching parenting skills.

3. medication follow-up.
4. depression screening.

Answer: 2

Rationale: Primary prevention activities are directed to healthy populations to provide information for developing skills that will result in preventing mental illness. The other options are secondary prevention activities.

Cognitive level: Application
Nursing process: Implementation
NCLEX: Psychosocial Integrity
See text page: 86

13. A Vietnamese immigrant is a student at the local community college nursing program. The nursing instructor is concerned because the student has poor eye contact and has difficulty asking the direct questions necessary for client assessment. The nursing instructor arranges for the student to be assessed by the nurse practitioner in the college health service. This action reflects
1. appropriate secondary prevention by the instructor.
2. insufficient understanding of the student's culture.
3. a violation of the student's civil rights.
4. prejudice and discrimination.

Answer: 2

Rationale: In the student's culture making eye contact can be perceived as disrespectful. In addition, asking direct questions may seem to the student to be intrusive and disrespectful. Option 1: This behavior is not symptomatic of psychiatric illness; thus referral is inappropriate. Option 3: Referral does not violate civil rights, although it is insensitive on the part of the nursing instructor. Option 4: No evidence exists that the instructor was prejudiced rather than uninformed.

Cognitive level: Analysis
Nursing process: Implementation
NCLEX: Psychosocial Integrity
See text pages: 87, 88

14. A client who has serious and persistent symptoms of schizophrenia lives in the community. On a home visit, the community psychiatric nurse case manager learns that the client:
_ Will begin attending an activities group at the mental health outreach center
_ Is worried that he may not have enough money to pay for the therapy
_ Does not know how to get from home to the outreach center
_ Has an appointment to have blood work at the same time the activities group meets

221

The task listed below that is outside the coordinating role of the nurse would be
1. negotiating the cost of therapy for the client.
2. rearranging conflicting care appointments.
3. arranging transportation to the outreach center.
4. monitoring to ensure that client needs are met.

Answer: 1
Rationale: The actions mentioned in options 2, 3, and 4 reflect the coordinating role of the community psychiatric nurse case manager. Negotiating the cost of therapy is an intervention the nurse would not be expected to undertake.
Cognitive level: Application
Nursing process: Implementation
NCLEX: Safe and Effective Care Environment
See text page: 89

15. The assessment data item more relevant for the community psychiatric health nurse than the hospital-based psychiatric nurse for planning client interventions is
1. history of mental illness in the family.
2. culturally related psychotropic dosing.
3. financial status of the client.
4. physical state of the client.

Answer: 3
Rationale: The financial status of the client determines the viability of certain interventions in the community but is of little or no concern when determining a program of in-hospital treatment. The family history of mental illness, the physical status of the client, and culturally related dosage differences for psychotropic drugs would be of equal concern to the nurse in the hospital and the nurse in the community.
Cognitive level: Application
Nursing process: Planning
NCLEX: Psychosocial Integrity
See text pages: 87, 88

16. The community psychiatric nurse is attempting to facilitate medication compliance for a client by having the physician prescribe depot medication that will be given by injection every 3 weeks at the community mental health outreach clinic. For this plan to be successful, what factor will the nurse assess as being of critical importance?
1. The attitude of significant others toward the client
2. Nutrition services in the client's neighborhood
3. A trusting relationship between the client and the nurse
4. The availability of transportation to the clinic

Answer: 4
Rationale: The ability of the client to get to the clinic is of paramount importance to the success of the plan.

The depot medication relieves the client of the necessity to take medication daily, but if he or she does not receive the injection at 3-week intervals, noncompliance will again be the issue. Options 1, 2, and 3: Attitude toward the client, trusting relationships, and nutrition are important but not fundamental to this particular problem.
Cognitive level: Analysis
Nursing process: Assessment
NCLEX: Safe and Effective Care Environment
See text pages: 86, 87

17. The community psychiatric nurse makes a home visit to see a client who is scheduled to receive home care. The nurse notes the client and family make poor eye contact and that the client and all members of the family deferred to the father to answer questions during the visit. In what sphere does the explanation for this observation probably reside?
1. Physical
2. Cultural
3. Environmental
4. Psychopathological

Answer: 2
Rationale: Eye contact and family patterns of authority are often culturally determined. The other options are much less likely to provide a plausible explanation of the observation. Option 1: All parties are physically able to communicate. Option 3: The environment is identical for all possible speakers. Option 4: No mention of psychopathology for any family members is given.
Cognitive level: Application
Nursing process: Assessment
NCLEX: Psychosocial Integrity
See text pages: 87, 88

18. Outcomes established with the mentally ill client in the community compared with those planned for a hospitalized client will
1. involve a longer time frame.
2. require more psychoeducation.
3. have greater focus on symptom absence.
4. be more concerned with medication management.

Answer: 1
Rationale: Community care is concerned with long-term outcomes, whereas hospital care is concerned with short-term outcomes. Options 2 and 4: Planning in either setting would be equally concerned with medication management and necessary psychoeducation. Option 3: Planning in either setting would probably not set goals for absence of symptoms, which might be unrealistic.
Cognitive level: Analysis

Nursing process: Planning
NCLEX: Psychosocial Integrity
See text page: 88

19. Nurse extenders in the hospital are called psychiatric technicians or nursing assistants. Whom should the nurse identify as extenders in community psychiatric care?
    1. Pharmacists
    2. Social workers
    3. Psychiatrists and psychologists
    4. Supportive or concerned acquaintances

Answer: 4
Rationale: Nurses in the community are often assisted by informal helpers such as the significant others of the client, the landlord, the local police, clergy, and other concerned volunteers. Community-based nurses and clients have less contact with the traditional members of the interdisciplinary team than do individuals in the hospital-based setting.
Cognitive level: Comprehension
Nursing process: Assessment
NCLEX: Safe and Effective Care Environment
See text page: 88

20. The client assessment finding that deserves priority intervention by the nurse working in the community setting is that the client
    1. receives Social Security disability income plus a small check from a trust fund.
    2. lives in an apartment with two clients who attend day hospital programs.
    3. has a sister who is interested and active in his care planning.
    4. purchases and uses marijuana on a frequent basis.

Answer: 4
Rationale: Clients who regularly buy illegal substances often become medication noncompliant. Medication noncompliance, along with the disorganizing influence of illegal drugs on cellular brain function, promotes relapse. Options 1, 2, and 3 do not suggest problems.
Cognitive level: Analysis
Nursing process: Planning
NCLEX: Safe and Effective Care Environment
See text pages: 86, 87

21. The client statements that identify aspects of nursing functions of high therapeutic value to a client being followed by an interdisciplinary community mental health team are "The nurse (more than one answer may be correct)
    1. talks in language I can understand."
    2. looks at me as a whole person with lots of needs."

    3. lets me do whatever I choose without interfering."
    4. helps me keep track of my medication."
    5. is willing to go on a date with me."

Answers: 1, 2, 4
Rationale: Each of the correct answers is an example of appropriate nursing foci: communicating at a level understandable to the client, using holistic principles to guide care, and providing medication supervision. Option 3 suggests a laissez faire attitude on the part of the nurse, when the nurse should provide thoughtful feedback and help clients test alternative solutions. Option 5 is a boundary violation.
Cognitive level: Analysis
Nursing process: Implementation
NCLEX: Safe and Effective Care Environment
See text pages: 88, 89

22. A client tells the nurse at the medication management clinic that she hasn't taken her antidepressant medication as the physician directed; she "forgets" the midday dose because she has lunch with friends and doesn't want to be different because she takes pills. The most appropriate intervention for the nurse would be to
    1. investigate the possibility of once-daily dosing.
    2. explain how taking each dose of medication on time relates to health maintenance.
    3. suggest she confide in a co-worker and ask if the co-worker would also take some sort of medication at noon.
    4. establish the nursing diagnosis of "noncompliance with medication regimen related to lack of knowledge" on the care plan.

Answer: 1
Rationale: Option 1 has the highest potential for helping the client achieve compliance. Many antidepressants can be administered by once-daily dosing, a plan that increases compliance. Option 2 is reasonable but would not achieve the goal because it does not address the issue of stigma. Option 3: The self-conscious client would not be comfortable doing this. Option 4: A better etiology statement would be related to social stigma.
Cognitive level: Analysis
Nursing process: Implementation
NCLEX: Psychosocial Integrity
See text page: 89

23. The community psychiatric nurse makes the assessment that, based on biological signs, a seriously and persistently mentally ill client with a mood disorder seems to be somewhat more depressed than on his previous clinic visit a month ago. The client, how-

ever, states he feels the same. The intervention that gives credence to the nurse's assessment while supporting client autonomy is to
1. arrange for a short hospitalization.
2. schedule weekly clinic appointments.
3. refer to the crisis intervention clinic.
4. call the client's family and ask them to observe the client closely.

Answer: 2

Rationale: Scheduling clinic appointments at shorter intervals will give the opportunity for more frequent assessment of symptoms and allow the nurse to use early intervention. Option 1 is wasteful of scarce resources. Option 3: If the client does not admit to having a crisis or problem this referral would be useless. Option 4: This may or may not produce reliable information.

Cognitive level: Analysis
Nursing process: Implementation
NCLEX: Psychosocial Integrity
See text page: 89

24. A client with serious mental illness lives alone in a neighborhood in which she is well accepted as someone who can baby-sit for an hour or two or who will help with housekeeping chores if someone is ill. The client receives depot medication injections but lately has missed regular clinic appointments, saying "My life is so busy I couldn't find time to come in." To prevent hospitalization associated with noncompliance with medication regimen, the community mental health nurse should arrange for
1. psychosocial club membership.
2. assertive community treatment.
3. an appointment with a nurse in private practice.
4. health maintenance organization authorization for changing to daily oral medication.

Answer: 2

Rationale: The assertive community treatment team could bring the client's medication to her in her neighborhood. Option 4: Depot medication is a strategy to reduce noncompliance and is often preferable to daily oral medication. Options 1 and 3 do not directly relate to the noncompliance problem.

Cognitive level: Application
Nursing process: Implementation
NCLEX: Safe and Effective Care Environment
See text pages: 92-94

25. In a rush of words, a client tells the community mental health nurse "Everything's a mess! I can't concentrate. My disability check didn't come. My roommate moved out and the rent is too much for me to

pay on my own. To top it all off, my therapist is moving out of state. I don't know where to turn and I feel as though I'm coming apart at the seams." A nursing diagnosis the nurse should consider for this client is
1. decisional conflict related to challenges to personal values.
2. spiritual distress related to ethical implications of treatment regimen.
3. anxiety related to changes perceived as threatening to psychological equilibrium.
4. deficient knowledge related to need to solve multiple problems affecting security needs.

Answer: 3

Rationale: Subjective and objective data obtained by the nurse suggest the client is experiencing anxiety caused by multiple threats to security needs. Option 1: Data are not present to suggest decisional conflict, ethical conflicts around treatment causing spiritual distress, or deficient knowledge.

Cognitive level: Analysis
Nursing process: Diagnosis
NCLEX: Psychosocial Integrity
See text pages: 87, 88

26. The client that a nurse would plan to refer to a partial hospitalization program is the individual who
1. spent yesterday in the 24-hour supervised crisis care center and continues to be actively suicidal.
2. has agoraphobia and panic episodes and needs psychoeducation for relaxationtherapy.
3. is well regulated on lithium and reports regularly for blood tests and clinic follow-up.
4. is being discharged from an alcohol detoxification unit. He states, "I'm not sure I can abstain after my wife goes to work in the morning."

Answer: 4

Rationale: This client could profit from the structure and supervision provided by spending the day at the partial hospitalization program. During the evening, at night, and on weekends his wife could assume responsibility for supervision. Option 1: This client would need hospitalization. Option 2: This client could be referred to home care. Option 3: This client could continue on the same plan.

Cognitive level: Analysis
Nursing process: Planning
NCLEX: Safe and Effective Care Environment
See text page: 90

27. For the client to be discharged from acute hospital care to clinical case management at home, care planning should be predicated on evidence that best outcomes will be produced by

1. weekly follow-up for 6 weeks, then every 2 weeks.
2. monthly follow-up for 6 months to 1 year.
3. no follow-up for 3 months, then quarterly visits.
4. referral to the assertive treatment team for daily contact.

Answer: 1

Rationale: Best outcomes are achieved when clients have regular, frequent follow-up in the community. Options 2 and 3 provide too little follow-up. Option 4 provides a more intensive follow-up than may be required.

Cognitive level: Analysis
Nursing process: Planning
NCLEX: Safe and Effective Care Environment
See text page: 90

CHAPTER 7

1. The cultural pattern highly valued in American society that often results in nurses of the dominant culture establishing unrealistic outcomes for clients of other cultural groups is
   1. interdependence.
   2. present orientation.
   3. using direct confrontation to solve problems.
   4. suspending one's own needs in favor of external obligations.

Answer: 3

Rationale: Directly confronting problems is a highly valued approach in the American culture; however, it is not part of many other cultures in which harmony and restraint are valued. American nurses mistakenly think that all clients are capable of taking direct action. Clients with other values will be unable to meet this culturally inappropriate outcome. Option 1: This cultural pattern is valued more by indigenous peoples. Option 2: Present orientation is not part of Western culture; it is seen more in the Hispanic tradition and indigenous cultures. Option 4: This pattern is seen more often in Eastern cultures.

Cognitive level: Comprehension
Nursing process: Planning
NCLEX: Psychosocial Integrity
See text pages: 102-105

2. The provision of culturally competent nursing care will be fostered when the nurse plans and implements care on the belief that
   1. a nursing goal is to foster assimilation and conformity.
   2. reading a handbook describing the practices of various cultures is sufficient.

3. the ability to work within the client's cultural context requires ongoing effort.
4. self-examination of attitudes toward various cultures promotes dehumanizing care.

Answer: 3

Rationale: Cultural competence requires health care providers to see themselves as becoming culturally competent rather than being culturally competent. This view requires the provider to continuously strive to work effectively within the cultural context of the client. Option 1: Assimilation and conformity may not be desired by the client. Option 2: Handbooks can be helpful but do not provide all knowledge. Option 4: This action should move the nurse toward providing more humanistic care rather than dehumanizing care.

Cognitive level: Application
Nursing process: Implementation
NCLEX: Psychosocial Integrity
See text pages: 109, 110

3. To provide culturally competent care after becoming familiar with the way of life of individuals of a particular culture, the nurse will
   1. accurately interpret the thinking of individual clients.
   2. anticipate how a client will perceive treatment interventions.
   3. need to identify strategies that fit within the cultural context of the clients.
   4. find it possible to devise interventions to reduce the client's ethnocentrism.

Answer: 3

Rationale: Cultural competence is a continual process of "becoming" as opposed to a state that is arrived at and maintained without ongoing effort. Culture is dynamic, diversified, and changing. The nurse must be prepared to gain cultural knowledge and then determine the nursing care measures that clients find acceptable and helpful. Option 1: Interpreting the thinking of individual clients cannot be done simply by having knowledge of the culture. Option 2: This may be true to some extent: however, because of individual thinking, it cannot be a certainty. Option 4: Reducing a client's ethnocentrism may not be a desired outcome.

Cognitive level: Application
Nursing process: Implementation
NCLEX: Psychosocial Integrity
See text page: 110

4. A clinical specialist supervises therapy for a 26-year-old African American client originally from Haiti who was admitted for depression. A staff nurse tells the clinical specialist that " The client can't

225

seem to express her feelings when I ask about them. She just looks down." The nurse adds, "But I've seen her talking to a young African American client, and she seems quite spontaneous." What remark by the clinical specialist would help the staff nurse develop cultural competence?

1. "Why not ask the other client to tell you what your client tells him. Once you have an opening, your client will become more spontaneous with you."
2. "Don't take it personally. African Americans often have a resentful attitude that takes weeks to overcome."
3. "She may have difficulty communicating her feelings in standard English. Have you considered using a cultural translator?"
4. "Most African Americans depend on the African American church for support. Why not ask her pastor to come in to pray with the two of you for the success of her treatment?"

Answer: 3

Rationale: Society expects a culturally diverse client to accommodate and use standard English. This may be virtually impossible during episodes of mental illness. Cultural translators can be helpful with language and helping the nurse to understand the Haitian worldview and cultural nuances.

Cognitive level: Application
Nursing process: Implementation
NCLEX: Psychosocial Integrity
See text pages: 111, 112

5. A Haitian client who has been diagnosed with depression tells the nurse that "There's nothing you can do. I'm being punished. The only thing I can do is see Sister Ondine. She's the only one who can take away curses." How might the culturally knowledgeable nurse assess the situation? The client

1. is feeling hopeless, helpless, and worthless related to some yet-to-be-established cause.
2. may have a delusion of persecution.
3. has probably been misdiagnosed.
4. may believe her distress resulted from a spell cast upon her.

Answer: 4

Rationale: Culturally diverse individuals of African American or Caribbean cultures who have a fatalistic attitude about illness may believe they are being punished for wrongdoing or that they are victims of witchcraft or voodoo. They are usually more reticent to share information about curses with therapists than the client in this scenario, however. Options 1 and 2: No data are present in the scenario to support

these assessments. Option 3: Misdiagnosis more commonly labels a client with depression as having schizophrenia.

Cognitive level: Analysis
Nursing process: Assessment
NCLEX: Psychosocial Integrity
See text page: 105

6. An African American client who is highly suspicious is given to angry outbursts and accusations that staff are discriminating against him when they remove possibly harmful objects from his possession according to hospital policy. An explanation that shows cultural awareness relating to the client's behavior is that it may be prompted by

1. feelings of powerlessness.
2. institutional discrimination.
3. fear of abandonment.
4. family solidarity.

Answer: 1

Rationale: The rules of the health care system often seem like added measures of oppression to African Americans, who respond with behavior designed to fend off feelings of powerlessness and vulnerability. The other options have no bearing on the situation.

Cognitive level: Analysis
Nursing process: Assessment
NCLEX: Psychosocial Integrity
See text page: 110

7. The nurse in the outpatient medication clinic has a full appointment book. A Hispanic American client misses his 10 AM appointment, arriving at 12:30 PM, and a Native American client does not keep her appointment at all. What understanding on the part of the nurse will lead to satisfactory planning? These culturally diverse clients are

1. members of cultural groups that have a different view of time.
2. immature and irresponsible in health care matters.
3. displaying passive-aggressive tendencies.
4. acting out feelings of anger toward the system.

Answer: 1

Rationale: Hispanic Americans and Native Americans traditionally treat time in a way unlike the "American" culture. They tend to be present-oriented; that is, they value the current interaction more than what is to be done in the future. Thus, if engaged in an activity, they may simply continue the activity and appear hours or days later for an appointment. Understanding this, the nurse can avoid feelings of frustration and anger when the nurse's future orientation comes into conflict with the client's present orientation.

Cognitive level: Application
Nursing process: Planning
NCLEX: Psychosocial Integrity
See text pages: 101, 102

8. A nurse is assigned to work with a single Asian American college student. The nurse tells a colleague that the client has very poor eye contact, and that no matter what strategies he uses to try to get her to meet his gaze, she will not look directly at him. Which of the following explanations would be possible reasons for the client's behavior? In some Asian cultures
   1. a strong cultural injunction exists against using assertive communication measures.
   2. looking directly at a person of the opposite sex indicates sexual interest.
   3. looking down signifies deference to authority.
   4. trancelike syndromes are common.

Answers: 1, 2, 3
Rationale: Options 1, 2, and 3 describe cultural beliefs often held by Asian American groups. They are each based on valuing concepts of respect and restraint. Although trancelike syndromes do occur among members of certain cultures, they are not related to this situation.

Cognitive level: Analysis
Nursing process: Assessment
NCLEX: Psychosocial Integrity
See text page: 103

9. The sibling of a client who is a single Asian American college student tells the nurse "My sister needs help for the pain in her back. She goes crazy—screaming and crying, like when they brought her to the hospital, from the hurt." What understanding on the part of the nurse will contribute to a culturally relevant care plan? The client
   1. will require a prolonged hospitalization to stabilize these symptoms.
   2. will probably respond best to a therapist who remains aloof and ungiving.
   3. may express emotional distress with physical symptoms and look to health professionals to treat the physical symptoms.
   4. has an independent worldview and must be treated without consideration to information given by family members.

Answer: 3
Rationale: The orientation that psychological problems are caused by a physical imbalance is prevalent

among Asian Americans. These clients often expect healers to focus on treatment of the physical symptoms and believe the psychological symptoms will then subside. Option 1: Hospitalization will likely be short. Option 2: The client will probably respond best to a therapist who is perceived as giving; thus giving a medication to treat the back pain would be expected by the client. Option 4: Asian Americans usually have strong family ties. Information from the family may be invaluable.

Cognitive level: Application
Nursing process: Planning
NCLEX: Psychosocial Integrity
See text pages: 105-108

10. The communication style that would be most effective for a culturally knowledgeable nurse to adopt during an assessment interview with a 40-year-old Native American client would be
    1. the frequent use of nonverbal behaviors such as gesturing, smiling, and making wry faces to express negatives.
    2. a loud voice, unbroken eye contact, minimal gesturing, and straight-to-the-point questions.
    3. to be open and friendly, ask direct questions, and touch the client's arm or hand occasionally for reassurance.
    4. a soft voice, breaking eye contact occasionally, with general leads and reflective techniques.

Answer: 4
Rationale: Native American culture stresses living in harmony with nature. Cooperative, sharing styles rather than competitive or intrusive approaches are preferred; thus the more passive style described in option 4 would be best received. The other options would be more effective to use with clients with a Western orientation.

Cognitive level: Application
Nursing process: Implementation
NCLEX: Psychosocial Integrity
See text pages: 110, 111

11. A Native American client describes having difficulty learning as a child, living on a reservation, and being sent away to the Native American boarding school. He began to use alcohol as a teenager to feel euphoria and escape the feelings of isolation. As an adult he states he feels "stupid and good for nothing." Gastritis forced him to give up drinking 10 years ago. Recently, he has found some comfort in tribal rituals. In planning care for this client the nurse should realize that he should be offered a program based on
    1. treatment for both depression and alcohol abuse.
    2. group discussion of posttraumatic stress disorder.

227

3. holistic principles.
4. psychoanalysis.

Answer: 3

Rationale: Native Americans, because of their beliefs in the interrelatedness of parts and about being in harmony with nature, respond best to a holistic approach. Option 1: No data are present to support dual diagnosis because the client has resolved the problem of excessive alcohol use. Option 2: No data are present to support a diagnosis of posttraumatic stress disorder. Option 4: Psychoanalysis is a long-term therapy that is very expensive. Cognitive therapy might be a better choice.

Cognitive level: Application
Nursing process: Planning
NCLEX: Psychosocial Integrity
See text page: 102

12. A Native American client describes having difficulty learning as a child, living on a reservation, and being sent away to the Native American boarding school. He began to use alcohol as a teenager to feel euphoria and escape the feelings of isolation. As an adult he states he feels "stupid and good for nothing." The nursing diagnosis a culturally competent nurse should consider developing for him is
    1. risk for other-directed violence.
    2. chronic low self-esteem.
    3. deficient knowledge.
    4. noncompliance.

Answer: 2

Rationale: The client has given several indications that he has chronic low self-esteem. Forming a positive self-image is often difficult for Native American individuals because these indigenous people must blend together both American and Native American worldviews. No defining characteristics are present for any of the other nursing diagnoses mentioned.

Cognitive level: Analysis
Nursing process: Diagnosis
NCLEX: Psychosocial Integrity
See text page: 109

13. To plan effective care, the nurse needs to understand that the family characteristic reflecting the worldview of Asian American and Hispanic American families that will most affect how decisions are made about care is
    1. the mother as head of the household.
    2. the father as the authority figure.
    3. giving considerable freedom to women.
    4. using emotional communication styles.

Answer: 2

Rationale: Both Asian American and Hispanic American families traditionally place the father in the position of power as the head of the household. Option 1: The mother is usually subservient to the father in these cultures. Option 3: Women are often placed in subservient roles, and adolescent girls are sheltered in both cultures. Option 4: Hispanic Americans may use a communication style that is high in affect, but Asian Americans are more likely to be reserved.

Cognitive level: Application
Nursing process: Planning
NCLEX: Psychosocial Integrity
See text page: 105

14. The client, a newly arrived Russian immigrant, was admitted to the mental health unit after creating a disturbance in a church while a funeral was taking place. During the admission interview he is loud, mixes English and Russian phrases, and makes gestures such as vigorously shaking his fist. The nurse responsible for admitting him should
    1. tell him she is going to ask him some questions that he must try to answer in English.
    2. defer the nursing admission interview until after the client has calmed down.
    3. request the assistance of a security guard.
    4. request the assistance of an interpreter.

Answer: 4

Rationale: A psychotic client who is mixing English and his or her native language cannot be accurately assessed by an English-speaking nurse who does not speak the other language. The care plan should be based on accurate assessment data; hence calling for an interpreter is necessary and expedient. Most hospitals have a list of individuals who are fluent in various languages and are willing to assist the medical staff. Option 1 will not produce the desired result if the client is disorganized and unable to comply. Option 2: Assessment information is necessary to obtain if at all possible. Deferring the interview should not be an initial option. Option 3: Data do not suggest the client is aggressive, although fist-shaking might be interpreted as aggressive in some cultural contexts.

Cognitive level: Application
Nursing process: Implementation
NCLEX: Psychosocial Integrity
See text page: 106

15. The statement relating to conceptions of self that will help a nurse accurately assess culturally diverse clients and plan care is
    1. The Western conception of self is the ego, the aspect of personality that mediates demands of the

id, the superego, and the environment. The definition of self in the interdependent worldview tradition is described as a web of relationships and expectations of the hierarchical group.

2. The conception of self of indigenous peoples is an unbounded ego interacting primarily with family. The Western self is defined in the context of collective family genealogy traced from male lineage over centuries.

3. The Western worldview views self as being independent and isolated from family and community. The Eastern worldview defines self in terms of the relationship with all of nature.

4. The Eastern worldview sees self as independent of family and social relationships, with little emphasis on duty. Western tradition views self as interdependent, interrelated, and connected with all ancestors and community.

Answer: 1

Rationale: The Western self is individual and focuses on articulation of one's own ideas, desires, and needs as well as on goal attainment and is consistent with an independent worldview. The interdependent worldview is exemplified in Asian cultures, in which self is incomplete and part of a cooperative hierarchical group of insiders with common needs, goals, and concerns. The Native American self also exemplifies an interdependent worldview with self linked with all other living things. Two other cultures that exemplify an interdependent worldview are the Arabic culture, in which self is viewed as part of a group that includes a lineage, and one's value is derived from the social unit, and the African culture, where self includes one's ancestors, nature, and community.

Cognitive level: Comprehension
Nursing process: Implementation
NCLEX: Psychosocial Integrity
See text pages: 101, 102

16. A Hispanic client whose only child died of pneumonia over a year ago states that she is unable to go about her usual home duties and community interactions because of debilitating headaches and backaches. The psychiatrist diagnoses depression. Her primary care nurse tells the clinical nurse specialist "I can't seem to help her. All she talks about are the headaches and the backaches." The clinical nurse specialist can foster the cultural competence of the nurse by saying
   1. "You need to be patient and let her take the lead."
   2. "You must take the lead and focus on the reason for her resistance."
   3. "In her culture, physical symptoms are idioms of distress expressing emotional pain."

4. "You might ask the client why she has chosen to grieve for her child in this particular way."

Answer: 3

Rationale: Nurses often need to be sensitized to client use of physical symptoms as a means of expressing psychological pain. Somatic equivalents are seen in clients of the Western culture as well.

Cognitive level: Application
Nursing process: Implementation
NCLEX: Psychosocial Integrity
See text pages: 106-108

17. A client who is Chinese American has been diagnosed with an anxiety disorder. The client tells the nurse she thinks her symptoms began when her energy became imbalanced. When the nurse asks what ideas the client has about ways of treating the imbalance, the nurse should expect the client to suggest a plan for
   1. eating special foods.
   2. taking antianxiety medication.
   3. undergoing cognitive behavior therapy.
   4. having a native healer perform a ritual.

Answer: 1

Rationale: The concept of energy imbalance as a source of illness is an explanatory model familiar to Asian cultures. A source of healing is dietary change to include either "hot" or "cold" foods to correct the imbalance. "Hot" and "cold" in this case do not refer to thermal properties of the foods. Option 2 would not be a first-line option for a client with an Eastern worldview. Herbal remedies are more in keeping with this worldview. Option 3: Cognitive therapy would not be a treatment suggested by a client with an Eastern worldview. Option 4: This remedy would be suggested by someone from an indigenous culture.

Cognitive level: Application
Nursing process: Planning
NCLEX: Psychosocial Integrity
See text page: 105

18. Which of the following tips would be useful to an American nurse preparing for a cross-cultural encounter with a female client from Japan? (More than one answer may be correct.)
   1. Anticipate diversity.
   2. Promote a feeling of acceptance.
   3. Learn what it means to be the client by assessing health beliefs.
   4. Facilitate communication by using direct eye contact and a handshake.
   5. Remember that all Eastern women adhere to the same cultural norms.

Answers: 1, 2, 3

Rationale: Options 1, 2, and 3 are helpful hints. Anticipating diversity puts the nurse in a position of guarding against stereotyping and opens the nurse to cultural awareness. Option 2: Promoting feelings of acceptance prevents cultural pain. Option 3: Learning about the position of the client facilitates empathy. Option 4: The least useful strategy would be to use direct eye contact and touch. In a cross-cultural encounter strategies known to be acceptable to the client are preferable. When particular strategies have not been identified, try to avoid offending the client. Direct eye contact and touch may be offensive to clients whose culture calls for more reserved cultural practices. Option 5: This stereotype may lead to culturally insensitive care decisions.

Cognitive level: Analysis
Nursing process: Implementation
NCLEX: Psychosocial Integrity
See text page: 105

19. A psychiatric nurse with 3 years of inpatient experience has been assigned to work in a medication follow-up clinic beginning Monday. The clinic sees culturally diverse clients. To prepare for work in the clinic it would be advisable for the nurse to
   1. review the literature on cultural differences in client responses to psychotropic medications.
   2. read a handbook on the various health beliefs of members of diverse cultures.
   3. contact the clinical nurse specialist for guidelines for cultural competence.
   4. take a course in psychopharmacology.

Answer: 1

Rationale: A nurse with 3 years' experience working on a mental health inpatient unit can be assumed to be familiar with the action and side effects of most commonly prescribed psychotropic medications. However, because culturally diverse clients are seen in the clinic, reviewing cultural differences in client response to these medications could be helpful. One such difference is the development of extrapyramidal side effects at lower drug doses in Asian clients. Options 2 and 3: Neither is sufficient to produce cultural competence. Option 4: This might be helpful in the long run, but the nurse begins work at the clinic on Monday.

Cognitive level: Application
Nursing process: Implementation
NCLEX: Physiological Integrity
See text page: 108

20. A mental health nurse with 3 years of inpatient experience is about to begin work in a medication follow-up clinic that serves a culturally diverse client population. Which way of sitting during an interview is most neutral and acceptable to people of most cultures?
   1. Legs crossed, leaning slightly backward in chair with one arm extended on the desk
   2. Feet on the floor and upper body leaning slightly forward toward client
   3. One leg crossed and the upper body turned slightly away from client
   4. Feet on the floor and arms crossed over chest

Answer: 2

Rationale: The correct pose is most neutral related to arms and legs. Leaning slightly forward denotes interest in the person toward which the nurse is inclined. Option 1: Leg crossing is not accepted in some cultures, and leaning backward suggests the individual is placing the barrier of space between self and the other person. Option 3: Crossing the leg to show the bottom of the foot is considered impolite in some cultures. Turning away suggests distancing. Option 4: Crossing the arms over the chest is considered a "closed" authoritarian posture.

Cognitive level: Application
Nursing process: Implementation
NCLEX: Psychosocial Integrity
See text page: 106

21. A client who is a believer in Ayurvedic medicine (traditional remedies) has agreed to take antidepressant medication but tells the nurse that she also wishes to treat her symptoms with healing practices consistent with her own beliefs. The priority question the nurse should ask the client is
   1. "Will be doing special breathing exercises?"
   2. "How will astrology figure into your treatment plan?"
   3. "What, if any, herbs do you plan to take?"
   4. "Will your treatment include yoga?"

Answer: 3

Rationale: The nurse needs to make sure that any herbs the client may take are not harmful when taken in conjunction with the prescribed antidepressants. Options 1, 2, and 4 are considered complementary treatments and are of somewhat less concern because they do not involve harmful interactions among ingested substances.

Cognitive level: Analysis
Nursing process: Assessment
NCLEX: Physiological Integrity
See text page: 105

22. According to the values of cultures whose members use folk healing practices, the factors most important for a nurse to possess include (more than one answer may be correct)
   1. ethnocentrism.
   2. cultural skill.
   3. cultural desire.
   4. cultural knowledge.
   5. academic credentials.
   6. respect for persons.

Answers: 2, 3, 4, 6
Rationale: Cultural skill allows the nurse to make culturally sensitive assessments and plan for care. Cultural desire refers to willingness to learn from the client. Cultural knowledge alerts the nurse to areas where cultural differences may be present, helps with understanding, and reduces misinterpretations. Respect for persons is important to members of all cultures and is part of cultural desire. Option 1: Ethnocentrism may result in imposing the nurse's cultural norms on a client. Option 5: Academic credentials are not of concern because curative factors in healing systems focusing on folk healing. More important are collaboration with cultural translators and extensive involvement with the family and the community when delivering education and making treatment plans.
Cognitive level: Application
Nursing process: Implementation
NCLEX: Safe and Effective Care Environment
See text pages: 106-110

23. The nurse is caring for a family in which four members have tuberculosis. The family describes its health system to the nurse, noting that shamanic healing is used. The nurse will have the greatest success in planning treatment if she creates a plan that uses antituberculin medication as well as
   1. services of a folk healer.
   2. behavior therapy.
   3. acupuncture.
   4. yoga.

Answer: 1
Rationale: Shamanic healing considers that all things have spirit. Healing practices include rituals, cleansings, and prayers delivered by a shaman or folk healer. Folk healing rituals can be successfully combined with Western medicine. Accommodating culture-specific interventions builds on client coping and healing systems. Option 2: Behavior therapy would be of less cultural significance to the family than folk healing. Options 3 and 4: These complementary therapies were not specifically described by the client as being part of her health system.

Cognitive level: Application
Nursing process: Planning
NCLEX: Psychosocial Integrity
See text page: 105

24. Which question would help the nurse assess feminist issues governing the availability of healing options for a woman of a culture with an Eastern interdependent worldview?
   1. "What does someone of your culture call this illness?"
   2. "How does someone with this illness usually behave?"
   3. "How does being a woman affect someone with this illness?"
   4. "How do people of your culture express dislike or displeasure?"

Answer: 3
Rationale: This question will help the nurse understand a woman's importance in the culture. In a culture in which women play a lesser role, healing options may not be readily available. Option 1: This question would help assess culture-bound illness. Option 2: This question relates to sick roles, pain expression, and predominant symptoms. Option 4: This question is more related to general cultural factors than women's issues.
Cognitive level: Analysis
Nursing process: Assessment
NCLEX: Psychosocial Integrity
See text pages: 100, 101

25. During the assessment interview the nurse has ascertained that the client follows cultural tradition and uses spiritual healing. The question that would help the nurse understand the healing options available as part of this health system is
   1. "What do people believe cause this illness?"
   2. "Do people shun or avoid someone who has this illness?"
   3. "Are any ceremonies or prayers used to treat this illness?"
   4. "What language do your people generally use when speaking among yourselves?"

Answer: 3
Rationale: Option 3 is the only question that directly addresses healing options.
Cognitive level: Analysis
Nursing process: Assessment
NCLEX: Psychosocial Integrity
See text pages: 111, 112

26. The hospice nurse planning care for four culturally diverse clients, each of whom has terminal cancer,

Chapter 7   Culturally Relevant Mental Health Nursing

should anticipate that the client who will wish to engage in end-of-life planning (such as making a will, a living will, and funeral arrangements) will be the client who is
1. a single Native American who had worked as a forest ranger.
2. a female immigrant from China who is an acupuncturist.
3. a refugee laborer from a war-torn Western African country.
4. a fourth-generation New England native who is an accountant.

Answer: 4
Rationale: This client would hold a Western worldview and value autonomy, independence, and self-reliance. He would see time as linear and would have an internal locus of control. Self-action would be a high priority. Options 1 and 3: The clients would hold indigenous worldviews. Option 2: The client would hold an Eastern worldview. For options 1, 2, and 3, the concept of person is defined more in relationship to others, and the locus of control is self-rooted in tradition or in natural forces. The need for independence and self-reliance is far less. Tradition, fate, or other forces are seen as being in control.
Cognitive level: Analysis
Nursing process: Planning
NCLEX: Psychosocial Integrity
See text page: 102

27. A health care aide caring for a mentally ill client receiving home care insists that the client must balance energy forces of his body by eating specific foods. The client tells the nurse that he "goes along with the diet to keep the aide happy." The community psychiatric nurse should assess this situation as demonstrating
1. biculturalism.
2. cultural imposition.
3. culture-bound syndrome.
4. preserve-accommodate-restructure phenomenon.

Answer: 2
Rationale: Cultural imposition occurs when a member of one culture forces a member of another culture to adhere to the certain cultural norms. Option 1 refers to the ability to move back and forth between traditional culture and a new culture. Option 3: A culture-bound illness refers to the behavior that one culture understands as illness but that is not so designated in other cultures. Option 4 refers to a framework for care planning that preserves helpful aspects of client culture, accommodates neutral practices, and restructures problematic patterns.

Cognitive level: Application
Nursing process: Assessment
NCLEX: Psychosocial Integrity
See text pages: 102-105

28. The nurse should be particularly alert to somatization of psychological distress among clients whose cultural beliefs include the idea that (more than one answer may be correct)
1. mental illness reflects badly on a family.
2. mental illness is a significant moral weakness.
3. everyone should plan for the future.
4. mind, body, and spirit are merged.
5. intergenerational conflict is to blame.

Answers: 1, 2, 4
Rationale: Physical symptoms are seen as more acceptable in cultural groups in which interdependence and harmony of the group are emphasized. Mental illness is often perceived as reflecting a failure of the entire family. In groups in which mental illness is seen as a moral weakness and both the individual and family are stigmatized, somatization of mental distress is better accepted. In groups in which mind, body, and spirit are holistically perceived, somatization of psychological distress is readily effected. Option 3: Somatization is seen among clients with both future and present orientation to time. Option 5: Intergenerational conflict has not been noted as a risk factor for somatization.
Cognitive level: Comprehension
Nursing process: Assessment
NCLEX: Psychosocial Integrity
See text pages: 106-109

29. A client has inferred that her symptoms of depression are related to an imbalance of yin and yang. A query that should elicit information to guide treatment and nursing care designed to accommodate the client's culture is
1. "Are you concerned about treatment in a hospital setting?"
2. "Are you willing to take Western medications to treat your illness?"
3. "Who should receive information about your health problems?"
4. "What foods should a person with this illness eat?"

Answer: 4
Rationale: Accommodation involves including neutral health practices in the client's plan of care. A diet that addresses correcting yin and yang imbalance would probably be psychologically helpful and would not be likely to interfere with Western medical

232

treatment with selective serotonin reuptake inhibitors. Options 1 and 3 are not relevant to accommodation of diverse cultural health practices. Option 2 would be more related to restructuring.
Cognitive level: Analysis
Nursing process: Assessment
NCLEX: Psychosocial Integrity
See text pages: 111, 112

30. The psychiatric home care nurse makes visits a Hispanic client being treated for depression. The client greets the nurse with a smile and eagerly offers to make coffee. The nurse initiates a handshake, politely refuses the coffee so as not to make work for the client, and suggests they talk about how the client is doing. During the session the nurse notes the client seems less spontaneous in affect and becomes more withdrawn. In analyzing the situation the nurse should correctly conclude that
   1. the client is experiencing rapid cycling.
   2. the client may feel rejected by the nurse.
   3. the nurse has broached a taboo topic.
   4. social touch is inappropriate for Hispanic clients.

Answer: 2
Rationale: In the Hispanic culture, good etiquette requires accepting offers of food and spending some time in small talk before getting down to business. The nurse behaved impolitely by the client's standards. Option 1: Rapid cycling is related to rapid mood swings of bipolar disorder. Option 3: Data are not present to suggest that the nurse touched on a taboo topic. Option 4: Clients of Hispanic culture engage in "high touch" behaviors.
Cognitive level: Analysis
Nursing process: Evaluation
NCLEX: Psychosocial Integrity
See text page: 103

CHAPTER 8

1. The intervention by a psychiatric nurse that implements the ethical principle of autonomy is when the nurse
   1. explores alternative solutions with the client, who later chooses one alternative.
   2. stays with a client who is demonstrating a high level of anxiety.
   3. intervenes when a self-mutilating client attempts to slash her wrists.
   4. suggests that two clients who were fighting be restricted to the unit.

Answer: 1
Rationale: Autonomy is the right to self-determination, that is, to make one's own decisions. By exploring

alternatives with the client, the client is better equipped to make an informed, autonomous decision. Options 2 and 3: These actions demonstrate beneficence and fidelity. Option 4 demonstrates the principles of fidelity and justice.
Cognitive level: Analysis
Nursing process: Implementation
NCLEX: Safe and Effective Care Environment
See text pages: 116, 117

2. The action by a psychiatric nurse that supports the client's right to be treated with dignity and respect is when the nurse
   1. addresses the client by his title and surname (e.g., Mr. Jones).
   2. discusses the client's condition with his physician as they have lunch in the cafeteria.
   3. tells the treatment team that the client is too drowsy to be consulted about the plan of care.
   4. strongly encourages the client to participate in recreational activities available on the unit.

Answer: 1
Rationale: A simple way of showing respect is to address the client by title and surname rather than assume that the client would wish to be called by his first name. Option 2 violates confidentiality. Option 3 violates client autonomy. Option 4 exemplifies beneficence and fidelity.
Cognitive level: Application
Nursing process: Implementation
NCLEX: Safe and Effective Care Environment
See text pages: 118, 119

3. Two psychotic clients in the inpatient unit get into fights when they are in the same room. During a team meeting, one nurse suggests the safety of the two clients is of paramount importance and that their treatment plans should call for both to be placed in seclusion to keep them from injuring each other. The suggestion is significant because it
   1. violates the civil rights of the two clients.
   2. reinforces the autonomy of the two clients.
   3. reveals that the nurse values the principle of justice.
   4. represents the intentional tort of battery.

Answer: 1
Rationale: Clients have a right to treatment in the least restrictive setting. Less restrictive measures should be tried first. Unnecessary seclusion may result in a charge of false imprisonment. Option 2: Seclusion removes the client's autonomy. Option 3: The principle by which the nurse is motivated is beneficence, not justice. Option 4: The tort represented is false imprisonment.

233

Cognitive level: Analysis
Nursing process: Planning
NCLEX: Safe and Effective Care Environment
See text page: 119

4. In a treatment team planning meeting a nurse states her concern about whether the staff is behaving ethically in using restraint to prevent one client from engaging in self-mutilating behavior when the care plan for another self-mutilating client calls for one-on-one supervision. The ethical principle that should govern the situation is
   1. beneficence.
   2. autonomy.
   3. fidelity.
   4. justice.

Answer: 4
Rationale: The nurse is concerned about justice, that is, fair treatment with the least restrictive methods for both clients. Option 1: Beneficence means promoting the good of others. Option 2: Autonomy is the right to make one's own decisions. Option 3: Fidelity is the observance of loyalty and commitment to the client.
Cognitive level: Analysis
Nursing process: Planning
NCLEX: Safe and Effective Care Environment
See text pages: 116, 117

5. Which of the following is an example of a tort?
   1. The primary nurse does not complete the plan of care for a client within 24 hours of the client's admission.
   2. The advanced practice nurse recommends that a client who is a danger to self and others be voluntarily admitted to the psychiatric unit.
   3. The treatment team changes a client's admission status from involuntary to voluntary after medication alleviates the client's hallucinations.
   4. The nurse decides to give a prn dose of neuroleptic drug to a client to prevent violent acting out because the unit is short staffed.

Answer: 4
Rationale: A tort is a civil wrong against a person that violates his or her rights. Giving unnecessary medication for the convenience of staff controls behavior in a manner similar to secluding a client; thus false imprisonment is a possible charge. The other options do not exemplify torts.
Cognitive level: Comprehension
Nursing process: NA
NCLEX: Safe and Effective Care Environment
See text pages: 124, 128

6. What is the legal significance of the nurse's action when a client verbally refuses his medication and the nurse gives the medication over the client's objection? The nurse
   1. can be charged with battery.
   2. can be charged with negligence.
   3. can be charged with malpractice.
   4. will face no charges.

Answer: 1
Rationale: Battery is an intentional tort in which one individual violates the rights of another through touching without consent. Forcing a client to take medication after the medication has been refused constitutes battery. The charge of battery, rather than negligence or malpractice, can be brought against the nurse.
Cognitive level: Analysis
Nursing process: Implementation
NCLEX: Safe and Effective Care Environment
See text page: 128

7. The nursing intervention that constitutes false imprisonment is:
   1. The client is confused and combative. He insists that no one can stop him from leaving. The nurse restrains him without a physician's order, then seeks the order.
   2. The client has been "pesky," seeking the attention of nurses in the nurses' station much of the day. Now the nurse escorts him to his room and tells him to stay there or he'll be put into seclusion.
   3. A psychotic client, admitted as an involuntary patient, runs out of the psychiatric unit. The nurse runs after him and succeeds in talking the client into returning to the unit.
   4. A client, hospitalized as an involuntary admission, attempts to leave the unit. The nurse calls the security team and, acting on established protocol, they prevent him from leaving.

Answer: 2
Rationale: False imprisonment involves holding a competent person against his or her will. Actual force is not a requirement of false imprisonment. The individual needs only to be placed in fear of imprisonment by someone who has the ability to carry out the threat. The client in option 1 is not competent, and the nurse is acting beneficently. The clients in options 3 and 4 have been admitted as involuntary clients and should not be allowed to leave without permission of the treatment team.
Cognitive level: Analysis
Nursing process: Assessment
NCLEX: Safe and Effective Care Environment
See text page: 128

8. The client the nurse should consider for involuntary commitment for psychiatric treatment is the client who
   1. is noncompliant with the medical regimen.
   2. broke the law by selling illegal drugs.
   3. threatens to harm himself and others.
   4. who is filing for bankruptcy.

Answer: 3
Rationale: Involuntary commitment protects clients who are dangerous to themselves or others and cannot care for their own basic needs. Involuntary commitment also protects other individuals in society. The behaviors described in the other options are not sufficient to require involuntary hospitalization.
Cognitive level: Analysis
Nursing process: Assessment
NCLEX: Safe and Effective Care Environment
See text pages: 120, 121

9. The nurse is planning care for a client who voluntarily admitted herself for treatment of mood disorder. The understanding that will serve as a basis for planning is that the client is
   1. considered incompetent.
   2. not considered dangerous to self or others.
   3. able to refuse antipsychotic medications.
   4. not subject to the least restrictive alternative doctrine.

Answer: 3
Rationale: Voluntary clients are considered competent and have the right to make treatment decisions. Option 1: Voluntary clients are considered competent. Option 2: Admission status is not a determinant of dangerousness. Option 4: All clients are subject to the least restrictive alternative doctrine.
Cognitive level: Application
Nursing process: Planning
NCLEX: Safe and Effective Care Environment
See text page: 120

10. Several nurses at Hospital X are concerned that agency policies related to restraint and seclusion and documentation practices are inadequate. The understanding about the relation of substandard institutional policies and individual nursing practice that should guide nursing practice is
    1. the policies do not absolve the individual nurse of the responsibility to practice according to professional standards of nursing care.
    2. agency policies are considered by the courts to be the legal standard by which the professional nurse must act and therefore override the American Nurses Association standards of care.

    3. in an institution with substandard policies, the nurse has a responsibility to inform the supervisor and leave the premises without delay.
    4. interpretation by the judicial system will be rendered on an individual basis and therefore cannot be predicted.

Answer: 1
Rationale: Nurses are professionally bound to uphold the American Nurses Association standards of practice regardless of lesser standards established by a health care agency or a state. Conversely, if the agency standards are higher than the American Nurses Association standards of practice, the agency standards must be upheld. The courts may seek to establish the standard of care through the use of expert witnesses when the issue is clouded.
Cognitive level: Analysis
Nursing process: Implementation
NCLEX: Safe and Effective Care Environment
See text page: 130

11. A newly admitted acutely psychotic client is a private client of the chief of staff and a private-pay client. To whom does the psychiatric nurse caring for the client owe the duty of care?
    1. Physician
    2. Hospital
    3. Client
    4. Profession

Answer: 3
Rationale: Although the nurse is accountable to the physician, the agency, the client, and the profession, the duty of care is owed to the client.
Cognitive level: Application
Nursing process: Implementation
NCLEX: Safe and Effective Care Environment
See text page: 129

12. An example of a breach of a client's constitutional right to privacy occurs when the nurse
    1. discusses the client's history with other staff during care planning.
    2. releases information to the client's employer without consent.
    3. documents the client's daily behaviors during hospitalization.
    4. asks the client's family to share information about prehospitalization behavior.

Answer: 2
Rationale: Release of information without client authorization violates the client's right to privacy. The other options are acceptable nursing practices.
Cognitive level: Application

Chapter 8   Legal and Ethical Guidelines for Safe Practice

13. A male adolescent was admitted to a psychiatric unit after a violent physical outburst. He asks the nurse to promise to keep confidential a plan he has to kill his father. The nurse should respond by saying
   1. "Those kinds of thoughts will make your hospitalization longer."
   2. "I can make that promise to you based on nurse-client privilege."
   3. "You really should share this thought with your psychiatrist."
   4. "I am obligated to share information with the treatment team."

Answer: 4

Rationale: Breach of nurse-client confidentiality does not pose a legal dilemma for nurses in these circumstances because a team approach to delivery of psychiatric care presumes communication of client information to other staff members to develop treatment plans and outcome criteria.

Cognitive level: Application
Nursing process: Implementation
NCLEX: Safe and Effective Care Environment
See text pages: 125, 126

14. A client approaches the unit charge nurse and states he wants to talk to the mental health advocate immediately about getting released. The unit has no pay phone and agency policy does not permit clients to enter the nurses' station. The nurse should
   1. tell the client to secure a physician's order to leave the unit to make the call.
   2. give the client a pen and paper and ask him to write the advocate.
   3. document the request in the client's medical record.
   4. call the advocate and convey the client's request.

Answer: 4

Rationale: The client has a constitutional right to freedom of speech. This includes the right to speak by telephone to outside parties such as a mental health advocate or lawyer. Immediately conveying the request for the client would be an acceptable action when a unit does not have a phone that can be used by clients. A cell phone would be another acceptable alternative. Option 1 poses a delay if the physician is not immediately available. Option 2: The mail poses a lengthy delay. Option 3: Documenting the request without acting on it is insufficient.

Cognitive level: Application
Nursing process: Implementation

NCLEX: Safe and Effective Care Environment
See text page: 118

15. A voluntary client on a psychiatric inpatient unit asks the nurse to get her the forms for discharge against medical advice so she can leave immediately. The best response for the nurse to make would be
   1. "I can't give you those forms without your physician's knowledge."
   2. "I'll get the forms for you and bring them to your room."
   3. "Your lawyer must get the forms for you from your doctor."
   4. "Please tell me how you came to the decision to leave treatment."

Answer: 4

Rationale: A client who has been voluntarily admitted as a psychiatric inpatient has the right to demand and obtain release in most states. However, as a client advocate, the nurse is responsible for weighing factors related to the client's wishes and best interests. By asking for information, the nurse may be able to help the client reconsider the decision. Option 1 is not a true statement. Option 2: Facilitating discharge without consent is not in the client's best interests before exploring the reason for the request.

Cognitive level: Application
Nursing process: Implementation
NCLEX: Safe and Effective Care Environment
See text page: 121

16. The family of a client whose health maintenance organization will not pay for continuing hospitalization is considering transfer of the client to a public mental hospital. They express concern that the client will be "warehoused and never get any treatment." The reply by the nurse that would be most helpful is
   1. "Under the law, treatment must be provided. Hospitalization without treatment violates client rights."
   2. "That's a justifiable concern because the right to treatment extends only to provision of food, shelter, and safety."
   3. "Much will depend on other clients because the right to treatment for a psychotic client takes precedence over the right to treatment of a client who is stabilized."
   4. "All clients in public hospitals have the right to choose both a primary therapist and a primary nurse."

Answer: 1

Rationale: The right to medical and psychiatric treatment was conferred on all clients hospitalized in public mental hospitals with the enactment of the federal Hospitalization of Mentally Ill Act in 1964. Option 2 supports the erroneous belief the family holds. Options 3 and 4: These stated provisions are not part of this or any other statute governing psychiatric care.

Cognitive level: Application
Nursing process: Implementation
NCLEX: Safe and Effective Care Environment
See text pages: 121, 122

17. What is the nurse's duty when a client tells the nurse he plans to kill his wife and her lover as soon as he is released from the hospital? The nurse must
   1. document this information in the client's record and report it to the physician and team.
   2. immediately call the client's wife and her lover to warn them.
   3. immediately call to warn the client's wife but not her lover.
   4. file a report with the local law enforcement authorities.

Answer: 1
Rationale: The professional responsibility of the staff nurse extends to reporting threats to injure others to the health care team and documenting the information in the client's record. Failure to do so would be considered substandard care. Options 2, 3, and 4: The physician or treatment team leader would be responsible for giving the warning to the various parties under threat and to law enforcement if deemed necessary.

Cognitive level: Application
Nursing process: Implementation
NCLEX: Safe and Effective Care Environment
See text pages: 125, 126

18. A client being treated in an alcohol rehabilitation unit reveals to the nurse that he feels "terrible guilt" for sexually abusing his 6-year-old stepdaughter before his admission. On the basis of state and federal laws, the best action for the nurse to take is to
   1. anonymously report the abuse through a phone call to the local child abuse hotline.
   2. respect nurse-client relationship confidentiality.
   3. file a written report on agency letterhead.
   4. report the finding to the district attorney.

Answer: 1
Rationale: Laws regarding child abuse reporting discovered by a professional during the suspected abuser's alcohol or drug treatment differ by state. Federal law supercedes state law and prohibits disclosure without a court order except in instances in which the re-

port can be made anonymously or without identifying the abuser as a client in an alcohol or drug treatment facility. Option 1 meets federal criteria. Option 2 does not accomplish reporting. Options 3 and 4 violate federal law.

Cognitive level: Analysis
Nursing Process: Implementation
NCLEX: Safe and Effective Care Environment
See text pages: 126, 127

19. The nurse volunteers for a committee that must develop hospital policy and procedure for implementing suicide precautions. Of the following resources, the one(s) that would provide the best guidance would be (more than one answer may be correct)
   1. the *DSM-IV-TR*.
   2. the state's Nurse Practice Act.
   3. the regulations that govern hospital licensure.
   4. a summary of common practices of several local hospitals.
   5. the American Nurses Association Scope and Standards of Practice for Psychiatric-Mental Health Nursing Practice.

Answers: 3, 5
Rationale: State regulations regarding hospital licensure provide information about the minimal standard. American Nurses Association national standards focus on elevating practice by setting high standards for nursing practice. Options 1 and 2 would not provide relevant information. Option 4 cannot be guaranteed to be helpful because the customs may or may not comply with laws or best practices.

Cognitive level: Analysis
Nursing process: Implementation
NCLEX: Safe and Effective Care Environment
See text page: 130

20. The wife of a client who has delusions of infidelity asks the nurse if any circumstances exist under which the treatment team is justified in violating the client's right to confidentiality. The nurse must reply that confidentiality may be violated
   1. under no circumstances.
   2. at the discretion of the psychiatrist.
   3. when questions are asked by law enforcement.
   4. if the client threatens the life of another person.

Answer: 4
Rationale: The duty to warn a person whose life has been threatened by a psychiatric client overrides the client's right to confidentiality. The right to confidentiality is not suspended at the discretion of the therapist or for legal investigations.

Cognitive level: Application

Chapter 8   Legal and Ethical Guidelines for Safe Practice

Nursing process: Implementation
NCLEX: Safe and Effective Care Environment
See text pages: 125, 126

21. The nurse caring for a 72-year-old client admitted for treatment of depression notes that the physician's order to begin therapy with an antidepressant calls for a dose greater than the usual adult dose. The nurse should
    1. consult a drug reference.
    2. implement the order.
    3. give the usual adult dose.
    4. hold the medication and consult the physician.

Answer: 4
Rationale: The dose of antidepressants for elderly clients is often less than the usual adult dose. The nurse should withhold the medication and consult the physician who wrote the order. The nurse's duty is to intervene and protect the client. Option 1 is unnecessary because the nurse already knows the dose is excessive. Option 2 is negligent. Option 3: A nurse without prescriptive privileges cannot change the dose.
Cognitive level: Application
Nursing process: Implementation
NCLEX: Safe and Effective Care Environment
See text pages: 130, 131

22. A client tells the nurse "When I saw my therapist yesterday, he stroked my breast and suggested that he will give me a pass to leave the hospital if I will meet him at his apartment." What action should the nurse take?
    1. None. Psychiatric clients are not reliable.
    2. Report the client's statements to the unit nurse manager.
    3. Discuss the statements with the medical director.
    4. Call the state medical board.

Answer: 2
Rationale: Reporting the client's statements is necessary. Investigation will determine whether the client's accusation is reliable. The agency chain of command should be used for reporting.
Cognitive level: Application
Nursing process: Implementation
NCLEX: Safe and Effective Care Environment
See text pages: 130, 131

23. A client became aggressive, struck another client, and required seclusion. The best documentation is
    1. "Client apparently doesn't like client X, as evidenced by his striking client X when client attempted to leave day room to go to bathroom.

Seclusion necessary at 2:15 PM. Plan: Maintain seclusion for 8 hours and keep this client and client X away from each other for 24 hours."
    2. "Seclusion ordered by Dr. at 2:15 PM when voices told the client to hit another client."
    3. "Client pacing, shouting at people not present in the environment. Chlorpromazine 50 mg administered po at 1 PM with no effect by 2 PM. At 2:15 PM client shouted that he would punch the first person who got near him, then struck client X on the jaw with his fist as client X walked out of day room to go to bathroom. Client physically restrained by staff and placed in seclusion by order of Dr. Y."
    4. "Seclusion ordered by Dr. Y for aggressive behavior, begun at 2:15 PM. Maintained for 2 hours without incident. Outcome: Client calmer."

Answer: 3
Rationale: Option 1 introduces the nurse's subjective views. Options 2 and 4 do not include necessary details. Documentation should include a description of behavior and verbalizations, interventions tried and their outcomes, and the name of the physician ordering the use of seclusion.
Cognitive level: Application
Nursing process: Implementation
NCLEX: Safe and Effective Care Environment
See text pages: 131, 132

24. A nursing intervention that violates the rights of the psychiatric client would be if the nurse
    1. imposes suicide precautions before the client has been interviewed by the physician.
    2. opens and reads mail the client has left at the nurse's station to be mailed.
    3. places the client's expensive watch in the hospital business office safe.
    4. reports overhearing the client tell a friend that he will spit out oral medication.

Answer: 2
Rationale: The client has the right to send and receive mail without interference.
    The other options are examples of good nursing judgment and do not violate the client's civil rights.
Cognitive level: Analysis
Nursing process: Implementation
NCLEX: Safe and Effective Care Environment
See text page: 118

25. A client demonstrating symptoms of psychosis asks a psychiatric technician "What's the matter with me?" The technician replies "Your wing nuts need tightening." Another technician states "Yeah, you're like a six-pack without the plastic holder." The client looks

perplexed and wanders off. The nurse who overheard the exchange will need to take action based on
1. violation of the client's right to be treated with dignity and respect.
2. the nursing obligation to report caregiver negligence.
3. preventing defamation of the client's character.
4. supervisory liability.

Answer: 1

Rationale: Clients have the right to be treated with dignity and respect. Clients should never be made the butt of jokes about their illness. Option 2: Client emotional abuse has been demonstrated, not negligence. Option 3: This example is not clearly defamation. Option 4: Client abuse, not supervisory liability, is the issue.

Cognitive level: Application
Nursing process: Implementation
NCLEX: Safe and Effective Care Environment
See text page: 118

26. On a day that the unit is short staffed the nurse assigns an orienting nursing assistant to provide one-to-one supervision for a suicidal client. The nursing assistant takes the client to the hospital coffee shop, where the client runs out of the hospital into the path of a speeding automobile and sustains permanent brain injury. The hospital investigation reveals the nursing assistant had not received training relative to suicide precautions or one-to-one supervision. The statement that best explains the liability of the nurse in this situation is that the nurse
1. is not liable because the nursing assistant provided the direct client supervision.
2. is vicariously responsible for the nursing assistant's actions because she delegated the responsibility.
3. is not accountable because she acted as an agent for the hospital.
4. is not accountable because the hospital should have provided adequate staff.

Answer: 2

Rationale: The nurse remains accountable for all tasks he or she delegates. The nurse should have determined the nursing assistant's competence to carry our the delegated task before leaving it in the assistant's hands. Option 3: Although the hospital will also be called to account, the nurse is accountable for delegated tasks. Option 4: Short-staffing is only one factor in the situation. The nurse is ultimately accountable for delegated tasks.

Cognitive level: Application
Nursing process: Implementation
NCLEX: Safe and Effective Care Environment
See text page: 127

27. The situations in which the nurse has a duty to intervene and report are when (more than one answer may be correct)
1. a peer is unable to write behavioral outcomes.
2. a physician consults the *Physician's Desk Reference* relative to dosing.
3. a peer arrives for duty in an alcohol-impaired state.
4. a team member has been discovered to have violated the boundaries of a vulnerable client.

Answers: 3, 4

Rationale: Both instances jeopardize client safety. Option 1 is of concern but can be resolved informally. Option 2 is acceptable practice.

Cognitive level: Analysis
Nursing process: Assessment
NCLEX: Safe and Effective Care Environment
See text pages: 130, 131

28. Situations that qualify as abandonment are when the nurse (more than one answer may be correct)
1. allows a client exhibiting mania to refuse hospitalization without taking further action.
2. terminates employment without referring a seriously mentally ill client for aftercare.
3. calls police to bring a suicidal client to the hospital after a suicide attempt.
4. refers a client with persistent paranoid schizophrenia to assertive community treatment.

Answers: 1, 2

Rationale: Abandonment arises when a nurse does not place a client safely in the hands of another health professional before discontinuing treatment. Options 3 and 4 provide for patient safety.

Cognitive level: Analysis
Nursing process: Assessment
NCLEX: Safe and Effective Care Environment
See text pages: 130, 131

29. A night shift nurse who usually works in labor and delivery is floated to a 30-bed inpatient psychiatric unit to be charge nurse. The staff consists of a licensed practical nurse and two aides. The nurse believes she is not competent to ensure safe client care because several clients are on suicide precautions, one is in seclusion, and an admission is arriving from the emergency department. Rank the actions the nurse should take in the order they should be performed.
1. Perform to the best of her ability with available resources.
2. Remain on duty until replaced.
3. Inform the immediate supervisor of the lack of experience and skills to provide safe care.

Chapter 8   Legal and Ethical Guidelines for Safe Practice

4. Ask for a replacement.
5. Document that she is working under protest and state the reasons.

Answer. 3, 4, 2, 5, 1

Rationale: The nurse has a duty to provide safe care according to American Nurses Association standards. If the nurse's experience is insufficient to allow her to provide safe interventions, her duty to clients is breached. The nurse must communicate this through the nursing chain of command and seek relief from unsafe working conditions. Option 3 communicates by using the chain of command. Option 4 requests replacement as remediation of the unsafe situation. Option 2 would leave clients in the hands of another professional who can provide safe care and avoids a charge of abandonment. Option 5: The nurse has a duty to document in writing unsafe conditions for client care and her actions to remediate the situation. Option 1: Performance according to the nurse's best judgment until replaced is required. This includes seeking clarification and validation.

Cognitive level: Analysis
Nursing process: Implementation
NCLEX: Safe and Effective Care Environment
See text pages: 127, 128

30. Staff nurse A goes off duty, having forgotten to document administration of a prn medication to a client. She calls the unit and asks staff nurse B to use his personal password to access the medical record and document the administration of the medication. Nurse B is not authorized to enter that client's computerized medical record. Nurse B should
   1. make an exception and fulfill the request.
   2. refer the matter to the charge nurse to resolve.
   3. report the request to the client's physician.
   4. seek access to the record from the hospital's information systems department.

Answer: 2

Rationale: At most hospitals, termination is a possible penalty for unauthorized entry into a client record. Referring the matter to the charge nurse will allow observance of hospital policy while ensuring that documentation occurs. Option 1 puts staff nurse B in jeopardy. Option 3 would be unnecessary. Option 4 would be unnecessary when the charge nurse can resolve the problem.

Cognitive level: Application
Nursing process: Implementation
NCLEX: Safe and Effective Care Environment
See text page: 132

31. The community mental health nurse has been working for 6 months to establish a trusting relationship with J, a delusional and suspicious client. J is fired from his job, has no money for medication, and decompensates within the span of 1 week. Should J be hospitalized or provided with medication and allowed to remain at home? The ethical principles affecting the decision are
   1. justice and truth.
   2. beneficence and autonomy.
   3. malfeasance and fidelity.
   4. confidentiality and negotiation.

Answer: 2

Rationale: The nurse's desire to do good (beneficence) is in conflict with the client's right to the least restrictive setting (autonomy). Option 1: Justice refers to treating clients fairly and equally. Truth refers to truth-telling or veracity. Option 3: Malfeasance refers to doing harm to the client, and fidelity refers to being loyal and committed to the client. Option 4: These choices are not ethical principles.

Cognitive level: Analysis
Nursing process: Planning
NCLEX: Safe and Effective Care Environment
See text pages: 116, 117

32. A client with bipolar disorder is monitored by the community mental health nurse. The client's mood disorder is under good control when the client takes the prescribed doses of lithium. The client tells the nurse she is pregnant as the result of her boyfriend committing date rape. The nurse makes the following assessments: lithium taken throughout pregnancy may result in a baby born with birth defects; the client is likely to have a relapse of her illness if she stops taking lithium; and the client is a devout Catholic who believes her boyfriend will marry her "even if he did get carried away" and care for their child. Which option would be congruent with the client's values and ethical beliefs?
   1. Continue lithium; deal with the issue of a baby with birth defects if it occurs.
   2. Continue lithium and encourage the client to undergo a therapeutic abortion.
   3. Discontinue lithium, use alternative medication, and prepare for hospitalization prn.
   4. Arrange for involuntary hospitalization for the duration of the pregnancy.

Answer: 3

Rationale: Discontinuing lithium will protect the fetus. Taking a "safe" or nonteratogenic psychotropic medication may avert decompensation, but preparing the client for the possibility of hospitalization in the event she becomes manic is ethical. Option 1 is in conflict with the client's plans to marry and care for the child. Option 2 is contrary to the client's religious beliefs. Option 4 violates the client's rights to the least restrictive treatment.

Cognitive level: Analysis
Nursing process: Planning
NCLEX: Psychosocial Integrity
See text pages: 117, 118

CHAPTER 9

1. The nurse notes the following entry on the client's plan of care: "Outcome: Client will demonstrate suicide self-control. Interventions: Initiate suicide precautions. Allow client to retain personal belongings. Allow client to leave unit unsupervised." Which principles of planning a nursing intervention to facilitate achievement of identified client outcomes are violated? (More than one answer may be correct.)
   1. Feasibility
   2. Evidence basis
   3. Appropriateness
   4. Within the capability of the nurse

Answers: 2, 3
Rationale: All interventions are not supported by evidence. Evidence supports removing personal property that can be used to attempt self-harm. Evidence also supports restricting the client to the unit and closely supervising client activity while on the psychiatric unit. If the client leaves the unit, staff would accompany the client on a one-to-one basis. The interventions are inappropriate because they do not provide a safe environment for the client. Option 1: The interventions are feasible although misguided. Option 4: The interventions are within the capability of the nurse, but a nurse using good judgment would question them.

Cognitive level: Analysis
Nursing process: Planning
NCLEX: Safe and Effective Care Environment
See text pages: 146-148

2. A new graduate with an associate's degree in nursing has just completed the new staff orientation to the psychiatric unit. The aspect of nursing care this nurse must have an advanced practice nurse perform is
   1. performing a mental health assessment interview.
   2. establishing a therapeutic relationship.
   3. individualizing a nursing care plan.
   4. prescribing psychotropic medication.

Answer: 4
Rationale: Prescriptive privileges are granted to masters-prepared nurse practitioners who have taken special courses on prescribing medication. The nurse pre-

pared at the basic level is permitted to perform mental health assessments, establish relationships, and provide individualized care planning.

Cognitive level: Application
Nursing process: Implementation
NCLEX: Safe and Effective Care Environment
See text page: 149

3. Admission data for a newly admitted client who is severely depressed reveal he has lost 20 pounds over the past month, has chronic low self-esteem, and has both the intent and a plan for committing suicide. He has been taking a selective serotonin reuptake inhibitor for 1 week without remission of symptoms. The priority nursing diagnosis is
   1. imbalanced nutrition: less than body requirements.
   2. chronic low self-esteem.
   3. risk for suicide.
   4. ineffective protection.

Answer: 3
Rationale: Risk for suicide is the priority diagnosis when the client has both suicidal ideation and has developed a plan to carry out the suicidal intent. Imbalanced nutrition and chronic low self-esteem are viable nursing diagnoses, but these problems do not affect client safety as urgently as would a suicide attempt. Ineffective protection would be of greater concern if the client were taking risperidone or an immune suppressant drug.

Cognitive level: Analysis
Nursing process: Diagnosis
NCLEX: Safe and Effective Care Environment
See text page: 145

4. Admission data for a newly admitted client who is severely depressed reveal he has lost 20 pounds over the past month, has chronic low self-esteem, and has both the intent and a plan for committing suicide. He has been taking a selective serotonin reuptake inhibitor for 1 week without remission of symptoms. The nurse must plan interventions directed toward meeting the client outcome: Client will refrain from gestures and attempts at killing self. The nursing intervention most directly related to this outcome is
   1. offer high-calorie fluids as between-meal nourishment.
   2. assist client to identify three personal strengths.
   3. observe client for therapeutic effects of psychotropic medication.
   4. implement suicide precautions.

Answer: 4
Rationale: Option 4 is the only option related to client safety. Option 1 relates to nutrition. Option 2 relates to self-esteem. Option 3 relates to medication therapy.

241

Cognitive level: Analysis
Nursing process: Planning
NCLEX: Safe and Effective Care Environment
See text pages: 146-148

5. The client's nursing diagnosis is disturbed sleep pattern related to anxiety. The desired outcome is that client will sleep for a minimum of 5 hours nightly by October 31. On November 1 review of sleep data for the 6 days of hospitalization shows the client sleeps an average of 4 hours nightly and takes a 2-hour afternoon nap. The outcome can be evaluated as
   1. consistently demonstrated.
   2. often demonstrated.
   3. sometimes demonstrated.
   4. never demonstrated.

Answer: 4
Rationale: Although the client is sleeping 6 hours daily, the total is not in one uninterrupted session at night. Therefore the outcome must be evaluated as never demonstrated.
Cognitive level: Analysis
Nursing process: Evaluation
NCLEX: Physiological Integrity
See text page: 149

6. The client's nursing diagnosis is disturbed sleep pattern related to anxiety. The desired outcome is that the client will sleep for a minimum of 5 hours nightly by October 31. On November 1 sleep data show the client sleeps an average of 4 hours nightly and takes a 2-hour afternoon nap. After the evaluation, the nurse should
   1. leave the care plan unchanged.
   2. remove the nursing diagnosis from the care plan.
   3. write a new nursing diagnosis that better reflects the problem and its cause.
   4 extend the time in which the goal is to be accomplished and examine interventions.

Answer: 4
Rationale: Sleeping a total of 5 hours at night is still a reasonable outcome. Extending the time frame for attaining the outcome is appropriate. Examining interventions might result in planning an activity during the afternoon rather than permitting a nap. Option 1 is inappropriate. At the very least, the time in which the outcome is to be attained must be extended. Option 2 could be used when the outcome goal has been met and the problem resolved. Option 3 is inappropriate because no other nursing diagnosis relates to the problem.
Cognitive level: Analysis

Nursing process: Evaluation
NCLEX: Safe and Effective Care Environment
See text page: 149

7. The nurse interviewed a client who participated reluctantly, answering questions with minimal responses and rarely making eye contact with the nurse. When documenting the baseline data obtained during the interview the nurse should include
   1. only data obtained from client verbal responses.
   2. a disclaimer that the client was uncooperative and provided minimal data.
   3. both the content derived from client subjective responses and a description of the client's behavior during the interview.
   4. speculation regarding the reason the client was unwilling to respond openly during the interview.

Answer: 3
Rationale: Both content and process of the interview should be documented. Option 1 provides a skewed picture of the client. Option 2 is subjectively worded. An objective description of client behavior would be preferable. Option 4: Speculation is inappropriate.
Cognitive level: Application
Nursing process: Assessment
NCLEX: Safe and Effective Care Environment
See text page: 142

8. The nurse performing the assessment interview for a client decides to have the client use the Zung Self-Report Inventory at the end of the interview. The functions accomplished with this tool include (more than one answer may be correct)
   1. identifying North American Nursing Diagnosis Association nursing diagnoses.
   2. obtaining data related to current symptoms of depression.
   3. establishing a baseline for evaluation of progress over time.
   4. comparing client responses with responses of others with depression.

Answers: 2, 3, 4
Rationale: A self-report rating scale is useful for obtaining data about the client's perception of illness at the beginning of treatment, and, with repeated administration, to provide information about progress over time. The data obtained also permit comparison for research purposes of client responses with those of groups of people with the same illness. This scale does not refer directly to nursing diagnoses, although data gathered may indirectly assist the nurse in formulating nursing diagnoses.

Cognitive level: Application
Nursing process: Assessment
NCLEX: Psychosocial Integrity
See text pages: 144, 145

9. Before interviewing a new client, the nurse is told by another health care worker, "I know that client. He's usually nutty as a fruitcake when he is admitted, and not much better when we discharge him." The nurse's responsibility is to
   1. accept the other worker's assessment as fact.
   2. form an impression based on the data he or she collects from all sources.
   3. validate the worker's impression by contacting the family and other secondary sources.
   4. discuss the worker's impression with the client during the course of the assessment interview.

Answer: 2
Rationale: Assessment should include data obtained from both the primary and reliable secondary sources. Biased assessments by others should be evaluated as objectively as possible by the nurse, bearing in mind the possible effects of countertransference on others' assessments.
Cognitive level: Application
Nursing process: Assessment
NCLEX: Psychosocial Integrity
See text pages: 140, 144

10. After a nurse has completed the assessment for a new client with a psychiatric disorder, data are analyzed to formulate nursing diagnoses. The information that will be conveyed by the nursing diagnoses includes (more than one answer may be correct)
    1. medical judgments about the disorder.
    2. unmet client needs present at the moment.
    3. supporting data that validate the diagnoses.
    4. probable causes that will be targets for nursing interventions.

Answers: 2, 3, 4
Rationale: Nursing diagnoses focus on phenomena of concern to nurses rather than on medical diagnoses.
Cognitive level: Application
Nursing process: Diagnosis
NCLEX: Psychosocial Integrity
See text page: 145

11. While working with a client to establish outcomes for treatment, the nurse believes that an outcome suggested by the client is not in the client's best interest. The best action for the nurse would be to
    1. remain silent.
    2. tell the client that the outcome is not realistic.

3. formulate a different, appropriate outcome for the client.
4. explore the consequences that might occur if the outcome is achieved.

Answer: 4
Rationale: The nurse should not impose outcomes on the client; however, the nurse has a responsibility to help the client evaluate what is in his or her best interests. Exploring possible consequences is an acceptable approach.
Cognitive level: Application
Nursing process: Planning
NCLEX: Psychosocial Integrity
See text pages: 146-148

12. A client lists the following problems: "I have no sense of self-worth. I constantly think negative thoughts about myself. I feel anxious and shaky all the time. Sometimes my mood is so low that I think I want to go to sleep and never wake up." The nursing interventions that should be accorded the highest priority relate to outcomes associated with
    1. self-esteem.
    2. anxiety self-control.
    3 depression self-control.
    4. suicide self-restraint.

Answer: 4
Rationale: The nurse would place a priority on monitoring and reinforcing suicide self-restraint because it relates directly and immediately to client safety. Client safety is always a priority concern. The nurse would also be expected to monitor and reinforce all client attempts to control anxiety, control depression, and develop self-esteem while giving priority attention to suicide self-restraint.
Cognitive level: Analysis
Nursing process: Planning
NCLEX: Safe and Effective Care Environment
See text page: 148

13. Select the best outcome for a client with the nursing diagnosis of impaired social interaction related to sociocultural dissonance, as evidenced by client stating "Although I'd like to, I don't join in because I don't speak the language so good." Client will
    1. cooperate with others.
    2. become more independent.
    3. express a desire to interact with others.
    4. consistently participate in unit group activity of his choice.

Answer: 4
Rationale: The outcome describes social involvement on the part of the client. Neither cooperation nor inde-

243

pendence has been an issue. The client has already expressed a desire to interact with others.
Cognitive level: Analysis
Nursing process: Planning (Outcome Identification)
NCLEX: Psychosocial Integrity
See text page: 146

14. Nursing behaviors associated with the implementation phase of the nursing process are concerned with
   1. gathering accurate and sufficient client-centered data.
   2. participating in mutual identification of client outcomes.
   3. carrying out interventions and coordinating care.
   4. comparing client responses and expected outcomes.

Answer: 3
Rationale: Nursing behaviors relating to implementation include considering available resources, performing care-giving interventions, finding alternatives when necessary, and coordinating care with other team members.
Cognitive level: Comprehension
Nursing process: Implementation
NCLEX: Safe and Effective Care Environment
See text page: 148

15. Which strategies would be helpful for the nurse to use when gathering assessment data about a client whose family has indicated that he is very suspicious and believes the FBI has him under surveillance? (More than one answer may be correct.)
   1. Ask the client to identify the problem as he sees it.
   2. Seek information about when the problem began.
   3. Listen to the client's theory about the cause of the problem.
   4. Tell the client his ideas are not realistic.
   5. Reassure the client of his safety.
   6. Tell the client that staff will control his behavior

Answers: 1, 2, 3, 5
Rationale: During the assessment interview the nurse should listen attentively and accept the client's statements in a nonjudgmental way. Because the client is suspicious and fearful, reassuring him of his safety may be helpful, although he is unlikely to trust the nurse so early in the relationship. Option 4 suggests to the client that the nurse is not willing to try to understand his views. Option 6 may be perceived as a threat.
Cognitive level: Application
Nursing process: Assessment
NCLEX: Safe and Effective Care Environment
See text pages: 140-143

16. Which statement made by a client during the initial assessment interview will provide the nurse with the best understanding of the client's current problem and reason for seeking treatment?
   1. "I can always trust my wife."
   2. "You never know who will turn against you."
   3. "I've been hearing the voices of my dead parents."
   4. "I wish I knew what I've done to deserve such bad luck."

Answer: 3
Rationale: Option 3 tells the nurse that the client is experiencing auditory hallucinations. The other statements are vague and do not clearly identify the client's chief symptom.
Cognitive level: Analysis
Nursing process: Assessment
NCLEX: Psychosocial Integrity
See text pages: 140-143

17. Which entry in the medical record will meet the requirement that the nurse must document with problem-oriented charting?
   1. "A: Client muttering to self as though answering an unseen person. P: Sensory perceptual alteration related to internal auditory stimulation. I: Client received prn fluphenazine po at 9 AM and went to room to lie down. E: Client calmer by 9:30 AM. Returned to community room to watch TV."
   2. "Agitated behavior. D: Client muttering to self as though answering an unseen person. A: Given Haldol 2 mg po and went to room to lie down. E: Client calmer. Returned to lounge to watch TV."
   3. "S: Client states 'I feel like I'm ready to blow up.' O: Pacing hall and mumbling to self as though answering an unseen person. A: Client is experiencing auditory hallucinations. P: Offered prn Haldol 2 mg po. I: 2 mg Haldol po administered. E: Client calmer. Returned to lounge and watched TV."
   4. "Client seen pacing hall and muttering to self as though answering an unseen person. Haldol 2 mg po administered at 9 AM with calming effect in 30 minutes. Stated he was no longer 'bothered by the voices.'"

Answer: 3
Rationale: Problem-oriented documentation uses the first letter of key words to organize data: S for subjective data, O for objective data, A for assessment, P for plan, I for intervention, and E for evaluation. Option 1 is an example of PIE charting. Option 2 is an example of focus documentation. Option 4 is an example of narrative documentation.

244

Cognitive level: Analysis
Nursing process: Implementation
NCLEX: Safe and Effective Care Environment
See text pages: 150, 151

18. A nurse is assigned to perform the assessment interview for a 65-year-old woman brought to the hospital emergency department by her 16-year-old granddaughter, who found her wandering around the yard of her suburban home, saying "I can't find my way home." The nurse finds the client to be so profoundly confused that she is unable to respond to or answer any questions posed. In this case the nurse should
    1. persevere and record the client's answers to questions on the agency assessment form.
    2. document the client's confusion and obtain as much data as possible from the granddaughter.
    3. ask a more experienced nurse to perform the interview.
    4. call for a mental health advocate to support the client's rights.

Answer: 2
Rationale: When the client (primary source) is unable to provide information, secondary sources should be used, in this case the granddaughter. Later, more data may be obtained from other relatives or neighbors who are familiar with the client. Option 3: An experienced nurse would probably do no better. Option 4 is unnecessary.
Cognitive level: Application
Nursing process: Assessment
NCLEX: Safe and Effective Care Environment
See text page: 144

19. A nurse is assigned to perform the assessment interview for a 65-year-old woman brought to the hospital emergency department by her 16-year-old granddaughter, who found her wandering around the yard of her suburban home, saying "I can't find my way home." The nurse finds the client to be so confused that she is unable to respond to or answer any questions posed. The nurse experiences feelings of profound sadness and reflects "She is like my grandmother: helpless." The feelings being experienced by the nurse can be assessed as
    1. autodiagnosis.
    2. countertransference.
    3. catastrophic reaction.
    4. defensive coping reaction.

Answer: 2
Rationale: Countertransference is the nurse's transference or response to a client that is based on the nurse's unconscious needs, conflicts, problems, or view of the world. Option 1: Autodiagnosis refers to

the nurse's self-monitoring and awareness of his or her own reactions. Option 3: A catastrophic reaction refers to an angry, sometimes violent reaction by a client with dementia. Option 4: The nurse is responding honestly rather than coping defensively.
Cognitive level: Application
Nursing process: Assessment
NCLEX: Safe and Effective Care Environment
See text page: 140

20. During the initial assessment interview the client becomes anxious and evasive when the nurse asks her if she has ever heard voices when no one else was around. The client asks, "What do you need to know that for?" The nurse should say
    1. "Please be honest about this," after repeating the question.
    2. "Sometimes questions seem highly personal, but we have our reasons for asking each one."
    3. "What purpose do you think we might have in asking about whether you hear voices?"
    4. "I can see this subject makes you uncomfortable. We can discuss it at another time."

Answer: 4
Rationale: The nurse should not try to pry information out of a client who is reluctant to give the information. The nurse should note the client's reaction to the question and carefully observe for behavioral signs that the client may be experiencing auditory hallucinations. Option 1 implies the client has been dishonest. Option 2 treats the client in a demeaning fashion. Option 3 is game playing.
Cognitive level: Application
Nursing process: Implementation
NCLEX: Psychosocial Integrity
See text page: 140

21. A 16-year-old client asks the nurse conducting the assessment interview "Why should I tell you anything? You'll just run back and tell my mother whatever you find out." The best reply for the nurse would be
    1. "That's not true. Whatever you tell me will be held in the strictest confidence."
    2. "Your mother may find out what you say, but is that really such a bad thing?"
    3. "Anything you say about feelings is confidential, but things like suicidal thinking must be reported to the treatment team."
    4. "It sounds as though you're not really ready to work on your problems and make changes."

Answer: 3
Rationale: The client has a right to know that most information will be held in confidence but that certain

Chapter 9   Assessment Strategies and the Nursing Process

material must be reported or shared with the treatment team, such as threats of suicide, homicide, use of illegal drugs, or issues of abuse. Option 1 is not strictly true. Option 2 will not inspire the confidence of the client. Option 4 is confrontational.

Cognitive level: Application
Nursing process: Implementation
NCLEX: Psychosocial Integrity
See text page: 140

22. The nurse interviewing an adolescent client should plan to use the HEADSSS interview topics to
    1. establish rapport.
    2. identify risk factors.
    3. identify treatment objectives.
    4. assess level of current cognitive functioning.

Answer: 2
Rationale: HEADSSS structures the interview to gather data useful in assessing risk factors. HEADSSS refers to home environment; education; activities; drug, alcohol, tobacco use; sexuality; suicide risk; and savagery (violence/abuse in the environment). Option 1: Rapport would be difficult to establish if only the HEADSSS interview is used. Option 3: Direct questions might better identify treatment objectives. Option 4: The mental status examination would be preferable.

Cognitive level: Comprehension
Nursing process: Assessment
NCLEX: Psychosocial Integrity
See text pages: 140, 141

23. When the nurse begins the assessment interview with a client, aged 62 years, she notes that the client gives answers to questions that seem somewhat vague or slightly unrelated to the question. The client also leans forward and frowns as she listens intently to the nurse. An appropriate question for the nurse to ask would be
    1. "I notice you frowning. Are you feeling annoyed with me?"
    2. "Are you able to hear clearly when I speak in this tone of voice?"
    3. "How can I make this interview a bit easier for you?"
    4. "You seem to be having some trouble focusing on what I'm saying. Is something distracting you?"

Answer: 2
Rationale: The client's behaviors indicate she may have difficulty hearing. Identifying any physical need the client may have at the onset of the interview and making accommodations are important considerations. Option 1: The nurse is jumping to conclusions. Option 3 may not elicit a concrete answer.

Option 4 is a way of asking about the presence of auditory hallucinations, which is not appropriate because the nurse has observed that the client seems to be listening intently to her.

Cognitive level: Application
Nursing process: Implementation
NCLEX: Safe and Effective Care Environment
See text page: 140

24. A nurse is reluctant to ask questions related to spiritual matters during client interviews. At what point in the interview could the nurse logically ask the question "Does your faith help you in stressful situations?" During the assessment of
    1. substance use and abuse.
    2. childhood growth and development.
    3. usual client coping strategies.
    4. self-assessment of strengths and weaknesses.

Answer: 3
Rationale: When discussing coping strategies the nurse might ask what the client does when he or she becomes upset, what usually relieves stress, and to whom the client goes to talk about problems. The question regarding whether the client's faith helps deal with stress fits well here. It would seem out of place if introduced during exploration of the other topics.

Cognitive level: Application
Nursing process: Assessment
NCLEX: Psychosocial Integrity
See text pages: 142-144

25. When a new client has been admitted to the unit, the nurse takes the client on a tour, tells the client about the rules of the unit that guide behavior and activities of daily living, and discusses the daily schedule. In doing this the nurse is engaged in
    1. counseling.
    2. health teaching.
    3. milieu management.
    4. psychobiological intervention.

Answer: 3
Rationale: Milieu management provides a therapeutic environment in which the client can feel comfortable and safe, while engaging in activities that meet the client's physical and mental health needs. Option 1: Counseling refers to activities designed to promote problem solving and enhanced coping and includes interviewing, crisis intervention, stress management, and conflict resolution. Option 2: Health teaching involves identifying health education needs and giving information about these needs. Option 4: Psychobiological interventions involve medication administration and monitoring response to medications.

Cognitive level: Comprehension
Nursing process: Implementation
NCLEX: Safe and Effective Care Environment
See text page: 148

CHAPTER 10

1. A client, brought to the emergency department after attempting suicide by taking an overdose of acetaminophen (Tylenol), has been lavaged. She appears tense, withdrawn, and frightened. The nurse tells her "I am Mr. G, a unit nurse. You seem to be tense and I'm wondering if you are feeling frightened. I'd like to sit here with you for a while." The behavior indicating that the nurse has entered into a therapeutic rather than social encounter with the client is:
   1. The statement of "I'd like to sit here with you . . ." is offering friendship.
   2. The statement of "I'd like to sit here with you . . ." is meeting the need for a time of quiet reflection.
   3. The statement of "You seem tense and I'm wondering if you are feeling frightened" seeks to identify emotional needs.
   4. The statement of "You seem tense and I'm wondering if you are feeling frightened" is interpreting her behavior.

Answer: 3
Rationale: Through the use of empathy the nurse is fostering trust and communication. Options 1 and 2: He is offering positive regard rather than friendship or a time for reflection. Option 4: His remarks are not interpretations.
Cognitive level: Application
Nursing process: Implementation
NCLEX: Psychosocial Integrity
See text page: 156

2. The statement showing that the nurse has empathy for a client who has recently made a suicide attempt is
   1. "It makes me sad to see you going through such anguish."
   2. "If you tell me what's troubling you, I will be glad to speak to the doctor for you."
   3. "You must have been very upset to do what you did today."
   4. "Suicide is a drastic solution to a problem that may not be a matter of life or death at all."

Answer: 3
Rationale: Empathy permits the nurse to see an event from the client's perspective, understand the client's feelings, and communicate this to the client. Option 1 is nurse centered, focusing on the nurse's feelings

rather than the client's. Option 2 is not empathetic but is a nontherapeutic action that promotes client dependence. Option 4 is a belittling statement.
Cognitive level: Application
Nursing process: Implementation
NCLEX: Psychosocial Integrity
See text page: 157

3. After several therapeutic encounters with a client who recently attempted suicide, the behavior that would cause the nurse to consider the possibility of countertransference is that
   1. the client's reactions toward the nurse seem realistic and appropriate.
   2. the client states the nurse is concerned about her, just like her father.
   3. the nurse develops a trusting relationship with the client.
   4. the nurse feels exceptionally happy when the client's mood begins to lift.

Answer: 4
Rationale: Strong positive or negative reactions to a client or overidentification with the client signals possible countertransference. Nurses must carefully monitor their own feelings and reactions to detect countertransference, then seek supervision. Option 1 describes a desirable outcome. Option 2 suggests transference. Option 3 describes a desirable outcome.
Cognitive level: Application
Nursing process: Assessment
NCLEX: Psychosocial Integrity
See text pages: 159-161

4. How should the nurse respond if a client asks him not to share information with others?
   1. "I will not share information with your family or friends without your permission. I will, however, need to share information that relates to your reason for being here with other staff who work with you."
   2. "The nice thing about a therapeutic relationship is that it is just between the nurse and the client. You will have to tell others whatever you want them to know about you and the problems that led to your hospitalization."
   3. "It really depends on what you choose to tell me. I will be glad to disclose at the end of each session what I will report to other staff."
   4. "I really cannot tell anyone about you. It will be as though I am talking about my own problems and we can help each other by keeping it between us."

Answer: 1
Rationale: A client has the right to know with whom the nurse will share information and that confidential-

247

ity will be protected. Option 2 is untrue. Although the relationship is primarily between the nurse and client, other staff need to know pertinent data. Option 3 is inappropriate, promotes incomplete disclosure on the part of the client, and requires daily renegotiation of an issue that should be resolved as the nurse-client contract is established. Option 4 presents an inappropriate picture of the nurse-client relationship, suggesting it is used for mutual problem solving. The relationship must be client centered.

Cognitive level: Application
Nursing process: Implementation
NCLEX: Psychosocial Integrity
See text page: 165

5. A client who recently attempted suicide talks with the nurse about wanting a day pass to go home. The nurse responds by telling the client that he will talk with the psychiatrist on her behalf. An accurate analysis of this interaction is that
    1. the nurse is modeling healthy behaviors for the client.
    2. the client has manipulated the nurse into acting on her behalf.
    3. role boundary blurring is occurring because the nurse behaves in an overly helpful way.
    4. The nurse is demonstrating both positive regard for the client and clinical competence in the nursing role.

Answer: 3
Rationale: Being overly helpful is a classic example of role boundary blurring. Option 1 does not reflect the modeling of healthy behavior. Option 2 suggests the client is manipulative but is without supportive assessment data. Option 4 is false because clinical competence does not embrace role boundary violations.

Cognitive level: Analysis
Nursing process: Assessment
NCLEX: Psychosocial Integrity
See text pages: 160, 161

6. Termination of the therapeutic nurse-client relationship with a client has been handled successfully when the nurse
    1. gives the client his personal telephone number and permission to call after discharge.
    2. avoids upsetting the client by focusing on other clients beginning 1 week before the client's discharge.
    3. discusses with the client the changes that have happened during their time together and evaluates outcome attainment.

4. offers to meet the client for coffee and conversation three times a week for 2 weeks after discharge.

Answer: 3
Rationale: Summarizing and evaluating progress help validate the experience for the client and the nurse and facilitate closure. Option 2: Termination must be discussed; avoiding discussion by spending little time with the client promotes feelings of abandonment. Options 1 and 4: Successful termination requires that the relationship be brought to closure without the possibility of dependency-producing ongoing contact.

Cognitive level: Analysis
Nursing process: Evaluation
NCLEX: Psychosocial Integrity
See text page: 167

7. A desirable outcome for the initial stage of a nurse-client relationship is that the client will demonstrate behaviors that indicate he or she has
    1. developed a greater sense of independence.
    2. developed rapport and trust with the nurse.
    3. developed self-responsibility.
    4. resolved transferences.

Answer: 2
Rationale: Development of rapport and trust is necessary before the relationship can progress to the working phase. Options 1, 3 and 4 would probably occur in the working phase.

Cognitive level: Application
Nursing process: Planning (Outcome Identification)
NCLEX: Psychosocial Integrity
See text page: 164

8. During which phase of the nurse-client relationship can the nurse anticipate that identified client issues will be explored and resolved?
    1. The working phase
    2. The identifying phase
    3. The dysfunctional phase
    4. The termination phase

Answer: 1
Rationale: During the working phase, the nurse strives to assist the client in making connections among dysfunctional behaviors, thinking, and emotions and offers support while alternative coping behaviors are tried. Option 2: No phase of the nurse-client relationship is identified as the identifying phase. Option 3: No phase of the nurse-client relationship is identified as the dysfunctional phase. Option 4: Identified issues should be explored and resolved before the termination phase.

Cognitive level: Application
Nursing process: Planning
NCLEX: Psychosocial Integrity
See text pages: 165, 166

9. At what point in the nurse-client relationship should the nurse plan to first address the issue of termination?
   1. In the working phase
   2. In the termination phase
   3. In the orientation phase
   4. When the client initially brings up the topic

Answer: 3
Rationale: The client has a right to know the conditions of the nurse-client relationship. If the relationship is to be time limited, the client should be informed of the number of sessions. If it is open ended, the termination date will not be known at the outset, and the client should know that the issue will be negotiated at a later date. Option 1: Termination is usually discussed during the orientation phase. Option 2: Termination is discussed from the outset. Option 4: The nurse is responsible for discussing termination early in the relationship.
Cognitive level: Application
Nursing process: Planning
NCLEX: Psychosocial Integrity
See text pages: 164, 165

10. A nurse introduces the matter of a contract during the first session because contracts
    1. specify what the nurse will do for the client.
    2. are indicative of the feeling tone established between the participants.
    3. are binding and prevent either party from prematurely ending the relationship.
    4. spell out the participation and responsibilities of both parties.

Answer: 4
Rationale: A contract emphasizes that the nurse works *with* the client rather than doing something *for* the client. "Working with" is a process that suggests each party is expected to participate and share responsibility for outcomes. Contracts do not, however, stipulate roles or feeling tone, and premature termination is forbidden.
Cognitive level: Application
Nursing process: Planning
NCLEX: Safe and Effective Care Environment
See text pages: 164, 165

11. During scheduled sessions the client frequently asks the nurse for cigarettes and money, implying that he will be more willing to talk with the nurse if the requested items are forthcoming. The nurse should assess this behavior as
    1. typical of transference reactions.
    2. indicative of feelings of insecurity.
    3. reflecting resistance to involvement.
    4. testing the nurse's clinical competence.

Answer: 4
Rationale: Clients often unconsciously use testing behaviors to determine whether the nurse is able to set limits or will abandon them if they behave in an unlikable way.
Cognitive level: Application
Nursing process: Assessment
NCLEX: Psychosocial Integrity
See text pages: 164-166

12. The remark by a client that would indicate passage into the working phase of the nurse-client relationship is
    1. "I don't have any problems."
    2. "It is so difficult for me to talk about problems."
    3. "I don't know how talking about things twice a week can help."
    4. "I think I would like to find a way to deal with my anger without blowing up."

Answer: 4
Rationale: Thinking about a more constructive approach to dealing with anger indicates a readiness to make a behavioral change. Behavioral change is associated with the working phase of the relationship. Option 1: Denial is often seen in the orientation phase. Option 2: This reaction is common early in the relationship before rapport and trust are firmly established. Option 3 is more typically a reaction during the orientation phase.
Cognitive level: Analysis
Nursing process: Assessment
NCLEX: Psychosocial Integrity
See text pages: 165, 166

13. The nurse attempts to explain to the family of a mentally ill client how the nurse-client relationship differs from other interpersonal relationships. The best explanation is that
    1. the focus is on the client; problems are discussed by the nurse and client; and solutions are implemented by the client.
    2. the focus shifts from nurse to client; advice is given by both parties; and solutions are implemented by each.
    3. the focus is socialization; mutual needs are met; and feelings are shared.
    4. the focus is creation of a partnership in which each member is concerned with growth and satisfaction of the other.

249

Answer: 1

Rationale: Options 2, 3, and 4 describe events that occur in social or intimate relationships. Only option 1 describes the elements of a therapeutic relationship.

Cognitive level: Application
Nursing process: Implementation
NCLEX: Psychosocial Integrity
See text pages: 167, 168

14. The nurse wishes to demonstrate genuineness within the context of the nurse-client relationship with his client who has been diagnosed with schizophrenia. The nurse will need to
   1. use extensive self-revelation in client interactions.
   2. encourage the client to depend on him for support and reassurance.
   3. consistently make value judgments about client behaviors.
   4. be aware of his own feelings and use congruent communication strategies.

Answer: 4

Rationale: Genuineness is a desirable characteristic involving awareness of one's own feelings as they arise and the ability to communicate them when appropriate. The other possible options are undesirable in a therapeutic relationship.

Cognitive level: Application
Nursing process: Implementation
NCLEX: Safe and Effective Care Environment
See text page: 157

15. The nurse caring for a withdrawn, suspicious client finds himself feeling angry with the client. The nurse should
   1. suppress the angry feelings.
   2. express the anger openly and directly.
   3. tell the nurse manager to assign the client to another nurse.
   4. discuss the anger with a clinician during a supervisory session.

Answer: 4

Rationale: The nurse is accountable for the relationship. Objectivity is threatened by strong positive or negative feelings toward a client. Supervision is necessary to work through countertransference feelings.

Cognitive level: Application
Nursing process: Implementation
NCLEX: Safe and Effective Care Environment
See text pages: 159, 160

16. The nurse wishes to enhance growth in her client by showing positive regard. The action consistent with this desire is

   1. administering daily medication as prescribed.
   2. making rounds according to the daily assignment.
   3. staying with the client when the client cries.
   4. taking a group of clients for a walk.

Answer: 3

Rationale: Options 1, 2, and 4 are tasks that could be part of an assignment and do not necessarily reflect positive regard. Staying with a crying client offers support and shows positive regard.

Cognitive level: Application
Nursing process: Implementation
NCLEX: Psychosocial Integrity
See text pages: 157, 158

17. A client says, "I've done a lot of cheating and manipulating in my relationships." A nonjudgmental response by the nurse would be
   1. "How do you feel about that?"
   2. "It's good that you realize this."
   3. "What a rotten way to behave."
   4. "Have you outgrown that immature behavior?"

Answer: 1

Rationale: Asking a client to reflect on feelings about his or her actions does not imply any judgment about those actions, and it encourages clients to explore feelings and values. Options 2, 3, and 4 offer negative judgments.

Cognitive level: Analysis
Nursing process: Implementation
NCLEX: Psychosocial Integrity
See text page: 158

18. A client states "I think people should be allowed to commit suicide without interference from others." A nurse replies "You're wrong! Nothing is ever so bad that dying is justified." What assessment about this interchange is accurate?
   1. The client is correct in his thinking.
   2. The nurse is correct.
   3. Neither person is totally correct.
   4. Differing values are reflected in the two statements.

Answer: 4

Rationale: Values guide beliefs and actions. The individuals stating their positions place different values on life and autonomy. Nurses must be aware of their own values and be sensitive to the values of others.

Cognitive level: Analysis
Nursing process: Assessment
NCLEX: Psychosocial Integrity
See text pages: 162, 163

19. The issues a nurse should plan to address during the first interview with a client with a psychiatric disorder include
   1. trust, congruence, attitudes, and boundaries.
   2. relationship parameters, the contract, confidentiality, and termination.
   3. transference, countertransference, intimacy, and developing resources.
   4. goals, resistance, unconscious motivations, and diversion.

Answer: 2

Rationale: Option 2 lists issues that should be considered during the orientation phase of the relationship. Options 1, 3, and 4 are issues that are dealt with later.

Cognitive level: Application
Nursing process: Planning
NCLEX: Psychosocial Integrity
See text pages: 164, 165

20. A peer mentions that a new nurse seems to be spending a lot of time with a young female client. The nurse visits the client before reporting for duty, seeks out the client for interactions during the shift, and makes sure to spend a few minutes with the client after going off duty. The new nurse was overheard giving the client's nurse therapist opinions about the client and the care plan. Yesterday, the new nurse brought the client a gift. Which assessment could be made? The new nurse is
   1. overinvolved.
   2. expressing anger.
   3. experiencing boredom.
   4. looking to be rescued.

Answer: 1

Rationale: There are no data to support options 2, 3, or 4. The nurse behavior described is typical of overinvolvement.

Cognitive level: Application
Nursing process: Assessment
NCLEX: Psychosocial Integrity
See text pages: 158, 159

21. A nursing behavior that shows the nurse values autonomy takes place when the nurse
   1. sets limits on a client's romantic overtures toward the nurse.
   2. suggests one-on-one supervision for a client who is suicidal.
   3. tells a client that his wife has called to say she will not be in during visiting hours.
   4. discusses alternatives available to a client and helps the client weigh the consequences of each.

Answer: 4

Rationale: A high level of valuing is acting on one's belief. Autonomy is supported when the nurse helps a client weigh alternatives and their consequences before the client makes a decision. Autonomy or self-determination is not the issue in any of the other behaviors.

Cognitive level: Application
Nursing process: Implementation
NCLEX: Psychosocial Integrity
See text pages: 162, 163

22. A nurse remarks to a peer that "All the literature tells nurses that relationships are facilitated by consistency. I wish someone would give me some concrete examples." Examples the nurse could cite include (more than one answer may be correct)
   1. having the same nurse care for a client on a daily basis.
   2. providing a schedule of client activities daily.
   3. setting a time for regular sessions with the client.
   4. encouraging the client to share initial impressions of staff.

Answers: 1, 2, 3

Rationale: Consistency implies predictability. Options 1, 2, and 3 help a client predict what will happen during each day and develop a greater degree of security and comfort. Encouraging a client to share initial impressions of staff has nothing to do with consistency and would not be considered a therapeutic intervention.

Cognitive level: Application
Nursing process: Implementation
NCLEX: Safe and Effective Care Environment
See text page: 168

23. The events listed below occurred in the first few days of the nurse-client relationship. The development of a positive relationship was hampered when the
   1. nurse had to cancel their second and third sessions because of short staffing.
   2. nurse let the client set the pace during the initial interview.
   3. client used the nurse as a sounding board while discussing recent work problems.
   4. nurse's initial impression was that the client would be interesting to work with.

Answer: 1

Rationale: Inconsistency and unavailability are specific factors that hamper the development of positive nurse-client relationships. The other events listed are considered positive indicators of a satisfying relationship.

Cognitive level: Analysis
Nursing process: Evaluation
NCLEX: Safe and Effective Care Environment
See text page: 168

Chapter 10   Developing Therapeutic Relationships

24. The client mentions to the nurse "I'm still on restriction to the unit and I'd really like to start attending off-unit activities. Would you ask the doctor to upgrade my privileges?" The best response for the nurse would be
1. "I'll be glad to mention it when I see the doctor later today."
2. "That's a good topic for you to take up with the doctor. You'll be meeting at 2 PM."
3. "Why are you asking me to do this when you're perfectly capable of speaking for yourself?"
4. "Do you think you are so unimportant that you can't speak to a doctor and that a nurse must intercede?"

Answer: 2
Rationale: Nurses should encourage clients to work at their optimal level of functioning. The nurse does not act for the client unless absolutely necessary. Acting for a client increases feelings of helplessness and dependency. Options 3 and 4 are pseudotherapeutic attempts that do nothing to develop the client's resources.
Cognitive level: Application
Nursing process: Implementation
NCLEX: Psychosocial Integrity
See text page: 168

25. A community mental health nurse has monitored a client in the community for the past 4 years. The nurse is moving out of the city and must terminate her relationship with the client. When the new nurse begins work with the client, what can he or she anticipate as the starting point for the relationship?
1. Beginning at the orientation phase
2. Resuming the working relationship
3. Entering into a social relationship
4. Returning to the emotional catharsis phase

Answer: 1
Rationale: After termination of a long-term relationship, the client and new nurse usually have to begin at ground zero, the orientation phase, to build a new relationship. If termination is successfully completed, the orientation phase sometimes progresses quickly to the working phase. Other times, even after successful termination, the orientation phase may be prolonged.
Cognitive level: Application
Nursing process: Assessment
NCLEX: Psychosocial Integrity
See text pages: 164, 165

26. The nurse tells a peer, "I feel really uncomfortable with the client and I find myself wanting to avoid both informal contacts on the unit and scheduled sessions." Without supervision, evidence suggests that the outcome of this relationship will be
1. growing interest and mutuality.
2. mutual withdrawal.
3. positive regard.
4. trust.

Answer: 2
Rationale: A nurse's negative preconceived ideas about a client and negative feelings toward the client usually result in frustration and mutual withdrawal. Supervision would cause the nurse to explore the origins of the feelings and make changes as necessary. The other options suggest positive outcomes, which rarely occur in the face of negative feelings on the part of the nurse.
Cognitive level: Comprehension
Nursing process: Evaluation
NCLEX: Psychosocial Integrity
See text page: 168

27. A nurse realizes that he believes he is the only one who truly understands a particular client and that other staff are too critical of the client. The nurse has identified a situation known as
1. boundary blurring.
2. sexual harassment.
3. positive regard.
4. egalitarianism.

Answer: 1
Rationale: When the role of the nurse and the role of the client shift, boundary blurring may arise. In this situation the nurse is becoming overinvolved with the client as a probable result of unrecognized countertransference. When boundary issues occur, the need for supervision exists. Option 2: The situation does not describe sexual harassment. Options 3 and 4: Data are not present to suggest positive regard or egalitarian behavior.
Cognitive level: Application
Nursing process: Evaluation
NCLEX: Safe and Effective Care Environment
See text pages: 158-161

CHAPTER 11

1. As a client converses with the nurse, she states "I dreamed I was stoned. When I woke up, I was feeling emotionally drained, as though I hadn't rested well." If the nurse needs clarification of "stoned," it would be appropriate to say
1. "It sounds as though you were quite uncomfortable with the content of your dream."

2. "Can you give me an example of what you mean by stoned?"
3. "I understand what you're saying. Bad dreams leave me feeling tired, too."
4. "So, all in all, you feel as though you had a rather poor night's sleep?"

Answer: 2

Rationale: The technique of exploring is useful because it helps the nurse examine meaning. Option 2 directly asks for clarification. Option 1 focuses on client feelings. Options 3 and 4 fail to clarify the meaning of the word in question.

Cognitive level: Application
Nursing process: Implementation
NCLEX: Psychosocial Integrity
See text page: 189

2. At the beginning of a clinical interview the nurse tells a teenaged client "While I'm here with you I will focus on the content and process of our communication as a participant observer." The client looks blankly at the nurse. The nurse can make the assessment that communication was not understood because of
   1. a personal factor: the use of terms not understood by the client.
   2. a social factor: the socioeconomic difference between nurse and client.
   3. an environmental factor: lack of privacy.
   4. incongruent verbal and nonverbal communication.

Answer: 1

Rationale: Various personal, environmental, and social factors may be responsible for ineffective communication. In this case, a personal factor is involved. The nurse used a highly technical explanation of his purpose for talking with the client. Data are not present in the scenario to support the choice of any other option.

Cognitive level: Application
Nursing process: Evaluation
NCLEX: Psychosocial Integrity
See text page: 178

3. The client remarks "My husband and I get along just fine. We usually agree on everything." As the client speaks her foot is moving continuously and she twirls a button on her blouse. What assessment can the nurse make? The client's communication is
   1. clear.
   2. explicit.
   3. inadequate.
   4. mixed.

Answer: 4

Rationale: Mixed messages involve the transmission of conflicting or incongruent messages by the speaker. The client's verbal message that all was well in the relationship was modified by the nonverbal behaviors denoting anxiety. Data are not present to support the choice of the verbal message being clear, explicit, or inadequate.

Cognitive level: Application
Nursing process: Assessment
NCLEX: Psychosocial Integrity
See text pages: 180, 181

4. A new nurse tells a mentor "I want to convey to my clients that I am interested in them and that I want to listen to what they have to say." The behaviors helpful in meeting the nurse's goal include the nurse (more than one answer may be correct)
   1. sitting behind a desk, facing the client.
   2. introducing herself to the client and identifying her staff role.
   3. using facial expressions that convey interest and encouragement.
   4. assuming an open body posture and sometimes mirror imaging.
   5. maintaining control of the topic under discussion by asking direct questions.

Answers: 2, 3, 4

Rationale: Options 2, 3, and 4 are helpful behaviors. Trust is fostered when the nurse introduces herself and identifies her role. Facial expressions that convey interest and encouragement support the nurse's verbal statements to that effect and strengthen the message. An open body posture conveys openness to listening to what the client has to say. Mirror imaging enhances client comfort. Option 1: The desk places a physical barrier between the nurse and client. A face-to-face stance should be avoided when possible and a less intense 90- or 120-degree angle used to permit either party to look away without discomfort. Option 5: Once introductions have been accomplished the nurse should turn the interview over to the client by using an open-ended question such as "Where should we start?"

Cognitive level: Application
Nursing process: Implementation
NCLEX: Psychosocial Integrity
See text pages: 172, 173

5. During the first interview with a restless young man, the nurse notices that he does not make eye contact throughout most of the interview. The nurse can correctly assume that

1. he is not to be trusted in what he says because he is evasive.
2. he is feeling sad and cannot look the nurse in the eye.
3. he is shy and the nurse must move slowly.
4. more information is needed to draw a conclusion.

Answer: 4

Rationale: The data presented are insufficient to draw a conclusion. The nurse must continue to gather information.

Cognitive level: Application
Nursing process: Assessment
NCLEX: Psychosocial Integrity
See text pages: 181, 184

6. Which statement made by a nurse during a nurse-client interaction may underrate a client's feelings and belittle his or her concerns?
   1. "You appear tense."
   2. "Everything will be all right."
   3. "I notice you are biting your lip."
   4. "I'm not sure I follow you."

Answer: 2

Rationale: Option 2 offers false reassurance. This is a nontherapeutic technique that suggests to a client that his or her views and feelings are not being taken seriously. Options 1, 3, and 4 use therapeutic techniques.

Cognitive level: Analysis
Nursing process: Evaluation
NCLEX: Psychosocial Integrity
See text pages: 191, 192

7. The nurse is talking with a young male client and has 5 minutes to go in the session with him. He has been silent and sullen most of the session and has been staring at the floor for the last 10 minutes. A troubled young woman comes to the door of the room and says to the nurse, "I really need to talk to you." The nurse should
   1. tell the woman she is busy at the present time.
   2. end the session and spend time with the young woman.
   3. invite the woman to sit down and join in the session with the other client.
   4. tell the woman that the session with this client will take 5 more minutes, after which the nurse will talk with her.

Answer: 4

Rationale: When a specific duration for sessions has been set, the nurse must adhere to the schedule. Leaving the first client would be equivalent to abandonment and would destroy any trust the client had in the nurse. Adhering to the contract demonstrates that the nurse can be trusted and that the client and the sessions are viewed as important. Option 1 preserves the nurse-client relationship with the young male client but may seem abrupt to the young female client. Option 2 abandons the young male client. Option 3 does not observe the contract with the young male client.

Cognitive level: Application
Nursing process: Implementation
NCLEX: Psychosocial Integrity
See text page: 177

8. Which remark by the nurse would be an appropriate way to begin a clinical interview session?
   1. "How shall we start today?"
   2. "Shall we talk about losing your privileges yesterday?"
   3. "What happened when your husband came to visit yesterday?"
   4. "Let's get started trying to unravel your marital relationship."

Answer: 1

Rationale: The interview is client centered; thus the issues are chosen by the client. The nurse assists the client by using communication skills and actively listening to provide opportunities for the client to reach goals. In options 2, 3, and 4 the nurse selects the topic.

Cognitive level: Application
Nursing process: Implementation
NCLEX: Psychosocial Integrity
See text page: 173

9. The nurse can best communicate to the client that she or he is interested in listening by
   1. restating the feeling or thought the client has expressed.
   2. making a judgment about the client's problem.
   3. asking a direct question, such as "Did you feel angry?"
   4. saying "I understand what you're saying."

Answer: 1

Rationale: Restating allows the client to validate the nurse's understanding of what has been communicated. Restating is an active listening technique. Option 2: Judgments should be suspended in a nurse-client relationship. Option 3: Closed-ended questions ask for specific information rather than showing understanding. Option 4 states that the nurse understands, but the client has no way of measuring the understanding.

Cognitive level: Application

Nursing process: Implementation
NCLEX: Psychosocial Integrity
See text page: 189

10. The client has disclosed several of his concerns and associated feelings. If the nurse wishes to seek clarification he could say
   1. "What are the common elements here?"
   2. "Tell me again."
   3. "Am I correct in concluding that . . ."
   4. "Tell me everything from the beginning."

Answer: 3
Rationale: Option 3 permits clarification to ensure that both the nurse and client share mutual understanding of the communication. Option 1 is a closed-ended question. Options 2 and 4 are implied questions.
Cognitive level: Application
Nursing process: Implementation
NCLEX: Psychosocial Integrity
See text pages: 189, 190

11. A client tells the nurse "I don't think I'll ever get out of here." A therapeutic response would be
   1. "You shouldn't talk that way. Of course you'll leave here!"
   2. "Everyone feels that way sometimes."
   3. "You don't think you're making progress?"
   4. "Keep up the good work and you certainly will."

Answer: 3
Rationale: In option 3 the nurse is reflecting by putting into words what the client is hinting. By making communication more explicit, issues are easier to identify and resolve. Options 1, 2, and 4 are nontherapeutic techniques. Option 1 is disapproving. Option 2 minimizes feelings. Option 4 is falsely reassuring.
Cognitive level: Application
Nursing process: Implementation
NCLEX: Psychosocial Integrity
See text pages: 191, 192

12. Documentation in a client's chart includes the following information: "Throughout a 5-minute interaction the client fidgeted and tapped his left foot, periodically covered his face with his hands, looked under his chair, all while stating he was enjoying spending time with this nurse." Of the following assessments, which is most accurate?
   1. The client is giving positive feedback about the nurse's communication techniques.
   2. The nurse is viewing the client's behavior through a cultural filter.

3. The client's verbal and nonverbal messages are incongruent.
   4. The client is demonstrating psychotic behaviors.

Answer: 3
Rationale: When a verbal message is not reinforced with nonverbal behavior, the message is confusing and incongruent. Some clinicians call it a "mixed message." Option 1 is an inaccurate statement. Option 2: A cultural filter determines what we will pay attention to and what we will ignore. This concept is not relevant to the situation presented. Option 4: Data are insufficient to draw this conclusion.
Cognitive level: Application
Nursing process: Assessment
NCLEX: Psychosocial Integrity
See text pages: 180, 181

13. The nurse finds himself feeling angry with a client. The nurse should
   1. tell the nurse manager to assign the client to another nurse.
   2. suppress the angry feelings.
   3. express the anger openly.
   4. discuss the anger with a clinician during a supervision session.

Answer: 4
Rationale: The nurse is accountable for the relationship. Objectivity is threatened by strong positive or negative feelings toward a client. Supervision is necessary to work through negative feelings. Option 1: This is not a first-line solution. Option 2: Suppression rarely results in a satisfactory outcome for client or nurse. Option 3: Open expression of anger will confuse a client who has been unaware of the nurse's feelings.
Cognitive level: Application
Nursing process: Implementation
NCLEX: Safe and Effective Care Environment
See text pages: 173-175

14. As she talks with a deeply depressed client, the nurse notices that the client is unable to maintain eye contact. The client drops her chin to her chest and looks down. The nurse has made an assessment of the client's
   1. nonverbal communication.
   2. mental status.
   3. nursing diagnosis.
   4. social skill.

Answer: 1
Rationale: Eye contact and body movements are considered nonverbal communication.

15. During a therapy session a client cries as the nurse explores the relationship of the client and her now-deceased mother. The client sobs "I shouldn't be blubbering like this." A response by the nurse that will hinder communication is
   1. "The relationship with your mother is very painful for you."
   2. "I can see that you feel sad about this situation."
   3. "Why do you think you are so upset?"
   4. "Crying is a way of expressing the hurt you're experiencing."

Answer: 3
Rationale: "Why" questions often imply criticism or seem intrusive or judgmental. They are difficult to answer; thus they are barriers to communication. The other options are therapeutic in nature.
Cognitive level: Application
Nursing process: Implementation
NCLEX: Psychosocial Integrity
See text page: 193

16. During the first interview with a woman who has just lost her son in a car accident, the nurse feels so sorry for the woman that she reaches out and touches her. The nurse's response
   1. is empathetic and will encourage the woman to continue to express her feelings.
   2. will be perceived by the client as intrusive and overstepping boundaries.
   3. is inappropriate because a "no touch" rule should be applied to all psychiatric clients.
   4. may be premature as the cultural and individual interpretation of touch is unknown.

Answer: 4
Rationale: Touch has various cultural and individual interpretations. Nurses should refrain from using touch until an assessment can be made regarding the way in which the client will perceive touch. The other options present prematurely drawn conclusions.
Cognitive level: Application
Nursing process: Evaluation
NCLEX: Psychosocial Integrity
See text page: 184

17. The nurse working with a young woman who is depressed tries to cheer the client by being casual and humorous. At one point the client smiles. What assessment can be made?

   1. The nurse has succeeded in reaching the client and is on the way to cheering her.
   2. The use of distraction and humor can be added to the intervention list in the plan of care.
   3. The nurse has identified an approach that may prove useful in other, similar situations.
   4. The nurse needs to seek supervision because the approach described is not acceptable.

Answer: 4
Rationale: Clinical supervision will review the nurse's actions and thoughts and help the nurse arrive at a more therapeutic approach. Attempts at cheering up a depressed client serve only to emphasize the disparity between the client's mood and that of others. Active listening should be the technique used by the nurse. Options 1, 2, and 3 suggest the approach is therapeutic when it is not.
Cognitive level: Application
Nursing process: Evaluation
NCLEX: Psychosocial Integrity
See text pages: 186-188

18. A male African American client says to a white male nurse "There's no sense in talking with you. You wouldn't understand because you live in a white world." The best response for the nurse would be to
   1. explain that the nurse can understand because everyone goes through the same experiences.
   2. ask the client to give an example of something he thinks the nurse wouldn't understand.
   3. reassure him that nurses are trained to deal with people from all cultures.
   4. gently change the subject to one that is less emotionally charged.

Answer: 2
Rationale: Having the client speak in specifics rather than globally will help the nurse understand the client's perspective. This approach will help the nurse draw out the client.
Cognitive level: Application
Nursing process: Implementation
NCLEX: Psychosocial Integrity
See text page: 189

19. A nurse working with a Filipino American client has noted that the client rarely makes eye contact during their interactions. The nurse hypothesizes that the reason for lack of eye contact is client low self-esteem and plans interventions designed to raise the client's self-esteem. After 3 weeks the client's eye contact has not improved. The nurse's clinical supervisor suggests that a problem exists with the assessment and plan. The most accurate formulation of the problem is

1. the client's poor eye contact is indicative of anger and hostility that are going unaddressed.
2. the client's eye contact should have been directly addressed by role playing to increase comfort with eye contact.
3. the nurse should have considered the client's culture during the assessment and before making a plan.
4. the nurse should not have independently embarked on assessment and planning.

Answer: 3
Rationale: The amount of eye contact a person engages in is often culturally determined. In some cultures eye contact is considered insolent, whereas in others eye contact is expected. Filipino Americans often prefer not to engage in direct eye contact.
Cognitive level: Analysis
Nursing process: Evaluation
NCLEX: Psychosocial Integrity
See text page: 184

20. When a Mexican American client and the primary nurse are sitting together, the client often takes the nurse's hand and holds it. The client also takes the nurse's hand or links her arm through the nurse's when they are walking. The nurse has made the assessment that the client is a lesbian and is quite uncomfortable with the behavior. Which of the following alternatives might be a more accurate assessment?
1. The client is accustomed to touch during conversation, as are members of many Hispanic subcultures.
2. The client understands that touch makes the nurse uncomfortable and controls the relationship based on that factor.
3. The client is afraid of being alone. When touching the nurse, the client is reassured that she is not alone.
4. The nurse is homophobic.

Answer: 1
Rationale: The most likely answer is that the client's behavior is culturally influenced. Hispanic women frequently touch women they consider to be their friends. Although the other options are possible, they are much less likely.
Cognitive level: Application
Nursing process: Assessment
NCLEX: Psychosocial Integrity
See text page: 184

21. A Puerto Rican American client uses dramatic body language whenever describing emotional discomfort. Of the possibilities below, which is most likely to be an accurate explanation of the client's behavior? The client
1. wishes to impress staff with her degree of emotional pain.
2. has a histrionic character disorder and uses this behavior habitually.
3. believes dramatic body language has high sexual appeal.
4. is a member of a culture in which dramatic body language is the norm.

Answer: 4
Rationale: Members of Hispanic American subcultures tend to use high affect and dramatic body language as they communicate. The other options are more remote possibilities.
Cognitive level: Application
Nursing process: Assessment
NCLEX: Psychosocial Integrity
See text pages: 183, 184

22. What would be the preferable remark for a student nurse to use after introductions have been made to begin the first nurse-client interview?
1. "So tell me, do you like having students here?"
2. "I'd like to have you tell me your problems."
3. "Perhaps you would like to begin by telling me about some of the stresses you've experienced recently."
4. "I read your chart and understand that you would like to focus on new ways to improve your self-esteem."

Answer: 3
Rationale: The nurse-client interview should be client centered and client paced. Option 3 is the least directive approach and turns the interview over to the client. Option 1 is student focused. Option 2 is a demand for immediate information. Option 4 takes the pacing of the interview away from the client.
Cognitive level: Application
Nursing process: Implementation
NCLEX: Psychosocial Integrity
See text page: 173

23. During a nurse-client interview the client attempts to shift the session focus from himself to the nurse by asking personal questions. The nurse should respond by saying
1. "You have no right to ask questions about my personal life."
2. "Nurses prefer to direct the interview."
3. "You've turned the tables on me."
4. "This time we spend together is for you to discuss your concerns."

Chapter 11   The Clinical Interview and Communication Skills

Answer: 4

Rationale: When a client chooses to focus on the nurse, the nurse should refocus the discussion back onto the client. Option 4 refocuses discussion in a neutral way. Option 1 shows indignation. Option 2 reflects superiority. Option 3 states the fact but does not refocus the interview.

Cognitive level: Application
Nursing process: Implementation
NCLEX: Psychosocial Integrity
See text page: 177

24. The nurse interviewing a client who is having difficulty staying focused could best help the client by saying
    1. "Go on."
    2. "What would you like to discuss?"
    3. "Tell me what is happening right now."
    4. "It seems as though you are having trouble staying focused."

Answer: 3

Rationale: Closed-ended questions may be necessary to elicit information from a client who is having difficulty concentrating.

Cognitive level: Application
Nursing process: Implementation
NCLEX: Psychosocial Integrity
See text page: 190

25. The nurse records the following data about a client: "Client has not spoken despite repeated efforts to elicit speech by nurse and other staff. Makes no eye contact and is inattentive to staff who attempt to engage him, gazing off to the side or looking upward rather than at speaker." A possible nursing diagnosis that deserves more investigation is
    1. defensive coping.
    2. risk for violence.
    3. decisional conflict.
    4. impaired verbal communication.

Answer: 4

Rationale: The defining characteristics are more related to the nursing diagnosis of impaired verbal communication than to the other nursing diagnoses.

Cognitive level: Analysis
Nursing process: Diagnosis
NCLEX: Psychosocial Integrity
See text page: 179

26. The remark by the nurse that gives the client verbal tracking feedback is
    1. "Describe your relationship with your wife."

2. "Am I correct in stating you are feeling angry with your wife?"
3. "You're saying you do not have a good relationship with your wife."
4. "Give me an example of not getting along with your wife."

Answer: 3

Rationale: Verbal tracking simply keeps track of what the client is saying. It is giving neutral feedback in the form of restating or summarizing what the client has said. Option 2 seeks validation. Options 1 and 4 are examples of exploring.

Cognitive level: Application
Nursing process: Implementation
NCLEX: Psychosocial Integrity
See text page: 183

27. A principle that should guide the nurse in determining the extent of silence to allow during client interview sessions is that
    1. the nurse is responsible for breaking silences.
    2. clients withdraw if silences are prolonged.
    3. silence provides meaningful moments for reflection.
    4. silence helps clients know that what they said was understood.

Answer: 3

Rationale: Silence can be helpful to both participants by giving each an opportunity to contemplate what has transpired, weigh alternatives, and formulate ideas. Option 1 is not a principle related to silences. Options 2 and 4 are not true statements. Feedback helps clients know they have been understood.

Cognitive level: Analysis
Nursing process: Implementation
NCLEX: Psychosocial Integrity
See text pages: 185, 186

28. During a session with a client who seems bewildered by his predicament, the nurse is conflicted about whether to provide advice. The rule of thumb that should be followed is that giving advice to a client
    1. is rarely helpful.
    2. fosters independence.
    3. lifts the burden of personal decision making.
    4. helps the client develop feelings of personal adequacy.

Answer: 1

Rationale: Giving advice fosters dependence on the nurse and interferes with the client's right to make personal decisions. It robs clients of the opportunity to weigh alternatives and develop problem-solving skills. Furthermore, it contributes to client feelings of personal inadequacy. It also keeps the nurse in control and feeling powerful.

Cognitive level: Comprehension
Nursing process: Implementation
NCLEX: Psychosocial Integrity
See text pages: 192, 193

29. The relationship between a nurse and a client as it relates to status and power is best described by the term
   1. symmetrical.
   2. complementary.
   3. incongruent.
   4. paralinguistic.

Answer: 2
Rationale: When a difference in power exists, as between a student and teacher or nurse and client, the relationship is said to be complementary. Symmetrical relationships exist between individuals of like or equal status. Incongruent and paralinguistic are not terms used to describe relationships.

Cognitive level: Comprehension
Nursing process: Assessment
NCLEX: Psychosocial Integrity
See text page: 178

30. A client seeks to elicit personal information about the nurse by asking several direct questions about the nurse's living arrangements. To refocus the interview the nurse should say
   1. "I am uncomfortable when you ask me personal questions, so please stop."
   2. "It seems a bit odd that you are focusing on me rather than on yourself."
   3. "Your questioning is manipulative and distracting us from our purpose."
   4. "This is your time to focus on your situation. Tell me about your concerns."

Answer: 4
Rationale: Option 4 restates the purpose of the interview, shifting the focus off the nurse and back to the client while remaining neutral. Option 1 remains nurse focused. Option 2 challenges the client. Option 3 is accusatory.

Cognitive level: Application
Nursing process: Implementation
NCLEX: Psychosocial Integrity
See text page: 177

CHAPTER 12

1. The daughter of a severely depressed client asks the nurse "What do you think about the relationship between depression and physical illness? Since my mother has been grieving over my father's death, she has been physically unwell. She has had a series of colds, an outbreak of shingles, and an episode of the flu." The answer that best reflects the current thinking about psychoimmunology is
   1. "It is probably a coincidence. Not much evidence is available that the stress of grieving makes one prone to physical illnesses."
   2. "Your observation might be explained by the fact you are paying more attention to your mother since your father died and you are noticing things such as minor illnesses."
   3. "The literature has not dwelt on the relation between mental state and the body other than to say that one influences the other."
   4. "The immune system is thought to respond to changes in brain chemistry by suppressing white blood cell production when the person experiences prolonged stress."

Answer: 4
Rationale: Option 4 best explains evidence-based thinking. Research indicates that stress can induce modulation of the immune system. Activation of the immune system sends proinflammatory cytokines to the brain. The brain, in turn, releases it own cytokines that signal the central nervous system to initiate myriad responses to stress. Alteration in neural activity in the brain can alter everything that flows from neural activity, including behavior, thought, and mood. Prolonged stress suppresses the immune system and lowers resistance to infections. The other options underplay the fact that evidence exists that partially explains the effect of stress on the immune system.

Cognitive level: Application
Nursing process: Implementation
NCLEX: Physiological Integrity
See text pages: 198-200

2. A client with emphysema who has severe shortness of breath and frequent hospitalizations often depends on her portable oxygen tank when she leaves her home. Recently she was tearful at a Better Breathers Group meeting because in the last 2 weeks she has not been able to go upstairs to her bedroom at night because of slight shortness of breath by the third step and fear of having severe breathing difficulty as she continues up the stairs. The group leader provides several suggestions and

259

Chapter 12   Understanding Stress and Holistic Approaches to Stress Management

arranges to teach the client guided imagery. What image would the client be encouraged to imagine?
1. A younger, healthier body that knows no exercise limitations.
2. Learning to sleep downstairs as an acceptable alternative to her bedroom.
3. Separating herself from and being free and independent from her oxygen tank.
4. Walking up the stairs in a relaxed manner with regular depth and rate of breathing.

Answer: 4
Rationale: The client has dysfunctional images of dyspnea and her ability to climb stairs. Guided imagery can help her replace the dysfunctional image with a positive coping image. Athletes have found that picturing successful images can enhance performance. Encouraging the client to imagine a regular breathing depth and rate will help improve oxygen—carbon dioxide exchange and help her achieve further relaxation. Options 1 and 3 are not as closely related to the stated problem as option 4. Option 2 introduces an entirely different resolution
Cognitive level: Application
Nursing process: Implementation
NCLEX: Psychosocial Integrity
See text page: 205

3. A nurse who leads group therapy for a group of depressed clients also plans to implement a plan of exercise for each client. The rationale to use when presenting this plan to the treatment team is that exercise
1. releases hormones called β-endorphins that have antidepressant and anxiolytic effects.
2. prevents damage from sympathetic nervous system overstimulation.
3. improves circulation and oxygenation to brain and body cells.
4. detoxifies the body by ridding it of metabolic wastes.

Answer: 1
Rationale: β-Endorphins produced during exercise result in improvement in mood and lowered anxiety. The other options are not accurate.
Cognitive level: Application
Nursing process: Implementation
NCLEX: Physiological Integrity
See text page: 205

4. A recent immigrant from Central America is brought to the clinic by her daughter, who has been a U.S. resident for 10 years. The daughter says the stress of immigration has made her mother unwell.

For which expression of stress should the nurse be alert during the assessment interview?
1. Moderate anxiety
2. Somatic complaints
3. Memory deficiencies
4. Sensory perceptual alterations

Answer: 2
Rationale: Many people from Central American cultures express distress in somatic terms. The other options are less likely to be observed.
Cognitive level: Application
Nursing process: Assessment
NCLEX: Psychosocial Integrity
See text pages: 200, 201

5. Which client will probably be at greatest risk for experiencing untoward effects of stress?
1. Mr. A, who sought medical help for his stress-related symptoms and follows a regimen of medication, proper diet, and rest.
2. Mr. B, who finds much satisfaction in implementing highly creative innovations in his work.
3. Mr. C, who can depend on the interested support of family, friends, and co-workers.
4. Mr. D, who chooses not to deal with the stress-producing situation.

Answer: 4
Rationale: Avoidance is a negative response to stress, predisposing the individual to the untoward effects of stress. Options 1, 2, and 3 present positive coping responses.
Cognitive level: Analysis
Nursing process: Assessment
NCLEX: Psychosocial Integrity
See text pages: 202, 203

6. A client states she is experiencing high stress. She is in a work environment in which her boss treats her "like a doormat." She states he thinks nothing of demanding that she stay overtime and work on Saturdays whenever he is "in the mood to work." A coping strategy the nurse might suggest using is
1. resigning the position.
2. learning to reframe the situation.
3. relying on the support of her family.
4. using assertiveness techniques.

Answer: 4
Rationale: The client is experiencing stress because her boss is violating her rights as an employee. Assertiveness techniques would help her stand up for her rights without being aggressive. Option 1 is a drastic option. Option 2 is not called for. Option 3 may not be effective.

Cognitive level: Application
Nursing process: Planning
NCLEX: Psychosocial Integrity
See text page: 207

7. According to the Life Changing Event Questionnaire the nurse can predict that a client will be prone to negative responses to stress if he or she has experienced
   1. a number of significant losses.
   2. a move within the same city or town.
   3. a change in religious beliefs.
   4. a promotion at work.

Answer: 1

Rationale: Deaths and other significant losses are high-scoring items on the questionnaire. A number of losses would suggest a high score and a greater propensity for difficulty.
Cognitive level: Application
Nursing process: Assessment
NCLEX: Psychosocial Integrity
See text page: 202

8. Of the four individuals described below, which client has the highest potential for attaining the outcome "the client will cope effectively with current stressors"?
   1. A, who "stews" about negative feelings and situations without taking action
   2. B, who blames himself for the situation, saying he acted "stupidly"
   3. C, who states he thinks things will eventually work out by themselves
   4. D, who sought help from siblings with whom he has close, conflict-free relationships

Answer: 4

Rationale: The use of high-quality social support is a positive response to stress likely to promote positive client outcomes. Clients A, B, and C are using the negative responses of avoidance, self-blame, and wishful thinking.
Cognitive level: Analysis
Nursing process: Evaluation
NCLEX: Psychosocial Integrity
See text page: 200

9. When including a 12-step program in a client's plan of care, the nurse can expect that stress mediators will include (more than one answer may be correct)
   1. social support.
   2. spiritual support.
   3. professional therapy.
   4. health-sustaining habits.

Answers: 1, 2, 4

Rationale: A 12-step program is a self-help program. Professional therapists do not provide the therapy; members do. Twelve-step programs provide social support in meetings and the sponsor program; spiritual support, as evidenced in the 12 steps; and health-sustaining habits such as abstinence from substances of abuse, pacing one's activities, and getting enough sleep. The 12-step programs rely on self-help principles rather than professional therapists.
Cognitive level: Application
Nursing process: Planning
NCLEX: Psychosocial Integrity
See text page: 200

10. A client tells the nurse that "My sister just never picks up colds or other illnesses that go around each year. The only difference between the two of us is that she is highly involved in her church, while I'm not very spiritual." The reply that shows the best understanding of psychoimmunology is
    1. "It is probably just a coincidence."
    2. "No correlation between spirituality and wellness exists."
    3. "Studies have shown that spiritual practices can enhance immune system function."
    4. "The mind and body are closely interrelated, so what you say may be true."

Answer: 3

Rationale: Studies have shown a positive correlation between spiritual practices and enhanced immune system function and sense of well-being. The other options downplay current research showing that spiritual practices can enhance the immune system.
Cognitive level: Application
Nursing process: Implementation
NCLEX: Physiological Integrity
See text page: 201

11. When the nurse asks the client to describe her social supports, the client gives the following information: she is divorced, has no siblings, her parents died last year, and she has contact with her former in-laws, who subtly blame her for the divorce. Regarding the relationship with her in-laws, the nurse can base plans on the knowledge that
    1. the in-laws offer the only opportunity to obtain social support for the client.
    2. low-quality support relationships often negatively affect coping in a crisis.
    3. her relationship with her in-laws can enhance the client's sense of control and competence.
    4. strong social support is of relatively little importance as a mediating factor.

Chapter 12   Understanding Stress and Holistic Approaches to Stress Management

Answer: 2

Rationale: High-quality social support enhances mental and physical health and acts as a significant buffer against distress. Low-quality support relationships are known to affect a person's coping effectiveness negatively.

Cognitive level: Application
Nursing process: Planning
NCLEX: Psychosocial Integrity
See text page: 200

12. A client who is experiencing great stress associated with a disturbing new diagnosis asks the nurse "Do you think saying a prayer would help?" The answer the nurse should give is
   1. "To be honest, prayer may be your only hope."
   2. "You may find prayer gives comfort and lowers your stress."
   3. "I could help you feel calmer by teaching you to meditate."
   4. "Guided imagery, progressive relaxation, and prayer have about the same degree of effectiveness."

Answer: 2

Rationale: Many clients find that spiritual measures, including prayer, are helpful in mediating stress. Studies have shown that spiritual practices can enhance the sense of well-being. When a client suggests a viable means of reducing stress, it should be supported by the nurse. Option 1 is pessimistic and would cause further distress. Option 3 suggests an alternative and implies that the nurse does not think prayer would be effective. Option 4 gives more information than the client is seeking.

Cognitive level: Application
Nursing process: Implementation
NCLEX: Psychosocial Integrity
See text page: 201

13. Rank the order in which a nurse, when teaching clients about the initial alarm reaction to stress, should present the following facts:
   1. The heart rate and blood pressure increase, airways dilate, and the liver releases glucose for fuel.
   2. The threat message goes to the hypothalamus, which communicates chemically with the pituitary gland.
   3. Adrenaline, noradrenaline, and other catecholamines enter the bloodstream.
   4. The initial alarm reaction, known as the fight or flight response, occurs when the individual perceives a threat to survival.
   5. Acetylcholine is released and activates hormones for the adrenal medulla.

Answer: 4, 2, 5, 3, 1

Rationale: The initial alarm reaction is known as the fight or flight response. It occurs when the individual perceives a threat to survival. The sympathetic nervous system is the pathway of stress responses. The threat message goes to the hypothalamus, triggering chemical communication with the pituitary gland. Acetylcholine is subsequently released and activates hormones for the adrenal medulla. Adrenaline, noradrenaline, and other catecholamines then enter the bloodstream, causing the heart rate and blood pressure to increase, airways to dilate, the liver to release glucose for fuel, blood flow to shift from smooth muscles to the digestive tract to skeletal muscles, and platelet aggregation to increase to aid blood clotting.

Cognitive level: Comprehension
Nursing process: Planning
NCLEX: Physiological Integrity
See text pages: 197, 198

14. When a client asks about the effects of long-term, sustained distress the nurse, basing a response on current research, should reply
   1. "Little is known about the long-term effects of stress on the body."
   2. "Hypertension, autoimmune disease, and obesity are proven to be stress related."
   3. "Research indicates depression and cognitive problems are related to effects of stress on the immune system."
   4. "Studies indicate stress acting on hypothalamic-pituitary-adrenal and sympathetic-adrenal medullary axes affects the immune system."

Answer: 4

Rationale: Stress causes the immune system to send chemical messages (proinflammatory cytokines) to the brain and that the brain then releases its own cytokines that signal the central nervous system to initiate responses to help the body adapt to stress. Research suggests that any process that alters neural activity in the brain can alter behavior, thought, and mood. Option 1 understates what is known. Options 2 and 3 overstate causation of these disorders.

Cognitive level: Application
Nursing process: Implementation
NCLEX: Physiological Integrity
See text pages: 198-200

15. On the basis of recent findings, which client could the nurse expect to have greater difficulty adjusting to life changes that have occurred over the past year?
   1. A, a 32-year-old woman who is pregnant, divorcing her husband, and changing residences

2. B, a 40-year-old man who has received a promotion and undertaken a weight loss program
3. C, a 45-year-old woman whose daughter left home to attend college and whose ill mother is moving in
4. D, a 67-year-old retired man who lost his home in a hurricane

Answer: 1

Rationale: The scores on the Life-Changing Events Questionnaire are the following: A, 151; B, 58; C, 100; and D, 95. The higher the score, the greater the stress placed on the individual. In addition, women assess and react to life stress events at a higher level than men. Men tend to underrate life change units by approximately 17%. Even when adjustments are made to the scores of the men, A still rates highest.

Cognitive level: Analysis
Nursing process: Assessment
NCLEX: Psychosocial Integrity
See text page: 202

16. The nurse planning to teach a client to use Benson's relaxation techniques to treat hypertension is essentially teaching the client to
   1. switch from the sympathetic mode of the autonomic nervous system to the parasympathetic mode.
   2. alter the internal state by acting on electronic signals related to physiologic processes.
   3. replace stress-producing activities with daily stress-reducing pleasant activities.
   4. reduce catecholamine production and produce β-endorphins.

Answer: 1

Rationale: When the sympathetic nervous system is operative, the individual experiences muscular tension and an elevated pulse, blood pressure, and respiratory rate. Relaxation is achieved when the sympathetic nervous system is quieted and the parasympathetic nervous system is operative. Option 2 is the basis for biofeedback, a behavioral approach to stress reduction. Option 3 is a cognitive approach called priority restructuring. Option 4 is the basis on which guided imagery, a behavioral approach to stress reduction, operates.

Cognitive level: Application
Nursing process: Implementation
NCLEX: Physiological Integrity
See text pages: 203-207

17. A client tells the nurse "I'm told that I should reduce the stress in my life, but I have no idea where to

start." The best suggestion for the nurse to make would be
   1. "Why not start by learning to meditate? That technique will cover everything."
   2. "In cases like yours, physical exercise works to elevate mood and reduce anxiety."
   3. "Most stress is related to conflicts in interpersonal relationships. You can work on becoming more assertive."
   4. "Keeping a journal can help you identify sources of stress by looking at activities that put a strain on energy or time or trigger anger or anxiety."

Answer: 4

Rationale: Journaling is the only option that will provide an opportunity for the client to identify stressful events or activities retrospectively. In the other options, the nurse is offering solutions without first assessing needs.

Cognitive level: Application
Nursing process: Implementation
NCLEX: Psychosocial Integrity
See text page: 206

18. A client tells the nurse "My doctor thinks my problems with stress relate to the negative way I think about things, and he wants me to learn a new way of thinking." The nurse should be prepared to help the client understand and apply a cognitive technique called
   1. priority restructuring.
   2. reframing/restructuring.
   3. guided imagery.
   4. assertiveness.

Answer: 2

Rationale: Cognitive reframing involves the individual reassessing a situation and changing his or her perception of the stress. The altered perception allows the individual to restructure the situation to one over which he or she can have a measure of control.

Option 1: Priority restructuring involves replacing stressful activities with pleasant activities and is not necessarily related to distorted or irrational cognitions. Option 3: Guided imagery is a behavioral technique. Option 4: Assertiveness focuses on standing up for one's rights without violating the rights of others. It is not necessarily related to distorted or irrational cognitions.

Cognitive level: Comprehension
Nursing process: Planning
NCLEX: Psychosocial Integrity
See text pages: 206, 207

19. A client tells the nurse that "I'm told that I should reduce the stress in my life, but I have no real idea

263

what things create stress for me and no idea of where to start." The nursing diagnosis the nurse should consider for this client is
1. ineffective coping.
2. defensive coping.
3. decisional conflict.
4. ineffective denial.

Answer: 1
Rationale: Only Option 1 relates to the data given. The definition of this nursing diagnosis is the inability to form a valid appraisal of the stressors, inadequate choices of practiced responses, or inability to use available resources. Option 2: Defensive coping involves projection of a falsely positive self-evaluation based on a self-protective pattern that defends against underlying perceived threats to positive self-regard. Option 3: Decisional conflict speaks to uncertainty about the course of action to be taken when the choice among competing actions involves risk, loss, or challenge to personal life values. Option 4: Ineffective denial suggests attempts to disavow the knowledge or meaning of an event to reduce anxiety, which lead to the detriment of health.
Cognitive level: Analysis
Nursing process: Diagnosis
NCLEX: Psychosocial Integrity
See text page: 202

20. A client tells the nurse "I've always been a religious person and I'm going to combat stress by spending more time in prayer each day." The nursing diagnosis that the nurse should consider establishing is
1. spiritual distress.
2. disturbed thought processes.
3. readiness for enhanced spiritual well-being.
3. ineffective therapeutic regimen management.

Answer: 3
Rationale: This nursing diagnosis is defined as ability to experience and integrate meaning and purpose in life through connectedness with self, others, art, music, literature, nature, or a power greater than self. The scenario provides no data to support the diagnoses in the other options.
Cognitive level: Analysis
Nursing process: Diagnosis
NCLEX: Psychosocial Integrity
See text page: 201

21. The client tells the nurse "I'll never be happy until I'm as successful as my older sister." The nurse asks the client to reassess this statement and reframe it. An acceptable reframed statement is
1. "I won't be happy until I make as much money as my sister."

2. "People should treat me as well as they treat my sister."
3. "I can find enjoyment in success at my own job level."
4. "I'm resigned to not being as smart or clever as my sister."

Answer: 3
Rationale: This reframed statement is positive and realistic. It speaks to finding satisfaction and happiness without measuring the self against another person. The other options show persistent negative, irrational thinking about the self compared with the sister.
Cognitive level: Analysis
Nursing process: Evaluation
NCLEX: Psychosocial Integrity
See text page: 207

22. A stress-laden client has elected to learn deep breathing as a means of reducing stress.
   Rank the order the nurse should give the following information when preparing a teaching plan:
1. Focus on your breathing; repeat the exercise for 2 to 5 minutes.
2. With each breath, pay attention to muscular sensations that accompany abdominal expansion.
3. Hold the breath for 3 seconds.
4. Find a comfortable position. Relax the shoulders and chest; let the body relax.
5. Take a deep breath through the nose, expanding the abdomen.
6. Exhale slowly through the nose, telling the body to relax.

Answer: 4, 5, 3, 6, 2, 1
Rationale: This sequencing of directions places the elements in the correct order and is easy to follow and remember.
Cognitive level: Application
Nursing process: Implementation
NCLEX: Health Promotion and Maintenance
See text page: 205

23. A client tells the nurse that one result of his chronic stress is that he has considerable fatigue. He has tried setting his alarm to give himself an extra 30 minutes of sleep each morning but feels no better. The nurse should suggest that
1. "You may need to speak to your doctor about taking a sedative."
2. "Keep doing what you have started. It takes a while to develop new sleep habits."
3. "Try going to bed a half hour earlier than usual and getting up at your regular time."
4. "Waking up to music, rather than an alarm, is often helpful in promoting relaxation."

Answer: 3

Rationale: Sleeping later in the morning is rarely helpful. It often disturbs circadian rhythms. Going to bed earlier and arising at the usual time alleviates fatigue more effectively. Option 1: Sedatives may disrupt sleep to a greater degree in the long run.

Option 2: This method results in circadian rhythm disturbance. Option 4 is not evidence based.

Cognitive level: Application
Nursing process: Implementation
NCLEX: Physiological Integrity
See text page: 208

24. A client who has been under stress for several years tells the nurse that "When a problem comes up, I just walk away from it because I don't know how to handle it. Then I feel worse because I didn't do anything." The client outcome the nurse should consider is
    1. comfort level.
    2. decision-making.
    3. anxiety self-control.
    4. acceptance: health status.

Answer: 2

Rationale: The client describes not knowing how to handle decision making and experiencing negative feelings as a result of an inability to make decisions. Decision making as an outcome is entirely relevant. The other options do not have the same degree of relevance.

Cognitive level: Analysis
Nursing process: Planning (Outcome Identification)
NCLEX: Psychosocial Integrity
See text page: 204

25. The nurse has worked for several weeks to teach a client to use assertiveness techniques.

    The remark by the client that the nurse should evaluate as demonstrating assertiveness is
    1. "I think you're a real jerk."
    2. "I wish I knew what the best course of action would be."
    3. "I wish I believed I have the right to refuse overtime."
    4. "When you shout at me, I feel embarrassed. Please lower your voice."

Answer: 4

Rationale: This technique is confrontationally assertive. It points out a fact and asks for a change of behavior. Option 1 is aggressive communication. Option 2 is passive/acquiescent. Option 3: This statement reflects doubt about personal rights, a block to assertiveness.

Cognitive level: Analysis
Nursing process: Evaluation
NCLEX: Psychosocial Integrity
See text page: 207

CHAPTER 13

1. The nurse wishes to teach an alternative coping strategy to a client who is currently experiencing severe anxiety. The nurse will first need to
   1. use measures designed to lower the client's anxiety.
   2. determine the mode of learning preferred by the client.
   3. devise outcomes and construct a teaching plan.
   4. assess the degree of trait anxiety present.

Answer: 1

Rationale: A client experiencing severe anxiety has a markedly narrowed perceptual field and difficulty attending to events in the environment. Thus a client experiencing severe anxiety will not learn readily. Options 2 and 3 are relevant to the task but are not the priority measure. Option 4: The nurse has already assessed the client's anxiety level.

Cognitive level: Analysis
Nursing process: Planning
NCLEX: Psychosocial Integrity
See text pages: 214, 215

2. A client approaches the nurse and blurts out "You've got to help me! Something terrible is happening. I'm falling apart. I can't think. My heart is pounding and my head is throbbing." The nurse responds "It's almost time for visiting hours. Let's get your hair combed." This interaction can be evaluated as
   1. a distracting technique to lower anxiety.
   2. bringing up an irrelevant topic.
   3. sensitive to physical needs.
   4. addressing false cognitions.

Answer: 2

Rationale: The nurse has closed off client-centered communication and introduced an irrelevant topic, a ploy designed to make the nurse, who is uncomfortable dealing with the client's severe anxiety, feel better.

Cognitive level: Evaluation
Nursing process: Evaluation
NCLEX: Physiological Integrity
See text page: 215

3. A client has been assessed as having moderate anxiety. He says "I feel undone." An appropriate response for the nurse would be
   1. "Why do you suppose you are feeling anxious?"
   2. "What would you like me to do to help you?"
   3. "I'm not sure I understand. Give me an example."
   4. "You need to get your feelings under control."

Answer: 3

Rationale: Increased anxiety results in scattered thoughts and an inability to articulate clearly. Clarifying helps

265

the client identify thoughts and feelings. Option 1 is a nontherapeutic question for which the client likely does not have an answer. Option 2: The client may be unable to determine this. Option 4 is a directive the client is probably unable to accomplish.
Cognitive level: Application
Nursing process: Implementation
NCLEX: Psychosocial Integrity
See text page: 215

4. A client is noted to have a high level of non-goal-directed motor activity, running from chair to chair in the solarium. He is wide eyed and seems terror stricken. He cries "They're coming! They're coming!" He neither follows staff direction nor responds to verbal efforts to calm him. The initial nursing intervention of highest priority is to
   1. provide for client safety.
   2. increase environmental stimuli.
   3. respect the client's personal space.
   4. encourage clarification of feelings.

Answer: 1
Rationale: Safety is of highest priority because the client experiencing panic is at high risk for self-injury related to increased non-goal-directed motor activity, distorted perceptions, and disordered thoughts. Option 2: The goal should be to decrease environmental stimuli. Option 3 is a lower priority than safety. Option 4: Clarification of feelings cannot take place until the level of anxiety is lowered.
Cognitive level: Analysis
Nursing process: Implementation
NCLEX: Safe and Effective Care Environment
See text pages: 216, 217

5. A client is noted to have a high level of non-goal-directed motor activity, running from chair to chair in the solarium. He is wide eyed and seems terror stricken. He cries "They're coming! They're coming!" He neither follows staff direction nor responds to verbal efforts to calm him. A nursing diagnosis of high priority is
   1. risk for injury.
   2. self-care deficit.
   3. disturbed energy field.
   4. impaired verbal communication.

Answer: 1
Rationale: A client experiencing panic-level anxiety is at high risk for self-injury related to increased non-goal-directed motor activity, distorted perceptions, and disordered thoughts. Data are not present to support the other nursing diagnoses.
Cognitive level: Analysis

Nursing process: Diagnosis
NCLEX: Safe and Effective Care Environment
See text pages: 216, 217

6. A secretary is asked by her boss to take on additional work. She initially agrees but feels resentful. A day later when the boss asks for the completed work, the secretary explains that she has been working on another priority job and hasn't been able to complete it. When asked several hours later, she states someone else was using the files and she hasn't been able to do the necessary research before typing the report. The secretary's behavior demonstrates
   1. acting out.
   2. projection.
   3. rationalization.
   4. passive aggression.

Answer: 4
Rationale: A passive-aggressive person deals with emotional conflict by indirectly and unassertively expressing aggression toward others. Compliance on the surface masks covert resistance. Resistance is expressed through procrastination, inefficiency, and stubbornness in response to assigned tasks.
Cognitive level: Application
Nursing process: Assessment
NCLEX: Psychosocial Integrity
See text page: 218

7. A client is undergoing a series of diagnostic tests. He insists nothing is wrong with him except a chest cold that he "can't shake off." His wife says he smokes and coughs a lot, has lost 15 pounds, and is easily fatigued. The defense mechanism the client is using is
   1. regression.
   2. displacement.
   3. denial.
   4. projection.

Answer: 3
Rationale: Denial is an unconscious blocking of threatening or painful information or feelings. Option 1: Regression involves using behaviors appropriate at an earlier stage of psychosexual development. Option 2: Displacement shifts feelings to a more neutral person or object. Option 4: Projection attributes one's own unacceptable thoughts or feelings to another.
Cognitive level: Application
Nursing process: Assessment
NCLEX: Psychosocial Integrity
See text page: 220

8. A client has had a series of diagnostic tests, although he protests that nothing is wrong with him except a chest cold that he "can't shake off." The diagnostic tests reveal a mass in the left upper lobe of the client's lung. He is scheduled to undergo a biopsy. When the nurse explains the procedure to him, he seems to have difficulty grasping what she is saying and asks questions such as "What do you mean I'm going to have surgery? What are they going to do?" His voice is tremulous. His respirations are noticeably rapid at 28 breaths/min, and his pulse is 110 beats/min. The nurse should assess the client's level of anxiety as
1. mild.
2. moderate.
3. severe.
4. panic.

Answer: 2
Rationale: Moderate anxiety causes the individual to grasp less information and reduces problem-solving ability to a less-than-optimal level. Option 1: Mild anxiety heightens attention and enhances problem solving. Option 3: Severe anxiety causes great reduction in the perceptual field. Option 4: Panic-level anxiety results in disorganized behavior.
Cognitive level: Application
Nursing process: Assessment
NCLEX: Psychosocial Integrity
See text page: 215

9. A client has a mass in the left upper lobe of his lung. He is scheduled to undergo a biopsy. When the nurse explains the procedure to him, he seems to have difficulty grasping what she is saying and asks questions such as "What do you mean I'm going to have surgery? What are they going to do?" His voice is tremulous. His respirations are noticeably rapid at 28 breaths/min, and his pulse is 110 beats/min. The client can be assessed as having a cognitive problem called
1. rationalization.
2. conversion.
3. introjection.
4. selective inattention.

Answer: 4
Rationale: Selective inattention means only certain things are understood or grasped unless they are brought to the client's attention. Options 1, 2, and 3 are defense mechanisms, not cognitive problems.
Cognitive level: Application
Nursing process: Assessment
NCLEX: Psychosocial Integrity
See text pages: 213, 214

10. A client has a mass in the left upper lobe of his lung. He is scheduled to undergo a biopsy. When the nurse explains the procedure to him, he seems to have difficulty grasping what she is saying and asks questions such as "What do you mean I'm going to have surgery? What are they going to do?" His voice is tremulous. His respirations are noticeably rapid at 28 breaths/min, and his pulse is 110 beats/min. The nursing diagnosis formulated for the client is anxiety related to impending biopsy, as evidenced by repeated questions and by voice tremors and elevated pulse and respirations. Outcomes the nurse should consider include (more than one answer may be correct)
1. compliance behavior.
2. anxiety self-control.
3. information processing.
4. aggression self-control.
5. social interaction skills.
6. adaptation to physical disability.

Answers: 2, 3
Rationale: When the client is able to control anxiety, he will be able to demonstrate comprehension and use of the information he is given. None of the other outcomes is directly related to the behaviors that support the nursing diagnosis.
Cognitive level: Application
Nursing process: Planning (Outcome Identification)
NCLEX: Psychosocial Integrity
See text page: 215

11. A client who is going to have a biopsy is demonstrating moderate anxiety, as exemplified by his inability to grasp information presented by the health care team. The nursing intervention that should be implemented is to
1. reassure the client that many treatments are available for a lung neoplasm.
2. describe the procedure again in a calm manner and with simple language.
3. tell the client that staff are prepared to help him in any way they can.
4. explain to the client that he should not keep his feelings to himself.

Answer: 2
Rationale: Giving information in a calm, simple manner will help the client grasp the important facts. Introducing extraneous topics, as in options 1, 3, and 4, will further scatter his attention.
Cognitive level: Application
Nursing process: Implementation
NCLEX: Psychosocial Integrity
See text page: 215

Chapter 13 Understanding Anxiety and Anxiety Defenses

12. While working with an anxious client, the nurse begins to feel tense and jittery and notices that she is having difficulty concentrating on what the client is telling her. How can this be explained? The nurse is experiencing
   1. introjected anxiety.
   2. secondary anxiety.
   3. empathized anxiety.
   4. maturational anxiety.

Answer: 3

Rationale: Anxiety is transmissible from one person to another through empathy, the ability to experience another's feelings. Option 1: Introjected anxiety is an illogical answer; introjection is a defense mechanism. Option 2: Secondary anxiety is associated with a physical disorder. Option 4: Maturational anxiety arises from a situation in which a threat is present to achievement of a developmental task.
Cognitive level: Analysis
Nursing process: Assessment
NCLEX: Safe and Effective Care Environment
See text page: 216

13. The nurse plans to encourage an anxious client to talk about his feelings and concerns. The rationale for this intervention is that
   1. offering hope allays the client's anxiety.
   2. concerns stated aloud become less overwhelming and can serve as the basis for problem solving.
   3. anxiety can be reduced by focusing on and validating what is occurring in the environment.
   4. encouraging clients to explore alternatives increases the sense of control and lessens anxiety.

Answer: 2

Rationale: All principles listed are valid, but the only principle directly related to the intervention of assisting the client to talk about his feelings and concerns is option 2.
Cognitive level: Application
Nursing process: Planning
NCLEX: Psychosocial Integrity
See text page: 215

14. A college student usually gets As but scored a C on a difficult examination. When he received the grade he felt nauseated and clammy and had difficulty comprehending what was written on the paper. A friend sensed his distress and touched him on the shoulder. The student jumped, looked dazed, and mumbled "They got the grade wrong," as he quickly walked away. What assessment can be made? The student is experiencing
   1. panic.

2. mild to moderate anxiety.
3. severe anxiety.
4. reaction formation.

Answer: 3
Rationale: The symptoms described are those of severe anxiety. The student seems to have a poor grasp of what is happening in the environment but is not totally disorganized as he would be with panic-level anxiety. His symptoms, however, are more severe than would be found in mild to moderate anxiety. Option 4: Reaction formation is a defense mechanism unrelated to what is described in the situation.
Cognitive level: Application
Nursing process: Assessment
NCLEX: Psychosocial Integrity
See text pages: 216, 217

15. A college student usually gets As but scored a C on a difficult examination. When he received the grade, he experienced anxiety. The best explanation for the student's reaction is that
   1. intense anger associated with the low grade gave rise to acute anxiety.
   2. fear of academic repercussions associated with a low grade prompted the response.
   3. the expectation of a high grade was unmet, precipitating a threat to self-esteem, causing anxiety.
   4. the physical symptoms and cognitive impairment are related to parasympathetic response.

Answer: 3
Rationale: The operational definition of anxiety suggests that an expectation or need is unmet, causing anxiety and prompting relief behavior. Options 1 and 2: The scenario does not support a rationale associated with anger or fear. Option 4: The responses associated with anxiety are related to sympathetic nervous system responses.
Cognitive level: Application
Nursing process: Assessment
NCLEX: Psychosocial Integrity
See text pages: 212, 213

16. A client is brought to the emergency department displaying disorganized behavior and incoherence after an acquaintance suggested a homosexual encounter. In which room should the nurse place the client until he can be seen by the physician?
   1. An interview room furnished with a desk and two chairs
   2. A small, empty storage room that has no windows or furniture
   3. The nurse's office, furnished with a desk, chairs, files, and bookcases

268

4. An examining room containing an examining table, instrument storage cabinets, a desk, and a chair

Answer: 1

Rationale: Individuals experiencing severe to panic-level anxiety require a safe environment that is quiet, non-stimulating, structured, and simple. Option 1 provides simplicity, few objects with which he could harm himself, and a small floor space in which the client can move about. Option 2 would be like a jail cell. Options 3 and 4 may be overstimulating and unsafe.

Cognitive level: Application
Nursing process: Implementation
NCLEX: Safe and Effective Care Environment
See text pages: 216, 217

17. A client is assessed as experiencing moderate anxiety. To reduce the client's level of anxiety as quickly as possible, the nurse should
   1. stay with him.
   2. tell him that help will come.
   3. tell him he will not be allowed to hurt anyone.
   4. question him to discover the events that led to his decompensation.

Answer: 1

Rationale: The presence of a caring person provides a link with reality. The nurse can offer structure and set limits when necessary. Option 2 implies that the nurse cannot provide assistance. Option 3 is a premature attempt to set physical limits. Option 4 is inappropriate when a client is highly disorganized.

Cognitive level: Application
Nursing process: Implementation
NCLEX: Safe and Effective Care Environment
See text page: 215

18. A client accompanied her boyfriend to the emergency department after the two had been in a motorcycle accident. The boyfriend was badly hurt, but the client had only minor cuts and bruises. The client appears confused and has trouble focusing on what the nurse is saying. She reports nausea and dizziness, has tachycardia, and is hyperventilating as the nurse interviews her. She tells the nurse that she feels as though something awful is going to happen. The nurse should assess the client's level of anxiety as
   1. mild.
   2. moderate.
   3. severe.
   4. panic.

Answer: 3

Rationale: The person whose anxiety is assessed as severe is unable to solve problems and may have a poor grasp of what is happening in the environment. Somatic symptoms such as those described are usually present. The individual with mild anxiety is only mildly uncomfortable and may even find his or her performance enhanced. The individual with moderate anxiety grasps less information about a situation and has some difficulty with problem solving. The individual in panic will demonstrate markedly disturbed behavior and may lose touch with reality.

Cognitive level: Application
Nursing process: Assessment
NCLEX: Psychosocial Integrity
See text pages: 214, 215

19. A client accompanied her boyfriend to the emergency department after the two had been in a motorcycle accident. The boyfriend was badly hurt, but the client had only minor cuts and bruises and was discharged. She mentioned to the nurse that since she was driving, she should have been the one to be injured. Twenty-four hours later, while visiting her boyfriend, the client reported that she was unable to move from her chair and unable to walk. Diagnostic workup revealed no physical reason for the problem. The anxiety relief behavior the client is demonstrating is
   1. acting out.
   2. somatization.
   3. withdrawal.
   4. problem solving.

Answer: 2

Rationale: Somatization is the expression of an emotional conflict in physical symptoms. The client manifests several physical symptoms associated with severe anxiety. Option 1: Acting out refers to behaviors such as anger, crying, laughter, and physical or verbal abuse. Option 3: Withdrawal is a reaction in which psychic energy is withdrawn from the environment and focused on the self in response to anxiety. Option 4: Problem solving takes place when anxiety is identified and the unmet need serving as the origin of the anxiety is met.

Cognitive level: Application
Nursing process: Assessment
NCLEX: Psychosocial Integrity
See text page: 218

20. A client who has been in an accident but is unhurt is displaying moderate anxiety, including scattering of attention, dizziness, nausea, tachycardia, and hyper-

Chapter 13   Understanding Anxiety and Anxiety Defenses

ventilation. The statement indicating that the nurse is reacting to the client's relief behavior rather than her needs is

1. "It must have been a frightening experience to be in an accident."
2. "Accidents can result in all kinds of feelings. It must have been scary."
3. "I'll stay with you in case you would like to share your feelings with me."
4. "There is nothing physically wrong with you. You need to stop breathing so rapidly."

Answer: 4

Rationale: In option 4 the nurse is addressing the client's hyperventilation and other somatic symptoms rather than her feelings about the accident. All other options address the client's feelings about the accident.

Cognitive level: Analysis
Nursing process: Implementation
NCLEX: Psychosocial Integrity
See text pages: 213, 214

21. Two staff nurses were considered for promotion. The promotion was announced by a memo on the unit bulletin board. When the nurse who was not promoted first read the memo and learned that the other nurse had received the promotion, she left the room in tears. This behavior is an example of

1. conversion.
2. regression.
3. introjection.
4. rationalization.

Answer: 2

Rationale: Crying is a regressive behavior. The ego returned to an earlier, comforting, and less mature way of behaving in the face of disappointment. Option 2: Conversion involves the unconscious transformation of anxiety into a physical symptom. Option 3: Introjection involves intense, unconscious identification with another person. Option 4: Rationalization involves the unconscious process of developing acceptable explanations to justify unacceptable ideas, actions, or feelings.

Cognitive level: Application
Nursing process: Assessment
NCLEX: Psychosocial Integrity
See text page: 218

22. A client who asked for and was refused a pass to leave the unit left the nurse's station and went to his room, where he slammed his closet door several times while looking for a sweater. This behavior exemplifies

1. displacement.
2. sublimation.

3. conversion.
4. reaction formation.

Answer: 1

Rationale: Displacement unconsciously transfers emotions associated with a person, object, or situation to another less threatening person, object, or situation. The client slammed doors instead of discharging his feelings against the individual who refused to give him the pass. Option 2: Sublimation is the unconscious process of substituting constructive activity for unacceptable impulses. Slamming of closet doors cannot be considered a constructive activity. Option 3: Conversion involves unconsciously transforming anxiety into a physical symptom. Option 4: Reaction formation keeps unacceptable feelings or behaviors out of awareness by using the opposite feeling or behavior.

Cognitive level: Application
Nursing process: Assessment
NCLEX: Psychosocial Integrity
See text page: 218

23. A client who asked for and was refused a pass to leave the unit left the nurse's station and went to his room, where he slammed his closet door several times while looking for a sweater. A nurse came into the room and remarked "You seem pretty angry." The client replied that he was not the least bit angry. In this instance the client is probably demonstrating

1. reaction formation.
2. rationalization.
3. compensation.
4. denial.

Answer: 4

Rationale: Denial involves an unconscious process of escaping an unpleasant reality by ignoring its existence; in this case the client ignores his true feelings. Option 1: Reaction formation is an unconscious process that would call for displaying a feeling that is the opposite of anger. Option 2: Rationalization involves justifying illogical or unreasonable ides, actions, or feelings by developing acceptable explanations that satisfy the listener and the self. Option 3: Compensation requires unconsciously making up for perceived deficits by excelling in another area to maintain self-esteem.

Cognitive level: Application
Nursing process: Assessment
NCLEX: Psychosocial Integrity
See text page: 220

24. A client tells the nurse "My new friend is the most perfect person one could imagine! I can't find a single flaw. He is kind, considerate, handsome—and he

puts me before anyone or anything else." The nurse should hypothesize that this client may be demonstrating
1. denial.
2. projection.
3. idealization.
4. compensation.

Answer: 3

Rationale: Idealization is an unconscious process that occurs when the individual attributes exaggerated positive qualities to another. Option 1: Denial is an unconscious process that would call for the nurse to ignore the existence of the situation. Option 2: Projection operates unconsciously and would result in blaming behavior. Option 4: Compensation would result in the nurse unconsciously attempting to make up for a perceived weakness by emphasizing a strong point.

Cognitive level: Application
Nursing process: Assessment
NCLEX: Psychosocial Integrity
See text page: 219

25. A client who was recently fired from his position tells the nurse "It was predictable. Ever since I discovered a way to save the company money, the boss has had it in for me. He knew I was smarter than he is, and he had to get rid of me." If the client actually believes this of the executive, who, in reality, knows little of the client, he is demonstrating
1. denial.
2. projection.
3. compensation.
4. reaction formation.

Answer: 2

Rationale: Projection results in unconsciously adopting blaming behavior. It allows people to attribute their own unacceptable attributes to other people. Option 1: Denial involves unconsciously determining to ignore the existence of an unpleasant reality. Option 3: Compensation would result in the client unconsciously attempting to emphasize a strong point in an attempt to make up for a perceived weakness. Option 4: Reaction formation would require the client to unconsciously adopt behavior that is the opposite of her actual feelings.

Cognitive level: Application
Nursing process: Assessment
NCLEX: Psychosocial Integrity
See text page: 219

26. When a talent show contestant lost to another singer, the contestant suddenly found she had lost her voice and was unable to congratulate the other singer. The mute contestant is probably demonstrating

1. denial.
2. somatization.
3. suppression.
4. repression.

Answer: 2

Rationale: Somatization unconsciously transforms anxiety into a physical symptom that has no organic basis. In this situation, the symptom resolves a conflict between the need to and the desire not to congratulate the other contestant. Option 1: Denial involves unconsciously determining to ignore the existence of an unpleasant reality. Option 3: Suppression consciously puts an event, idea, or feeling out of awareness. Option 4: Repression unconsciously puts an event, idea, or feeling out of awareness.

Cognitive level: Application
Nursing process: Assessment
NCLEX: Psychosocial Integrity
See text page: 218

27. Two staff nurses were considered for promotion to head nurse. The nurse who was not promoted initially experienced feelings of loss, but as the weeks went on she went out of her way to be supportive of the new head nurse and help make the transition smooth. She offered to take on additional responsibility to help out and was heard encouraging others. She told a friend "I feel good about the way things are turning out. I have an investment in this unit and want the best for our staff." The phenomenon occurring has its basis in
1. altruism.
2. suppression.
3. displacement.
4. passive aggression.

Answer: 1

Rationale: Altruism is the mechanism by which an individual deals with emotional conflict by meeting the needs of others and receiving gratification vicariously or from the responses of others. Option 2: Suppression is conscious denial of a disturbing feeling or situation. Option 3: Displacement transfers emotions associated with a particular person or event to another person or situation that is less threatening. Option 4: Passive aggression occurs when an individual deals with emotional conflict by indirectly and unassertively expressing aggression toward others.

Cognitive level: Application
Nursing process: Assessment
NCLEX: Psychosocial Integrity
See text page: 217

28. A rather unattractive woman repeatedly tells her husband that although she is not beautiful, she is smart. This is an example of an attempt at
1. repression.
2. compensation.
3. identification.
4. devaluation.

Answer: 2

Rationale: Compensation is an unconscious process that allows us to make up for deficits in one area by excelling in another area to raise self-esteem. Option 1: Repression unconsciously puts an idea, event, or feeling out of awareness. Option 3: Identification is an unconscious mechanism calling for imitation of mannerisms or behaviors of another. Option 4: Devaluation occurs when the individual attributes negative qualities to self or others.

Cognitive level: Application
Nursing process: Assessment
NCLEX: Psychosocial Integrity
See text pages: 220, 221

29. A woman speaking of a rival for her husband's affection says in a gushy, syrupy voice "She is a lovely person. I simply adore her." The woman may be demonstrating
1. reaction formation.
2. denial.
3. projection.
4. repression.

Answer: 1

Rationale: Reaction formation is an unconscious mechanism that keeps unacceptable feelings out of awareness by using the opposite behavior. Instead of saying how much she hates the "other woman," she praises her. Option 2: Denial operates unconsciously to allow an anxiety-producing idea, feeling, or situation to be ignored. Option 3: Projection involves unconsciously disowning an unacceptable idea, feeling, or behavior by attributing it to another. Option 4: Repression involves unconsciously placing an idea, feeling, or event out of awareness.

Cognitive level: Application
Nursing process: Assessment
NCLEX: Psychosocial Integrity
See text page: 218

30. The husband who is sexually inadequate and blames it on his partner, saying she is unattractive and that her manner is to blame, may be demonstrating
1. rationalization.
2. regression.
3. compensation.
4. introjection.

Answer: 1

Rationale: Rationalization involves unconsciously making excuses for one's behavior, inadequacies, or feelings. Option 2: Regression involves the unconscious use of a behavior from an earlier stage of emotional development. Option 3: Compensation involves making up for deficits in one area by excelling in another area. Option 4: Introjection is an unconscious, intense identification with another person.

Cognitive level: Application
Nursing process: Assessment
NCLEX: Psychosocial Integrity
See text page: 218

31. A client who is a university student states that before taking an examination he feels a heightened sense of awareness and a sense of restlessness. The nurse can correctly assess the client's situation as
1. possible hypoglycemia.
2. possible hyperthyroidism.
3. mild depression.
4. mild anxiety.

Answer: 4

Rationale: Mild anxiety is rarely obstructive to the task at hand. It may be helpful to the client by promoting study and making him more aware of the nuances of questions. The other problems mentioned have quite different symptoms.

Cognitive level: Application
Nursing process: Assessment
NCLEX: Psychosocial Integrity
See text page: 213

32. A client who is a university student states that before taking an examination he feels a heightened sense of awareness and a sense of restlessness. The nursing intervention most suitable for assisting the client is to
1. explain his symptoms as resulting from mild anxiety and discuss the helpful aspects of mild anxiety.
2. advise the client to discuss his experience with a physician or psychologist.
3. offer to obtain an order for an anxiolytic to be used when necessary.
4. listen without comment.

Answer: 1

Rationale: Teaching about symptoms of anxiety, their relation to precipitating stressors, and, in this case, the positive effects of anxiety will serve to reassure the client. Options 2 and 3 imply a serious problem. Option 4 will do no harm but deprives the client of health teaching.

Cognitive level: Application

33. An anxious client who receives anxiolytic medication every 6 hours prn is in the corridor pacing. He grabs the arms of anyone who comes along and asks "When can I have medication?" His voice is high pitched and shaky. His respiratory rate is rapid. His assigned nurse should intervene by
   1. ascertaining when the client's medication is due and informing him.
   2. sending him to his room to lie down for half an hour.
   3. joking with him to reduce tension.
   4. suggesting that he watch television.

Answer: 1
Rationale: Medication should be given promptly when a client is experiencing severe anxiety. The client should be told when his next dose will be forthcoming and reassured that it will be given promptly. This intervention can be helpful in lowering his present state of anxiety. Options 2 and 4: Sending the client away to lie down or to watch television will not lower his anxiety. However, staying with him could be helpful. Option 3: Joking is inappropriate because the severely anxious client has difficulty processing information and will be unable to differentiate joking from fact.
Cognitive level: Application
Nursing process: Implementation
NCLEX: Psychosocial Integrity
See text page: 216

34. If a cruel and abusive man rationalizes his behavior, he would most characteristically say
   1. "I don't know why it happens."
   2. "That person shouldn't have provoked me."
   3. "I'm really a coward who is afraid of being hurt."
   4. "I have poor impulse control."

Answer: 2
Rationale: Rationalization consists of justifying one's unacceptable behavior by developing explanations that satisfy the teller and attempt to satisfy the listener. The abuser is suggesting that the abuse is not his fault and would not have occurred except for the provocation by the other person.
Cognitive level: Application
Nursing process: Assessment
NCLEX: Psychosocial Integrity
See text page: 218

35. A 10-year-old child, who has been placed in a foster home after being removed from parental contact be-

cause of abuse, demonstrates a high level of apprehension and overreaction to environmental stimuli. The foster parents ask the nurse what measures they can use to help the child. The nurse should recommend (more than one answer may be correct)
   1. using a calm manner and low voice.
   2. avoiding repetition in what is said to the child.
   3. structuring and maintaining simplicity in the environment.
   4. minimizing opportunities for exercise and play.
   5. explaining and reinforcing reality to avoid distortions.

Answers: 1, 3, 5
Rationale: The child can be hypothesized to have moderate to severe trait (chronic) anxiety. A calm manner will calm the child. A simple, structured, predictable environment is less anxiety provoking and will reduce overreaction to stimuli.

Calm, simple explanations that reinforce reality validate the environment. Option 2: Repetition is often needed when the individual is unable to concentrate because of elevated levels of anxiety. Option 4: Opportunities for play and exercise should be provided as avenues to reduce anxiety. Physical movement helps channel and lower anxiety. Play helps by allowing the child to act out concerns.
Cognitive level: Application
Nursing process: Implementation
NCLEX: Psychosocial Integrity
See text page: 216

36. A client with severe anxiety who has been pacing the hall suddenly begins to run, shouting "I'm going to explode!" over and over. The nurse who has been walking with him should
   1. run after the client and call out for the client to stop running.
   2. capture him in a basket hold when he runs back up the hall.
   3. Ask "I'm not sure what you mean. Give me an example."
   4. assemble a show of force and state "We will help you regain control."

Answer: 4
Rationale: Safety needs of the client and other clients are a priority. The client is less likely to hurt himself or others when several staff take responsibility for providing limits.

The explanation given the client should be simple and neutral. Simply being told that others can provide the control he is losing may be sufficient to help the client regain control. Option 1: Running after the client will increase his anxiety. Option 2: More than one staff member will be needed to provide physical limits if they become necessary.

Option 3 would be futile; a client in panic processes information poorly.

Cognitive level: Application
Nursing process: Implementation
NCLEX: Safe and Effective Care Environment
See text page: 216

37. A client being treated on an outpatient basis for generalized anxiety disorder reports "I have a little difficulty falling asleep but then I sleep soundly for about 7 hours. I do not worry excessively about what is going on in my life anymore, and I'm able to enjoy spending time with friends and relatives. For the past 3 weeks I've been able to use relaxation to stop the episodes of racing pulse and thinking I'm going to die." The nurse should evaluated the outcome, anxiety self-control, as
   1. seldom demonstrated.
   2. sometimes demonstrated.
   3. often demonstrated.
   4. consistently demonstrated.

Answer: 4
Rationale: Being able to consistently control the anxiety response (e.g., elevated blood pressure, pulse, respiration, dilated pupils, sweating) is the most definitive indicator of anxiety self-control. Adequate nightly sleep and maintenance of social relationships also suggest the client is making progress toward anxiety self-control. Lack of exaggerated concerns about life events is also an indicator of decreased anxiety.

Cognitive level: Analysis
Nursing process: Evaluation
NCLEX: Physiological Integrity
See text page: 223

CHAPTER 14

1. The psychiatric home care nurse visits a client who tells the nurse that he experiences palpitations, difficulty breathing, and a sense of overwhelming dread whenever he leaves his home. This problem began after he was robbed on his way to work. He has been unable to go to his office for more than a month. The nurse recognizes this problem as
   1. mysophobia.
   2. claustrophobia.
   3. acrophobia.
   4. agoraphobia.

Answer: 4
Rationale: *Agoraphobia* refers to the client's fear of open spaces. Option 1: Mysophobia refers to fear of dirt or germs. Option 2: Claustrophobia refers to fear of closed spaces. Option 3: Acrophobia refers to fear of heights.

Cognitive level: Application
Nursing process: Assessment
NCLEX: Psychosocial Integrity
See text page: 234

2. A client who has been unable to leave his home for more than a month because of symptoms of severe anxiety tells the nurse "I know it's probably crazy, but I just can't bring myself to leave my apartment alone. And I can't expect somebody to take me to work every day." The nurse can make the assessment that the client
   1. knows his symptom is unrealistic.
   2. is misinterpreting reality.
   3. is seeking sympathy.
   4. is depersonalizing.

Answer: 1
Rationale: Symptoms of anxiety disorders are often recognized by the client as strange and nonadaptive and are sources of dissatisfaction to the client. Options 2 and 3: The client is interpreting reality appropriately and does not seem to be attempting to elicit sympathy from the nurse. Option 4: The scenario does not give evidence of depersonalization (experiencing feelings of unreality or alienation).

Cognitive level: Application
Nursing process: Assessment
NCLEX: Psychosocial Integrity
See text pages: 239, 240

3. A client who has been unable to leave his home for more than a month because of symptoms of severe anxiety asks the nurse "Don't you agree that not being able to go out is pretty stupid?" The most therapeutic reply is
   1. "No, I do not think it's stupid."
   2. "Many individuals share this situation with you."
   3. "You feel stupid because you're afraid to leave home?"
   4. "I guess some people might say that being housebound is pretty strange."

Answer: 3
Rationale: This response will allow the nurse to validate the possibility that the client is dissatisfied with being unable to control his symptom and suggests openness to listening to feelings of powerlessness. The nurse should neither agree nor disagree with the

client. Clarifying his own thinking is more important for the client.
Cognitive level: Application
Nursing process: Implementation
NCLEX: Psychosocial Integrity
See text pages: 248, 249

4. A client who has been unable to leave his home for more than a month because of symptoms of severe anxiety tells the nurse "I know it's probably crazy, but I just can't bring myself to leave my apartment alone." An appropriate nursing intervention for the nurse to include in the nursing care plan is to
   1. teach the client to use positive self-talk.
   2. assist the client to apply for disability benefits.
   3. reinforce the irrationality of the client's fears.
   4. advise the client to accept the situation and use a companion.

Answer: 1
Rationale: This intervention, a form of cognitive restructuring, replaces negative thoughts such as "I can't leave my apartment" with positive thoughts such as "I can control my anxiety." This technique helps the client gain mastery over his symptoms. The other options reinforce the sick role.
Cognitive level: Application
Nursing process: Implementation
NCLEX: Psychosocial Integrity
See text page: 233

5. A client is seeking treatment for a specific phobia: fear of cats. The nurse in the anxiety disorders clinic has established the nursing diagnosis of anxiety related to exposure to phobic object (cats). A realistic indicator for the outcome anxiety self-control would be that within 10 days, the client will
   1. avoid the feared object whenever possible.
   2. face the feared object without supportive assistance.
   3. state that the fear of cats is unrealistic and inappropriate.
   4. practice relaxation techniques and report decreased physiological sensations associated with thoughts of the feared object.

Answer: 4
Rationale: When the client is able to relax in the presence of thoughts, pictures, or the phobic object, the client will begin to experience a sense of control over the phobia. Option 1 is unrelated to anxiety self-control. Option 2 probably cannot be achieved within 10 days. Option 3: Intellectual understanding does not automatically convey behavioral change associated with anxiety self-control.
Cognitive level: Application

Nursing process: Planning (Outcome Identification)
NCLEX: Psychosocial Integrity
See text page: 243

6. Which piece of subjective data obtained during the nurse's psychosocial assessment of a client experiencing severe anxiety would indicate the possibility of obsessive-compulsive disorder?
   1. "I have to keep checking to see where my car keys are."
   2. "My legs feel weak most of the time."
   3. "I'm afraid to go out in public."
   4. "I keep reliving the rape."

Answer: 1
Rationale: Recurring doubt (obsessive thinking) and the need to check (compulsive behavior) suggest obsessive-compulsive disorder. The repetitive behavior is designed to decrease anxiety but fails and must be repeated. Option 2 is more in keeping with a somatoform disorder. Option 3 is associated with agoraphobia and option 4 with posttraumatic stress disorder.
Cognitive level: Application
Nursing process: Assessment
NCLEX: Psychosocial Integrity
See text page: 235

7. The nurse interviewing a client with suspected posttraumatic stress disorder should be alert to findings indicating the client (more than one answer may be correct)
   1. experiences flashbacks.
   2. demonstrates hypervigilance.
   3. feels detached, estranged, or empty inside.
   4. feels driven to repeat ritualistic behaviors.
   5. avoids people and places that arouse painful memories.
   6. experiences sympathetic nervous system symptoms suggestive of a heart attack.

Answers: 1, 2, 3, 5
Rationale: These assessment findings are consistent with the symptoms of posttraumatic stress disorder according to the *DSM-IV-TR*. Option 4 is consistent with obsessive-compulsive disorder and option 6 with panic attack.
Cognitive level: Application
Nursing Process: Assessment
NCLEX: Psychosocial Integrity
See text page: 236

8. When the psychiatrist prescribes alprazolam (Xanax) for the acute anxiety experienced by a client with agoraphobia, health teaching should include instructions to

Chapter 14 Anxiety Disorders

1. eat a tyramine-free diet.
2. report drowsiness.
3. avoid alcoholic beverages.
4. adjust dose and frequency of ingestion based on anxiety level.

Answer: 3

Rationale: Drinking alcohol or taking other anxiolytics along with the prescribed benzodiazepine should be avoided because depressant effects of both drugs will be potentiated. Option 1: Tyramine-free diets are necessary only with monoamine oxidase inhibitors. Option 2: Drowsiness is an expected effect and needs to be reported only if it is excessive. Option 4: Clients should be taught not to deviate from the prescribed dose and schedule for administration.

Cognitive level: Application
Nursing process: Planning
NCLEX: Physiological Integrity
See text pages: 246, 247

9. Which statement made by a client who has agoraphobia and does not leave her home identifies the thinking typical of a client with this disorder?
    1. "I know I'll get over not wanting to leave home soon; it just takes time."
    2. "When I have a good incentive to go out, I'll be able to do it."
    3. "My husband and kids tell me they like it now that I stay home."
    4. "Being afraid to go out seems ridiculous, but I can't go out the door."

Answer: 4

Rationale: The individual who is agoraphobic generally acknowledges that the behavior is not constructive and that he or she does not really like it. The symptom is ego dystonic. However, the client will state he or she is unable to change the behavior. Options 1 and 2: Agoraphobics are not optimistic about change. Option 3: Most families are dissatisfied with the behavior.

Cognitive level: Application
Nursing process: Assessment
NCLEX: Psychosocial Integrity
See text pages: 233, 234

10. For the client whose nursing diagnosis is powerlessness related to an inability to control compulsive cleaning, the nurse must understand that the client uses the cleaning to
    1. temporarily reduce anxiety.
    2. gain a feeling of superiority.
    3. receive praise from friends and family.
    4. ensure the health of household members.

Answer: 1

Rationale: The primary gain achieved from the client's use of these rituals is anxiety relief. Unfortunately, the anxiety relief is short lived and the client must frequently repeat the ritual. The other options are not related to the dynamics of compulsive behavior.

Cognitive level: Analysis
Nursing process: Planning
NCLEX: Psychosocial Integrity
See text pages: 234, 235

11. For the client with ritualistic hand washing and an identified outcome of the use of more effective coping patterns, the nurse should use the intervention of
    1. allowing the client to set own hand-washing schedule.
    2. encouraging the client to participate in unit activities.
    3. encouraging the client to discuss hand washing in all groups.
    4. focusing on the client's symptoms rather than on the client.

Answer: 2

Rationale: Because obsessive-compulsive clients become overly involved in the rituals, promotion of involvement with other people and activities is necessary to improve coping. Daily activities prevent constant focus on anxiety and symptoms. The other interventions focus on the compulsive symptom.

Cognitive level: Application
Nursing process: Implementation
NCLEX: Psychosocial Integrity
See text pages: 234, 235

12. For the client with compulsive hand washing, which outcome indicator can be used to evaluate that social interaction is occurring? The client
    1. asks for anxiolytic medication when anxiety increases.
    2. spends time talking to staff and clients in the lounge area.
    3. decreases the amount of time spent hand washing.
    4. sleeps 7 to 8 hours nightly.

Answer: 2

Rationale: The behavior that indicates improved social interaction is spending more time interacting with others. The other indicators are desirable but not related to improved social interaction.

Cognitive level: Analysis
Nursing process: Evaluation
NCLEX: Psychosocial Integrity
See text pages: 234, 235

13. The plan of care for a client with obsessive-compulsive disorder relative to self-esteem enhancement should include (more than one answer may be correct)
    1. encouraging the client to identify and reinforce strengths.
    2. encouraging the client to examine negative self-perceptions.
    3. encouraging the use of as-needed anxiolytic medication.
    4. assisting the client to identify positive responses from others.
    5. refraining from giving praise to the client for accomplishments.
    6. discouraging experiences that increase client autonomy.

Answers: 1, 2, 4
Rationale: Self-identification of strengths that can subsequently be reinforced by the nurse builds esteem and promotes self-acceptance. Examining negative self-perceptions permits reframing in positive ways. Identifying positive responses from others helps the client see self in a more positive light. Option 3: This intervention is not directly related to self-esteem enhancement. Option 5: Clients should receive realistic praise. Option 6: Realistic levels of client autonomy should be encouraged because autonomy can be esteem enhancing.
Cognitive level: Application
Nursing process: Implementation
NCLEX: Psychosocial Integrity
See text page: 237

14. The nurse caring for a client who has been diagnosed as having generalized anxiety disorder tells a preceptor "I find myself feeling uncomfortable and anxious around the client. When he starts trembling and perspiring and pacing, I find myself with cold, clammy hands and my pulse races. I start worrying whether I will be able to help him stay in control." In such an interaction the client will most likely experience
    1. fatigue.
    2. claustrophobia.
    3. increased anxiety.
    4. improved self-esteem.

Answer: 3
Rationale: Anxiety is transmissible interpersonally. The client who "tunes in" to the nurse's anxiety usually experiences heightening of his or her own anxiety. Option 1: The client's immediate reaction would be heightened anxiety rather than fatigue. Option 2: Claustrophobia is rarely the outcome of empathized

anxiety. Option 4: Improved self-esteem would not result from empathic anxiety.
Cognitive level: Application
Nursing process: Assessment
NCLEX: Psychosocial Integrity
See text pages: 239, 240

15. A client who is a recovering alcoholic has been diagnosed as having panic attacks. The psychiatrist mentions plans to treat the client with daily doses of medication. Of the medications listed below, for which drug should the nurse plan client teaching?
    1. Paroxetine (Paxil)
    2. Alprazolam (Xanax)
    3. Chlorpromazine (Thorazine)
    4. Propranolol (Inderal)

Answer: 1
Rationale: Selective serotonin reuptake inhibitors are first-line drugs for the treatment of panic disorder. Both paroxetine and sertraline are approved by the Food and Drug Administration for treatment of panic disorder. Selective serotonin reuptake inhibitors are nonaddicting and have a relatively low incidence of unpleasant side effects. Also useful are tricyclic antidepressants, such as imipramine, which are more useful than the benzodiazepines because they are nonaddicting. Option 2: Alprazolam is a benzodiazepine and would not be the drug of choice for a client who has a problem of chemical dependency. Option 3: Chlorpromazine is a neuroleptic and not useful for treating panic disorder. Propranolol is more often used in the treatment of social phobias.
Cognitive level: Application
Nursing process: Planning
NCLEX: Physiological Integrity
See text page: 246

16. When the nurse diagnoses that a client is experiencing panic-level anxiety, an intervention that should be immediately implemented is to
    1. teach relaxation techniques.
    2. administer anxiolytic medication.
    3. provide calm, brief, directive communication.
    4. gather a show of force in preparation for physical control.

Answer: 3
Rationale: Calm, brief, directive verbal interaction can help the client gain control of overwhelming feelings and impulses related to anxiety. Option 1: Clients experiencing panic-level anxiety are unable to focus on reality; thus learning is virtually impossible. Option 2 should be considered if option 3 is ineffective. Option 4: Although the client is disorganized, violence may not

277

be imminent, ruling out this option until other less-restrictive measures are proven ineffective.
Cognitive level: Application
Nursing process: Implementation
NCLEX: Psychosocial Integrity
See text page: 243

17. A client with moderate to severe anxiety associated with generalized anxiety disorder can be assessed as successfully lowering her anxiety level to mild when she
   1. asks "What's the matter with me?"
   2. stays in her room and paces.
   3. states she is uninterested in eating.
   4. can concentrate on what the nurse is saying.

Answer: 4
Rationale: The ability to concentrate and attend to reality is increased slightly in mild anxiety and decreased in moderate, severe, and panic-level anxiety. Option 1: Clients with high levels of anxiety often ask this question. Option 2: This behavior suggests moderate anxiety. Option 3 is not necessarily a criterion for evaluation of anxiety.
Cognitive level: Application
Nursing process: Evaluation
NCLEX: Psychosocial Integrity
See text page: 235

18. A veteran of the Gulf War has intrusive thoughts of missiles screaming toward her and exploding. She reexperiences feelings of terror first experienced in combat. These recurrent events are part of
   1. obsessive-compulsive disorder.
   2. generalized anxiety disorder.
   3. panic disorder with agoraphobia.
   4. posttraumatic stress disorder.

Answer: 4
Rationale: *DSM-IV-TR* criteria mention reexperiencing the traumatic event as consistent with posttraumatic stress disorder. These symptoms are not part of the clinical manifestations of obsessive-compulsive disorder, generalized anxiety disorder, or agoraphobia.
Cognitive level: Application
Nursing process: Assessment
NCLEX: Psychosocial Integrity
See text page: 236

19. A client reveals that he becomes panic stricken when he sees a dog. The nurse can assess this behavior as being consistent with
   1. social phobia.
   2. specific phobia.
   3. agoraphobia.
   4. generalized anxiety disorder.

Answer: 2
Rationale: Intense, persistent fear of an object is a clinical manifestation of a specific phobia. Option 1: Social phobias involve fear of a social situation. Option 3: Agoraphobia involves fear of an environment from which escape would be difficult. Option 4: Generalized anxiety disorder involves generalized anxiety rather than a specific fear.
Cognitive level: Application
Nursing process: Assessment
NCLEX: Psychosocial Integrity
See text page: 234

20. A client tells the nurse he cannot go out on a date because he might have to eat something in front of others. He reveals that he is afraid that someone will laugh at the way he eats or that he will spill food and be laughed at. The nurse can assess this behavior as being consistent with
   1. social phobia.
   2. specific phobia.
   3. agoraphobia.
   4. posttraumatic stress disorder.

Answer: 1
Rationale: Fear of a potentially embarrassing situation is called a social phobia. Option 2: Specific phobias are fears of specific objects, such as dogs. Option 3: Agoraphobia is fear of a place in the environment. Option 4: Posttraumatic stress disorder is associated with a major traumatic event.
Cognitive level: Application
Nursing process: Assessment
NCLEX: Psychosocial Integrity
See text page: 234

21. A client believes doorknobs are "filthy" with bacteria, and he must clean each knob three times before he can touch it or must use a paper towel to avoid putting his fingers in contact with the knob. The nurse must make the assessment that this behavior serves the purpose of reducing
   1. sexual ideation.
   2. anxiety.
   3. guilt.
   4. hallucinations.

Answer: 2
Rationale: The client's behavior is termed a compulsion. Compulsions serve the purpose of temporarily relieving anxiety. Option 1: Obsessions may involve sexual ideation, but the purpose of compulsions is to relieve anxiety. Option 3: Guilt may be obsessive in nature, but compulsive behavior serves the purpose of relieving anxiety. Option 4: Compulsive does not reduce hallucinations.

278

Cognitive level: Application
Nursing process: Assessment
NCLEX: Psychosocial Integrity
See text pages: 234, 235

22. When working with a client with posttraumatic stress disorder who has frequent flashbacks as well as persistent symptoms of arousal, effective nursing interventions would include (more than one answer may be correct)
    1. encouraging repression of memories associated with the traumatic event.
    2. explaining that physical symptoms are related to the psychological state.
    3. teaching stress management techniques.
    4. discussing possible meanings of the event.
    5. advising the use of alcohol as adjunctive sedation.

Answers: 2, 3, 4
Rationale: The goal of treatment for posttraumatic stress disorder is to come to terms with the event rather than repress it; thus option 4 is correct and option 1 is incorrect. Option 2 will help the client understand the mind-body relation and the fact that relaxation, breathing exercises, and imagery can be helpful in symptom reduction (option 3). Option 5 is inadvisable. Substance abuse is often a comorbidity with posttraumatic stress disorder because the client seeks to self-medicate.
Cognitive level: Application
Nursing process: Implementation
NCLEX: Psychosocial Integrity
See text page: 236

23. The nurse has a client who checks and rechecks her home in response to an obsessive thought that her house will burn down. The nurse and client explore the likelihood that the house will actually burn. The client states this event is not likely. This counseling demonstrates principles of
    1. desensitization.
    2. cognitive restructuring.
    3. relaxation technique.
    4. flooding.

Answer: 2
Rationale: Cognitive restructuring involves the client in testing automatic thoughts and drawing new conclusions. Option 1: Desensitization involves graduated exposure to a feared object. Option 3: Relaxation training teaches the client to produce the opposite of the stress response. Option 4: Flooding exposes the client to a large amount of an undesirable stimulus in an effort to extinguish the anxiety response.

Cognitive level: Application
Nursing process: Implementation
NCLEX: Psychosocial Integrity
See text page: 244

24. When a client asks what causes his panic attacks, the nurse should reply that research gives evidence to support the theory that panic disorders have their etiology in
    1. faulty learning.
    2. traumatic events.
    3. genetic-biological factors.
    4. developmental fixations.

Answer: 3
Rationale: Panic attacks can be caused by the introduction of various chemicals into the body, thus supporting a biological theory of etiology. Clients experiencing panic attacks frequently have close relatives who experience panic attacks, a finding that suggests a genetic tie.
Cognitive level: Application
Nursing process: Implementation
NCLEX: Psychosocial Integrity
See text pages: 229, 230

25. For planning purposes, the nurse caring for a client with a social phobia should know that an effective treatment for this disorder is
    1. analysis.
    2. thought stopping.
    3. cognitive therapy.
    4. response prevention.

Answer: 3
Rationale: Cognitive therapy assists the client to identify automatic, negative beliefs that cause anxiety, reevaluate the situation, and replace negative self-talk with supportive ideas. Option 1: Analysis is expensive, requires years of commitment, and may not be effective. Options 2 and 4: Thought stopping and response prevention are more useful to treat obsessive-compulsive disorder.
Cognitive level: Application
Nursing process: Planning
NCLEX: Psychosocial Integrity
See text page: 244

26. When interviewing and planning care for a client with fear of public speaking, the nurse must be aware that social phobias are often treatable with
    1. neuroleptics.
    2. β-blockers.
    3. tricyclic antidepressants.
    4. monoamine oxidase inhibitors.

279

Answer: 2

Rationale: β-Blockers such as propranolol are often effective in preventing symptoms of anxiety associated with social phobias. Option 1: Neuroleptics are major tranquilizers and not useful in treating social phobias. Option 3: Tricyclic antidepressants are rarely used because of their side-effect profile. Option 4: Monoamine oxidase inhibitors are used for depression and only by individuals who can observe the special diet required.

Cognitive level: Application
Nursing process: Planning
NCLEX: Physiological Integrity
See text page: 245

27. A client tells the nurse that she wants her physician to prescribe diazepam (Valium) for anxiety reduction. The physician has prescribed buspirone (BuSpar). The nurse's reply should be based on the knowledge that buspirone
   1. can be administered prn.
   2. does not predispose the client to blood dyscrasias.
   3. is not habituating.
   4. is faster acting.

Answer: 3

Rationale: Buspirone is considered effective in the long-term management of anxiety because it is not habituating. Options 1 and 4: Because it is long acting, it is not valuable as a prn medication or a fast-acting medication. Option 2: This fact is of lesser relevance in the decision to prescribe buspirone.

Cognitive level: Application
Nursing process: Implementation
NCLEX: Physiological Integrity
See text page: 247

28. An insurance agent who is sitting in his office after returning from a physical examination in which he was pronounced "in good health" suddenly experiences a feeling of terror. His heart pounds, he feels as though he cannot breathe, and he cannot focus on what is being said to him. Several earlier episodes and the fear of their repetition had prompted the visit to the doctor. This experience should be assessed as a possible
   1. panic attack.
   2. phobic reaction.
   3. dissociative reaction.
   4. obsessive-compulsive crisis.

Answer: 1

Rationale: According to the *DSM-IV-TR,* panic attacks cause symptoms of sympathetic nervous system arousal and occur without warning, as described in the scenario. Option 2: A phobic reaction involves excessive fear. Option 3: A dissociative reaction involves separation of an event from conscious awareness. Option 4: No disorder is known as an obsessive-compulsive crisis.

Cognitive level: Application
Nursing process: Assessment
NCLEX: Psychosocial Integrity
See text page: 232

29. The nurse planning health teaching for a client with generalized anxiety disorder who is taking lorazepam (Ativan) should include information about the need for (more than one answer may be correct)
   1. a tyramine-free diet.
   2. caffeine restriction.
   3. use of care with machinery.
   4. avoidance of alcohol and other sedatives.

Answers: 2, 3, 4

Rationale: Caffeine is a central nervous system stimulant that acts as an antagonist to the benzodiazepine lorazepam. Daily caffeine intake should be reduced to the amount contained in one cup of coffee. Benzodiazepines are sedatives, thus the importance of exercising caution when driving or using machinery and the importance of not using other central nervous system depressants such as alcohol or sedatives to avoid potentiation. Option 1: Benzodiazepines do not require a special diet.

Cognitive level: Application
Nursing process: Planning
NCLEX: Health Promotion and Maintenance
See text page: 247

30. The care plan for an engineer with agoraphobia includes increasing self-esteem with cognitive restructuring. When the client tells the nurse "I'm not smart enough to get that job," the nurse should say
   1. "It must be difficult to be in that position."
   2. "You should not demean your abilities."
   3. "Let's think about what you just said."
   4. "You seem intelligent to me."

Answer: 3

Rationale: Cognitive restructuring calls for the client to examine automatic negative thoughts about himself and replace them with more realistic evaluations of his own abilities. The other options would not promote examination of the negative thinking exhibited by the client.

Cognitive level: Application
Nursing process: Implementation
NCLEX: Psychosocial Integrity
See text page: 244

31. A client with generalized anxiety disorder and depression comes to the anxiety disorders clinic displaying severe anxiety. Of the medications listed in the client's medical record, which one, with an appropriate order, can be given as a prn anxiolytic?
1. Buspirone (BuSpar)
2. Lorazepam (Ativan)
3. Phenytoin (Dilantin)
4. Fluoxetine (Paxil)

Answer: 2

Rationale: Lorazepam is a benzodiazepine used to treat anxiety. It may be given as a prn medication. Option 1: Buspirone has a long action and is not useful as a prn drug. Option 3: Phenytoin is an anticonvulsant. Option 4: Fluoxetine is a selective serotonin reuptake inhibitor used to treat the client's depression.

Cognitive level: Application
Nursing process: Implementation
NCLEX: Physiological Integrity
See text pages: 246, 247

32. A client has generalized anxiety disorder but is otherwise healthy. He is receiving buspirone daily. The topic that would be excluded from the health teaching plan is
1. the importance of daily aerobic exercise.
2. avoidance of foods and drinks containing caffeine.
3. effects and side effects of buspirone.
4. how to prevent the occurrence of flashbacks.

Answer: 4

Rationale: Flashbacks are not part of the symptom picture of generalized anxiety disorder. All other topics are appropriate health teaching for this client.

Cognitive level: Application
Nursing process: Planning
NCLEX: Health Promotion and Maintenance
See text page: 247

33. The nurse teaches a client to snap a rubber band on her wrist whenever an obsessive thought enters her mind. This technique, designed to interrupt obsessive thinking, can be identified as
1. modeling.
2. flooding.
3. desensitization.
4. thought stopping.

Answer: 4

Rationale: Thought stopping uses techniques such as rubber band snapping, saying "stop" aloud, and stomping one's foot to interrupt obsessive thinking. Option 1: Modeling involves the therapist acting as a role model to demonstrate an appropriate

behavior. Option 2: Flooding exposes a client to a large amount of a feared stimulus in an effort to extinguish the anxiety response. Option 3: Desensitization involves gradual exposure to a feared stimulus.

Cognitive level: Application
Nursing process: Implementation
NCLEX: Psychosocial Integrity
See text page: 244

34. Two forms of therapy that call for the nurse to plan for an initial rise in client anxiety level are
1. relaxation training and meditation.
2. flooding and response prevention.
3. anxiolytic therapy and β-blocker use.
4. modeling and cognitive restructuring.

Answer: 2

Rationale: Flooding introduces a phobic client to the feared stimulus in continual large doses, and response prevention requires a client with obsessive-compulsive disorder to avoid performing the ritual that relieves anxiety. Both cause an initial rise in anxiety before the anxiety level is reduced. The goal of options 1 and 3 is anxiety reduction without initial anxiety increase. Option 4: Modeling will not cause an initial rise in anxiety, and cognitive restructuring is performed in a nonthreatening way.

Cognitive level: Application
Nursing process: Planning
NCLEX: Psychosocial Integrity
See text page: 244

35. A nurse has been counseling a client with generalized anxiety disorder to increase the client's anxiety self-control. The client has identified several stressful situations that cause physical and psychological manifestations of anxiety. The indicator the nurse should monitor relative to the Nursing Outcomes Classification outcome of anxiety self-control is
1. plans coping strategies for stressful situations.
2. identifies situations that precipitate hostility.
3. refrains from destroying property.
4. identifies alternatives to aggression.

Answer: 1

Rationale: This indicator is directly related to having identified situations that precipitate anxiety. The other options are indicators of aggression self-control.

Cognitive level: Analysis
Nursing process: Planning (Outcome Identification)
NCLEX: Psychosocial Integrity
See text page: 237

36. A client with severe obsessive-compulsive symptoms will be admitted to the hospital for a short stay

Chapter 14   Anxiety Disorders

for assessment and initiation of therapy with a selective serotonin reuptake inhibitor. The assessments of critical importance include (more than one answer may be correct)
1. anxiety level.
2. sleep pattern.
3. elimination.
4. nutritional status.
5. hygiene and grooming.
6. presence of delusions and hallucinations.

Answers: 1, 2, 3, 4, 5

Rationale: Options 2 through 5 are important because each may be adversely affected by the client's excessive use of ritualistic behaviors. A baseline anxiety level must be established for later comparison. When the drug therapy is initiated, the anxiety level may rise before the desired effect of anxiety reduction is accomplished. Option 6: The client is not expected to demonstrate either delusions or hallucinations.
Cognitive level: Analysis
Nursing process: Assessment
NCLEX: Physiological Integrity
See text pages: 239-241

37. An assessment question that would be highly appropriate to ask a client with possible generalized anxiety disorder would be
1. "Have you been a victim of a crime or seen someone badly injured or killed?"
2. "Do you feel especially uncomfortable in social situations involving people?"
3. "Do you repeatedly do certain things over and over again?"
4. "Do you find it difficult to control your worrying?"

Answer: 4

Rationale: Clients with generalized anxiety disorder frequently engage in excessive worrying. They are less likely to engage in ritualistic behavior, fear social situations, or have been involved in a highly traumatic event.
Cognitive level: Analysis
Nursing process: Assessment
NCLEX: Psychosocial Integrity
See text page: 240

38. Assessment questions that would be highly appropriate to ask a client with possible obsessive-compulsive disorder would be (more than one answer may be correct)
1. "Have you been a victim of a crime or seen someone badly injured or killed?"
2. "Do you feel especially uncomfortable in social situations involving people?"
3. "Do you do certain things over and over again?"
4. "Do you find it difficult to keep certain thoughts out of awareness?"
5. "Do you have to do things in a certain way to feel comfortable?"

Answers: 3, 4, 5

Rationale: These questions refer to obsessive thinking and compulsive behaviors. Option 1 is more pertinent to a client with suspected posttraumatic stress disorder. Option 2 is more relevant for a client with suspected social phobia.
Cognitive level: Analysis
Nursing process: Assessment
NCLEX: Psychosocial Integrity
See text page: 240

39. A client with obsessive-compulsive disorder spends 2 hours each morning checking and rechecking her home before leaving for work, then comes home on the lunch hour and spends more than an hour rechecking faucets, stove burners, appliances, window and door locks, and so forth. The checking continues after work and during the evening. The client spends so much time in ritualistic behavior that grooming is poor and social activities are nonexistent. Nursing diagnoses the nurse can immediately rule out include (more than one answer may be correct)
1. ineffective role performance relative to time spent in rituals.
2. impaired environmental interpretation syndrome relative to confusion.
3. ineffective coping relative to use of compulsive behavior.
4. social isolation relative to excessive use of time to perform rituals.
5. defensive coping relative to feelings of superiority to others.
6. dressing/grooming self-care deficit relative to time spent in rituals.

Answers: 2, 5

Rationale: Impaired environmental interpretation syndrome refers to consistent lack of orientation to person, place, time. Defensive coping is defined as repeated projection of falsely positive self-evaluation based on a self-protective pattern that defends against underlying perceived threats to positive self-regard. The other options are relevant to the scenario.
Cognitive level: Analysis
Nursing process: Diagnosis
NCLEX: Psychosocial Integrity
See text pages: 234, 235

40. A client with obsessive-compulsive disorder spends 2 hours each morning checking and rechecking her home before leaving for work, then comes home on the lunch hour and spends more than an hour rechecking faucets, stove burners, appliances, window and door locks, and so forth. The checking continues after work and during the evening. The client spends so much time in ritualistic behavior that grooming is poor and social activities are nonexistent. Indicators for measuring progress should include
1. adequate grooming achieved daily.
2. participation in a social activity 30 minutes per day.
3. refraining from checking more than once when leaving home.
4. calling to request that a neighbor to check the home in her absence.

Answers: 1, 2, 3
Rationale: Individualized indicators that show the client is spending less time in checking rituals and using more time for activities of daily living and social/recreational activities indicate progress toward the outcome of symptom control. Option 4 suggests symptom control is still tenuous.
Cognitive level: Analysis
Nursing process: Planning (Outcome Identification)
NCLEX: Psychosocial Integrity
See text pages: 234, 235

41. A nurse is counseling a client with an anxiety disorder by using cognitive therapy strategies. She gives the client a homework assignment to keep a diary in which he records the symptoms of anxiety he experiences and the events that transpired just before the onset of symptoms. The rationale for this strategy is
1. to keep the client intellectually occupied to prevent dwelling on physiologic phenomena.
2. to link symptoms with precipitating events, which provides a basis for discussion and reframing.
3. that anxiety gives rise to automatic, negative cognitions that must be analyzed.
4. that antecedent events have less to do with the anxiety onset than internal events.

Answer: 2
Rationale: Reframing is necessary for change. It permits the client to see situations in a new way and move away from the use of automatic, negative thinking. The other options are not reasonable explanations of the use of a diary to support cognitive reframing.
Cognitive level: Comprehension
Nursing process: Implementation
NCLEX: Psychosocial Integrity
See text page: 244

CHAPTER 15

1. The medical-surgical nurse working with a client who has a somatoform disorder will find planning is facilitated by the understanding that the client will probably
1. readily seek psychiatric counseling.
2 be difficult to convince to seek psychiatric help.
3. attend psychotherapy sessions without encouragement.
4. be eager to discover the true reasons for his or her physical symptoms.

Answer: 2
Rationale: Clients with somatoform disorders go from doctor to doctor trying to establish a physical cause for their symptoms. When a psychological basis is suggested and a referral for counseling is offered, these clients reject both. Thus, options 1, 3, and 4 are incorrect.
Cognitive level: Application
Nursing process: Planning
NCLEX: Psychosocial Integrity
See text pages: 258, 262

2. A client has been diagnosed as having blindness related to conversion disorder. She displays indifference regarding the conversion symptom. The nurse states "I can't understand why the client doesn't seem more anxious about her symptom." The understanding that should guide planning is that the
1. client is suppressing her true feelings.
2. client's anxiety has been relieved through the physical symptom.
3. client's needs are met during hospitalization, so she has no need to be anxious.
4. client does not wish to display her actual fear.

Answer: 2
Rationale: Psychoanalytical theory suggests conversion reduces anxiety through production of a physical symptom that is symbolically linked to an underlying conflict. Option 1: Conversion, not suppression, is the operative defense mechanism in this disorder. Option 3: This explanation oversimplifies the dynamics, suggesting that only dependency needs are of concern. Option 4: This option suggests conscious motivation, but conversion operates unconsciously.
Cognitive level: Application
Nursing process: Planning
NCLEX: Psychosocial Integrity
See text page: 259

3. A client has blindness related to conversion disorder. To help the client eat, the nurse should

Chapter 15 Somatoform and Dissociative Disorders

1. establish a "buddy" system with other clients who can feed the client at each meal.
2. expect the client to feed self after explaining the arrangement of the food on the tray.
3. see to the needs of other clients in the dining room, then feed this client.
4. direct the client to locate items on the tray independently and feed self unassisted.

Answer: 2

Rationale: The client is expected to maintain some level of independence by feeding self, while the nurse is supportive in a matter-of-fact way. Options 1 and 3 support dependency. Option 4 offers little support.

Cognitive level: Application
Nursing process: Implementation
NCLEX: Psychosocial Integrity
See text page: 262

4. A client with blindness related to conversion disorder tells the nurse "I'm really popular here in the hospital. Lots of doctors and nurses stop by to check on my blindness and the other patients are really interested in it, too. Too bad people outside the hospital don't find me so interesting." On the basis of this statement, the nurse should continue to gather assessment data to support the nursing diagnosis of
1. social isolation.
2. chronic low self-esteem.
3. interrupted family processes.
4. ineffective health maintenance.

Answer: 2

Rationale: The client mentions that her symptoms make her more interesting to people, inferring that she is uninteresting and unpopular without the symptoms, thus supporting the nursing diagnosis of chronic low self-esteem. Defining characteristics for the other nursing diagnoses are not present in the scenario.

Cognitive level: Analysis
Nursing process: Diagnosis
NCLEX: Psychosocial Integrity
See text pages: 256, 257

5. To best assist a client with a somatoform disorder, a nursing intervention of high priority that should be planned is
1. shift focus from somatic symptoms to feelings.
2. imply that somatic symptoms are not real.
3. help client suppress feelings of anger.
4. investigate each physical symptom as it is offered.

Answer: 1

Rationale: Shifting the focus from somatic symptoms to feelings or to neutral topics conveys interest in the client as a person rather than as a condition. The

need to gain attention with the use of symptoms is reduced over the long term. Option 2 destroys trust. Option 3: A desired outcome would be that client would express feelings, including anger if it is present. Option 4: Once physical symptoms have been investigated, they do not need to be reinvestigated each time the client reports them.

Cognitive level: Analysis
Nursing process: Planning
NCLEX: Safe and Effective Care Environment
See text page: 263

6. A client who is concerned that she may have serious heart disease seeks help at the mental health center after a referral from the internist who told her that she has no physical illness. The client reports she has had tightness in her chest and the sensation of her heart missing a beat. Because of her concern over her symptoms, she has missed much time from work over the past 2 years. Her social life has been severely restricted because she believes she must rest each evening. The client can be assessed as having symptoms consistent with
1. somatization disorder.
2. dysthymic disorder.
3. antisocial disorder.
4. hypochondriasis.

Answer: 4

Rationale: Hypochondriasis, according to the *DSM-IV-TR,* involves preoccupation with fears of having a serious disease even when evidence to the contrary is available. The preoccupation causes impairment in social or occupational functioning. Option 1: Somatization disorder involves a variety of physical symptoms. Option 2: Dysthymic disorder is a disorder of lowered mood. Option 3: Antisocial disorder applies to a personality disorder in which the individual has little regard for the rights of others.

Cognitive level: Application
Nursing process: Assessment
NCLEX: Psychosocial Integrity
See text pages: 258, 259

7. The nurse assessing a client with a somatoform disorder is most likely to note that the client
1. readily sees a relation between symptoms and interpersonal conflicts.
2. rarely derives personal benefit from the symptoms.
3. has little difficulty communicating emotional needs.
4. has altered comfort and activity needs.

Answer: 4

Rationale: The client frequently has altered comfort and activity needs associated with the symptoms he or she displays (fatigue, insomnia, weakness, tension, pain, etc.). In addition, hygiene, safety, and security needs may also be compromised. Option 1: The client is rarely able to see a relation between symptoms and events in his or her life, which is readily discernable to health professionals. Option 2: Clients with somatoform disorders often derive secondary gain from their symptoms. Option 3: Clients with somatoform disorders have considerable difficulty identifying feelings and conveying emotional needs to others.

Cognitive level: Application
Nursing process: Assessment
NCLEX: Physiological Integrity
See text page: 260

8. To plan effective care for clients with somatoform disorders, the nurse must understand that the clients may have difficulty giving up the symptoms because they
   1. are generally ego dystonic.
   2. can be voluntarily controlled.
   3. provide relief of anxiety.
   4. have a physiological basis.

Answer: 3

Rationale: At the unconscious level, the client's primary gain from the symptoms is anxiety relief. Considering that the symptoms actually make the client more psychologically comfortable and may also provide secondary gain, clients frequently fiercely cling to the symptoms. Option 1: The symptoms tend to be ego syntonic. Option 2: The symptoms are not under voluntary control. Option 4: The symptoms are not physiologically based.

Cognitive level: Application
Nursing process: Planning
NCLEX: Psychosocial Integrity
See text page: 260

9. The client with somatoform pain disorder reveals to the nurse that he has begun to question why God has chosen to have him lead the life of an invalid who is unable to provide for his family. He states that he believes the burden placed on his spouse and his children may be even greater than the burden he must bear. He blames God for punishing his "innocent family." Select the nursing diagnoses that could be developed for the client. (More than one answer may be correct.)
   1. Spiritual distress
   2. Self-care deficit
   3. Decisional conflict
   4. Ineffective role performance

Answers: 1, 4

Rationale: The client's verbalization is consistent with spiritual distress. Moreover, his description of being unable to provide for and burdening his family suggests ineffective role performance. Data are not provided to support diagnoses of self-care deficit or decisional conflict.

Cognitive level: Analysis
Nursing process: Diagnosis
NCLEX: Psychosocial Integrity
See text page: 261

10. A client with somatization has an established nursing diagnosis of interrupted family processes related to client's symptoms. The client's spouse and children assume roles and tasks that previously belonged to the client. An appropriate outcome for the client is that the client will
   1. demonstrate resumption of former roles and tasks.
   2. assume roles and functions of other family members.
   3. focus energy on problems occurring in the family.
   4. rely on family members to meet all client needs.

Answer: 1

Rationale: The client with somatization has typically adopted a sick role in the family, characterized by dependence. Increasing independence and resumption of former roles are necessary to change this pattern. The other options are inappropriate outcomes.

Cognitive level: Application
Nursing process: Planning (Outcome Identification)
NCLEX: Psychosocial Integrity
See text pages: 261, 262

11. A client who is 5 feet 7 inches tall and weighs 160 pounds believes that her size-9 feet are enormous compared with the rest of her body. She has visited orthopedic surgeons to see if surgery to reduce the length of her feet is possible. She spends hours trying to buy shoes that make her feet look smaller, and she prefers social interactions where she can sit with her feet concealed under a table. The nurse can assess that the client's symptoms are consistent with
   1. hypochondriasis.
   2. somatoform pain disorder.
   3. body dysmorphic disorder.
   4. depersonalization disorder.

Answer: 3

Rationale: Body dysmorphic disorder refers to preoccupation with some imagined defect in appearance in a normal-appearing person. The client's feet are proportional to the rest of her body. Option 1: Hypochondriasis involves misinterpreting physical

Chapter 15   Somatoform and Dissociative Disorders

symptoms as signs of a serious medical disorder. Option 2: Somatoform pain disorder involves the presence of pain not associated with a medical disorder. Option 4: Depersonalization disorder involves alteration in perception of self, such as feeling mechanical or unreal.

Cognitive level: Application
Nursing process: Assessment
NCLEX: Psychosocial Integrity
See text page: 259

12. The data element obtained during nursing assessment that supports the presence of a fugue state is that the client states he
   1. cannot recall why he is living in his present location.
   2. feels as if he is living in a fuzzy dream state.
   3. feels very anxious about his problems.
   4. feels that different parts of him are at war.

Answer: 1
Rationale: The client in a fugue state frequently relocates and assumes a new identity while not recalling his previous identity or where he lived in the past. Option 2 is more consistent with depersonalization disorder. Option 3 is consistent with generalized anxiety disorder. Option 4 is consistent with feelings experienced with dissociative identity disorder.

Cognitive level: Application
Nursing process: Assessment
NCLEX: Psychosocial Integrity
See text page: 266

13. The client lives with her roommate in a condominium. She tells the nurse that her roommate has urged her to seek a therapist's advice about episodes of strange behavior observed by the roommate but that the client cannot remember. The roommate has observed her leaving the condo wearing seductive clothing, quite different from her usual wardrobe, and returning 12 to 24 hours later, after which she sleeps for 8 to 12 hours. Episodes have also occurred in which the client and her roommate have argued about household matters and the client has gone to sit on the floor in the corner of the kitchen. While seated there she has spoken like a young child. The client's problem can be assessed as being consistent with *DSM-IV-TR* criteria for
   1. antisocial personality.
   2. borderline personality.
   3. dissociative identity disorder.
   4. body dysmorphic disorder.

Answer: 3
Rationale: Dissociative identity disorder involves the existence of two or more distinct subpersonalities,

each with its own patterns of relating, perceiving, and thinking. At least two of the subpersonalities take control of the person's behavior but leave the individual unable to remember the periods of time in which the subpersonality was in control. Option 1: Antisocial personality disorder features include impulsive, irresponsible behaviors, little concern for the rights of others, inability to empathize, and failure to learn from experience. Option 2: Borderline personality disorder features include intense, stormy relationships, idealization/devaluation, impulsivity, self-mutilation, and fear of abandonment. Option 4: Body dysmorphic disorder involves excessive concern with an imagined defect in a part of the body.

Cognitive level: Application
Nursing process: Assessment
NCLEX: Psychosocial Integrity
See text pages: 266, 267

14. A client who lives with her roommate in a condominium seeks advice about episodes of strange behavior observed by the roommate but that the client cannot remember. The roommate has observed her leaving the condo wearing seductive clothing, quite different from her usual wardrobe, and returning 12 to 24 hours later, after which she sleeps for 8 to 12 hours. Episodes have also occurred in which the client and her roommate have argued about household matters and the client has gone to sit on the floor in the corner of the kitchen. While seated there she has spoken like a young child. The nurse should assess that the ego defense mechanism responsible for the client's condition is most likely
   1. rationalization.
   2. dissociation.
   3. projection.
   4. symbolization.

Answer: 2
Rationale: Dissociation involves the splitting off from awareness of an event or series of events, thus explaining the client's inability to remember the episodes described by the roommate. Dissociated processes (memories and feelings) may take on a separate existence, becoming a subpersonality.

Cognitive level: Application
Nursing process: Assessment
NCLEX: Psychosocial Integrity
See text pages: 266, 267

15. A client's roommate has observed the client behaving in uncharacteristic ways, but the client cannot remember the episodes. During the assessment, which question should the nurse omit as irrelevant?

1. "Are you sexually promiscuous?"
2. "Are your memories of childhood clear and complete, or do you have many blank spots?"
3. "Have you ever found new things in your belongings that you cannot remember buying?"
4. "Have you ever found yourself someplace and did not know how you got there?"

Answer: 1

Rationale: This question would probably produce defensiveness on the part of the client. If a subpersonality acts out sexually, the main personality is probably not aware of the behavior. All other questions would be pertinent.

Cognitive level: Application
Nursing process: Assessment
NCLEX: Psychosocial Integrity
See text pages: 266-268

16. For a client with dissociative identity disorder, the nursing diagnosis of disturbed personal identity most likely has an etiology statement of "related to
   1. poor impulse control."
   2. chronic low self-esteem."
   3. unresolved childhood abuse issues."
   4. high risk for self-directed violence."

Answer: 3

Rationale: Nearly all clients with multiple personality disorder resulting in disturbance of personal identity have a history of having been abused in childhood. None of the other etiology statements are relevant.

Cognitive level: Analysis
Nursing process: Diagnosis
NCLEX: Psychosocial Integrity
See text pages: 264, 266, 267

17. For the client with dissociative amnesia, an appropriate indicator for the outcome of cognition (demonstrate ability to execute complex mental processes) is that the client will
   1. verbalize feelings of safety.
   2. function independently.
   3. regularly attend diversional activities.
   4. describe previously forgotten experiences.

Answer: 4

Rationale: The ability to recall previously repressed or dissociated material is an indication that the client is integrating identity and memory. Option 1: A client may verbalize feeling safe but may be disoriented and have memory deficits. Option 2: A client may be able to function independently on a basic level without being able to remember significant information. Option 3: Attending activities is possible without being able to remember antecedent events.

Cognitive level: Application
Nursing process: Planning (Outcome Identification)
NCLEX: Psychosocial Integrity
See text page: 265

18. Establishing a therapeutic relationship with a client with a dissociative disorder may be more difficult for the nurse than establishing a relationship with a psychotic client because the client with a dissociative disorder
   1. seems haughty, distant, and aloof.
   2. has symptoms that may seem contrived.
   3. seems too needy, overwhelming the nurse.
   4. seeks enormous amounts of secondary gain.

Answer: 2

Rationale: The nurse often questions the genuineness of the behaviors of a client with dissociative disorder. They may seem sensational, exaggerated, and not authentic. Option 1: The client with a dissociative disorder often appears withdrawn and vague. Options 3 and 4 are not typical of clients with dissociative disorders.

Cognitive level: Application
Nursing process: Implementation
NCLEX: Psychosocial Integrity
See text pages: 268, 269

19. The nurse who is counseling a client with a dissociative disorder should understand that the assessment of highest priority is
   1. risk for self-harm.
   2. cognitive functioning.
   3. identification of drug abuse.
   4. readiness to reestablish identity or memory.

Answer: 1

Rationale: Assessments that relate to client safety take priority. Clients with dissociative disorders may be at risk for suicide or self-mutilation, so the nurse must be alert for hints of hopelessness, helplessness and worthlessness, low self-esteem, and impulses to self-mutilate. The other options are important assessments but rank beneath safety.

Cognitive level: Application
Nursing process: Implementation
NCLEX: Safe and Effective Care Environment
See text page: 268

20. A client states "I feel detached and weird all the time. It's as though I'm looking at life through a cloudy window. Everything seems unreal. These feelings really get in the way of working and studying." The nurse can assess that the client is experiencing

Chapter 15 Somatoform and Dissociative Disorders

1. depersonalization disorder.
2. body dysmorphic disorder.
3. dissociative amnesia.
4. hypochondriasis.

Answer: 1

Rationale: The *DSM-IV-TR* description of depersonalization disorder states that it involves a persistent or recurrent experience of feeling detached from and outside one's mental processes or body. Although reality testing is intact, the experience causes significant impairment in social or occupational functioning and distress to the individual. Option 2: Body dysmorphic disorder involves preoccupation with a body part the individual believes to be distorted. Option 3: Dissociative amnesia involves memory loss. Option 4: Hypochondriasis involves interpretation of body sensations as symptomatic of a serious illness.

Cognitive level: Analysis
Nursing process: Assessment
NCLEX: Psychosocial Integrity
See text page: 265

21. The nursing assistant remarks to the nurse, "The client with amnesia looks together, but when I talk to her she seems rather vague. What should I be doing for her?" The best reply would be
    1. "Give her lots of space to test her independence."
    2. "Whenever you think she needs direction, use short, simple sentences."
    3. "Spend as much time with her as you can and ask questions about her recent life."
    4. "Keep her busy and make sure she doesn't take naps during the day."

Answer: 2

Rationale: Disruptions in ability to perform activities of daily living, confusion, and anxiety are often apparent in clients with amnesia. Offering simple directions to promote activities of daily living and reduce confusion helps increase feelings of safety and security. Option 1: This option does not provide the structure or support often required by clients with amnesia. Option 3: Probing is not a recommended strategy for a client with amnesia. Option 4: Clients with amnesia need a balanced activity schedule that allows for rest because they often feel fatigued.

Cognitive level: Application
Nursing process: Implementation
NCLEX: Psychosocial Integrity
See text page: 270

22. The husband of a client who has been diagnosed with severe depersonalization disorder asks the nurse if he is in any way at fault for his wife's ill-ness. He states their relationship is mutually supportive and no trauma has recently occurred. The nurse's reply should be predicated on the knowledge that this disorder is thought to be related to
    1. faulty learning.
    2. genetic predisposition.
    3. childhood emotional abuse.
    4. the intentional production of symptoms.

Answer: 3

Rationale: Depersonalization is sometimes preceded by severe stress; however, many authorities believe depersonalization disorder is associated with childhood emotional abuse. Options 1, 2, and 4 have not been implicated as causative factors.

Cognitive level: Application
Nursing process: Implementation
NCLEX: Psychosocial Integrity
See text page: 265

23. To plan effective nursing care for a client with somatization disorder, the nurse should be aware that the etiology of somatoform disorders may be related to
    1. faulty perceptions and assessments of body sensations.
    2. traumatic memories of childhood events.
    3. culture-bound phenomena.
    4. depressive equivalents.

Answer: 1

Rationale: Structural or functional abnormalities of the brain have been suggested to lead to the somatoform disorders, resulting in disturbed processes of perception and interpretation of bodily sensations. Furthermore, cognitive theorists believe clients misinterpret the meaning of certain bodily sensations and then become excessively alarmed by them. Option 2: Traumatic childhood events are related to the dissociative disorders. Option 3: Culture-bound phenomena may explain the prevalence of some symptoms but cannot explain the cause. Option 4: Somatoform disorders are not seen to be another facet of depression; however, depression may coexist with a somatoform disorders.

Cognitive level: Application
Nursing process: Planning
NCLEX: Psychosocial Integrity
See text page: 258

24. To assess clients effectively, the nurse must understand that an essential difference between somatoform disorders and dissociative disorders is
    1. symptoms of somatoform disorders are under voluntary control, whereas symptoms of dissociative disorders are unconscious and automatic.

2. symptoms of dissociative disorders are precipitated by psychological factors, whereas symptoms of somatoform disorders are related to stress.
3. dissociative disorders involve stress-related disruptions of memory, consciousness, or identity, whereas somatoform disorders involve expression of psychological stress through somatic symptoms.
4. symptoms of dissociative disorders are individually determined and related to childhood sexual abuse, whereas symptoms of somatoform disorders are culture bound.

Answer: 3

Rationale: Option 3 is the only fully accurate statement. Option 1: Somatoform symptoms are not under voluntary control. Option 2 points out a similarity. Option 4 incorrectly suggests that all somatoform symptoms are culture bound.
Cognitive level: Application
Nursing process: Assessment
NCLEX: Psychosocial Integrity
See text pages: 252-273

25. Which of the following areas would be more relevant to the assessment of a client with somatoform disorder than for a client with dissociative disorder?
    1. Voluntary control of symptoms
    2. Ability to perform self-care activities
    3. Effect of symptoms on family processes
    4. Use of alcohol, psychoactive drugs, and prescription anxiolytics

Answer: 2

Rationale: Voluntary control of symptoms is an important feature in differentiating somatoform disorder from malingering and factitious disorder but is less relevant to the assessment of dissociative symptoms. The other options should be included in the assessment for both types of disorders.
Cognitive level: Application
Nursing process: Assessment
NCLEX: Psychosocial Integrity
See text page: 260

26. Which assessment data would help the health care team distinguish symptoms of conversion from symptoms of hypochondriasis?
    1. Results of diagnostic testing
    2. Voluntary control of symptoms
    3. Client's cognitive style
    4. Secondary gains

Answer: 3

Rationale: The cognitive style of clients with hypochondriasis tends to be more anxious and displays more obsessive attention to detail, whereas the client with conversion exhibits a more dramatic style of communicating and may exhibit unconcern for the symptom.
Cognitive level: Application
Nursing process: Assessment
NCLEX: Psychosocial Integrity
See text page: 260

27. The emotional reaction that nurses who counsel clients with somatoform disorder are most likely to experience is
    1. fear and anxiety.
    2. pleasure and interest.
    3. frustration and resentment.
    4. sympathy and desire to rescue.

Answer: 3

Rationale: Many nurses consider it unsatisfying to work with a client with somatoform disorder. The client's resistance makes for slow progress. Medical-surgical nurses often feel as though they are wasting their time on a client with no organic basis for his or her symptoms. The other options are less likely reactions to these difficult clients.
Cognitive level: Application
Nursing process: Assessment
NCLEX: Psychosocial Integrity
See text pages: 260, 261

28. A client with depersonalization disorder tells the nurse "It's starting again. I feel as though I'm going to float away." The nurse should help the client by
    1. advising her to begin meditating.
    2. administering an as-needed anxiolytic.
    3. helping her visualize a pleasant scene.
    4. staying with her to help her focus on the here and now.

Answer: 4

Rationale: Talking with someone who can help the client focus on reality allows the client to interrupt the stimulus to dissociate. Options 1, 2, and 3 foster detachment.
Cognitive level: Application
Nursing process: Implementation
NCLEX: Psychosocial Integrity
See text page: 265

29. A client with somatoform pain disorder who has been in treatment for 4 weeks tells the clinic nurse that although he still has a considerable amount of pain, he notices it less and is able to perform more

Chapter 15   Somatoform and Dissociative Disorders

activities of daily living. The nurse should evaluate the treatment plan as
1. unsuccessful.
2. minimally successful.
3. partially successful.
4. totally successful.

Answer: 3
Rationale: Decreased preoccupation with symptoms and increased ability to perform activities of daily living suggest partial success of the treatment plan. Total success is rare because of client resistance.
Cognitive level: Analysis
Nursing process: Evaluation
NCLEX: Psychosocial Integrity
See text page: 259

30. Outcomes for health promotion and maintenance for clients with somatoform and dissociative disorders can be considered attained when clients
1. identify stressors associated with symptom formation.
2. keep a detailed daily journal of events and feelings.
3. make contact with a number of different health care agencies.
4. schedule regular physicals, screening tests, and dental care.

Answer: 4
Rationale: Most health care visits by clients with somatoform and dissociative disorders are illness related. Regular dental and medical examinations and screenings are part of health promotion and maintenance. Options 1 and 2 are not relevant to health promotion. Option 3 suggests uncoordinated care.
Cognitive level: Analysis
Nursing process: Evaluation
NCLEX: Psychosocial Integrity
See text page: NA

31. The treatment modality the nurse should recommend to help a client with chronic pain disorder cope more effectively is
1. flooding.
2. relaxation techniques.
3. response prevention.
4. systematic desensitization.

Answer: 2
Rationale: Pain is increased when the client has muscle tension. Relaxation can diminish the client's perceptions of the intensity of pain. The other options are modalities useful in treating selected anxiety disorders.
Cognitive level: Application

Nursing process: Planning
NCLEX: Psychosocial Integrity
See text page: 263

32. A client believes she has a brain tumor despite numerous diagnostic tests that show no evidence of a tumor. She tells the nurse "People with brain tumors vomit. Yesterday I vomited all day. I know I have a brain tumor." The approach that fosters cognitive restructuring is
1. "You do not have a brain tumor. The more you talk about it, the more it reinforces your illogical thinking. We'll talk about something else."
2. "Let's see if there are any other possible explanations for your vomiting."
3. "How worried you seem! Let's talk about how you're feeling."
4. "What interpersonal problems have you had recently?"

Answer: 2
Rationale: Questioning the evidence is a cognitive restructuring technique. Learning that headaches, visual disturbances, weakness, and vomiting can have causes other than the feared disease can be helpful in changing distorted perceptions. Option 1 does not foster questioning on the part of the client. Option 3 is empathetic, but does not foster restructuring. Option 4 queries, but not with an appropriate focus.
Cognitive level: Application
Nursing process: Implementation
NCLEX: Psychosocial Integrity
See text page: 264

33. A client who is being counseled for somatoform pain disorder states he believes his pain is the result of an undiagnosed injury. He adds that he cannot adhere to his plan for care involving performing own activities of daily living, walking 20 minutes daily, and using pain medication only at bedtime. Desired outcomes for the client include (more than one answer may be correct)
1. compliance behavior.
2. anxiety self-control.
3. risk control—drug use.
4. spiritual health.

Answers: 1, 3
Rationale: The client should ideally develop compliance behaviors that allow him to adhere to his plan for care. The risk for the excessive use of pain medication must also be controlled. The other options are less directly related to the scenario.
Cognitive level: Analysis
Nursing process: Planning (Outcome Identification)

290

34. A client who is being counseled for somatoform pain disorder states he believes his pain is the result of an undiagnosed injury. He adds that he cannot adhere to his plan for care involving performing own activities of daily living, walking 20 minutes daily, and using pain medication only at bedtime. He states he feels "like a baby" because his wife and children must provide so much care for him. The nurse understands that it is important to assess
1. mood.
2. cognitive style.
3. secondary gain.
4. identity and memory.

Answer: 3

Rationale: Secondary gain should be assessed. The client's dependency needs may be being met through care from his family. When secondary gains are prominent, the client is more resistant to giving up the symptom. Option 1 is an important concern, but the scenario does not allude to a problem of mood. Option 2: Cognitive style and identity and memory assessment (option 4) are of lesser concern because the client's diagnosis has been established.

Cognitive level: Analysis
Nursing process: Assessment
NCLEX: Psychosocial Integrity
See text page: 260

35. A college senior comes to the mental health clinic with the chief complaint that "My face is so ugly I can't go out in public." Assessment reveals she has no actual disfigurement and is of average attractiveness. She tells the nurse that she goes to class wearing a scarf draped across her lower face but is concerned that she will be unable to interview for positions after graduation because of her ugly appearance. The client's symptoms are consistent with the clinical picture of
1. dissociative identity disorder.
2. body dysmorphic disorder.
3. hypochondriasis.
4. malingering.

Answer: 2

Rationale: Body dysmorphic disorder involves preoccupation with an imagined defect in appearance. Option 1: Dissociative identity disorder involves the existence of two or more distinct subpersonalities, each with its own patterns of relating, perceiving, and thinking. Option 3: Hypochondriasis is defined by preoccupation with fears of having a serious dis-

ease or the idea that one has a serious disease. Option 4: Malingering is defined as intentionally producing symptoms for a personal gain.

Cognitive level: Analysis
Nursing process: Assessment
NCLEX: Psychosocial Integrity
See text page: 259

CHAPTER 16

1. A physical therapist recently convicted of multiple counts of Medicare fraud is brought to the emergency department after taking an overdose of sedatives. He tells the nurse "Sure I overbilled. Why not? Everybody takes advantage of the government. They have too many rules. No one can abide by all of them." These statements can be assessed as showing
1. glibness and charm.
2. superficial remorse.
3. lack of guilt feelings.
4. excessive suspiciousness.

Answer: 3

Rationale: Rationalization is being used to explain behavior and deny wrongdoing. Option 2: The individual who does not believe he or she has done anything wrong will not manifest anxiety, remorse, or guilt about the act. Options 1 and 4: The client's remarks cannot be assessed as charming, and lack of trust and concern that others are determined to harm him are not shown.

Cognitive level: Application
Nursing process: Assessment
NCLEX: Psychosocial Integrity
See text page: 282

2. The intervention appropriate for an antisocial client with a nursing diagnosis of ineffective coping related to manipulation of others is to
1. refer requests and questions related to care to the primary nurse.
2. provide negative reinforcement for acting-out behavior.
3. ignore, rather than confront, inappropriate behavior.
4. encourage the client to discuss feelings of fear and inferiority.

Answer: 1

Rationale: Manipulative clients frequently make requests of many different staff, hoping one will give in. Having one decision maker provides consistency and avoids the potential for playing one staff member against another. Option 2: Positive reinforcement of appropriate behaviors is more effective.

Option 3: Judicious use of confrontation is necessary. Option 4: Antisocial clients rarely have these feelings.
Cognitive level: Application
Nursing process: Implementation
NCLEX: Psychosocial Integrity
See text page: 289

3. A nursing strategy that makes limit setting better accepted by clients with personality disorders is to first
   1. confront the client with the inappropriateness of the behavior.
   2. explore with the client the underlying dynamics of the behavior.
   3. reflect back to the client an understanding of the client's distress.
   4. state a value judgment regarding the behavior and its consequences.

Answer: 3
Rationale: Setting limits is better accepted by clients if staff first use empathetic mirroring without making a value judgment, which are suggested in options 1 and 4. Option 2 has little to do with client acceptance of limits.
Cognitive level: Analysis
Nursing process: Implementation
NCLEX: Psychosocial Integrity
See text pages: 292, 293

4. An appropriate outcome for a client with a personality disorder with a nursing diagnosis of ineffective coping related to use of manipulation would be that the client will
   1. identify when angry.
   2. use manipulation only to get legitimate needs met.
   3. acknowledge manipulative behavior when it is called to his or her attention.
   4. accept the decision that staff will fulfill a client request within an hour rather than immediately.

Answer: 3
Rationale: This is an early outcome that paves the way for later taking greater responsibility for controlling manipulative behavior. Option 1 relates to anger and aggression control. Option 2: This outcome is inappropriate. The client would ideally use assertive behavior to promote need fulfillment. Option 4: This outcome relates to impulsivity and immediacy control.
Cognitive level: Analysis
Nursing process: Planning (Outcome Identification)
NCLEX: Psychosocial Integrity
See text page: 288

5. An antisocial client tells Nurse A "You're a much better nurse than Nurse B said you were." The client tells Nurse B "Nurse A's upset with you for some reason." To Nurse C the client states "You'd like to think you're perfect, but I've seen three of your mistakes this morning." These interactions can be assessed as
   1. seductive.
   2. detached.
   3. guilt producing.
   4. manipulative.

Answer: 4
Rationale: Clients manipulate and control staff in various ways. By keeping staff off balance or fighting among themselves, the antisocial person is left to operate as he or she pleases. Option 1: Seductive behavior has sexual connotations. Option 2: The client is displaying the opposite of detached behavior. Option 3: Guilt is a factor only in the interaction with Nurse C.
Cognitive level: Application
Nursing process: Assessment
NCLEX: Psychosocial Integrity
See text page: 286

6. The nurse reports to the interdisciplinary team that an antisocial client lies to other clients, verbally abuses a client with Alzheimer's disease, flatters his primary nurse, and is detached and superficial during counseling sessions. The behavior that most clearly warrants limit setting is
   1. lying to other clients.
   2. flattering the nurse.
   3. verbal abuse of another client.
   4. detached superficiality during counseling.

Answer: 3
Rationale: Limits must be set in areas in which the client's behavior affects the rights of others. Limiting verbal abuse of another client is a priority intervention. The other concerns should be addressed during therapeutic encounters.
Cognitive level: Analysis
Nursing process: Planning
NCLEX: Safe and Effective Care Environment
See text page: 292

7. A client with personality disorder seemed intelligent to the nurse. He said all the right things but often failed to follow through. One evening he did not return after going out on a pass. The police later brought him back to the hospital acutely intoxicated. The nurse seemed dismayed and remarked "I thought he was making such good progress." The nurse was probably experiencing

292

1. guilt.
2. anger.
3. helplessness.
4. disappointment.

Answer: 4

Rationale: Inexperienced nurses often have high expectations for the progress of antisocial clients. Their initial reaction to continuing acting-out behaviors is often disappointment. The scenario does not establish guilt, anger, or helplessness as being experienced by the nurse.

Cognitive level: Application
Nursing process: Assessment
NCLEX: Safe and Effective Care Environment
See text page: 286

8. A client remanded by the court after his wife had him jailed for battery told the judge how sorry he was and suggested he needed psychiatric help. His history reveals acting-out behaviors as an adolescent and several adult arrests. The nurse interviews him about his relationship with his wife. The statement that would be most characteristic of the thinking of an individual with an antisocial personality is
    1. "I've done some stupid things in my life, but I've learned a lesson."
    2. "I'm feeling terrible about the way my behavior has hurt my family."
    3. "I have a quick temper, but I can usually keep it under control."
    4. "I hit her because she nags at me. She deserves it when I beat her up."

Answer: 4

Rationale: The antisocial client often impulsively acts out feelings of anger and feels no guilt or remorse. Option 1: Antisocial clients rarely seem to learn from experience. Option 2: Antisocial clients rarely feel true remorse. Option 3: Antisocial clients have problems with anger management and impulse control.

Cognitive level: Application
Nursing process: Assessment
NCLEX: Psychosocial Integrity
See text page: 282

9. The priority nursing diagnosis to formulate for a client with antisocial personality disorder who has made threats against staff, ripped objects off walls, and thrown objects during 4 hours of hospitalization is
    1. disturbed sensory perception: auditory hallucinations.
    2. risk for other-directed violence.
    3. ineffective denial.
    4. social isolation.

Answer: 2

Rationale: The use of violence against property along with threats to harm staff make this diagnosis the

priority. Option 1: Antisocial clients rarely have psychotic symptoms. Option 3: When antisocial client use denial, they use it effectively. Option 4: Rarely are antisocial clients social isolates; instead, they develop superficial relationships.

Cognitive level: Application
Nursing process: Diagnosis
NCLEX: Safe and Effective Care Environment
See text page: 287

10. When a client with a personality disorder uses manipulation as a way of getting needs met, the staff agree to consider limit setting as an intervention. This intervention diminishes manipulative behavior because
    1. it indulges the client's wishes.
    2. it provides an outlet for feelings of anger and frustration.
    3. external controls are necessary while internal controls are being developed.
    4. the client's anger and anxiety will be decreased if staff assume responsibility for the client's behavior.

Answer: 3

Rationale: A lack of internal controls leads to manipulative behaviors such as lying, cheating, conning, and flattering. To protect the rights of others, external controls must be consistently maintained until the client is able to behave appropriately.

Cognitive level: Application
Nursing process: Planning
NCLEX: Psychosocial Integrity
See text page: NA

11. The emotional response by a nurse to a client with antisocial personality disorder that would be most obstructive to care is
    1. a negative response, because of the client's ability to evoke frustration and anger.
    2. a negative response, because behaviors are related to sensitive areas of moral values.
    3. a negative response, because the client criticizes the abilities of staff members.
    4. a positive response, because client motivation for behavioral change is satisfying.

Answer: 4

Rationale: Most nurses recognize negative feelings toward clients and monitor associated behaviors; thus effective care can be preserved. When positive countertransference occurs, self-assessment may be more difficult. Believing that a client with antisocial personality disorder is motivated to change can hinder care-giving because motivation for change is usually nonexistent. Nursing assessment and evaluation will be inaccurate and interventions may be inappropriate.

293

12. The most challenging nursing intervention with clients with personality disorders who use manipulation for getting needs met is
    1. supporting behavioral change.
    2. using aversive therapy.
    3. maintaining consistent limits.
    4. monitoring suicide attempts.

Answer: 3

Rationale: Maintaining consistent limits is by far the most difficult intervention because of the client's superior skills at manipulation. Options 1 and 4: Supporting behavioral change and monitoring client safety are less difficult tasks. Option 2: Aversive therapy would probably not be part of the care plan because positive reinforcement strategies for acceptable behavior seem to be more effective than aversive techniques.

Cognitive level: Application
Nursing process: Implementation
NCLEX: Safe and Effective Care Environment
See text pages: 292, 293

13. A physician mentions to a nurse that a newly admitted client is impulsive. The nurse should assess for behavior characterized by
    1. adherence to a strict moral code.
    2. manipulative, controlling strategies.
    3. postponing gratification to an appropriate time.
    4. little time elapsed between thought and action.

Answer: 4

Rationale: The impulsive individual acts in haste without taking time to consider the consequences of the action. None of the other options describes impulsivity.

Cognitive level: Application
Nursing process: Assessment
NCLEX: Psychosocial Integrity
See text page: 293

14. The client tells the nurse "I get into trouble because I have hair-trigger responses. I shoot from the hip. Lots of times that gets me into a mess." A therapeutic response would be
    1. "Let's consider the advantages of being able to stop and think before acting."
    2. "It sounds as though you've developed some insight into your situation."
    3. "I'll bet you have some interesting stories to share about overreacting."

    4. "It's good that you're showing readiness for behavioral change."

Answer: 1

Rationale: The client is showing openness to learning techniques for impulse control. One technique is to teach the client to stop and think before acting impulsively. The client can then be taught to evaluate outcomes of possible actions and choose an effective action. Option 2 is pseudotherapeutic. Option 3 shifts the encounter to a social level. Option 4 is judgmental.

Cognitive level: Application
Nursing process: Implementation
NCLEX: Psychosocial Integrity
See text page: 293

15. The nurse who assesses a client diagnosed as having paranoid personality disorder is most likely to describe the client as
    1. superficially charming.
    2. intense and impulsive.
    3. guarded and suspicious.
    4. friendly and open.

Answer: 3

Rationale: Clients with paranoid personality disorder are highly mistrustful of others. They expect to be exploited or wronged by others without justification. Option 1: Antisocial clients display superficial charm. Option 2: Borderline clients are intense and impulsive. Option 4: Well-adjusted individuals display friendly openness.

Cognitive level: Application
Nursing process: Assessment
NCLEX: Psychosocial Integrity
See text page: 287

16. While the nurse at the personality disorders clinic is interviewing a client, the client constantly scans the environment and frequently interrupts to ask what the nurse means by certain words or phrases. The nurse notes that the client is very sensitive to the nurse's nonverbal behavior. His responses are often argumentative, sarcastic, and hostile. He suggests that he is being hospitalized so "they can exploit me." The nurse can make the assessment that the client's behaviors are most consistent with the clinical picture of
    1. paranoid personality disorder.
    2. histrionic personality disorder.
    3. avoidant personality disorder.
    4. narcissistic personality disorder.

Answer: 1

Rationale: The behaviors described are consistent with the clinical picture given in the *DSM-IV-TR*. Option 2: The client with histrionic personality disorder would

be flamboyant and attention seeking. Option 3: The client with avoidant personality disorder would be excessively anxious and hypersensitive. Option 4: The client with narcissistic personality disorder would be grandiose and disparaging of others.
Cognitive level: Analysis
Nursing process: Assessment
NCLEX: Psychosocial Integrity
See text page: 288

17. The nurse caring for the client with a paranoid personality disorder tells the advanced practice nurse "I tried being caring and nurturing, but the client just kept telling me to stay away." The advanced practice nurse can be helpful by advising "Clients with paranoid personality disorders respond best to
   1. a cynical, joking approach."
   2. interpretation of their behaviors."
   3. a neutral but courteous and concerned manner."
   4. active friendliness, but they require a longer time to establish a relationship than you allowed."

Answer: 3
Rationale: A detached, neutral, straightforward, and courteous approach is most effective. Option 1 is never appropriate. Option 2 would be a counterproductive approach. Option 4: A warm, actively pursuant approach will be interpreted as intrusive and threatening by the suspicious client.
Cognitive level: Application
Nursing process: Implementation
NCLEX: Psychosocial Integrity
See text page: 288

18. The client with a paranoid personality disorder is described as haughty, aloof, and superior acting in addition to being highly suspicious. Whenever the nurse interacts with this client, she describes feelings of being belittled. The nurse adds "Sometimes I'd like to tell the client 'I don't think you're so hot, either.'" The nurse's mentor would correctly advise
   1. "Feel free to show the client you feel angry."
   2. "The relationship will deteriorate if you retaliate."
   3. "Tell the client the belittling behavior hurts your feelings."
   4. "You need to get some distance from the client. Stay away for a day or two."

Answer: 2
Rationale: Courtesy, honesty, and respect are the cardinal rules in treating a paranoid individual. Option 1: The nurse cannot act out countertransference reactions. The goal is to make the client feel comfortable and secure in his or her surroundings. Retaliation and rejection thwart that goal. Option 3 is inappropriate

advice. Option 4 promotes withdrawal from the client. The behavior is inconsistent with earlier behavior and would destroy trust.
Cognitive level: Application
Nursing process: Implementation
NCLEX: Safe and Effective Care Environment
See text page: 288

19. To plan effective interventions the nurse should understand that the underlying reason a client with paranoid personality disorder is so critical of others probably lies in the client's
   1. need to set limits.
   2. use of intellectualization to protect against anxiety.
   3. inflexible view of the environment.
   4. projection of self-hate, hurt, and rage.

Answer: 4
Rationale: Projection allows the client to disown negative feelings about self and see these feelings as being directed at self from an outside source (the nurse). The client then can justifiably retaliate by being hostile to the nurse. To realize that the client is accusing the nurse of his or her own faults makes the criticism easier to manage without retaliation. The other options are not related to the dynamics of critical behaviors on the part of the client.
Cognitive level: Application
Nursing process: Assessment
NCLEX: Psychosocial Integrity
See text page: NA

20. A client with paranoid personality disorder is noted to sit alone in a corner of the unit living room. When anyone approaches, the client is haughty or simply ignores the other person. When staff invite her to join an activity, she tells them "I do not care to be with people who do not like me." A nursing diagnosis that should be considered is
   1. fear.
   2. activity intolerance.
   3. powerlessness.
   4. impaired social interaction.

Answer: 4
Rationale: Impaired social interaction is a state in which an individual participates in an insufficient (or excessive) quantity or quality of social exchange. A defining characteristic is dysfunctional interaction with others. The client's suspiciousness, rigidity, and distortions of reality related to projection are responsible.
Cognitive level: Analysis
Nursing process: Diagnosis
NCLEX: Psychosocial Integrity
See text page: 287

Chapter 16   Personality Disorders

21. A client with borderline personality disorder has had 21 admissions to the mental health unit, each precipitated by a suicide attempt, usually resulting in superficial cuts on the arm. On this admission the client has developed a relationship with a highly supportive nurse. The client has progressed to having a pass to spend an afternoon in a nearby shopping mall. The nurse is shocked when the emergency department calls to say that the client had just been brought in with multiple self-inflicted lacerations. The nurse asks a peer, "Why? Everything was going well. How could she do this to me?" What response by the other nurse reflects understanding of the client's borderline disorder?

1. "I know what you mean. You put a lot of energy into working with this client. It must be disappointing to have her do something like this."
2. "I could have told you this would happen. A client like this always gets you in the end. I hope this will teach you not to get so involved."
3. "I know the client's behavior seems personal, but it's really not. Clients with borderline disorder act out to relieve anxiety, and I suspect having the pass provoked a great deal of anxiety."
4. "I wonder if all this could have been avoided if I'd clued you in on the client. This is a usual pattern for her. She burned me once, too, when I first worked here."

Answer: 3
Rationale: This is the only statement that addresses what would be the priority nursing diagnosis, risk for self-directed violence, and gives a possible reason for the client's acting out. The other statements are countertransference reactions.
Cognitive level: Application
Nursing process: Implementation
NCLEX: Safe and Effective Care Environment
See text page: 282

22. A client with borderline personality disorder lacerated her wrists while out on a pass. For future planning, staff should consider that the reason for the self-mutilation is probably related to

1. an inherited disorder that manifests itself as an incapacity to tolerate stress.
2. fear of abandonment associated with movement toward autonomy and independence.
3. use of projective identification and splitting to bring anxiety to manageable levels.
4. a constitutional inability to regulate affect, predisposing to psychic disorganization.

Answer: 2
Rationale: Fear of abandonment is a central theme for most clients with borderline personality disorder.

This fear is often exacerbated when borderline clients experience success or growth. Options 1 and 4 are not evidence based. Option 3 is unrelated to fear of abandonment.
Cognitive level: Application
Nursing process: Planning
NCLEX: Psychosocial Integrity
See text page: 282

23. A client with borderline personality disorder has lacerated her wrists. The physician orders daily dressing changes for the lacerations. The nurse performing this care should

1. encourage the client to express anger.
2. provide care in a matter-of-fact manner.
3. be kindly, sympathetic, and concerned.
4. offer to listen to the client's feelings about cutting.

Answer: 2
Rationale: A matter-of-fact approach does not provide the client with positive reinforcement for self-mutilation. The goal of providing emotional consistency is supported by this approach. All other options provide positive reinforcement of the behavior.
Cognitive level: Application
Nursing process: Implementation
NCLEX: Safe and Effective Care Environment
See text pages: 292, 293

24. The nurse has recently set limits for a client with borderline personality disorder. The client tells the nurse "You used to care about me. I thought you were wonderful. Now I can see I was mistaken. You're hateful." This outburst can be assessed as

1. splitting.
2. denial.
3. reaction formation.
4. separation-individuation strategies.

Answer: 1
Rationale: Splitting involves loving a person, then hating the person because the client is unable to recognize that an individual can have both positive and negative qualities. Option 2: Denial is unconsciously motivated refusal to belief something. Option 3: Reaction formation involves unconsciously doing the opposite of a forbidden impulse. Option 4: Separation-individuation strategies refer to childhood behaviors related to developing independence from the caregiver.
Cognitive level: Application
Nursing process: Assessment
NCLEX: Psychosocial Integrity
See text pages: 279, 280

25. The characteristic in individuals with personality disorders that makes it most necessary for staff to schedule frequent meetings is
1. flexibility and adaptability to stress.
2. ability to achieve true intimacy.
3. ability to evoke interpersonal conflict.
4. inability to develop trusting relationships.

Answer: 3

Rationale: Frequent team meetings are held to counteract the effects of the client's attempts to split staff and set them against one another, causing interpersonal conflict. Option 1: Clients with personality disorder are inflexible and demonstrate maladaptive responses to stress. Options 2 and 4: Clients with personality disorder are usually unable to develop true intimacy with others and are unable to develop trusting relationships. The problem with trust exists but is not the characteristic that requires frequent staff meetings.

Cognitive level: Application
Nursing process: Assessment
NCLEX: Safe and Effective Care Environment
See text pages: 275-277

26. The commonality a nurse would be most likely to assess when working with clients with personality disorders is that client
1. demonstrates behavior that causes little distress to self or others.
2. has self-esteem issues despite outward confidence.
3. does not experience real distress from symptoms.
4. invariably becomes psychotic under stress.

Answer: 2

Rationale: Self-esteem issues are present despite patterns of withdrawal, grandiosity, suspiciousness, or unconcern. They seem to relate to early life experiences and are reinforced through unsuccessful experiences in loving and working. Option 1: Personality disorders involve lifelong, inflexible, dysfunctional, and deviant patterns of behavior causing distress to others and in some cases to self. Option 2: Clients with personality disorder may experience very real anxiety and distress when stress levels rise. Option 4 is untrue. Some individuals may decompensate and show psychotic behavior under stress, but not all clients with personality disorder become psychotic under stress.

Cognitive level: Application
Nursing process: Assessment
NCLEX: Psychosocial Integrity
See text pages: 275-277

27. The priority intervention for the nurse working with a client with schizotypal personality disorder is

1. respecting client need for social isolation.
2. teaching the client not to dress oddly.
3. preventing the client from violating the nurse's rights.
4. keeping emotional distance so as not to be exploited.

Answer: 1

Rationale: Clients with schizotypal personality disorder are eccentric and often display perceptual and cognitive distortions. They are suspicious of others and have considerable difficulty trusting. They become highly anxious and frightened in social situations, thus the need to respect their desire for social isolation. Option 2 is not the priority intervention. Options 3 and 4: Clients with schizotypal personality disorder rarely engage in behaviors that violate the nurse's rights or exploit the nurse.

Cognitive level: Application
Nursing process: Implementation
NCLEX: Safe and Effective Care Environment
See text page: 288

28. A client tells the nurse that he is planning to hire a private detective to follow his wife, who he believes is having an extramarital affair. The nurse assesses him to be suspicious; the client looks behind the door to be sure no one is eavesdropping and asks the nurse what she did with his medical record after he left. The behaviors manifested by the client can be assessed as being most consistent with the clinical picture of
1. antisocial personality disorder.
2. schizoid personality disorder.
3. paranoid personality disorder.
4. obsessive-compulsive personality disorder.

Answer: 3

Rationale: *DSM-IV-TR* criteria for paranoid personality disorder include suspiciousness, lack of trust in others, fear of confiding in others, fear that personal information will be used against the individual, holding grudges, and interpreting remarks as being demeaning or threatening. Option 1: The client with antisocial personality disorder is aggressive, manipulative, and exploitative. Option 2: The client with schizoid personality disorder is avoidant and reclusive. Option 4: The client with obsessive-compulsive personality disorder is a perfectionist and is rigid and preoccupied with details and control issues.

Cognitive level: Analysis
Nursing process: Assessment
NCLEX: Psychosocial Integrity
See text page: 281

297

29. A street person is brought to the hospital after having been badly beaten. She is states the hospital is the "gateway to hell." She is withdrawn and does not want to talk with anyone. She is thought to have a schizoid personality disorder. The approach most useful for working with this client is to
   1. seek detailed information about what happened to help the client see her role in causation.
   2. simply and clearly tell her what is going to be done before taking any action.
   3. alternate between being warm and friendly and neutral and businesslike.
   4. try to inject a bit of humor into the situation to relieve tension.

Answer: 2

Rationale: When a client is having difficulty understanding reality, the nurse should communicate in clear, simple, concise language. Option 1 is inappropriate for a client unable to test reality accurately. Option 3 hinders establishment of trust. Option 4 is inappropriate for a client unable to test reality accurately.

Cognitive level: Application
Nursing process: Implementation
NCLEX: Psychosocial Integrity
See text page: 280

30. A worker is characterized by her co-workers as "painfully shy" and lacking in self-confidence. Her co-workers say she stays in her cubicle all day, never coming out for breaks or lunch. One day after falling on the ice in the parking lot, she goes to the nurse's office, where she apologizes for falling and mentions that she hopes the company will not fire her for being so clumsy. This worker's behavior could best be assessed as
   1. avoidant.
   2. dependent.
   3. histrionic.
   4. paranoid.

Answer: 1

Rationale: Patients with avoidant personality disorder are timid, socially uncomfortable, and withdrawn and avoid situations in which they might fail. They believe themselves to be inferior and unappealing. Option 2: Individuals with dependent personality disorder are clinging, needy, and submissive. Option 3: Individuals with histrionic personality disorder are seductive, flamboyant, shallow, and attention seeking. Option 4: Individuals with paranoid personality disorder are suspicious, hostile, and project blame.

Cognitive level: Application
Nursing process: Assessment
NCLEX: Psychosocial Integrity
See text page: 284

31. The nurse in the emergency department tells the daughter of a client that her 86-year-old mother has had a stroke. The daughter tearfully asks the nurse "Who will take care of me now?" When the nurse explores this query, the daughter mentions that her mother always tells her what job to take, what clothes to buy and wear, and what to have for lunch. The daughter states that she needs someone to direct her and reassure her when she gets anxious. This behavior could best be assessed as
   1. histrionic.
   2. dependent.
   3. narcissistic.
   4. borderline.

Answer: 2

Rationale: The main characteristic of the dependent personality is a pervasive need to be taken care of that leads to submissive behaviors and fear of separation. Option 1: Histrionic behavior is characterized by flamboyance, attention seeking, and seductiveness. Option 3: Narcissistic behavior is characterized by grandiosity and exploitive behavior. Option 4: Clients with borderline personality disorder demonstrate separation anxiety, impulsivity, and splitting.

Cognitive level: Analysis
Nursing process: Assessment
NCLEX: Psychosocial Integrity
See text page: 290

32. For which of the following behaviors would limit setting be most essential? The client
   1. clings to the nurse and asks for advice about inconsequential matters.
   2. is flirtatious and provocative toward staff members of the opposite sex.
   3. displays hypervigilance and refuses to attend unit activities.
   4. urges a suspicious client to hit anyone who stares at him.

Answer: 4

Rationale: This is a manipulative behavior. Because manipulation violates the rights of others, limit setting is absolutely necessary. Furthermore, limit setting is necessary in this case because the safety of two other clients is at risk. Limit setting may occasionally be used with dependent (option 1) and histrionic behavior (option 2), but other therapeutic techniques are also useful. Option 3: The need for limit setting is not demonstrated; rather, the need to develop trust is central to client compliance.

Cognitive level: Application
Nursing process: Planning
NCLEX: Safe and Effective Care Environment
See text page: 282

33. Place the steps for limit setting in the most desirable order.
1. With client input, identify undesirable client behavior.
2. Discuss concerns about behavior with client.
3. Together establish what behavior is desirable in a given situation.
4. Jointly establish consequences for nonoccurrence of desired behavior.
5. Monitor for occurrence and nonoccurrence of desired behaviors.
6. Communicate expectations and consequences to the client in simple terms.

Answer: 2, 1, 3, 4, 6, 5
Rationale: This sequence of steps is logical and involves the client in the process.
Cognitive level: Application
Nursing process: Planning
NCLEX: Safe and Effective Care Environment
See text page: 292

34. When told that he is scheduled to interview a client with narcissistic personality disorder, the nurse can anticipate the assessment findings will include the following: client
1. is charming, dramatic, seductive; seeks admiration.
2. is preoccupied with minute details; is a perfectionist.
3. describes difficulty being alone; shows indecision, submissiveness.
4. is grandiose, self-important, and has a sense of entitlement.

Answer: 4
Rationale: According to the *DSM-IV-TR,* the characteristics described in option 4 are consistent with narcissistic personality disorder. Option 1 describes a client with histrionic personality disorder. Option 2 describes an individual with obsessive-compulsive personality disorder. Option 3 describes an individual with dependent personality disorder.
Cognitive level: Application
Nursing process: Assessment
NCLEX: Psychosocial Integrity
See text page: 289

35. The statement made by a client with borderline personality disorder that indicates the treatment plan is effective is
1. "I think you are the best nurse on the unit."
2. "I hate my doctor. He never gives me what I ask for."
3. "I feel empty and want to cut myself so I called you."
4. "I'm never going to get high on drugs again."

Answer: 3
Rationale: Seeking a staff member instead of impulsively self-mutilating shows an adaptive coping strategy. Option 1 demonstrates idealization. Option 2 demonstrates devaluation. Option 4 demonstrates wishful thinking.
Cognitive level: Analysis
Nursing process: Evaluation
NCLEX: Safe and Effective Care Environment
See text page: 295

36. A client diagnosed with antisocial personality disorder is admitted to the forensic unit. Characteristic behaviors for which the nurse should be alert include (more than one answer may be correct)
1. aggression.
2. callous attitude.
3. reclusive behavior.
4. anxiety.
5. clinginess.
6. perfectionism.

Answer: 1, 2
Rationale: The antisocial individual characteristically demonstrates manipulative, exploitative, aggressive, callous, and guilt-instilling behaviors. Option 3: Antisocial individuals are more extroverted than reclusive. Option 4: Antisocial individuals rarely show anxiety. Option 5: Antisocial individuals rarely demonstrate clinging or dependent behaviors. Option 6: Antisocial individuals are more impulsive than perfectionist.
Cognitive level: Analysis
Nursing process: Assessment
NCLEX: Psychosocial Integrity
See text page: 289

37. A client with borderline personality disorder has been hospitalized several times after self-mutilating episodes. The client has been assessed as demanding, impulsive, and immature. The client has entered dialectical behavior therapy on an outpatient basis. The priority focus for counseling is
1. anger control assistance.
2. risk for self-mutilation.
3. risk for trauma.
4. powerlessness.

Answer: 2
Rationale: Risk for self-mutilation is a nursing diagnosis relating to client safety needs and is therefore of high priority. Options 1 and 4: Anger control assistance and powerlessness may be appropriate foci for therapeutic work but are not the priority. Option 3: Risk for trauma implies accidental injury, which is

299

not the case for the client with borderline personality disorder.

Cognitive level: Analysis
Nursing process: Diagnosis
NCLEX: Safe and Effective Care Environment
See text page: 287

38. A client with borderline personality disorder has been hospitalized several times after self-mutilating episodes and suicide attempts. The client has entered dialectical behavior therapy on an outpatient basis. During therapy, the advanced practice nurse has been counseling her regarding self-harm behavior management. Today the client called the nurse and reported that she is "feeling empty and anxious" and wants to cut her arms. The nurse should
   1. arrange for emergency in-patient hospitalization.
   2. send her to the crisis intervention unit for 8 to 12 hours.
   3. assist the client to identify the trigger situation and choose a coping strategy.
   4. advise the client to take an anxiolytic to decrease anxiety level and go to sleep.

Answer: 3
Rationale: The client has responded appropriately to the urge to harm herself by calling a helping individual. A component of dialectical behavior therapy is telephone access to the therapist for "coaching" during crises. The nurse can assist the client to choose an alternative to self-mutilation. Options 1 and 2: The need for a protective environment may not be necessary if the client is able to use cognitive strategies to determine a coping strategy that will reduce the urge to mutilate. Option 4: Taking a sedative and going to sleep should not be the first-line intervention because sedation may reduce the client's ability to weigh alternatives to mutilating behavior.

Cognitive level: Application
Nursing process: Implementation
NCLEX: Safe and Effective Care Environment
See text pages: 293, 295

39. A client with borderline personality disorder has been hospitalized several times after self-mutilating episodes and suicide attempts. The client has entered dialectical behavior therapy on an outpatient basis. During the sessions the client reveals she is mildly depressed and angry with the way her life is going. The psychiatrist suggests use of medication. For which type of medication should the nurse prepare a teaching plan?
   1. Selective serotonin reuptake inhibitors (SSRIs)
   2. Antipsychotics

3. Benzodiazepines
4. Monoamine oxidase inhibitors

Answer: 1
Rationale: SSRIs are used to treat depression. Many clients with borderline personality disorder are fearful of taking something over which they have little control. The presence of side effects makes medications even more objectionable. Because SSRIs have a good side-effect profile, the client is more likely to comply with the medication. Options 2 and 3: Low-dose antipsychotics or anxiolytics are not supported by the data given in the scenario. Option 4: Monoamine oxidase inhibitors require great diligence in adherence to a restricted diet and are therefore rarely used for clients who are impulsive.

Cognitive level: Application
Nursing process: Planning
NCLEX: Health Promotion and Maintenance
See text page: 293

40. A teacher comes to the mental health clinic saying a co-worker recently confronted her about behaviors that are annoying to other co-workers. Because of the confrontation, the client has experienced moderate to severe levels of anxiety. The co-worker told the client that others find her very difficult because she is a perfectionist and micromanages the tasks of others on the teaching team, always demanding that things should be done according to her plans. The co-worker mentioned that the client made everyone feel as though everything they tried was inadequate, and that her co-workers feel frustrated and angry about her need to control. The client states she likes her co-workers and only wanted to help them be successful. The nurse realizes the client's behaviors are most consistent with
   1. obsessive-compulsive personality disorder.
   2. narcissistic personality disorder.
   3. histrionic personality disorder.
   4. schizoid personality disorder.

Answer: 1
Rationale: The need to control at the expense of flexibility and openness, along with patterns of preoccupation with orderliness and perfectionism, is consistent with obsessive-compulsive personality disorder. Option 2: Narcissistic personality disorder involves grandiosity, the need for admiration, and lack of empathy. Option 3: Histrionic personality disorder involves excessive emotionality and attention seeking. Option 4: Schizoid personality disorder involves detachment from social relationships and a restricted range of expression in interpersonal settings.

Cognitive level: Application

300

Nursing process: Assessment
NCLEX: Psychosocial Integrity
See text page: 285

CHAPTER 17

1. A client, age 18 years, is referred to the mental health center by the primary care physician. The following history is given. The client and her mother began to visit colleges to which the client had applied. When not traveling, the client spent the summer cooking gourmet meals for her family. Eventually, the mother noticed that the client was eating only tiny portions of the food, saying she wasn't hungry because she had tasted while she cooked. She began wearing several layers of loose clothing, saying she liked the style. At summer's end the client had a physical examination for the school sports program. Her weight had dropped from 130 to 95 pounds and she had amenorrhea. The history and symptoms are most consistent with the medical diagnosis of
   1. anorexia nervosa.
   2. bulimia nervosa.
   3. binge eating.
   4. eating disorder not otherwise specified.

Answer: 1
Rationale: Overcontrol of eating behaviors, extreme weight loss, amenorrhea, preoccupation with food, and wearing several layers of loose clothing to appear larger are part of the clinical picture of an individual with anorexia nervosa. Option 2: The bulimic individual usually is near normal weight. Option 3: The binge eater is often overweight. Option 4: The client with eating disorder not otherwise specified may be obese.
Cognitive level: Analysis
Nursing process: Assessment
NCLEX: Psychosocial Integrity/Physiological Integrity
See text page: 302

2. A client, age 18 years, is referred to the mental health center by the primary care physician. The following history is given. The client and her mother began to visit colleges to which the client had applied. When not traveling, the client spent the summer cooking gourmet meals for her family. Eventually, the mother noticed that the client was eating only tiny portions of the food, saying she wasn't hungry because she had tasted while she cooked. She began wearing several layers of loose clothing, saying she liked the style. At summer's end the client had a physical examination for the school sports program. Her weight had dropped

from 130 to 95 pounds and she had amenorrhea. The psychiatric nurse clinical specialist focused on the client's feelings about her role in choosing a college as well as concerns about assuming an autonomous adult role as she prepared for college. The theory of the etiology of eating disorders that guides the nurse is the
   1. psychological model.
   2. sociocultural model.
   3. multidimensional model.
   4. neurobiological model.

Answer: 1
Rationale: One psychological model (Bruch) suggests that girls who develop anorexia perceive themselves as ineffectual, passive, and unable to assert their will. Efforts to separate and lead an autonomous life lead to self-starvation and a distorted sense of being powerful. Option 2: The sociocultural model focuses on cultural factors that lead to efforts to restrict weight. Option 3: The multidimensional model does not exist. Option 4: The neurobiological model focuses neuroendocrine causation.
Cognitive level: Application
Nursing process: Assessment
NCLEX: Psychosocial Integrity
See text page: 301

3. A client referred to the eating disorders clinic has lost 35 pounds during a summer spent looking at colleges and cooking gourmet meals for her family. She was referred by her physician, who was alarmed by her weight loss. To assess the client's eating patterns, the nurse should ask
   1. "Do you often feel fat?"
   2. "Who plans the family meals?"
   3. "What do you eat in a typical day?"
   4. "What do you think about your present weight?"

Answer: 3
Rationale: Although all the questions might be appropriate to ask, only option 3 focuses on the client's eating patterns. Option 1 focuses on distortions in body image. Option 2 is unrelated to eating pattern. Option 4 explores the client's feelings about weight.
Cognitive level: Application
Nursing process: Assessment
NCLEX: Physiological Integrity
See text pages: 304, 307

4. A client referred to the eating disorders clinic has lost 35 pounds during the summer and has developed amenorrhea. Physical manifestations of anorexia nervosa for which the nurse should assess include (more than one answer may be correct)

1. peripheral edema.
2. parotid swelling.
3. constipation.
4. hypotension.
5. dental caries.
6. lanugo.

Answers: 1, 3, 4, 6

Rationale: Peripheral edema is often present because of hypoalbuminemia. Constipation related to starvation is often present. Hypotension is often present because of dehydration. Lanugo is often present and is related to starvation. Option 2: Parotid swelling is associated with bulimia. Option 5: Dental caries are associated with bulimia.

Cognitive level: Application
Nursing process: Assessment
NCLEX: Physiological Integrity
See text page: 302

5. A client referred to the eating disorders clinic has been diagnosed as having anorexia nervosa. History reveals she virtually stopped eating 5 months ago and has lost 25% of her body weight. When the nurse questions her about her present weight and what she thinks about her appearance, the response that would be most consistent with the medical diagnosis is
   1. "I'm fat and ugly."
   2. "What I think about myself is my business."
   3. "I'm grossly underweight, but thin is interesting."
   4. "I'm a few pounds overweight, but I can live with it."

Answer: 1

Rationale: Untreated clients with anorexia nervosa do not recognize their thinness. They perceive themselves to be overweight and unattractive. Option 2: The client with anorexia will usually tell people perceptions of self. Option 3: The client with anorexia does not recognize his or her thinness. Option 4: The client with anorexia does not recognize the thinness and will persist in trying to lose more weight.

Cognitive level: Analysis
Nursing process: Assessment
NCLEX: Psychosocial Integrity
See text page: 302

6. A client referred to the eating disorders clinic has been diagnosed as having anorexia nervosa. History reveals she virtually stopped eating 5 months ago and has lost 25% of her body weight. Lab tests reveal hypokalemia. On the basis of what is currently known about the client, the nursing diagnosis that can be established is

1. adult failure to thrive related to abuse of laxatives, as evidenced by electrolyte imbalances.
2. disturbed energy field related to physical exertion in excess of energy produced through caloric intake, as evidenced by weight loss.
3. ineffective health maintenance related to self-induced vomiting, as evidenced by swollen parotid glands.
4. imbalanced nutrition: less than body requirements related to refusal to eat, as evidenced by loss of 25% of body weight.

Answer: 4

Rationale: The client's history supports this nursing diagnosis. Options 1, 2, and 3: Data are not present that the client uses laxatives, induces vomiting, or exercises excessively.

Cognitive level: Analysis
Nursing process: Diagnosis
NCLEX: Physiological Integrity
See text page: 307

7. A client has been diagnosed with anorexia nervosa. She will be treated as an outpatient. A desired outcome related to the nursing diagnosis of "imbalanced nutrition: less than body requirements" would be that within 1 week, the client will
   1. gain 1 pound.
   2. gain 3 pounds.
   3. exercise 1 hour daily.
   4. take a laxative every 3 days.

Answer: 1

Rationale: Only option 1 can be accomplished within 1 week when the client is an outpatient. Option 2: Greater weight gain may be an outcome with hospitalization. Options 3 and 4 are not desirable.

Cognitive level: Application
Nursing process: Planning (Outcome Identification)
NCLEX: Physiological Integrity
See text page: 308

8. What nursing intervention should be planned related to the outcome that a client with anorexia nervosa will gain 1 to 2 pounds per week?
   1. Assessing for depression and suicidal ideation
   2. Observing for adverse side effects of refeeding
   3. Communicating empathy for the client's feelings
   4. Directing the client to balance energy expenditure and caloric intake

Answer: 2

Rationale: The nursing intervention of observing for adverse side effects of refeeding most directly relates to the goal of weight gain. Options 1 and 3 would re-

late to goals dealing with coping. Option 4 is an inappropriate intervention.
Cognitive level: Application
Nursing process: Planning
NCLEX: Physiological Integrity
See text page: 308

9. A client with anorexia nervosa is particularly resistant to the idea of weight gain. What is the rationale for establishing a contract with the client in which she agrees to participate in measures designed to produce a specified weekly weight gain?
   1. Because severe anxiety concerning eating is to be expected, objective and subjective data must be routinely collected.
   2. A team approach to planning the diet ensures that physical and emotional needs will be met.
   3. Client involvement in decision making increases sense of control and promotes compliance with treatment.
   4. Because of increased risk of physical problems with refeeding, client permission is essential.

Answer: 3
Rationale: A sense of control for the client is vital to the success of therapy. A diet that controls weight gain can allay client fears of too-rapid weight gain. Option 1: Data collection is not the reason for contracting. Option 2: A team approach is wise but is not a guarantee that needs will be met. Option 4: Permission for treatment is a separate issue. The contract for weight gain is an additional aspect of treatment.
Cognitive level: Application
Nursing process: Planning
NCLEX: Psychosocial Integrity
See text page: 314

10. The nursing care plan contains the direction "observe for refeeding syndrome." The nurse should closely monitor for complications associated with
    1. renal dysfunction.
    2. central nervous system dysfunction.
    3. endocrine dysfunction.
    4. cardiovascular dysfunction.

Answer: 4
Rationale: Refeeding resulting in too-rapid weight gain can overwhelm the heart, resulting in cardiovascular collapse; thus focused assessment becomes a necessity to ensure client physiological integrity. The other body systems are not initially involved in the refeeding syndrome.
Cognitive level: Application
Nursing process: Assessment

NCLEX: Physiological Integrity
See text page: 308

11. The psychiatric clinical nurse specialist decides to use cognitive therapy techniques as she works with a client with anorexia nervosa. Which statement by the nurse is consistent with the use of cognitive therapy principles?
    1. "What are your feelings about not eating the food that you prepare?"
    2. "You seem to feel much better about yourself when you eat something."
    3. "It must be difficult to talk about private matters to someone you just met."
    4. "Being thin doesn't seem to solve your problems; you're thin now and are still unhappy."

Answer: 4
Rationale: Option 4 is the only strategy that attempts to question the client's distorted thinking.
Cognitive level: Application
Nursing process: Implementation
NCLEX: Psychosocial Integrity
See text page: 309

12. A 20-year-old college student who transferred from a community college in her hometown to a university 100 miles from home had been emotionally close to her mother and sister. When she transferred she broke up with her boyfriend of 2 years. She was slow to make new friends at the university. Gradually, she began to eat whenever she felt blue. She consumed large quantities of food nightly and then induced vomiting. The binge-purge cycles continued until they began to interfere with her schoolwork. She sought help from the university health clinic. During the initial interview, what other issue should the nurse address in addition to the binge-purge syndrome?
    1. Study habits
    2. School activities
    3. Losses
    4. Student aid

Answer: 3
Rationale: The client has a significant history of losses: her mother and sister are no longer available as supports, and she has terminated the relationship with her boyfriend. Feelings of loss and depression are often associated with bulimia. The other options are of lesser relevance.
Cognitive level: Application
Nursing process: Assessment
NCLEX: Psychosocial Integrity
See text pages: 300, 301

303

13. What behavior might signal that the nurse treating a client with bulimia nervosa is experiencing rescue feelings?
1. The nurse's comments are nonjudgmental.
2. The nurse refers the client to a self-help group for individuals with eating disorders.
3. The nurse teaches the client to recognize signs of increasing anxiety and ways to intervene.
4. The nurse assesses the client's problem as poor eating habits and gives her a diet to follow.

Answer: 4
Rationale: Rescue feelings stem from the nurse's wish to take over for or control a client who is recognized by the nurse as feeling out of control. When a nurse experiences rescue feelings, the nurse tries to provide simple answers rather than use a problem-solving approach and focus on the client's feelings of shame and low self-esteem. The other options reflect appropriate interventions that do not signal a particular need for supervision.
Cognitive level: Application
Nursing process: Assessment
NCLEX: Safe and Effective Care Environment
See text page: 307

14. A nursing diagnosis formulated for a client with bulimia nervosa was ineffective coping related to feelings of loneliness and isolation, as evidenced by use of overeating as a comfort measure followed by self-induced vomiting. The outcome related to this nursing diagnosis is that within 2 weeks the client will
1. appropriately express angry feelings.
2. verbalize two positive things about self.
3. verbalize the importance of eating a balanced diet.
4. identify two alternative methods of coping with loneliness and isolation.

Answer: 4
Rationale: The outcome of identifying alternative coping strategies is most directly related to the diagnosis of ineffective coping. The other options are outcomes that might be used for other nursing diagnoses.
Cognitive level: Application
Nursing process: Planning (Outcome Identification)
NCLEX: Psychosocial Integrity
See text page: 312

15. Which nursing intervention is of highest priority for a client with bulimia nervosa?
1. Assist the client in identifying triggers to binge eating
2. Provide remedial consequences for weight loss
3. Assess for signs of impulsive eating
4. Explore needs for health teaching

Answer: 1
Rationale: For most clients with bulimia nervosa, certain situations trigger the urge to binge. Purging then follows bingeing. Often the triggers are anxiety-producing situations. Identification of triggers makes it possible to break the binge-purge cycle. Because binge eating and purging directly affect physical status, the need to promote physical safety assumes highest priority.
Cognitive level: Analysis
Nursing process: Planning
NCLEX: Psychosocial Integrity
See text pages: 316, 317

16. A client is an outpatient at the eating disorders clinic. Her diagnosis is eating disorder not otherwise specified, related to binge eating. Her friend told the nurse "I can't believe she's so heavy. When we're together, I never see her eat." This alerts the nurse to the possibility that the client engages in the eating behavior of
1. purging.
2. eating in secret.
3. excessive exercise.
4. use of eating rituals.

Answer: 2
Rationale: Binge eating most often occurs in secret. Options 1 and 3 are consistent with weight loss and thinness. Option 4: Rituals are not implicated by the friend's statement.
Cognitive level: Application
Nursing process: Assessment
NCLEX: Psychosocial Integrity
See text pages: 314, 315

17. An obese client with the diagnosis of eating disorder not otherwise specified, related to binge eating, had been under a great deal of stress at work. She worked long hours to make up for a staff shortage. When she went home, she propped her feet up in front of the television and ate until she went to bed. She felt too exhausted to exercise. She gained 25 pounds in 1 month. At 5 feet tall, she weighs 175 pounds. One of the desired outcomes for the client is to replace binge eating by recognizing the anxiety that precedes it and reducing the anxiety with a constructive strategy. Of the following interventions, which would address the outcome?
1. Teach stress reduction techniques such as relaxation and imagery.
2. Explore the client's need to single-handedly make up for a staff shortage.
3. Explore ways in which the client may feel in control of her environment.

4. Encourage the client to attend a support group such as Overeaters Anonymous.

Answer: 1

Rationale: Teaching alternative stress reduction techniques that may be substituted for overeating most directly addresses the goal of replacing binge eating with a constructive anxiety-releasing activity. The other options offer interventions that better relate to other outcomes.

Cognitive level: Application
Nursing process: Planning
NCLEX: Psychosocial Integrity
See text pages: 318-320

18. As a client admitted to the eating disorders unit undresses, she removes layer after layer of clothing. The nurse realizes that she is extremely thin. Her skin has a yellow cast, her hair is limp and dry, and her body is covered by fine, downy hair. Her weight is 70 pounds and her height is 5 feet 4 inches. The client remains quiet and sullen during the physical assessment. Which of the following should be recorded in the nurse's written documentation?
   1. Amenorrhea
   2. Alopecia
   3. Lanugo
   4. Stupor

Answer: 3

Rationale: The fine, downy hair noted by the nurse is called lanugo. It is frequently seen in clients with anorexia nervosa. None of the other conditions can be supported by the data the nurse has gathered.

Cognitive level: Application
Nursing process: Assessment
NCLEX: Physiological Integrity
See text page: 302

19. A client being admitted to the eating disorders unit has a yellow cast to her skin, her hair is limp and dry, and her body is covered by fine, downy hair. Her weight is 70 pounds and her height is 5 feet 4 inches. She remains quiet and sullen during the physical assessment, but does say "I don't intend to eat until I lose enough weight to look thin." An initial nursing diagnosis for the client would be
   1. disturbed body image related to weight loss.
   2. anxiety related to fear of weight gain.
   3. ineffective coping related to lack of conflict resolution skills.
   4. imbalanced nutrition: less than body requirements related to self-starvation.

Answer: 4

Rationale: The physical assessment by the nurse revealed cachexia; thus, the diagnosis of imbalanced nutrition. No defining characteristics support the other diagnoses.

Cognitive level: Analysis
Nursing process: Diagnosis
NCLEX: Physiological Integrity
See text page: 307

20. The nurse responsible for conducting group therapy on the eating disorders unit schedules the sessions immediately after meals for the primary purpose of
   1. promoting processing of anxiety associated with eating.
   2. shifting the clients' focus from food to psychotherapy.
   3. preventing the use of maladaptive behavior such as purging.
   4. focusing on weight control mechanisms and food preparation.

Answer: 1

Rationale: Eating produces high anxiety for all clients with eating disorders. Anxiety levels must be lowered if the client is to be successful in attaining therapeutic goals. Options 2 and 4 are not desirable. Option 3 is an outcome that is subsumed under the primary purpose.

Cognitive level: Application
Nursing process: Planning
NCLEX: Safe and Effective Care Environment
See text pages: 308, 315-318

21. Nursing physical assessment of a bulimic client often reveals
   1. prominent parotid glands.
   2. peripheral edema.
   3 thin, brittle hair.
   4. amenorrhea.

Answer: 1

Rationale: Prominent parotid glands are associated with repeated vomiting. The other options are signs of anorexia nervosa and are not usually seen in bulimia.

Cognitive level: Application
Nursing process: Assessment
NCLEX: Physiological Integrity
See text page: 311

22. From a cognitive perspective, the characteristic the nurse is most likely to assess in a client with an eating disorder is
   1. carefree flexibility.
   2. open displays of emotion.
   3. rigidity, perfectionism.
   4. high spirits and optimism.

Answer: 3

Chapter 17   Eating Disorders

Rationale: Rigid thinking, inability to demonstrate flexibility, and difficulty changing cognitions are characteristic of clients with eating disorders. Each of the other options is rarely seen in a client with an eating disorder, for which inflexibility, controlled emotions, and pessimism are more the rule.

Cognitive level: Application
Nursing process: Assessment
NCLEX: Psychosocial Integrity
See text page: 309

23. Assuming all data have been collected for a client with an eating disorder, which item signals to the nurse that the client should be hospitalized for treatment?
  1. Pulse less than 60 beats/min
  2. Weight 15% below ideal weight
  3. Urine output less than 30 mL/hr
  4. Serum potassium 3.4 mEq/L

Answer: 3

Rationale: Severely reduced urinary output indicates dehydration, reduced kidney function, or retention caused by cardiac malfunction. Option 1: Many normal people have bradycardia. Option 2: Weight loss of more than 30% of ideal body weight would call for hospitalization. Option 4: This potassium level is within the normal range.

Cognitive level: Analysis
Nursing process: Assessment
NCLEX: Physiological Integrity
See text page: 304

24. The statement the nurse is most likely to hear during an interview session from a client with an eating disorder is
  1. "I'm thin for my height."
  2. "I'm fat and ugly."
  3. "I have nice eyes."
  4. "My mother is very attuned to my needs."

Answer: 2

Rationale: Clients with eating disorders have distorted body images and usually see themselves as overweight, even when their weight is woefully subnormal. Option 1 is therefore incorrect. Option 3: Poor self-image precludes making positive statements about self. Option 4: Many clients with eating disorders see supportive others as intrusive and out of tune with their needs.

Cognitive level: Application
Nursing process: Assessment
NCLEX: Psychosocial Integrity
See text page: 309

25. The nursing diagnosis more relevant for a client with anorexia nervosa who restricts intake and is 20% below normal weight than for a 130-pound client with bulimia nervosa who purges is
  1. powerlessness.
  2. disturbed body image.
  3. imbalanced nutrition: less than body requirements.
  4. ineffective coping.

Answer: 3

Rationale: The client with bulimia nervosa usually maintains a close-to-normal weight, whereas the client with anorexia nervosa may approach starvation. Options 1, 2, and 4 may be appropriate for clients with either anorexia nervosa or bulimia nervosa.

Cognitive level: Analysis
Nursing process: Diagnosis
NCLEX: Physiological Integrity
See text page: 307

26. The theme that might be expected to occur during family therapy with two parents, two siblings, and a teen client with anorexia nervosa who engages in provocative behaviors is
  1. building stable coalitions.
  2. interpreting negative messages as positive.
  3. competition of the client with the father.
  4. lack of trust in the client by the family.

Answer: 4

Rationale: The theme of lack of trust in the client by the family is frequently noted when the client does provocative things such as going to the bathroom and remaining there after meals. The client is unable to fathom the concern of the family about possible purging behaviors. Option 1: The client frequently shifts coalitions. Option 2: The client perceives positive messages as negative. Option 3: The client usually competes with the mother.

Cognitive level: Application
Nursing process: Assessment
NCLEX: Psychosocial Integrity
See text page: 310

27. When the nurse finds a client with anorexia nervosa vigorously exercising before she has gained the agreed-on weekly weight gain, the nurse should state
  1. "It bothers me to see you exercising. You'll lose more weight."
  2. "You and I will have to sit down and discuss this problem."
  3. "According to our agreement, no exercising is permitted until you have gained a specific amount of weight."
  4. "Let's discuss the relation between exercise and weight loss and how that affects your body."

306

Answer: 3

Rationale: Treatment plans have specific goals for weight restoration. Exercise is limited to promote weight gain. Clients must be held accountable for required behaviors.

Cognitive level: Application
Nursing process: Implementation
NCLEX: Physiological Integrity
See text page: 312

28. When an anorexic client is admitted for treatment, the milieu should provide (more than one answer may be correct)
    1. flexible meal times.
    2. adherence to a selected menu.
    3. observation during and after meals.
    4. unscheduled weight checks.
    5. monitoring during bathroom trips.
    6. privileges correlated with affective display.

Answers: 2, 3, 5

Rationale: Priority milieu interventions support restoration of weight and normalization of eating patterns. This requires close supervision of the client's eating and prevention of exercise, purging, and so forth. Menus are strictly adhered to. Observation is maintained during and after meals to prevent throwing away food or purging. All trips to the bathroom are monitored. Option 1: Mealtimes are precisely observed, not flexible. Option 4: Weighing is performed on a regular schedule. Option 6: Privileges are correlated with weight gain and treatment plan compliance.

Cognitive level: Application
Nursing process: Implementation
NCLEX: Safe and Effective Care Environment
See text pages: 308, 309

29. Which statement made by a client with an eating disorder reflects understanding of the condition rather than a cognitive distortion?
    1. "Gaining 1 pound is as much of a disaster as gaining 100 pounds."
    2. "I was happy when I was a size 4, so I must diet to that size."
    3. "Bingeing is the only way I can soothe myself."
    4. "I've been coping with disappointment by overeating."

Answer: 4

Rationale: This statement reflects understanding of the condition. Cognitive distortions often used by clients with eating disorders include "catastrophizing" (option 1), overgeneralization (option 2), all-or-none thinking (option 3), personalization, and emotional reasoning.

Cognitive level: Application
Nursing process: Assessment
NCLEX: Psychosocial Integrity
See text page: 309

30. A client with anorexia nervosa being treated on an outpatient basis has begun refeeding. Between the first and second appointments the nurse assesses that the client has gained 8 pounds. The nurse should
    1. praise the client for the weight gain.
    2. assess lung sounds and extremities.
    3. suggest use of an exercise program.
    4. establish a higher target for weight gain for the next week.

Answer: 2

Rationale: Weight gain of more than 2 to 5 pounds weekly may overwhelm the heart's capacity to pump, leading to cardiac failure. The nurse must assess for signs of pulmonary edema and congestive heart failure. The other options are undesirable because they increase the risk for cardiac complications.

Cognitive level: Application
Nursing process: Assessment
NCLEX: Physiological Integrity
See text pages: 315-318

31. Which statement made by the mother of a teen with anorexia nervosa would signal the nurse that teaching needs exist?
    1. "Will treatment affect her number one standing on the gymnastics team?"
    2. "We'll find the money for family counseling if it is needed."
    3. "The entire family has benefited from improved eating habits."
    4. "We'll work out our differences without getting into power struggles."

Answer: 1

Rationale: This remark suggests the mother places a high value on her child's gymnastics standing, which to a great extent depends on thinness. The other options suggest thinking synchronous with therapeutic goals.

Cognitive level: Analysis
Nursing process: Assessment
NCLEX: Psychosocial Integrity
See text page: 310

32. While providing health teaching for a client with binge-purge bulimia nervosa, the nurse should prioritize information about
    1. self-monitoring of daily food and fluid intake.
    2. establishing the desired daily weight gain.
    3. symptoms of hypokalemia.
    4. self-esteem maintenance.

Chapter 17   Eating Disorders

Answer: 3

Rationale: Hypokalemia results from potassium loss associated with vomiting. Physiological integrity can be maintained if the client can self-diagnose potassium deficiency and adjust the diet or seek medical assistance. Option 1: This option is not useful if the client purges. Option 2: Daily weight gain may not be desirable for a client with bulimia nervosa. Option 4: Self-esteem is an identifiable problem but is of lesser priority than the risk for hypokalemia.

Cognitive level: Application
Nursing process: Implementation
NCLEX: Physiological Integrity
See text pages: 316, 317

33. An appropriate intervention to undertake for a client with bulimia nervosa who binges and purges is to teach the client
   1. not to skip meals or restrict food.
   2. to eat a small meal after purging.
   3. eat a large breakfast but no lunch and concentrate intake after 4 PM.
   4. substitute laxative use once daily to replace induced vomiting.

Answer: 1

Rationale: One goal of health teaching is normalization of eating habits. Food restriction and skipping meals lead to rebound bingeing. Option 2 will probably perpetuate the need to induce vomiting. Option 3 will lead to late-day bingeing. Option 4 is highly undesirable.

Cognitive level: Application
Nursing process: Implementation
NCLEX: Health Promotion and Maintenance
See text pages: 312, 313

34. The statement by a nurse caring for a client with an eating disorder that signals a need for supervision is
   1. "I am working to encourage the client to be healthier."
   2. "I understand that the client is terrified of gaining weight."
   3. "The client's perfectionism and resistance often make me angry."
   4. "I have had to make sure I do not come across as a parent figure."

Answer: 3

Rationale: Frustration is common when client personality traits of perfectionism, obsessive thinking, and the need to control therapy are present. Anger and frustration signal a need for supervision. Options 1 and 4 are appropriate. Option 2 is empathetic and important to reflect to the client.

Cognitive level: Analysis
Nursing process: Assessment
NCLEX: Safe and Effective Care Environment
See text page: 307

35. One bed is available for admitting a client with an eating disorder. Of the following clients, who should be admitted? The client whose weight dropped from
   1. 150 to 100 pounds over a 4-months period, with the following vital signs: temperature, 35.9° C; pulse, 38 beats/min; blood pressure, 60/40 mm Hg.
   2. 120 to 90 pounds over a 3-month period, with the following vital signs: temperature, 36° C; pulse, 50 beats/min; blood pressure, 70/50 mm Hg.
   3. 110 to 70 pounds over a 4-month period, with the following vital signs: temperature 36.5° C; pulse, 60 beats/min; blood pressure, 80/66 mm Hg.
   4. 90 to 78 pounds over a 5-month period, with the following vital signs: temperature, 3;7° C; pulse, 62 beats/min; blood pressure, 74/48 mm Hg.

Answer: 1

Rationale: Physical criteria for hospitalization include weight loss of more than 30% of body weight within 6 months, temperature below 36° C (hypothermia), heart rate less than 40 beats/min, and systolic blood pressure less than 70 mm Hg.

Cognitive level: Analysis
Nursing process: Assessment
NCLEX: Physiological Integrity
See text page: 304

36. Disturbed body image has been established as a nursing diagnosis for a client with an eating disorder. The outcome indicator most appropriate to monitor is
   1. weight, muscle, and fat congruence with height, frame, age, and sex.
   2. calorie intake within required parameters of treatment plan.
   3. weight at established normal range for the client.
   4. client satisfaction with body appearance.

Answer: 4

Rationale: Body image disturbances are considered improved or resolved when the client is consistently satisfied with his or her own appearance and body function. This is a subjective consideration. The other indicators are more objective but less related to the nursing diagnosis.

Cognitive level: Application
Nursing process: Planning (Outcome Identification)
NCLEX: Psychosocial Integrity
See text page: 308

1. A client, age 56 years, became severely depressed when the last of her six children moved out of the home 4 months ago. Since then she has neglected to care for herself, lost weight, and repeatedly states "No one cares about me anymore." Before the onset of symptoms she had been a meticulous housekeeper, was neatly groomed, and often participated in community activities. She was noncompliant with tricyclic antidepressant therapy, so admission to the mental health unit was sought. After her admission, the client repeatedly tells nursing staff "No one cares about me. I'm not worth anything." A helpful response by the nurse would be
 1. "I care about you, and I want to try to help you get better."
 2. "Things will look brighter soon. Everyone feels down once in a while."
 3. "It is difficult for others to care about you when you say the same negative things over and over."
 4. "I'll sit with you for 10 minutes, I'll return for 10 minutes at lunchtime, and again at 2:30 this afternoon."

Answer: 4

Rationale: Spending time with the client at intervals throughout the day shows acceptance by the nurse and will help the client establish a relationship with the nurse. Setting definite times for the therapeutic contacts and keeping the appointments shows predictability on the part of the nurse, an element that fosters trust building. Option 1 is difficult for a profoundly depressed person to believe. Option 2 provides trite reassurance. Option 3 is counterproductive. The client is essentially unable to say positive things at this point.

Cognitive level: Application
Nursing process: Implementation
NCLEX: Psychosocial Integrity
See text pages: 339, 400

2. A client, age 56 years, became severely depressed when the last of her six children moved out of the home 4 months ago. Since then she has neglected to care for herself, sleeps poorly, lost weight, and repeatedly states "No one cares about me anymore. I'm not worth anything." After hospitalization the nursing diagnosis of situational low self-esteem related to feelings of abandonment has been established. An appropriate intermediate outcome would be "Client will
 1. verbalize realistic positive things about self by (date)."
 2. agree to take antidepressant medication regularly by (date)."

 3. initiate social interaction with another person daily by (date)."
 4. identify two personal behaviors that might push others away by (date)."

Answer: 1

Rationale: Low self-esteem is reflected by making consistently negative statements about self and self-worth. Replacing negative cognitions with more realistic appraisals of self is an appropriate intermediate outcome. Option 2 should be a short-term outcome. Options 3 and 4 are not as clearly related to the nursing diagnosis.

Cognitive level: Analysis
Nursing process: Planning (Outcome Identification)
NCLEX: Psychosocial Integrity
See text page: 338

3. A client, age 56 years, became severely depressed when the last of her six children moved out of the home 4 months ago. Since then she has neglected to care for herself, sleeps poorly, lost weight, and repeatedly states "No one cares about me anymore. I'm not worth anything." After hospitalization the nursing diagnosis of situational low self-esteem related to feelings of abandonment was identified. The nurse wishes to reinforce the client's self-esteem by acknowledging the improvement in her personal appearance. She's wearing a new dress and has combed her hair. The most appropriate remark would be
 1. "You look nice this morning."
 2. "I like the dress you're wearing."
 3. "What brought about this glamorous transformation?"
 4. "You're wearing a new dress."

Answer: 4

Rationale: Depressed clients usually see the negative side of things. The meaning of compliments may be altered to "I didn't look nice yesterday" or "They didn't like my other dress." Neutral comments such as an observation avoid negative interpretations.

Cognitive level: Application
Nursing process: Implementation
NCLEX: Psychosocial Integrity
See text page: 340

4. A client, age 56 years, became severely depressed when the last of her six children moved out of the home 4 months ago. Since then she has neglected to care for herself, sleeps poorly, lost weight, and repeatedly states "No one cares about me anymore. I'm not worth anything." An inappropriate intervention to include in the client's care plan is

1. observe and record sleep pattern nightly.
2. weigh weekly and observe eating patterns.
3. monitor bowel movements daily and evaluate need for laxatives.
4. provide activities that involve concentration and fine motor skills.

Answer: 4

Rationale: The activities that should be provided for a severely depressed client call for minimal concentration and involve gross motor skills rather than fine motor skills.

The other interventions related to physiological integrity are appropriate.

Cognitive level: Application
Nursing process: Planning
NCLEX: Physiological Integrity
See text page: 339

5. Planned interventions for a severely depressed client should include
   1. allowing the client to remain alone if he or she prefers.
   2. careful unobtrusive observation around the clock.
   3. encouraging the client to spend a major portion of each day in bed.
   4. opportunities to assume a leadership role in the therapeutic milieu.

Answer: 2

Rationale: Approximately two thirds of depressed people contemplate suicide. Depressed clients who exhibit feelings of worthlessness are at higher risk. Regular planned observations of the depressed client may prevent a suicide attempt on the unit.

Cognitive level: Application
Nursing process: Planning
NCLEX: Physiological Integrity
See text page: 339

6. Making use of evidence-based research, the advanced practice nurse who provides counseling to severely depressed clients should choose to address the negative thought patterns of these clients by using
   1. psychoanalytic therapy.
   2. desensitization therapy.
   3. cognitive behavioral therapy.
   4. alternative and complementary therapies.

Answer: 3

Rationale: Cognitive behavioral therapy attempts to alter the client's dysfunctional beliefs by focusing on positive outcomes rather than negative attributions. The client is also taught the connection between thoughts and resultant feelings. Research shows that cognitive behavioral therapy involves the formation of new connections between nerve cells in the brain and that it is at least as effective as medication. Evidence is not present to support superior outcomes for the other psychotherapeutic modalities mentioned.

Cognitive level: Application
Nursing process: Planning
NCLEX: Psychosocial Integrity
See text page: 341

7. The feelings most commonly experienced by a nurse working with a depressed client include
   1. a sense of satisfaction in seeing rapid improvement of client mood.
   2. gratification when client appreciation is openly expressed.
   3. frustration with client resistance.
   4. disinterest in client situation.

Answer: 3

Rationale: Depressed clients often seem to reject the overtures of staff and seem to resist change despite the nurse's best efforts. Feelings of anxiety, frustration, incompetence, and even helplessness may be engendered in the nurse. Supervision can help the nurse develop realistic expectations for the client and the nurse. Options 1 and 2: Pleasurable feelings are rarely the outcome of working with a depressed client. Option 4: Withdrawal and disinterest in the client on the part of the nurse are attributable to frustration with the client.

Cognitive level: Comprehension
Nursing process: Assessment
NCLEX: Safe and Effective Care Environment
See text pages: 336, 337

8. A nurse can deal preventively with the potential for experiencing negative feelings while working with a severely depressed client by (more than one response may be correct)
   1. understanding the part neurotransmitters play in depression.
   2. establishing realistic expectations for the client and self.
   3. focusing as little as possible on feelings toward the client.
   4. disregarding empathic information originating in the client.

Answers: 1, 2

Rationale: Understanding that neurotransmitter dysfunction is a greater causative factor in client depressive symptoms than client choice makes what appears to be client resistance less personal. Keeping expectations realistic decreases feelings of helplessness and contributes to the maintenance of self-esteem.

Option 3: Self-assessment of feelings toward the client is appropriate and necessary. Option 4: Awareness of empathic messaging originating in the client is essential because it is a clue to what the client is experiencing.
Cognitive level: Application
Nursing process: Implementation
NCLEX: Safe and Effective Care Environment
See text pages: 336, 337

9. A depressed client who is taking a tricyclic antidepressant tells the nurse "I don't think I can keep taking these pills. They make me very dizzy, especially when I stand up." The nurse should
   1. explain how to mange hypotension and reassure that side effects go away after several weeks.
   2. tell the client that the side effects are a minor inconvenience compared with feelings of depression.
   3. withhold the drug and have the physician examine the client.
   4. perform a mental status examination on the client.

Answer: 1
Rationale: Drowsiness, dizziness, and postural hypotension usually subside after the first few weeks of therapy with tricyclic antidepressants. Postural hypotension can be managed by teaching the client to stay well hydrated and rise slowly. Knowing these facts may be enough to convince the client to remain medication compliant. Option 2 would not be a convincing reason to remain on the medication. Option 3 is unnecessary. Independent nursing action is called for. Option 4 is unnecessary.
Cognitive level: Application
Nursing process: Implementation
NCLEX: Physiological Integrity
See text page: 348

10. A depressed client is receiving imipramine (Tofranil) 300 mg daily. The side effect of this drug for which the nurse should seek medical attention for the client is
    1. dry mouth.
    2. blurred vision.
    3. nasal congestion.
    4. urinary retention.

Answer: 4
Rationale: All the side effects mentioned are the result of the anticholinergic effects of the drug. Only urinary retention and severe constipation warrant immediate medical attention. Bethanechol may be given to promote urination, or urinary catheterization may be necessary. Dry mouth, blurred vision, and nasal congestion may be less troublesome as therapy continues.

Cognitive level: Application
Nursing process: Assessment
NCLEX: Physiological Integrity
See text pages: 345-348

11. A student nurse caring for a depressed client reads in the client's medical record: "This client clearly shows the vegetative signs of depression." The nursing diagnoses that most clearly relate to the vegetative signs include (more than one answer may be correct)
    1. imbalanced nutrition: less than body requirements.
    2. chronic low self-esteem.
    3. disturbed sleep pattern.
    4. sexual dysfunction.
    5. self-care deficit.
    6. constipation.

Answer: 1, 3, 4, 5, 6
Rationale: Vegetative signs of depression are alterations in body processes necessary to support life and growth, such as eating, sleeping, elimination, and sexual activity. These diagnoses are more closely related to vegetative signs than diagnoses associated with feelings about self (option 2).
Cognitive level: Application
Nursing process: Assessment
NCLEX: Physiological Integrity
See text page: 338

12. When the spouse of a client diagnosed with dysthymia asks what the major difference is between dysthymia and major depressive disorder, the nurse can point out that in major depressive disorder
    1. the symptoms persist for 2 or more years.
    2. evidence of an earlier hypomanic episode is present.
    3. evidence of persistent suicidal ideation is always present.
    4. the client does not give a history of feeling depressed for years.

Answer: 4
Rationale: Dysthymia is characterized by a chronic depressive syndrome usually present for many years. The depressive mood disturbance cannot be distinguished from the person's usual pattern of functioning. Option 1: Persistence of symptoms occurs in dysthymia. Option 2: This is true of bipolar disorder. Option 3: This is not universally true for major depressive disorder.
Cognitive level: Application
Nursing process: Implementation
NCLEX: Health Promotion and Maintenance
See text page: 329

311

13. A nurse working with a severely depressed client who displays withdrawn behavior and marked psychomotor retardation is at risk for feelings of
    1. overinvolvement.
    2. guilt and despair.
    3. interest and pleasure.
    4. incompetence and frustration.

Answer: 4

Rationale: Nurses may have expectations for self and clients that are not wholly realistic, especially regarding the client's progress toward health. Unmet expectations result in feelings of incompetence, anger, or frustration. Option 1: Nurses rarely become overinvolved with depressed clients because of the client's resistance. Option 2 might be seen when the nurse experiences client feelings as a result of empathy. Option 3: Interest is possible, but most nurses do not find working with depressed clients a pleasurable experience.

Cognitive level: Application
Nursing process: Assessment
NCLEX: Safe and Effective Care Environment
See text pages: 336, 337

14. Information given to a depressed client and family when the client begins selective serotonin reuptake inhibitor antidepressant therapy should include the directive to
    1. avoid exposure to bright sunlight.
    2. report increased suicidal thoughts.
    3. restrict sodium intake to 1 gm daily.
    4. maintain a tyramine-free diet.

Answer: 2

Rationale: Some evidence indicates that suicidal ideation may worsen at the beginning of antidepressant therapy; thus close monitoring is necessary. Options 1 and 3 are unnecessary. Option 4: Tyramine restriction is associated with monoamine oxidase inhibitor therapy.

Cognitive level: Application
Nursing process: Planning
NCLEX: Health Promotion and Maintenance
See text page: 342

15. A depressed client is to have his first electroconvulsive therapy session tomorrow morning. The interventions that would routinely be implemented in preparing the client for treatment include (more than one answer may be correct)
    1. administering pretreatment medication as ordered 30 to 45 minutes before treatment.
    2. withholding food and fluids for a minimum of 6 hours before treatment.

    3. removing dentures, glasses, contact lenses, and hearing aids.
    4. restraining the client in bed with padded limb restraints.

Answers: 1, 2, 3

Rationale: Options 1, 2, and 3 reflect routine electroconvulsive therapy preparation, which is similar to preoperative preparation: sedation and anticholinergic medication before anesthesia, maintaining nothing-by-mouth status to prevent aspiration during and after treatment, airway maintenance, and general safety by removal of prosthetic devices. Option 4: Restraint is not part of pretreatment protocol.

Cognitive level: Application
Nursing process: Implementation
NCLEX: Physiological Integrity
See text page: 351

16. A depressed client who is scheduled to receive electroconvulsive therapy this morning asks the nurse "How is this treatment supposed to help me?" The best reply would be "Electroconvulsive therapy
    1. probably increases the availability of brain neurotransmitters."
    2. makes you confused and you forget why you're feeling depressed."
    3. serves as a punishment so your own conscience can stop punishing you."
    4. works by opening your mind to learning and applying new coping skills."

Answer: 1

Rationale: This answer supports the biochemical theory of the cause of depression. The other remarks distort information from other etiological theories.

Cognitive level: Application
Nursing process: Implementation
NCLEX: Psychosocial Integrity
See text page: NA

17. The priority nursing interventions for the period immediately after electroconvulsive therapy treatment focus on
    1. establishing random eye movement latency.
    2. supporting physiological stability.
    3. reducing disorientation and confusion.
    4. assisting the client in identifying and testing negative cognitions.

Answer: 2

Rationale: During the immediate posttreatment period, the client is recovering from general anesthesia, hence the need to establish and support physiological stability. Option 1 is neither possible nor a priority. Option 3 is an acceptable intervention but not the priority.

Option 4 is inappropriate in the immediate posttreatment period because the client may be confused.

Cognitive level: Application
Nursing process: Implementation
NCLEX: Physiological Integrity
See text page: 351

18. A client is being treated for depression with phenelzine (Nardil). The indicator that would be useful to monitor the outcome "client will understand the potential side effects of monoamine oxidase inhibitor (MAOI) antidepressants" is that the client
1. wears supportive shoes.
2. elevates legs when sitting.
3. eats at Chinese restaurants.
4. avoids over-the-counter medications.

Answer: 4

Rationale: Over-the counter medicines may contain vasopressor agents or tyramine, a substance that must be avoided when the client takes MAOI antidepressants. Medications for colds, allergies, or congestion or any preparation that contains ephedrine, phenylephedrine, or phenylpropanolamine may precipitate a hypertensive crisis. Options 1 and 2: MAOI antidepressant therapy is unrelated to the need for specific shoe types or leg elevation. Option 3: This is undesirable. Chinese dishes often contain fermented soy products, which are high in tyramine. MAOIs interact with tyramine-containing foods to produce dangerously high blood pressure.

Cognitive level: Evaluation
Nursing process: Planning (Outcome Identification)
NCLEX: Physiological Integrity
See text pages: 349-351

19. A client who became severely depressed after losing her job tells the nurse that she is not worth the time the nurse spends with her. The client often mentions that she is "the worst person in the world." On the basis of these data, the nursing diagnosis that should be considered for this client is
1. powerlessness.
2. defensive coping.
2. situational low self-esteem.
3. disturbed personal identity.

Answer: 3

Rationale: The client's statements express feelings of worthlessness and most clearly relate to the nursing diagnosis of situational low self-esteem. Insufficient information exists to lead to other diagnoses.

Cognitive level: Analysis
Nursing process: Diagnosis
NCLEX: Psychosocial Integrity
See text pages: 337, 338

20. A severely depressed client shows vegetative signs of depression. Interventions to be implemented include (more than one answer may be correct)
1. monitoring food and fluid intake.
2. offering laxatives as needed.
3. providing a quiet sleep environment.
4. doubling the daily caffeine intake.
5. restricting intake of processed foods.

Answers: 1, 2, 3

Rationale: Options 1, 2, and 3 promote a normal elimination pattern. Option 4: Increasing the intake of stimulants such as caffeine may make the client feel jittery and anxious when the client is already feeling unwell. Option 5: No indication exists that processed foods should be restricted.

Cognitive level: Application
Nursing process: Planning
NCLEX: Physiological Integrity
See text page: NA

21. A depressed client does not converse except when addressed, and then only in monosyllables. The nurse wishes to show nonjudgmental acceptance and support for the client. This can best be done by
1. asking the client direct questions.
2. phrasing questions to require yes or no answers.
3. using platitudes to reduce guilt feelings.
4. stating observations.

Answer: 4

Rationale: Making observations about neutral topics such as the environment draws the client into the reality around him or her but places no burdensome expectations for answers on the client. Acceptance and support are shown by the nurse's presence. Option 1: Direct questions may make the client feel that the encounter is an interrogation. Option 2: Open-ended questions are preferable if the client is able to participate in dialogue. Option 3: Platitudes are never acceptable. They minimize client feelings and can increase feelings of worthlessness.

Cognitive level: Application
Nursing process: Implementation
NCLEX: Psychosocial Integrity
See text page: 340

22. If a nurse assesses that a profoundly depressed client has diurnal variation, a schedule should be planned that
1. calls for the client to be awakened early in the morning to participate in exercise.
2. places activities during the part of the day the client is most energetic.
3. permits the client freedom of choice.
4. concentrates activities after lunch.

313

Answer: 2

Rationale: Diurnal variation means the client feels better and has more energy at a certain time of the day. Activities should be planned for this period of higher functioning because the client is better able to participate at that time. Option 1: The client may not function optimally in the early morning. Option 3: Depressed clients usually need a schedule because decision making is difficult. Option 4: This may or may not coincide with client's period of higher functioning.

Cognitive level: Application
Nursing process: Planning
NCLEX: Physiological Integrity
See text page: 339

23. Which observations, if documented in the medical record, would indicate that the treatment plan of a severely depressed client has been effective?
    1. "Slept 6 hours uninterrupted, sang with activity group, anticipates seeing grandchild."
    2. "Slept 10 hours, attended craft group, stated his "project is a mess, just like me.""
    3. "Slept 5 hours, personal hygiene adequate with assistance, weight loss of 1 pound."
    4. "Slept 7 hours, states he feels tired all the time, preoccupied with perceived inadequacies."

Answer: 1

Rationale: Sleeping 6 hours, participating with a group, and anticipating an event are all positive events. All the other options show at least one negative finding.

Cognitive level: Analysis
Nursing process: Evaluation
NCLEX: Psychosocial Integrity/Physiological Integrity
See text page: 353

24. An appropriate nursing intervention for an agitated, depressed client who paces the corridor hour after hour is to
    1. restrain the client in a chair.
    2. seclude the client as needed.
    3. provide a simple monotonous task.
    4. explain that pacing produces fatigue.

Answer: 3

Rationale: Providing a simple monotonous task may reduce the amount of pacing. Options 1 and 2: Restraint and seclusion are punitive. Option 4: Explanations may not be comprehended when concentration is poor.

Cognitive level: Application
Nursing process: Implementation
NCLEX: Physiological Integrity
See text page: 339

25. A depressed client repeatedly tells staff that he's a bad person and that he has cancer. Diagnostic tests reveal no cancer. The priority nursing diagnosis for this client would be
    1. social isolation.
    2. risk for self-directed violence.
    3. impaired verbal communication.
    4. ineffective health maintenance.

Answer: 2

Rationale: A depressed client who feels so worthless that she believes she deserves cancer is at risk for suicide. The nursing diagnosis of risk for self-directed violence takes priority over the other diagnoses listed.

Cognitive level: Analysis
Nursing process: Diagnosis
NCLEX: Safe and Effective Care Environment
See text page: 338

26. Which beverage available on the unit should the nurse select for a between-meal supplement for a depressed client with a nursing diagnosis of imbalanced nutrition: less than body requirements when the client refuses solid food?
    1. Tomato juice
    2. Orange juice
    3. Hot tea
    4. Milk

Answer: 4

Rationale: Milk is the only beverage listed that provides protein, fat, and carbohydrates. In addition, milk is fortified with vitamins.

Cognitive level: Application
Nursing process: Implementation
NCLEX: Physiological Integrity
See text page: 341

27. Of the following clients on a medical-surgical unit, which one should be observed most closely by staff for symptoms of depression?
    1. L, age 36 years, married, diagnosis of laparoscopic cholecystectomy
    2. M, age 42 years, single, diagnosis of postoperative bilateral vein ligation
    3. T, age 24 years, married, diagnosis of infectious hepatitis
    4. C, age 38 years, divorced, diagnosis of testicular carcinoma

Answer: 4

Rationale: This client has an illness with a high component of associated loss and is likely to be at greatest risk for depression and suicidal ideation.

314

Cognitive level: Analysis
Nursing process: Assessment
NCLEX: Safe and Effective Care Environment
See text page: 331

28. A disheveled, severely depressed client with psychomotor retardation has not showered for several days. The nurse should
   1. avoid forcing the issue.
   2. firmly and neutrally assist the client to shower.
   3. calmly tell the client that he or she must shower or be secluded.
   4. bring the issue up at the community meeting.

Answer: 2
Rationale: When clients are unable to perform self-care activities, staff must assist them rather than ignore the issue (option 1). Being better groomed increases self-esteem. Options 3 and 4 are punitive.
Cognitive level: Application
Nursing process: Implementation
NCLEX: Psychosocial Integrity
See text page: 341

29. During assessment, the nurse is most likely to find the attitude of the depressed client toward his illness to be
   1. "It's just a matter of time and I'll be well."
   2. "If I ignore this, it will go away."
   3. "I can fight this and lick it."
   4. "I deserve to be this way."

Answer: 4
Rationale: Depressed clients feel worthless and often believe they deserve to have "bad" things happen. Option 1: Depressed clients are usually hopeless. Option 2: Depressed clients are not optimistic. Option 3: Depressed clients usually feel helpless.
Cognitive level: Application
Nursing process: Assessment
NCLEX: Psychosocial Integrity
See text pages: 334-336

30. A depressed client is being seen in the clinic and treated with selective serotonin reuptake inhibitors (SSRIs). She tells the nurse that she has some pills that she previously took for depression and that they are called MAOIs. She tells the nurse she thinks she should start taking them right now instead of her current medication. The most important information the nurse should convey is
   1. the need to have her blood pressure carefully monitored.
   2. that the SSRI antidepressant will be more effective as the weeks go by.
   3. the dietary restrictions required to take MAOIs.
   4. the risk of a serious reaction if she stops the SSRIs and begins the MAOIs.

Answer: 4
Rationale: The client is at risk for a hypertensive crisis if she takes MAOIs and SSRIs without an appropriate washout period. The duration of the washout period is determined by the half-life of the SSRI. The other options are of lesser relevance.
Cognitive level: Application
Nursing process: Implementation
NCLEX: Health Promotion and Maintenance
See text pages: 349-351

31. A client being treated for major depression is the CEO of her own business. She has received 12 electroconvulsive therapy sessions and has remained in the hospital 4 days after the last treatment while her SSRI dose was being adjusted. The client has been counseled not to make a major business decision for a month. The rationale for this counseling is that
   1. SSRIs may cause confusion related to the limitation of tyramine in the diet.
   2. SSRIs alter catecholamine levels, causing recurrent depressive symptoms.
   3. the client may have temporary memory impairment associated with electroconvulsive therapy.
   4. the client needs time to reorient to a pressured work schedule.

Answer: 3
Rationale: Recent memory impairment is often present during and for a short time after electroconvulsive therapy. An inappropriate business decision might be made because of forgotten important details. Options 1 and 2 are untrue statements. Option 4 is less relevant than option 3.
Cognitive level: Application
Nursing process: Implementation
NCLEX: Health Promotion and Maintenance
See text page: 351

32. A nurse teaching a client about a tyramine-restricted diet would approve a meal consisting of
   1. mashed potatoes, ground beef patty, corn, green beans, and apple pie.
   2. avocado salad, ham, creamed potatoes, asparagus, and chocolate cake.
   3. noodles with cheddar cheese sauce, smoked sausage, lettuce salad, and yeast rolls.
   4. macaroni and cheese, hot dogs, banana bread, and caffeinated coffee.

315

Answer: 1

Rationale: This meal contains little tyramine. Vegetables and fruits contain little or no tyramine, and fresh ground beef and apple pie should be safe. The other meals contain various amounts of tyramine-rich foods or foods that contain vasopressors: avocados, ripe bananas (banana bread), sausages/hot dogs, smoked meat (ham), cheddar cheese, yeast, caffeine drinks, and chocolate.

Cognitive level: Application
Nursing process: Implementation
NCLEX: Health Promotion and Maintenance
See text page: 349

33. A client being treated with paroxetine (Paxil) 50 mg po daily for depression reports to the clinic nurse that he took a few extra tablets earlier in the day and "feels bad" now. The nurse should assess (more than one answer may be correct)
   1. vital signs.
   2. for increased suicidal ideation.
   3. for presence of abdominal pain and diarrhea.
   4. for hyperactivity or feelings of restlessness.

Answers: 1, 3, 4

Rationale: The client is taking the maximum dose of this SSRI and has ingested an additional unknown amount of the drug. Central serotonin syndrome must be considered. Symptoms include abdominal pain, diarrhea, tachycardia, elevated blood pressure, hyperpyrexia, increased motor activity, and muscle spasms. Central serotonin syndrome may progress to a full medical emergency if not treated early. Option 2: Although assessing for suicidal ideation is never inappropriate, in this situation physiological symptoms should be the initial focus.

Cognitive level: Analysis
Nursing process: Assessment
NCLEX: Physiological Integrity
See text page: 344

34. A client who has been taking fluoxetine (Prozac) 60 mg daily for the past 6 months tells the nurse at the medication follow-up clinic that he is considering stopping pharmacotherapy. He states his mood is fine, and now that he is living normally his wife is concerned that he has no sexual drive. The nurse's response should be predicated on knowledge that
   1. sexual dysfunction is an expected side effect to which the client must adjust.
   2. morning dosing will alleviate the problem and foster late evening sexual activity.
   3. the problem is usually relationship-oriented and requires couples therapy.

4. switching to mirtazapine (Remeron) may restore sexual function.

Answer: 4

Rationale: Mirtazapine, an atypical antidepressant that blocks serotonin, is an α_2 adenoreceptor antagonist that blocks histamine, thus enhancing both nonadrenergic and serotonergic transmitters. It is often effective in restoring SSRI-induced sexual dysfunction. The other options reflect incorrect information.

Cognitive level: Comprehension
Nursing process: Implementation
NCLEX: Physiological Integrity
See text page: 346

35. A client being treated for depression has been taking 300 mg amitriptyline (Elavil) daily for nearly a year. She calls her case manager at the mental health clinic, stating she stopped taking her antidepressant 2 days ago and has developed something like the "flu," with cold sweats, nausea, a rapid heartbeat, and terrible nightmares when she sleeps. The nurse should advise the client
   1. to go to the nearest emergency department immediately.
   2. not to be alarmed and to take two aspirin and drink plenty of fluids.
   3. to take one dose of the tricyclic antidepressant and come to the clinic to see the physician.
   4. to resume taking the tricyclic antidepressant for 2 weeks and then discontinue again.

Answer: 3

Rationale: The client has symptoms associated with abrupt withdrawal of the tricyclic antidepressant. Taking a dose of the drug will ameliorate the symptoms. Seeing the physician will allow her to discuss the advisability of going off the medication and to be given a gradual withdrawal schedule if discontinuation is the decision. Option 1: This situation is not a medical emergency. Option 2: The situation calls for medical advice. Option 4 would produce the same symptoms she currently has.

Cognitive level: Application
Nursing process: Implementation
NCLEX: Physiological Integrity
See text page: 348

36. A 26-year-old woman who gave birth to a normal newborn 1 month ago reports she "simply cannot cope" with her situation. She is unable to sleep, eats little, and says she feels like a failure because she can't take care of her baby. She has been thinking her baby is "the devil's spawn" and the root of her problems. She sits and stares into space, her face a

worried, perplexed mask. The priority nursing diagnosis for the client is
1. disturbed sleep pattern.
2. disturbed thought processes.
3. situational low self-esteem.
4. risk for other-directed violence.

Answer: 4

Rationale: When the mother with depression of postpartum onset has ruminations or delusional thoughts about the infant, the risk for harming the infant is increased; thus it becomes the priority diagnosis. The other diagnoses are relevant but are of lower priority.

Cognitive level: Analysis
Nursing process: Diagnosis
NCLEX: Safe and Effective Care Environment
See text page: 330

37. A depressed client tells the nurse "The bad things that happen are always my fault." To assist the client to reframe this overgeneralization, the nurse should respond
   1. "I really doubt that one person can be blamed for all the bad things that happen."
   2. "You are being exceptionally hard on yourself when you imply you are a jinx."
   3. "What about the good things that happen; are any of them ever your fault?"
   4. "Let's look at one bad thing that happened to see if another explanation exists."

Answer: 4

Rationale: By questioning a faulty assumption, the nurse can help the client look at the premise more objectively and reframe it to a more accurate representation of fact. Option 1 casts doubt but does not require the client to evaluate the statement. Option 2 states a fact but does not require the client to evaluate the statement. Option 3 shifts the focus slightly and would probably elicit a "no" from the client.

Cognitive level: Application
Nursing process: Implementation
NCLEX: Psychosocial Integrity
See text page: 340

38. A severely depressed client with psychomotor retardation has begun activities therapy. His schedule is: 9 AM, ceramics; 10 AM, exercise group; 11 AM to noon, open; noon, lunch. The nurse creating the client's schedule should opt to fill the hour block from 11 AM to noon with
   1. group therapy.
   2. a rest period.
   3. reminiscence group.
   4. individual counseling.

Answer: 2

Rationale: Severely depressed clients have anergia (little mental or physical energy) and are readily fatigued. Psychomotor retardation also takes its toll. After 2 hours of activity the client may be simply too tired to gain anything from a therapy group. The client should be allowed to rest and have therapy scheduled later in the day.

Cognitive level: Analysis
Nursing process: Planning
NCLEX: Physiological Integrity
See text page: 341

39. Indicators suggesting that outcomes are being attained for a client with depression with melancholic features include (more than one answer may be correct)
   1. delusions consistently absent.
   2. echopraxia consistently absent.
   3. weight stable at preillness level.
   4. sleeping 7 hours nightly.
   5. diurnal variation marked.

Answers: 3, 4

Rationale: Melancholic features include anorexia or weight loss, diurnal variation of feeling worse in the morning, and early morning awakening. Thus a stable weight and sleeping 7 hours nightly are indicators that client outcomes are being met. Option 1: Delusions are associated with depression with psychotic features. Option 2: Echopraxia is associated with depression with catatonic features. Option 5: Marked diurnal variation suggests an unmet outcome. Diurnal variation should be consistently absent.

Cognitive level: Application
Nursing process: Evaluation
NCLEX: Physiological Integrity
See text page: 329

40. The admitting note describes a client with depression as having anergia and anhedonia. The nurse should plan measures to (more than one answer may be correct)
   1. channel excessive energy.
   2. reduce guilty ruminations.
   3. accommodate psychomotor retardation.
   4. instill a sense of hopefulness.

Answers: 3, 4

Rationale: Anergia refers to a lack of energy. Anhedonia refers to the inability to find pleasure or meaning in life; thus planning should include measures to accommodate psychomotor retardation and instill hopefulness. Option 1: Anergia is lack of energy, not

317

excessive energy. Option 2: Anhedonia does not necessarily imply the presence of guilty ruminations.

Cognitive level: Application
Nursing process: Planning
NCLEX: Psychosocial Integrity
See text pages: 334-336, 339

41. A middle-aged client who has been treated for depression with SSRIs and cognitive behavioral therapy has identified that passivity probably contributed to her depression. The nurse can appropriately suggest
    1. social skills training.
    2. use of complementary therapy.
    3. relaxation training classes.
    4. learning desensitization techniques.

Answer: 1
Rationale: Social skills training is helpful in treating and preventing the recurrence of depression. Training focuses on assertiveness training and coping skills that lead to positive reinforcement from others. Option 2 refers to adjunctive therapies such as herbals. Option 3: Assertiveness would be of greater value than relaxation training because passivity has been identified as a concern. Option 4: Desensitization is used in treatment of phobias.

Cognitive level: Application
Nursing process: Planning
NCLEX: Psychosocial Integrity
See text pages: 341, 342

CHAPTER 19

1. Three policemen bring a client to the mental health unit for admission. She had been directing traffic on a busy city street and shouting rhymes such as "to work, you jerk, for perks" and making obscene gestures at cars that came too close to her. When her husband was contacted at work, he reported that his wife had stopped taking her lithium 3 weeks ago and had not slept or eaten for 3 days, telling her husband she was "too busy." When making an assessment, the two features characteristic of the disorder the nurse can identify are
    1. increased muscle tension and anxiety.
    2. cognitive deficit and low mood.
    3. poor judgment and hyperactivity.
    4. vegetative signs and poor grooming.

Answer: 3
Rationale: Hyperactivity (directing traffic) and poor judgment (putting herself in a dangerous position) are characteristic of manic episodes. None of the

other characteristics is specifically alluded to in this scenario.

Cognitive level: Application
Nursing process: Assessment
NCLEX: Psychosocial Integrity
See text page: 364

2. A client, brought to the mental health unit by police, had been directing traffic and shouting rhymes on a busy city street. Her husband reported that she had stopped taking her lithium 3 weeks ago and had not slept or eaten for 3 days. She was dressed in a red leotard, an exercise bra, and an assortment of chains and brightly colored scarves on her head, waist, wrists, and ankles. Her first words to the nurse were "I'll punch you, munch you, crunch you," as she danced into the room, shadow boxing. Then she shook the nurse's hand and said gaily, "We need to become better acquainted. I have the world's greatest intellect and you are probably an intellectual midget." The nurse should assess the client's mood as
    1. irritable and belligerent.
    2. excessively happy and confident.
    3. unstable and unpredictable.
    4. highly suspicious and haughty.

Answer: 3
Rationale: The client has demonstrated angry behavior and pleasant, happy behavior within seconds of each other. Mood swings are often rapid and seemingly without understandable reason in manic clients. Options 1 and 2 are not entirely correct. Option 4 is not described in the scenario.

Cognitive level: Application
Nursing process: Assessment
NCLEX: Psychosocial Integrity
See text pages: 362, 364

3. Three policemen bring a client to the mental health unit. She had been directing traffic and shouting rhymes on a busy city street. Her husband reported that the client had stopped taking her lithium 3 weeks ago and had not slept or eaten for 3 days. Which behaviors listed below will be of priority concern as the nurse begins a care plan for the client?
    1. Bizarre, colorful, inappropriate dress
    2. Grandiose thinking, poor concentration
    3. Insulting, provocative behavior directed at staff
    4. Hyperactivity, ignoring eating and sleeping

Answer: 4
Rationale: Hyperactivity, poor nutrition, hydration, and not sleeping take priority in terms of the needs listed above because they threaten the physical integrity of

318

the client. The other behaviors are less threatening to the client's life.
Cognitive level: Analysis
Nursing process: Assessment
NCLEX: Safe and Effective Care Environment
See text page: 364

4. A client with bipolar disorder who became hyperactive after discontinuing lithium has not eaten or slept for 3 days. Which of the following nursing diagnoses would be of priority importance?
   1. Ineffective coping
   2. Risk for injury
   3. Caregiver role strain
   4. Impaired social interaction

Answer: 2

Rationale: Although each of the nursing diagnoses listed is appropriate for a client having a manic episode, the priority lies with the client's physiological safety. Hyperactivity and poor judgment put the client at high risk for injury.
Cognitive level: Analysis
Nursing process: Diagnosis
NCLEX: Safe and Effective Care Environment
See text page: 368

5. A client with bipolar disorder who became hyperactive after discontinuing lithium has not eaten or slept for 3 days. Mood and behavior are labile, changing rapidly from playful to aggressive. If the client threatens to hit another client or a staff member, which response would constitute an appropriate intervention?
   1. "Stop that! No one did anything to provoke an attack by you."
   2. "If you try that one more time, you will be placed in seclusion immediately."
   3. "Do not hit me/him/her. If you are unable to control yourself, we will help you."
   4. "You know we will not let you hit anyone! Why do you continue such self-defeating behavior?"

Answer: 3

Rationale: When the client is unable to control his or her behavior and violates or threatens to violate the rights of others, limits must be set in an effort to deescalate the situation. Limits should be set in simple, concrete terms. Option 1 does not offer appropriate assistance to the client. Option 2 threatens the client with seclusion as punishment. Option 4 asks a rhetorical question.
Cognitive level: Application
Nursing process: Implementation
NCLEX: Safe and Effective Care Environment
See text pages: 374, 375

6. A client with bipolar disorder who relapsed after discontinuing lithium has lost 5 pounds in the 4 days since hospitalization. The nursing diagnosis of "imbalanced nutrition: less than body requirements related to caloric intake insufficient to balance energy expenditure associated with hyperactivity" has been established. The short-term indicator that should be used to evaluate progress toward the desired outcome of "intake will be sufficient to maintain weight within normal range for height and age" is
   1. while in the acutely manic state, the client will drink 8 ounces of high-calorie, high-protein drink hourly throughout the day.
   2. the client will display consistently nonviolent behavior toward others on the unit within 1 week with the aid of medications and nursing interventions.
   3. the client will have competent medical assistance and legal protection when signing any document regarding personal matters during hospitalization.
   4. the client will consistently wear appropriate attire for age and sex within 1 week while on the psychiatric unit.

Answer: 1

Rationale: High-calorie, high-protein food supplements will provide the additional calories needed to offset the client's extreme hyperactivity. The other indicators are related to other nursing diagnoses that might be established for a manic client.
Cognitive level: Application
Nursing process: Planning (Outcome Identification)
NCLEX: Physiological Integrity
See text page: 367

7. A client with bipolar disorder who had a relapse after discontinuing lithium has orders for chlorpromazine (Thorazine) four times daily and twice-daily lithium. The nurse's planning will be aided if he understands that use of the phenothiazine will
   1. bring hyperactivity under rapid control.
   2. enhance the antimanic action of lithium.
   3. minimize the side effects of lithium.
   4. be used for long-term control of hyperactivity.

Answer: 1

Rationale: Manic symptoms are controlled by lithium only after a therapeutic serum level is attained. Because this takes several days to accomplish, a drug with rapid onset is necessary to reduce the hyperactivity initially. Options 2 and 3: Phenothiazines neither enhance lithium's antimanic activity nor minimize the side effects. Option 4: Lithium will be used for long-term control.
Cognitive level: Application

319

Nursing process: Planning
NCLEX: Physiological Integrity
See text pages: 370, 373

8. A manic client has been diagnosed as a "rapid cycler." The psychiatrist decides to prescribe an anticonvulsant medication that has been found to have mood-stabilizing properties. To prepare health teaching materials, the drug the nurse should anticipate being prescribed is
   1. sulindac (Clinoril).
   2. carbamazepine (Tegretol).
   3. clonidine (Catapres).
   4. chlorpromazine (Thorazine).

Answer: 2
Rationale: Some clients with bipolar disorder, especially those who have only short periods between episodes, have a favorable response to the anticonvulsants carbamazepine and valproate. Carbamazepine seems to work better in clients with rapid cycling and in severely paranoid, angry manic clients.

Cognitive level: Application
Nursing process: Planning
NCLEX: Health Promotion and Maintenance
See text page: 373

9. The husband of a bipolar client asks the nurse what causes manic disorder. The nurse should respond that the actual cause has not been determined but that
   1. several factors, including heredity, may have roles.
   2. excess norepinephrine is probably a major factor.
   3. brain structures have been altered by stress early in life.
   4. bipolar clients may have excess dopamine receptors.

Answer: 1
Rationale: The best explanation at this time is that bipolar disorder is most likely caused by an interplay of complex independent variables. Various theories implicate genetics, endocrine imbalance, early stress, and neurotransmitter imbalances.

Cognitive level: Application
Nursing process: Implementation
NCLEX: Health Promotion and Maintenance
See text pages: 361, 362

10. The spouse of a client with bipolar disorder asks what evidence supports the possibility of genetic transmission of bipolar disorders. The best response would be
    1. "A higher proportion of clients with bipolar disorders is found among creative writers."
    2. "A higher rate of relatives with bipolar disorder is found among clients with bipolar disorder."
    3. "A higher rate of relatives of clients with bipolar disorder respond in an exaggerated way to daily stress."
    4. "More individuals with bipolar disorder come from higher socioeconomic and educational backgrounds."

Answer: 2
Rationale: Evidence of genetic transmission is supported when twins or relatives of clients with a particular disorder also show an incidence of the disorder that is higher than the incidence in the general public. The other options do not support the theory of genetic transmission of bipolar disorder.

Cognitive level: Application
Nursing process: Implementation
NCLEX: Health Promotion and Maintenance
See text page: 361

11. A client with bipolar disorder is commanding another client to "Get me that book; take this other stuff out of here," and so forth. The nurse wants to interrupt this behavior without entering into a power struggle with the client. The best approach would be to use
    1. humor: "How much are you paying servants these days?"
    2. distraction: "Let's go to the dining room for a snack."
    3. limit setting: "You must stop ordering other clients around."
    4. honest feedback: "Your behavior is annoying other clients."

Answer: 2
Rationale: The distractibility characteristic of manic episodes can assist the nurse to direct the client toward more appropriate, constructive activities without entering into power struggles. Humor usually backfires by either encouraging the client or inciting anger. Limit setting and honest feedback may seem heavy handed to a labile client and may incite anger.

Cognitive level: Application
Nursing process: Implementation
NCLEX: Psychosocial Integrity
See text page: 368

12. The nurse in the medication clinic receives the following lithium level for a client: 1.0 mEq/L. The nurse should assess this as
    1. within therapeutic limits.
    2. below therapeutic limits.

320

3. above therapeutic limits.
4. completely incorrect because of inaccurate testing.

Answer: 1

Rationale: Normal range for a blood sample taken 8 to 12 hours after the last dose of lithium is 0.4 to 1.0 mEq/L.

Cognitive level: Analysis
Nursing process: Assessment
NCLEX: Physiological Integrity
See text page: 372

13. During a manic episode a newly admitted client who is displaying hyperactive, restless, and disorganized behavior goes into the dining room and begins to throw food and dishes. Verbal intervention is ineffective. The client's behavior is determined to pose a substantial risk of harm to others. Seclusion is instituted for the primary purpose of
1. maintaining a safe milieu for other clients.
2. reducing environmental stimuli that negatively affect the client.
3. reinforcing limit setting, enabling the client to learn to follow unit rules.
4. protecting the client's biological integrity until medication can take effect.

Answer: 2

Rationale: Seclusion is used when less restrictive measures have failed to help the client maintain control. One of its benefits is to reduce overwhelming environmental stimuli affecting an extremely distractible individual.

Cognitive level: Application
Nursing process: Planning
NCLEX: Safe and Effective Care Environment
See text pages: 374, 375

14. When a client displaying acute mania is admitted to a psychiatric unit, what initial nursing intervention should be planned?
1. Allowing the client to act out feelings because a safe environment can be provided
2. Providing verbal instructions to the client to try to remain calm
3. Being accessible to set limits on client behavior as necessary
4. Restraining the client to reduce hyperactivity and aggression

Answer: 3

Rationale: This intervention provides support through the nurse's presence and provides structure as necessary while the client's control is tenuous. Option 1:

Acting out may lead to loss of behavioral control. Option 2: Client will probably be unable to focus on instruction and comply. Option 4: Restraint is used only after other interventions have proved ineffective.

Cognitive level: Application
Nursing process: Planning
NCLEX: Psychosocial Integrity
See text page: 370

15. At a unit meeting, staff discuss the decor for a special bedroom for a manic client. The best suggestion from among those listed below is
1. an extra-large window with a view of the street.
2. brightly colored walls and print drapes.
3. deep colors for walls and upholstery.
4. neutral walls with pale, coordinated accessories.

Answer: 4

Rationale: The environment for a manic client should be as simple and nonstimulating as possible. Manic clients are highly sensitive to environmental distractions and stimulation.

Cognitive level: Application
Nursing process: Implementation
NCLEX: Safe and Effective Care Environment
See text page: 370

16. A client displaying acute mania has driven staff to the end of their tolerance by noon. The client has joked, manipulated, insulted, and fought his way through the morning. Staff are feeling defensive and exhausted. The best action to take is to
1. call the physician to come to the unit to evaluate the client and write a seclusion order.
2. seclude the client, then call the physician to come to the unit to write a seclusion order.
3. hold a staff meeting to discuss staff consistency and limit-setting approaches.
4. explain to the client that his behavior is unacceptable and seek his cooperation.

Answer: 3

Rationale: When staff members are at their wits' end, the client has succeeded in keeping the environment unsettled and avoided outside controls on behavior. Staff meetings can help minimize staff splitting and feelings of anger, helplessness, confusion, and frustration.

Cognitive level: Application
Nursing process: Implementation
NCLEX: Safe and Effective Care Environment
See text page: 370

Chapter 19   Mood Disorders: Bipolar

17. A client displaying acute mania undresses in the day room and dances about. The best intervention would be to
   1. quietly ask the client "Why don't you put your clothes on?"
   2. tell the client firmly to "Stop dancing and put on your clothing."
   3. let the client stay in the day room and move the other clients to a recreation area.
   4. put a blanket around the client and, with several staff, walk with the client to her room.

Answer: 4
Rationale: Clients must be protected from the embarrassing consequences of their poor judgment whenever possible. Protecting the client from public exposure by matter-of-factly covering the client and removing her from the area with a sufficient number of staff to avoid argument and provide control is an effective approach.
Cognitive level: Application
Nursing process: Implementation
NCLEX: Psychosocial Integrity
See text page: 370

18. A client displaying behaviors consistent with acute mania approaches the nurse, waves a newspaper, and says "I need to make a phone call right this minute. I need to call this department store while their sale is going on. I am going to order 10 dresses and four pairs of shoes." The most appropriate intervention would be for the nurse to
   1. tell the client she is not allowed to use the phone until she is in better control.
   2. suggest the client have someone shop for her and bring purchases to the unit.
   3. ask whether the client has enough money to pay for the purchases.
   4. invite the client to go to her room to see a new fashion magazine.

Answer: 4
Rationale: Situations such as this offer an opportunity to use the client's distractibility to staff's advantage. Clients become frustrated when staff deny requests (option 1) that the client sees as entirely reasonable. Distracting the client can avoid power struggles. Option 2 would not satisfy the client's need for immediacy and would ultimately result in the extravagant expenditure. Option 3 would likely precipitate an angry response.
Cognitive level: Application
Nursing process: Implementation
NCLEX: Psychosocial Integrity
See text page: 370

19. Lithium citrate 600 mg 3 times daily po is ordered for a client with acute mania who is being treated as an outpatient. The client calls the mental health nurse, stating he is nauseated. To lessen the nausea, the nurse can suggest that the lithium can be taken with
   1. meals.
   2. an antacid.
   3. an antiemetic.
   4. a large glass of juice.

Answer: 1
Rationale: Some clients find taking lithium with meals diminishes nausea. The other options are less helpful.
Cognitive level: Application
Nursing process: Implementation
NCLEX: Physiological Integrity
See text page: 373

20. A health teaching plan for a client taking lithium should include instructions to
   1. maintain normal salt and fluids in the diet.
   2. drink twice the usual daily amount of fluid.
   3. double the lithium dose if diarrhea or vomiting occurs.
   4. avoid eating aged cheese, processed meats, and red wine.

Answer: 1
Rationale: Sodium depletion and dehydration increase the chance for development of lithium toxicity. The other options offer inappropriate information.
Cognitive level: Application
Nursing process: Planning
NCLEX: Health Promotion and Maintenance
See text page: 373

21. A nursing diagnosis relevant for both the client with depression and the client with acute mania is
   1. deficient diversional activity.
   2. defensive coping.
   3. sleep pattern disturbance.
   4. excess fluid volume.

Answer: 3
Rationale: Physical needs of clients with mood disorders include sleep pattern disturbances. Assessment data should be routinely gathered about this possible problem. Option 1 is more relevant for clients with depression. Option 2 is more relevant for clients with mania. Option 4 is less relevant for clients with mood disorders than is fluid volume deficit.
Cognitive level: Analysis
Nursing process: Diagnosis
NCLEX: Physiological Integrity
See text page: 368

22. Appropriate plans to suggest to the family of a bipolar client who is being treated as an outpatient during a hypomanic episode include (more than one answer may be correct)
 1. providing structure.
 2. limiting credit card access.
 3. encouraging group social interaction.
 4. suggesting limiting work to half-days.

Answers: 1, 2
Rationale: A client with hypomania is expansive, grandiose, labile, uses poor judgment, spends inappropriately, and is overstimulated by a busy environment. Providing structure would help the client maintain appropriate behavior. Financial irresponsibility may be avoided by limiting access to cash and credit cards. Option 3: Group socialization should be kept to a minimum to reduce stimulation. Option 4: Leave of absence from work will be necessary to limit stimuli and prevent problems associated with poor judgment and inappropriate decision-making that accompany hypomania.
Cognitive level: Application
Nursing process: Planning
NCLEX: Psychosocial Integrity
See text page: 365

23. Of the dinner menus below, which one is best suited for a bipolar client with acute mania?
 1. Broiled chicken breast on a roll, an ear of corn, and an apple
 2. Spaghetti and meatballs, salad, and a banana
 3. Beef and vegetable stew, a roll, and chocolate pudding
 4. Goulash, green beans, and flavored gelatin with whipped cream

Answer: 1
Rationale: These foods provide adequate nutrition, but more importantly they are finger foods that the hyperactive client could "eat on the run." The foods listed in the other options cannot be eaten without utensils.
Cognitive level: Application
Nursing process: Implementation
NCLEX: Physiological Integrity
See text page: 369

24. During periods of laughter, talkativeness, and banter, a client with manic behavior is noted to abruptly become irritable. Such changes in mood should be assessed as
 1. dissociation.
 2. lability.
 3. undoing.
 4. flight of ideas.

Answer: 2
Rationale: The mood of the manic client is often unstable. Rapid mood shifts are called mood lability. Options 1 and 3: Dissociation and undoing are ego defense mechanisms. Option 4: Flight of ideas is a speech pattern in which speech is delivered rapidly and with abrupt changes of topic.
Cognitive level: Application
Nursing process: Assessment
NCLEX: Psychosocial Integrity
See text pages: 362-364

25. An appropriate outcome for the treatment plan of a client with grandiose thinking associated with acute mania would be that the client will demonstrate
 1. a more optimistic outlook.
 2. uncompromised sleep.
 3. interest in his or her environment.
 4. distorted thought self-control.

Answer: 4
Rationale: The desired outcome is that the client will be able to control the grandiose thinking associated with acute mania as evidenced by making realistic comments about self, abilities, and plans. Options 1 and 3: Clients with acute mania are already unduly optimistic as a result of their use of denial, and they are overly interested in their environment. Option 2: Uncompromised sleep is a desired outcome but is not related to distorted thought processes.
Cognitive level: Application
Nursing process: Planning (Outcome Identification)
NCLEX: Psychosocial Integrity
See text page: 367

26. Which observations, if documented in the medical record, would indicate that the treatment plan for a client with acute mania has been effective?
 1. "Converses appropriately, clothing matched, participates in activities."
 2. "Irritable, suggestible, distractible, napped for 10 minutes in afternoon."
 3. "Attention span short, writing copious notes, intrudes in conversations."
 4. "Heavily made up, seductive toward male staff, pressured speech."

Answer: 1
Rationale: The descriptors given indicate the client is functioning at an optimal level, using appropriate behavior, and thinking without becoming overstimulated by unit activities. Options 2, 3, and 4 reflect manic behavior.
Cognitive level: Analysis
Nursing process: Evaluation
NCLEX: Psychosocial Integrity
See text page: 381

323

27. A manic client dances around the unit, seldom sits, monopolizes conversations, interrupts, and intrudes. The nursing intervention that will best promote the outcome that the client will consistently demonstrate energy conservation is
1. monitoring physiological functioning.
2. supervising personal hygiene.
3. observing for mood changes.
4. providing a subdued environment.

Answer: 4

Rationale: All the options are reasonable interventions with a client with acute mania, but option 4 directly relates to the outcome of energy conservation by providing a subdued environment that will decrease stimulation and help balance activity and rest.

Cognitive level: Application
Nursing process: Planning
NCLEX: Physiological Integrity
See text page: 370

28. A client with acute mania is a business executive. He tells the nurse that his job is only his cover, that he's really the right-hand man to the president of the United States and that he has been sent to this city to reorganize the FBI and CIA. A desired outcome for this client is that he will
1. use his executive skills to organize unit activities.
2. consistently display distorted thought self-control.
3. demonstrate acceptance of unit policies.
4. act out feelings.

Answer: 2

Rationale: The client's reality testing is poor, as evidenced by the grandiose ideas he verbalizes. An appropriate outcome is the control of distorted thinking and maintenance of reality-based thinking. The other outcomes are not desirable.

Cognitive level: Application
Nursing process: Planning (Outcome Identification)
NCLEX: Psychosocial Integrity
See text page: 367

29. A male client displaying acute mania has disrobed in the hall three times in 2 hours. The nurse should
1. direct the client to wear his clothes at all times.
2. ask if the client finds the clothes bothersome.
3. tell the client he is embarrassing the women.
4. arrange for one-on-one supervision.

Answer: 4

Rationale: A client who repeatedly disrobes despite verbal limit setting needs more structure. One-on-one supervision may provide the necessary structure. Option 1 has not proven successful. Option 2 serves

no purpose. Option 3 will not make a difference to the client whose grasp of social behaviors is impaired by the illness.

Cognitive level: Application
Nursing process: Implementation
NCLEX: Safe and Effective Care Environment
See text page: 370

30. A client displaying acute mania is found pacing atop the pool table in the recreation room. She waves a cue in one hand and gestures that she'll throw the pool balls if anyone comes near her. The priority intervention is to
1. get her down off the table.
2. tell her she will be taken to seclusion.
3. clear the room of all clients.
4. assemble a show of force.

Answer: 3

Rationale: The safety of the other clients in the room is of primary importance. Once other clients are out of the room, a plan for controlling this client can be implemented.

Cognitive level: Analysis
Nursing process: Assessment
NCLEX: Safe and Effective Care Environment
See text page: 369

31. After hospital discharge, a priority intervention that should be planned for a family and the client with bipolar disorder who is taking antimanic medication is
1. decreasing physical activity.
2. increasing food and fluids.
3. meeting self-care needs.
4. psychoeducation.

Answer: 4

Rationale: Options 1, 2, and 3: During the continuation phase of treatment for bipolar disorder, the physical needs of the client are not as important an issue as they were during the acute episode. After hospital discharge, treatment focuses on maintaining medication compliance and preventing relapse, both of which are fostered by ongoing psychoeducation.

Cognitive level: Application
Nursing process: Planning
NCLEX: Health Promotion and Maintenance
See text pages: 368, 369

32. The physician prescribes chlorpromazine 150 mg orally 3 times daily and lithium 300 mg twice daily for a bipolar client. The nurse should plan interventions for
1. depressed mood.
2. increased anxiety.

3. confusion.
4. thirst and dry mouth.

Answer: 4
Rationale: Lithium and chlorpromazine both cause thirst and dry mouth. Sugarless gum and adequate fluid intake will be helpful to the client. The other options are not expected reactions to either drug.
Cognitive level: Application
Nursing process: Planning
NCLEX: Physiological Integrity
See text page: 372

33. The client receiving lithium should be assessed for
    1. alopecia, purpura, and drowsiness.
    2. pharyngitis, mydriasis, and dystonia.
    3. diaphoresis, weakness, and nausea.
    4. ascites, dyspnea, and edema.

Answer: 3
Rationale: The symptoms listed in option 3 are early signs of lithium toxicity. All other problems mentioned are unrelated to lithium therapy.
Cognitive level: Application
Nursing process: Assessment
NCLEX: Physiological Integrity
See text page: 372

34. A client with bipolar disorder tells the nurse "I am so ashamed of being bipolar. When I'm manic my behavior is so bizarre that it embarrasses my family. Even when I take my medication every day, it's no guarantee that I will not have a relapse. I am like a stone around my wife's neck, dragging the family down." These statements support the nursing diagnoses of
    1. defensive coping and ineffective denial.
    2. chronic low self-esteem and powerlessness.
    3. impaired social interaction and social isolation.
    4. impaired adjustment and parental role conflict.

Answer: 2
Rationale: Chronic low self-esteem and powerlessness are interwoven in the client's statements. No data support the other diagnoses.
Cognitive level: Analysis
Nursing process: Diagnosis
NCLEX: Psychosocial Integrity
See text page: 367

35. During the maintenance phase of treatment a client asks the nurse "Do I have to keep taking this lithium even though my mood is stable now?" The most appropriate response is
    1. "You will be able to stop the medication at the end of the month."

2. "Usually clients take medication for approximately 6 months after discharge."
3. "It is odd that the physician has not already discontinued your medication."
4. "Taking the medication each day helps prevent relapses and recurrences."

Answer: 4
Rationale: Bipolar clients may be maintained on lithium indefinitely to prevent recurrences. Helping the client understand this need will promote medication compliance. Option 1: This is untrue. Option 2: Medication will be taken over a longer period. Option 3: It is expected that the client will take medication for a long time.
Cognitive level: Application
Nursing process: Implementation
NCLEX: Psychosocial Integrity
See text page: 367

36. During an episode of acute mania a newly admitted client who is displaying hyperactive, restless, and disorganized behavior goes into the dining room and begins to throw food and dishes. Verbal intervention is ineffective and seclusion is instituted. The items of documentation that should be included in the medical record include (more than one answer may be correct)
    1. 1750: Client entered dining room and began to shout and randomly throw food and dishes at walls and other clients.
    2. Continued to throw items despite limit setting and verbal redirection. Client refused to leave dining room.
    3. Client's behavior determined to pose a substantial risk of harm to others. Client escorted to seclusion without a struggle by four staff.
    4. Seclusion explained. Harmful items removed from room and person per unit protocol.
    5. 1800: prn lorazepam (Ativan) administered IM.
    6. 1815: Vital signs: blood pressure, 120/85 mm Hg; pulse, 90 beats/min; respirations, 22 breaths/min. Client lying on mattress. Chanting profanity.

Answers: 1, 2, 3, 4, 5, 6
Rationale: All items should be included in the medical record. Options 1 and 2 provide essential information explaining the client's behavior and need for the environmental simplification provided by seclusion. Option 3 provides a rationale for seclusion and describes the process of secluding the client. Option 4 reiterates elements of the agency protocol designed to support client psychosocial and biophysical safety. Option 5 documents medication administration. Option 6 documents client physical status and behavior.
Cognitive level: Analysis
Nursing process: Implementation
NCLEX: Safe and Effective Care Environment
See text pages: 374, 375

325

37. A bipolar client being maintained on lithium calls the nurse at the clinic to say he has had severe diarrhea for 4 days. He mentions that he feels very weak and "kind of staggers" when he walks. He states his usual hand tremor has gotten worse. The nurse should advise

1. having someone bring the client to the clinic immediately.
2. restricting food and fluids for 24 hours and staying in bed.
3. drinking a large glass of water with 1 teaspoon of salt added.
4. taking over-the-counter antidiarrheal medication hourly until the diarrhea subsides.

Answer: 1

Rationale: The symptoms described suggest lithium toxicity. The client should have a lithium level drawn and may require further treatment. Because neurological symptoms are present, the client should not drive and should be accompanied by another person. Options 2, 3, and 4: These will not ameliorate the client's symptoms.

Cognitive level: Application
Nursing process: Implementation
NCLEX: Physiological Integrity
See text page: 372

38. A bipolar client with acute mania has been verbally abusive to staff since admission 3 hours ago. He tells the admitting nurse she'd probably make a better call girl than a nurse and refuses to answer assessment questions, saying "If you can't work with patients they'll eventually fire you." The nurse should

1. explain to the client that she holds a degree in nursing and is entirely competent.
2. tell the client his behavior is unacceptable and requires an apology.
3. state she will return in a few minutes to continue the interview.
4. tell the client she will report his behavior to the physician.

Answer: 3

Rationale: Angry verbal attacks against staff by clients with mania are commonplace. Staff must realize verbal attacks are part of illness behavior rather than personal in nature. Arguing, explaining, calling for apologies are counterproductive behaviors. Remaining neutral and allowing a cooling-down period will serve the nurse well. Because the client's mood is labile, the client may be willing to continue the assessment when the nurse returns.

Cognitive level: Application
Nursing process: Implementation
NCLEX: Psychosocial Integrity
See text page: 366

39. The medical record of a client about to be admitted to the inpatient unit states the client is diagnosed as having bipolar I disorder. The nurse should expect the client to display symptoms of

1. rapid cycling.
2. major depression or acute mania.
3. major depression or hypomania.
4. hypomania or minor depression.

Answer: 2

Rationale: Bipolar I disorder is diagnosed when the client has had one episode of mania alternating with major depression. Option 1: Bipolar I disorder may or may not be rapid cycling in nature. Option 3 describes bipolar II disorder. Option 4 describes cyclothymia.

Cognitive level: Application
Nursing process: Assessment
NCLEX: Psychosocial Integrity
See text page: 360

40. The statement by a client in the continuation phase of treatment for bipolar disorder that indicates need for planned intervention is

1. "It is difficult to live down all the crazy stuff I did during my last episode."
2. "I am getting better at problem-solving thanks to the group I attend on Tuesdays."
3. "Using a financial counselor to help manage my debts is keeping me solvent."
4. "I drank a lot when I relapsed, but Alcoholics Anonymous helps me manage stress without drinking."

Answer: 1

Rationale: The only option in which the client identifies a problem that is not being adequately addressed is option 1, reconciling illness behaviors. Ongoing therapy may be called for to address these issues.

Cognitive level: Analysis
Nursing process: Assessment
NCLEX: Psychosocial Integrity
See text pages: 359, 360

CHAPTER 20

1. A salesman has had difficulty holding a job because he accuses co-workers of conspiring to take his sales. Today, he argued with several office mates and threatened to kill one of them. The police were called, and he was brought to the mental health center for evaluation. He has had previous admissions to the unit for stabilization of symptoms of paranoid schizophrenia. When the nurse meets him, he points at staff in the nursing station and states loudly "They're all plotting to destroy me. Isn't that true?"

An appropriate response for the nurse would be
1. "No, that is not true. People here are trying to help you if you will let them."
2. "Everyone here is trying to help you. No one wants to harm you."
3. "Thinking that people want to destroy you must be very frightening."
4. "That is absurd. Staff are health care workers, not members of the mob."

Answer: 3
Rationale: Resist focusing on content; instead, focus on the feelings the client is expressing. This strategy prevents arguing about the reality of delusional beliefs. Such arguments increase client anxiety and the tenacity with which the client holds to the delusion. The other options focus on content and provide opportunity for argument.
Cognitive level: Application
Nursing process: Implementation
NCLEX: Psychosocial Integrity
See text page: 401

2. A newly admitted client diagnosed with paranoid schizophrenia is hypervigilant and constantly scans the environment. He states that he saw two doctors talking in the hall and knows they were plotting to kill him. The nurse may correctly assess this behavior as
1. an idea of reference.
2. a delusion of infidelity.
3. an auditory hallucination.
4. echolalia.

Answer: 1
Rationale: Ideas of reference are misinterpretations of the verbalizations or actions of others that give special personal meanings to these behaviors; for example, seeing two people talking, the individual assumes they are talking about him or her. The other behaviors do not correspond with the scenario.
Cognitive level: Application
Nursing process: Assessment
NCLEX: Psychosocial Integrity
See text page: 392

3. A newly admitted client diagnosed with paranoid schizophrenia believes co-workers are "out to get" him and has stated he thinks two doctors on the unit are plotting to kill him. How does the client perceive the environment?
1. Supportive
2. Dangerous
3. Disorganized
4. Bizarre

Answer: 2
Rationale: The client sees his world as hostile and dangerous. This assessment is important because the nurse can be more effective by using empathy to respond to the client. Data are not present to support any of the other options.
Cognitive level: Analysis
Nursing process: Assessment
NCLEX: Psychosocial Integrity
See text page: 392

4. Family members of a client newly diagnosed with paranoid schizophrenia state that they do not understand what caused the client's illness. The nurse's response should be predicated on the
1. neurobiological-genetic model.
2. stress model.
3. family theory model.
4. developmental model.

Answer: 1
Rationale: Compelling evidence exists that schizophrenia is a neurological disorder probably related to neurochemical abnormalities, neuroanatomical disruption of brain circuits, and genetic vulnerability. Options 2, 3, and 4: Stress, family disruption, and developmental influences may contribute but are not considered single etiologies.
Cognitive level: Application
Nursing process: Implementation
NCLEX: Physiologic Integrity
See text pages: 386, 387

5. A client was admitted to the mental health unit after arguing with co-workers and threatening to kill them. He is diagnosed with paranoid schizophrenia. On the unit he is aloof and suspicious. He mentioned that two physicians he saw talking were plotting to kill him. On the basis of data gathered at this point, two nursing diagnoses the nurse should consider are
1. disturbed thought processes and risk for other-directed violence.
2. spiritual distress and social isolation.
3. risk for loneliness and deficient knowledge.
4. disturbed personal identity and noncompliance.

Answer: 1
Rationale: Delusions of persecution and ideas of reference support a nursing diagnosis of disturbed thought processes. Risk for other-directed violence is substantiated by the client's feeling endangered by persecutors. Fearful individuals may strike out at perceived persecutors or may attempt self-harm to get away from persecutors. Data are not present to support the diagnoses in the other options.

327

Cognitive level: Analysis
Nursing process: Diagnosis
NCLEX: Psychosocial Integrity
See text pages: 396, 397

6. When a client diagnosed with paranoid schizophrenia was discharged from the unit 6 months ago, the plan was for him to take chlorpromazine (Thorazine) 300 mg po daily. He tells the nurse he stopped taking his pills after a few months because they made him feel like a "zombie." The common side effects the nurse should validate with the client include
   1. sweating, nausea, and diarrhea. ·
   2. sedation and muscle stiffness.
   3. headache, watery eyes, and runny nose.
   4. mild fever, sore throat, and skin rash.

Answer: 2
Rationale: Phenothiazines often produce sedation and extrapyramidal side effects such as stiffness and gait disturbance, effects the client might describe as making him feel like a "zombie." The side effects mentioned in the other options are usually not associated with phenothiazine therapy or would not have the effect described by the client.
Cognitive level: Application
Nursing process: Assessment
NCLEX: Physiological Integrity
See text pages: 405, 407

7. When a client with paranoid schizophrenia has a recurrence of positive symptoms after stopping his antipsychotic medication to be free of its orthostatic side effect, he is readmitted to the mental health unit. The physician orders the resumption of medication. The nurse adds the nursing diagnosis of "noncompliance with antipsychotic medication regimen related to side effects" to the client's care plan. What measure should the nurse suggest to the client?
   1. Ask the physician about prescribing an anticholinergic drug such as trihexyphenidyl(Artane).
   2. Chew sugarless gum or use sugarless hard candy to moisten oral mucous membranes.
   3. Reduce dosage by 5 mg daily if side effects recur.
   4. Wear elastic support hose, stay hydrated, and rise slowly from the lying or sitting position.

Answer: 4
Rationale: Orthostasis produces dizziness or fainting when moving from a lying or seated position to a standing position. This can be effectively combated by rising slowly. The use of support hose may also be helpful to prevent pooling of blood in the lower extremities. Options 1 and 2 are unnecessary. Anticholinergic side effects are not the problem. Option 3 The client

should be taught not to discontinue or adjust the dose of the medication, but rather to report annoying side effects to the physician or nurse.
Cognitive level: Application
Nursing process: Implementation
NCLEX: Physiological Integrity
See text page: 409

8. The nurse spends several sessions with a client with paranoid schizophrenia and the client's family to help them understand the importance of the client regularly taking antipsychotic medication. The client repeatedly states he does not like taking pills, and family members say they feel helpless to foster his compliance. The treatment strategy the nurse should discuss with the physician is
   1. use of an antipsychotic decanoate preparation.
   2. adjunctive use of amitriptyline (Elavil).
   3. use of benzodiazepines such as diazepam (Valium).
   4. use of chlordiazepoxide (Librium).

Answer: 1
Rationale: Medications such as fluphenazine decanoate and haloperidol decanoate are long-acting forms of antipsychotic medication. They are given by depot injection every 2 to 4 weeks, thus reducing daily opportunities for noncompliance. The other options do not address the client's dislike of taking pills.
Cognitive level: Application
Nursing process: Planning
NCLEX: Safe and Effective Care Environment
See text page: 407

9. A client's nursing care plan includes assessment for auditory hallucinations. Indicators that suggest the client may be hallucinating include
   1. aloofness, haughtiness, and suspicion.
   2. elevated mood, hyperactivity, and distractibility.
   3. performing rituals and avoiding open places.
   4. darting eyes, tilted head, and mumbling to self.

Answer: 4
Rationale: Clues to hallucinations include eyes looking around the room as though to find the speaker; tilting the head to one side as though listening intently; and grimacing, mumbling, or talking aloud as though responding conversationally to someone.
Cognitive level: Application
Nursing process: Assessment
NCLEX: Psychosocial Integrity
See text page: 393

10. A client, newly diagnosed with paranoid schizophrenia, is delusional, withdrawn, and aloof. One of

328

her nursing diagnoses is deficient diversional activity. An activity that would be appropriate to plan for the client early in the course of her hospital stay is
1. a basketball game.
2. ping-pong with another client.
3. a paint-by-number project.
4. a card game with three other clients.

Answer: 3

Rationale: Solitary, noncompetitive activities that require concentration are best while the client is overtly psychotic. Having to concentrate minimizes hallucinatory and delusional preoccupation. Options 1, 2, and 4 are all competitive.
Cognitive level: Application
Nursing process: Planning
NCLEX: Safe and Effective Care Environment
See text page: 400

11. A client is admitted to the in-patient unit in the withdrawn phase of catatonic schizophrenia. He is completely stuporous. While giving care to the client, the nurse must
   1. explain care activities in simple, explicit terms as though expecting a response.
   2. maintain a quiet, nonstimulating atmosphere, speaking as little as possible to the client.
   3. provide high levels of sensory stimulation by using conversation, the radio, and television.
   4. address negativism by asking the client to do exactly the opposite of what is desired.

Answer: 1

Rationale: Although the withdrawn, catatonic client may appear stuporous, he may be aware of everything going on around him. The client should be treated as though he can see and hear and as though he will respond normally. Option 2: The client needs contact with the nurse on a frequent basis. Option 3: Excessive auditory stimulation can be a disorganizing influence. Option 4: This is nontherapeutic.
Cognitive level: Application
Nursing process: Implementation
NCLEX: Safe and Effective Care Environment
See text page: 414

12. A client with catatonic schizophrenia exhibits little spontaneous movement and demonstrates waxy flexibility. The client's needs of priority importance are
   1. physical.
   2. psychosocial.
   3. safety and security.
   4. self-actualization.

Answer: 1

Rationale: Physical needs must be met to preserve life. A client who is semistuporous must be fed by hand or tube, toileted, given range-of-motion exercises, and so forth to preserve physiological integrity. Safety needs rank second to physical needs. Higher level needs are of lesser concern.
Cognitive level: Analysis
Nursing process: Assessment
NCLEX: Safe and Effective Care Environment
See text page: 414

13. A client with catatonic schizophrenia is semistuporous, demonstrating little spontaneous movement and waxy flexibility. The client's self-care activities of daily living have been assessed as severely compromised. An appropriate outcome would be that the client will
   1. demonstrate increased interest in the environment by the end of week 1.
   2. perform self-care activities with coaching by the end of week 1.
   3. gradually assume the initiative in self-care by the end of week 2.
   4. accept tube feeding without objection by day 2.

Answer: 2

Rationale: Outcomes related to self-care deficit nursing diagnoses should deal with increasing ability to perform self-care tasks independently, such as feeding, bathing, dressing, and toileting. Performing the tasks with coaching by nursing staff denotes improvement over the complete inability to perform the tasks. Option 1 is not directly related to self-care activities. Option 3 is difficult to measure. Option 4 is related to maintenance of nutrition.
Cognitive level: Application
Nursing process: Planning (Outcome Identification)
NCLEX: Psychosocial Integrity
See text page: 414

14. A catatonic client admitted in a stuporous condition begins to demonstrate increased motor activity. He sometimes walks slowly around the unit without interacting. One day the nurse observes him standing immobile, facing the wall with one arm bent behind his back and the other extended in a Nazi-like salute. He remains immobile in that position for 15 minutes, moving only when the nurse gently lowers his arm. This phenomenon is termed
   1. echolalia.
   2. waxy flexibility.
   3. depersonalization.
   4. thought withdrawal.

Answer: 2

Rationale: Waxy flexibility is the ability to hold distorted postures for extended periods of time, as though the client were molded in wax. Option 1: Echolalia is a speech pattern. Option 3: Depersonalization refers to a feeling state. Option 4: Thought withdrawal refers to an alteration in thinking.
Cognitive level: Application
Nursing process: Assessment
NCLEX: Physiological Integrity
See text page: 394

15. A highly suspicious client who has delusions of persecution about being poisoned has refused all hospital meals for 3 days. Assuming all interventions listed are possible, the one likely to be most acceptable to the client is
   1. allowing the client to contact a local restaurant to deliver his meals.
   2. offering to taste each portion on the tray for the client.
   3. allowing the client supervised access to lobby food machines.
   4. providing tube feedings or total parenteral nutrition.

Answer: 3
Rationale: The client who is delusional about his food being poisoned is likely to believe restaurant food might still be poisoned and to say that the staff member tasting the food has taken an antidote to the poison before tasting. Attempts to tube feed or give nutrition intravenously are seen as aggressive and usually promote violence. Clients perceive foods in sealed containers, packages, or natural shells as being safer.
Cognitive level: Application
Nursing process: Planning
NCLEX: Psychosocial Integrity
See text page: 414

16. To establish a relationship with a severely withdrawn schizophrenic client being cared for at home by a supportive family, the most realistic plan would be for the community mental health nurse to
   1. visit daily for 4 days, then every other day for 1 week; stay with client for 20 minutes, accept silence; state when the nurse will return.
   2. arrange to spend 1 hour each day with the client, with the focus on asking questions about what the client is thinking or experiencing; avoid silences.
   3. visit twice daily; sit beside the client with hand on the client's arm; leave if the client does not respond within 10 minutes.
   4. visit every other day; remind the client of the nurse's identity; tell the client he may use the time to talk or the nurse will work on reports.

Answer: 1
Rationale: Severe constraints on the community mental health nurse's time will probably not allow more time than what is mentioned in option 1, yet important principles can be used. A severely withdrawn client should be met "at the client's own level," with silence accepted. Short periods of contact are helpful to minimize both the client's and the nurse's anxiety. Predictability in returning as stated will help build trust. Option 2: An hour may be too long to sustain a home visit with a withdrawn client, especially if the nurse persists in leveling a barrage of questions at the client. Option 3: Twice-daily visits are probably not possible, and leaving after 10 minutes would be premature. Touch may be threatening. Option 4: Working on reports suggests the nurse is not interested in the client.
Cognitive level: Application
Nursing process: Planning
NCLEX: Safe and Effective Care Environment
See text pages: 399, 400

17. The nurse attempting to establish a relationship with a severely withdrawn schizophrenic client tells a preceptor that her frustration level is rising daily because the client turns his head away each time she sits down near him. The nurse states "I am beginning to wonder what is wrong with me as a nurse." The preceptor could be most helpful by explaining that withdrawn clients with schizophrenia
   1. universally fear sexual involvement with therapists.
   2. are socially disabled by the positive symptoms of schizophrenia.
   3. exhibit a high degree of hostility by demonstrating rejecting behavior.
   4. avoid relationships because they become anxious with emotional closeness.

Answer: 4
Rationale: When an individual is suspicious and distrustful and perceives the world and the people in it as potentially dangerous, withdrawal into an inner world can be a defense against uncomfortable levels of anxiety. When someone attempts to establish a relationship with such a client, the client's anxiety rises until trust is established. The truth of option 1 is not borne out by the evidence. Options 2 and 3: These options are not considered true in most cases.
Cognitive level: Application
Nursing process: Implementation
NCLEX: Safe and Effective Care Environment
See text pages: 394, 395

18. A newly admitted client with schizophrenia approaches the unit nurse and says "The voices are

bothering me. They are yelling and telling me I am bad. I have got to get away from them." The most helpful reply for the nurse to make would be

1. "Do you hear the voices often?"
2. "Do you have a plan for getting away from the voices?"
3. "I'll stay with you. Focus on what we are talking about, not the voices. "
4. "Forget the voices and ask some other clients to play cards with you."

Answer: 3

Rationale: Staying with a distraught client who is hearing voices serves several purposes: ongoing observation, the opportunity to provide reality orientation, a means of helping dismiss the voices, the opportunity of forestalling an action that would result in self-injury, and general support to reduce anxiety. Option 1 is not particularly relevant at this point. Option 2 is relevant for assessment purposes but is less helpful than option 3. Option 4 shifts responsibility for intervention from the nurse to the client and other clients.

Cognitive level: Application
Nursing process: Implementation
NCLEX: Psychosocial Integrity
See text page: 401

19. A client with schizophrenia who has received chlorpromazine (Thorazine) 200 mg po 4 times daily for 3 weeks has symptoms of a shuffling, propulsive gait, a masklike face, and drooling. These symptoms should be assessed as
1. hepatocellular effects.
2. pseudoparkinsonism.
3. tardive dyskinesia.
4. akathisia.

Answer: 2

Rationale: Pseudoparkinsonism induced by antipsychotic medication mimics the symptoms of Parkinson's disease. It frequently appears within the first month of treatment. Hepatocellular effects would produce abnormal liver test results. Tardive dyskinesia produces involuntary tonic muscular spasms. Akathisia produces symptoms of motor restlessness.

Cognitive level: Application
Nursing process: Assessment
NCLEX: Physiological Integrity
See text pages: 405-411

20. A client with schizophrenia is admitted to the psychiatric unit in an acutely disturbed, violent state. He is given several doses of haloperidol (Haldol) and becomes calm and approachable. During rounds, the nurse notices the client has his head rotated to one side in a stiffly fixed position. His lower jaw is thrust forward and he is drooling. He appears severely anxious. The client has
1. a dystonic reaction.
2. tardive dyskinesia.
3. waxy flexibility.
4. akathisia.

Answer: 1

Rationale: Acute dystonic reactions involve painful contractions of the tongue, face, neck, and back. Opisthotonos and oculogyric crisis may be observed. Dystonic reactions are considered emergencies requiring immediate intervention. Option 2: Tardive dyskinesia involves involuntary spasmodic muscular contractions that involve the tongue, fingers, toes, neck, trunk, or pelvis. It appears after prolonged treatment. Option 3: Waxy flexibility is a symptom seen in catatonic schizophrenia. Option 4: Akathisia is evidenced by internal and external restlessness, pacing, and fidgeting.

Cognitive level: Analysis
Nursing process: Assessment
NCLEX: Physiological Integrity
See text pages: 405-411

21. The nurse who observes a client prescribed haloperidol who has his head rotated to one side in a stiff, fixed position with his lower jaw thrust forward and drool coming from his mouth should intervene by
1. obtaining an order to administer diphenhydramine (Benadryl) 50 mg IM.
2. reassuring the client that the symptoms will subside if he relaxes.
3. administering trihexyphenidyl (Artane) 5 mg orally.
4. administering atropine 2 mg subcutaneously.

Answer: 1

Rationale: Diphenhydramine, trihexyphenidyl, benztropine, and other anticholinergic medications may be used to treat dystonias, but because the client is drooling the nurse must assume swallowing is difficult, if not impossible. Therefore oral medication is not an option. Medication should be administered intramuscularly. In this case the option given is diphenhydramine.

Cognitive level: Application
Nursing process: Implementation
NCLEX: Physiological Integrity
See text page: 409

22. A client received maintenance doses of trifluoperazine (Stelazine) 30 mg po daily for 1.5 years. The clinic nurse notes the client is grimacing and seems to be constantly smacking her lips. Her neck and

331

shoulders twist in a slow, snakelike motion. The nurse should suspect the presence of
1. agranulocytosis.
2. tardive dyskinesia.
3. Tourette's syndrome.
4. anticholinergic effects.

Answer: 2

Rationale: Tardive dyskinesia is a neuroleptic-induced condition involving the face, trunk, and limbs. Involuntary movements such as tongue thrusting; licking; blowing; irregular movements of the arms, neck, and shoulders; rocking; hip jerks; and pelvic thrusts are seen. These symptoms are frequently not reversible even when the drug is discontinued. The scenario does not present evidence consistent with the other disorders mentioned. Option 1: Agranulocytosis is a blood disorder. Option 3: Tourette's syndrome is a condition in which tics are present. Option 4: Anticholinergic effects include dry mouth, blurred vision, flushing, constipation, and dry eyes.

Cognitive level: Application
Nursing process: Assessment
NCLEX: Physiological Integrity
See text page: 409

23. The nurse is sitting with a client diagnosed as having schizophrenia, disorganized type, who starts to laugh uncontrollably, although the nurse has not said anything funny. The nurse should say
1. "Please share the joke with me."
2. "Why are you laughing?"
3. "I don't think I said anything funny."
4. "You're laughing. Tell me what's happening."

Answer: 4

Rationale: The client is likely laughing in response to inner stimuli such as hallucinations or fantasy. Moller suggests focusing on the hallucinatory clue (the client's laughter) and eliciting the client's observation. The other options are less useful in eliciting a response. Option 1: No joke may be involved. Option 2: "Why" questions are difficult to answer. Option 3: The client is probably not focusing on what the nurse said in the first place.

Cognitive level: Application
Nursing process: Implementation
NCLEX: Psychosocial Integrity
See text pages: 393, 401

24. The nurse is told that a client with disorganized schizophrenia is being admitted to the unit. The nurse should expect the client to demonstrate
1. highly suspicious, delusional behavior.
2. extremes of motor activity and excitement to stupor.

3. social withdrawal and ineffective communication.
4. severe anxiety and ritualistic behavior.

Answer: 3

Rationale: Clients with disorganized schizophrenia demonstrate the most regressed and socially impaired behaviors of the schizophrenias. Communication is often incoherent, with silly giggling and loose associations predominating. Option 1 relates more to paranoid schizophrenia. Option 2 relates to catatonic schizophrenia. Option 4 is seen with obsessive-compulsive disorder.

Cognitive level: Application
Nursing process: Assessment
NCLEX: Psychosocial Integrity
See text page: 413

25. The wife of a client with schizophrenia is worried about her 17-year-old daughter and asks the nurse what symptoms mark the prodromal stage of schizophrenia. The nurse should respond by listing behaviors such as
1. withdrawal, misinterpreting, poor concentration, and preoccupation with religion.
2. auditory hallucinations, ideas of reference, thought insertion, and broadcasting.
3. stereotyped behavior, echopraxia, echolalia, and waxy flexibility.
4. loose associations, concrete thinking, and echolalia neologisms.

Answer: 1

Rationale: Options 2, 3, and 4 each list the positive symptoms of schizophrenia that might be apparent during the acute stage of the illness. Prodromal symptoms, the symptoms that are present before the development of florid symptoms, are listed in option 1.

Cognitive level: Application
Nursing process: Implementation
NCLEX: Health Promotion and Maintenance
See text page: 389

26. Which findings listed in the medical record of a client with schizophrenia indicate a neurological origin for schizophrenia?
1. A hostile, overinvolved parent and a weak, uninvolved parent
2. Enlarged or asymmetrical ventricles, cortical atrophy
3. Presence of ambivalence and flattened affect
4. Presence of delusions and hallucinations

Answer: 2

Rationale: Only option 2 relates to neurological findings. Options 3 and 4 refer to symptoms. Option 1 refers to family dynamics.

Cognitive level: Analysis
Nursing process: Assessment
NCLEX: Physiological Integrity
See text page: 387

27. The physician prescribes risperidone for a client with schizophrenia who displays delusions, hallucinations, apathy, and social isolation. Which symptoms should be monitored to evaluate improvement?
    1. Positive symptoms
    2. Negative symptoms
    3. Disorganized symptoms
    4. Both positive and negative symptoms

Answer: 4
Rationale: The atypical antipsychotic medications target both the negative and positive symptoms of schizophrenia, an obvious advantage over the standard antipsychotics; thus both sets of symptoms should be the foci of evaluation. No specific subset of disorganized symptoms is available.
Cognitive level: Analysis
Nursing process: Evaluation
NCLEX: Psychosocial Integrity
See text page: 405

28. A client with the diagnosis of schizophrenia, disorganized type, approaches the nurse and says "It's beat, it's eat. No room. The cat." The nurse can correctly assess this verbalization as
    1. neologisms.
    2. ideas of reference.
    3. thought broadcasting.
    4. associative looseness.

Answer: 4
Rationale: Looseness of association refers to jumbled thoughts that are often incoherently expressed to the listener. Option 1: Neologisms are newly coined words. Option 2: Ideas of reference are a type of delusion. Option 3: Thought broadcasting is the belief that others can hear one's thoughts.
Cognitive level: Application
Nursing process: Assessment
NCLEX: Psychosocial Integrity
See text pages: 392, 393

29. A client with schizophrenia has received standard antipsychotics for a year. His hallucinations are less intrusive, but the client remains apathetic, has poverty of thought, cannot work, and is socially isolated. To address these symptoms, the nurse might expect the psychiatrist to prescribe
    1. haloperidol (Haldol).
    2. olanzapine (Zyprexa).

    3. diphenhydramine (Benadryl).
    4. chlorpromazine (Thorazine).

Answer: 2
Rationale: Olanzapine is an atypical antipsychotic that targets both positive and negative symptoms of schizophrenia. Options 1 and 4 are standard antipsychotics that target only positive symptoms. Option 3 is an antihistamine.
Cognitive level: Application
Nursing process: Planning
NCLEX: Physiological Integrity
See text page: 405

30. The family of a client with acute symptoms of schizophrenia knows nothing about the client's illness and the role the family can play in his recovery. The nurse should recommend that they attend
    1. psychoanalytic group therapy.
    2. a psychoeducational group.
    3. transactional therapy.
    4. family therapy.

Answer: 2
Rationale: A psychoeducational group explores the causes of schizophrenia, the role of medication, the importance of medication compliance, support for the ill member, and hints for living with a schizophrenic person. Such a group can be of immeasurable practical assistance to the family. The other types of therapy do not focus on psychoeducation.
Cognitive level: Application
Nursing process: Implementation
NCLEX: Health Promotion and Maintenance
See text pages: 402, 403

31. Select the outcomes most appropriate for a client in phase III of treatment of schizophrenia who displays many negative symptoms of the disorder. The client will (more than one answer may be correct)
    1. take medication as ordered.
    2. maintain a regular sleep pattern.
    3. use alcohol and caffeine as desired.
    4. participate in self-care skills training.

Answers: 1, 2, 4
Rationale: The stabilization phase of schizophrenia is seen when the client is well enough to be maintained in the community. It is a time for consolidating gains, learning relapse prevention (options 1 and 2), and promoting adaptation to deficits that still exist (option 4). Option 3: Use of alcohol, caffeine, and other recreational drugs should be discouraged because these substances interfere with therapeutic medication effects.

333

Cognitive level: Application
Nursing process: Planning (Outcome Identification)
NCLEX: Psychosocial Integrity
See text page: 398

32. The family of a client with schizophrenia who has been stable for a year reports to the community mental health nurse that the client reports feeling tense and having difficulty concentrating. He sleeps only 3 to 4 hours nightly and has begun to talk about "volmers" hiding in the warehouse where he works and undoing his work each night. The nurse can correctly assess this information as an indication of
   1. medication noncompliance.
   2. the need for psychoeducation.
   3. chronic deterioration.
   4. relapse.

Answer: 4
Rationale: Signs of potential relapse include feeling tense, difficulty concentrating, trouble sleeping, increased withdrawal, and increased bizarre or magical thinking.
   Option 1: Medication noncompliance may not be implicated. Relapse can occur even when the client is taking medication regularly. Option 2: Psychoeducation is better delivered when the client's symptoms are stable. Option 3: Chronic deterioration is not the most viable explanation.
Cognitive level: Application
Nursing process: Assessment
NCLEX: Physiological Integrity
See text pages: 399, 400

33. A client with schizophrenia begins to talk about "volmers" hiding in the warehouse where he works and undoing his work each night. The term "volmers" should be assessed as
   1. a neologism.
   2. concrete thinking.
   3. thought insertion.
   4. an idea of reference.

Answer: 1
Rationale: A neologism is a newly coined word having special meaning to the client. "Volmer" is not a known word. Option 2: Concrete thinking refers to the inability to think abstractly. Option 3: Thought insertion refers to the idea that the thoughts of others are being planted in one's mind. Option 4: Ideas of reference are a type of delusion in which trivial events are given personal significance.
Cognitive level: Application
Nursing process: Assessment
NCLEX: Psychosocial Integrity
See text pages: 392, 393

34. A client with schizophrenia anxiously describes seeing the left side of her body merge with the wall as she walked down the corridor and of seeing her face appear and disappear in the bathroom mirror. As the nurse listens she should
   1. sit close to the client on the bed.
   2. place an arm protectively around the client's shoulders.
   3. place a hand on the client's arm and exert light pressure.
   4. maintain the normal social interaction distance from the client.

Answer: 4
Rationale: The client is describing phenomena that indicate personal boundary difficulties. The nurse should maintain appropriate social distance from the client and not touch her because the client is anxious about her inability to maintain ego boundaries and merging or being swallowed by the environment. Physical closeness or touch could precipitate panic.
Cognitive level: Application
Nursing process: Implementation
NCLEX: Psychosocial Integrity
See text pages: 393, 394

35. A frightened, delusional client tells the nurse "I can't go to activities. When I am in a room with a lot of people I can feel them sucking my thoughts out of my head." The nurse can correctly assess this as
   1. anhedonia.
   2. concrete thinking.
   3. thought withdrawal.
   4. associative looseness.

Answer: 3
Rationale: Thought withdrawal is defined as a delusional belief that someone or something is removing thoughts from the client's mind. Option 1: Anhedonia is the inability to experience pleasure. Option 2: Concrete thinking refers to the inability to use abstraction. Option 4: Associative looseness refers to a lack of ties between thoughts, leading to jumbled thinking.
Cognitive level: Application
Nursing process: Assessment
NCLEX: Physiological Integrity
See text pages: 391, 392

36. A client with schizophrenia who admits to auditory hallucinations anxiously tells the nurse "The voice is telling me to do things." The priority assessment question the nurse should ask is
   1. "Do you recognize the voice speaking to you?"
   2. "How long has the voice been directing your behavior?"

334

3. "Does what the voice tell you to do frighten you?"
4. "What is the voice telling you to do?"

Answer: 4

Rationale: Learning what a command hallucination is telling the client to do is important because the command often places the client or others at risk for harm. Command hallucinations can be terrifying and may pose a psychiatric emergency. The other queries are of lesser importance than identifying the command.

Cognitive level: Application
Nursing process: Assessment
NCLEX: Safe and Effective Care Environment
See text page: 393

37. A client standing in the dining room is experiencing auditory hallucinations commanding him to strangle someone. His behavior and verbalizations indicate he is experiencing severe to panic level anxiety. Put each of the nursing interventions in the order they should be undertaken.
    1. Send another staff member to report the situation and obtain a prn medication.
    2. Assure the client that staff will help him resist the command.
    3. Take the client to a quiet, secure environment.
    4. Clear the dining room of other clients.
    5. Explain that the medication will stop the voices, then administer the drug.

Answer: 2, 4, 1, 3, 5

Rationale: This sequence supports client self-control to resist the command, protects other clients from potential harm, secures help from another while allowing the nurse to remain with the client to provide structure and set limits, removes client to a safer, less confusing environment, explains therapeutic use of medication, and limits the possibility of the client perceiving the medication as punishment.

Cognitive level: Analysis
Nursing process: Implementation
NCLEX: Safe and Effective Care Environment
See text page: NA

38. The physician is considering changing the antipsychotic medication for a client with schizophrenia who is troubled by the extrapyramidal symptoms of his current medication, haloperidol, and who seems to be becoming less motivated and more withdrawn. For planning purposes the nurse can assume that the physician will probably choose
    1. chlorpromazine (Thorazine).
    2. clozapine (Clozaril).
    3. olanzapine (Zyprexa).
    4. fluoxetine (Prozac).

Answer: 3

Rationale: Olanzapine is an atypical antipsychotic that produces few extrapyramidal side effects and is effective in treating both positive and negative symptoms of schizophrenia. Option 1: This drug often produces EPS. It is not effective in treating negative symptoms. Option 2: Clozapine would not be the drug of choice because of the danger of agranulocytosis. Option 4: Fluoxetine is a selective serotonin reuptake inhibitor antidepressant.

Cognitive level: Application
Nursing process: Planning
NCLEX: Physiological Integrity
See text page: 412

39. A client receiving risperidone (Risperdal) reports severe muscle stiffness mid-morning. During lunch he has difficulty swallowing food and is noted to drool. When vital signs are taken at 4 PM he is noted to be diaphoretic, with a temperature elevation of 38.4° C, pulse of 110 beats/min, and blood pressure of 150/90 mm Hg. The nurse should suspect
    1. agranulocytosis and institute reverse isolation.
    2. cholestatic jaundice and begin a high-protein, high-cholesterol diet.
    3. tardive dyskinesia and withhold the next dose of medication.
    4. neuroleptic malignant syndrome and notify physician stat.

Answer: 4

Rationale: Taking an antipsychotic medication coupled with the presence of extrapyramidal symptoms such as severe muscle stiffness and difficulty swallowing, hyperpyrexia, and autonomic symptoms (pulse elevation) suggest neuroleptic malignant syndrome, a medical emergency. The symptoms given in the scenario are not consistent with the medical problems listed in options 1, 2, or 3.

Cognitive level: Analysis
Nursing process: Assessment
NCLEX: Physiological Integrity
See text page: 409

40. A client with schizophrenia tells the nurse "Everyone must listen to me. I am the redeemer. I will bring peace to the world." From this the nurse can determine that an appropriate nursing diagnosis to be completed is
    1. disturbed sensory perception: auditory.
    2. risk for other-directed violence.
    3. chronic low self-esteem.
    4. noncompliance: medication.

Answer: 3

335

Rationale: The client's grandiose delusion is based on reaction formation to actual feelings of low self-esteem. The scenario does not provide sufficient data to support the other diagnoses.
Cognitive level: Analysis
Nursing process: Diagnosis
NCLEX: Psychosocial Integrity
See text pages: 391, 392, 396, 397

41. A client with many positive symptoms of schizophrenia whose behavior is disorganized and who is highly anxious tells the nurse in the psychiatric emergency department "You have got to help me. I do not know what is going on. I think someone is trying to wipe me out. I have to get a gun." The client, a college student, lives alone and has no family or support system in the immediate area. He has not left his room in 2 weeks, has not eaten in several days, and is unkempt. Of the available treatment settings, the nurse should recommend
   1. acute hospitalization for 4 to 5 days.
   2. partial hospitalization for 2 weeks.
   3. day treatment for 4 weeks.
   4. home treatment for 6 weeks.

Answer: 1
Rationale: A short-term hospital stay would probably serve the client best. Medication can be started, the inpatient milieu can provide structure, observation can be ongoing, interpersonal support can be provided, physical needs can be met, and the safety of client and others preserved. The client has no support system to provide care at home, and both partial hospitalization and day treatment would leave the client without structure and support for at least 12 hours daily.
Cognitive level: Analysis
Nursing process: Planning
NCLEX: Safe and Effective Care Environment
See text pages: 399, 400

42. A client with schizophrenia tells the nurse "I eat skiller. Tend to end. Easter. It blows away. Get it?" The best response for the nurse to make would be
   1. "Nothing you are saying is clear."
   2. "Your thoughts are very disconnected."
   3. "Try to organize your thoughts and then tell me again."
   4. "I am having difficulty understanding what you are saying."

Answer: 4
Rationale: When a client's speech is loosely associated, confused, and disorganized, pretending to understand is useless. The nurse should tell the client that she is having difficulty understanding what the client is saying. If a theme is discernable, ask the

client to talk about the theme. The other options tend to place blame for the poor communication with the client. Option 4 places the difficulty with the nurse rather than being accusatory.
Cognitive level: Application
Nursing process: Implementation
NCLEX: Psychosocial integrity
See text pages: 401, 402

43. The physician and advanced practice nurse are considering which antipsychotic medication to prescribe for a client with schizophrenia who demonstrates auditory hallucinations, apathy, anhedonia, and poor social functioning. The client is overweight and has hypertension. Bearing these facts in mind, the drug the nurse should advocate would be
   1. clozapine (Clozaril).
   2. ziprasidone (Geodon).
   3. olanzapine (Zyprexa).
   4. aripiprazole (Abilify).

Answer: 4
Rationale: Aripiprazole is a new atypical antipsychotic effective against both positive and negative symptoms of schizophrenia. It causes little or no weight gain and no increase in glucose, high- or low-density lipoprotein cholesterol, or triglycerides, making it a reasonable choice for a client with obesity or heart disease. Option 1: Clozapine may produce agranulocytosis, making it a poor choice as a first-line agent. Option 2: Ziprasidone may prolong the QT interval, making it a poor choice for a client with cardiac disease. Option 3: Olanzapine fosters weight gain.
Cognitive level: Analysis
Nursing process: Planning
NCLEX: Physiological Integrity
See text page: 406

44. A male client diagnosed with paranoid schizophrenia angrily tells the male nurse "You act like a homosexual. None of the men trust you or want to be around you." The nurse, who is heterosexual, is perplexed by the client's statements and discusses the event with his mentor. The most likely analysis of the event is
   1. the client was unleashing unconscious, hostile feelings toward the nurse.
   2. the client was demonstrating reaction formation in response to feelings of abandonment.
   3. dwelling on others' shortcomings puts them on the defensive.
   4. the client was projecting homosexual urges.

Answer: 4
Rationale: Clients with paranoid ideation unconsciously use the defense mechanism projection to deal with

336

unacceptable, anxiety-producing ideas and impulses, in this case homosexual urges. Option 1: Although the behavior seems hostile, the projection is homosexual urges rather than hostility. Option 2: Clients who exhibit paranoid ideation usually fear abandonment, but this situation does not represent reaction formation to abandonment feelings. Option 3: Although this statement about defensive behavior is true, it is not the correct analysis of the behavior described in the scenario.

Cognitive level: Analysis
Nursing process: Assessment
NCLEX: Psychosocial Integrity
See text page: 414

45. Which client with schizophrenia would be expected to have the lowest score in global assessment of functioning?
    1. Client A, aged 39 years, who had paranoid ideation develop at age 35 years.
    2. Client B, aged 40 years, who has had disorganized schizophrenia since age 18 years.
    3. Client C, diagnosed as catatonic at age 24 years, who has been stable for 3 years.
    4. Client D, aged 19 years, diagnosed with undifferentiated schizophrenia at age 17 years.

Answer: 2
Rationale: Disorganized schizophrenia represents the most regressed and socially impaired of all the schizophrenias. Client B could logically be expected to have the lowest global assessment of functioning. In addition, the client has been ill for a number of years. Option 1: Client A could be expected to have the highest score because paranoid schizophrenia of short duration may be less impairing than other types. Option 3: Client C has been stable more than 3 years, suggesting higher functional ability. Option 4: Client D has been ill only 2 years, and disability in undifferentiated schizophrenia remains fairly stable over time.

Cognitive level: Application
Nursing process: Assessment
NCLEX: Psychosocial Integrity
See text pages: 412, 414-416

CHAPTER 21

1. A widow, aged 72 years, lives alone and is visited weekly by her son. She takes digoxin, hydrochlorothiazide, and an antihypertensive drug. She also has a prescription for diazepam (Valium) as needed for moderate to severe anxiety. When the son visited today he found his mother confused. Her speech was thick and slurred and she had an unsteady gait. She

was taken to the emergency department, and hospital admission followed. The nurse assessed the client as having several cognitive problems, including memory and attention deficits and fluctuating levels of orientation. The nurse confirms that the client's symptoms developed over a 2-day period. The client's symptoms are most characteristic of
    1. delirium.
    2. dementia.
    3. amnestic syndrome.
    4. Alzheimer's disease.

Answer: 1
Rationale: Delirium is characterized by an abrupt onset of fluctuating levels of awareness, clouded consciousness, perceptual disturbances, and disturbed memory and orientation. Options 2 and 4: The onset of dementia or Alzheimer's disease, a type of dementia, is more insidious. Option 3: Amnestic syndrome involves memory impairment without other cognitive problems.

Cognitive level: Analysis
Nursing process: Assessment
NCLEX: Physiological Integrity
See text pages: 423, 424

2. A client with fluctuating levels of awareness, confusion, and disturbed orientation shouts "The bugs, they are crawling on my legs! Get them off me!" The nurse can assess this behavior as indicating that the client is experiencing
    1. aphasia.
    2. dystonia.
    3. tactile hallucinations.
    4. mnemonic disturbance.

Answer: 3
Rationale: The client feels bugs crawling on her legs, even though no sensory stimulus is actually present. This description coincides with the definition of a hallucination, a false sensory perception. Tactile hallucinations may be part of the symptom constellation of delirium. Option 1: *Aphasia* refers to a speech disorder. Option 2: *Dystonia* refers to excessive muscle tonus. Option 3: Mnemonic disturbance is associated with dementia rather than delirium.

Cognitive level: Application
Nursing process: Assessment
NCLEX: Physiological Integrity
See text page: 426

3. The most appropriate response for the nurse to make when a client with fluctuating levels of consciousness, disturbed orientation, and perceptual alterations begs to have someone get the bugs off her would be

1. "There are no bugs on your legs. Your imagination is playing tricks on you."
2. "Try to relax. The crawling sensation will go away sooner if you can relax."
3. "Don't worry, I will have someone stay here and brush away the bugs for you."
4. "I don't see any bugs, but I know you are frightened so I will stay with you."

Answer: 4

Rationale: When hallucinations are present, the nurse should acknowledge the client's feelings and state the nurse's perception of reality, but not argue. Staying with the client increases feelings of security, reduces anxiety, offers the opportunity for reinforcing reality, and provides a measure of physical safety. Option 1 does not support the client emotionally. Option 2 makes the client responsible for self-soothing. Option 3 supports the perceptual distortions.

Cognitive level: Application
Nursing process: Implementation
NCLEX: Safe and Effective Care Environment
See text pages: 426, 427

4. The nursing diagnosis established for a client with fluctuating levels of consciousness, disturbed orientation, and visual and tactile hallucinations that should be given priority is
   1. bathing/hygiene self-care deficit related to altered cerebral function, as evidenced by confusion and inability to perform personal hygiene tasks.
   2. risk for injury related to altered cerebral function, as evidenced by sensory perceptual alterations and unstable gait.
   3. disturbed thought processes related to altered cerebral function resulting from medication intoxication, as evidenced by confusion, disorientation, and hallucinations.
   4. fear related to sensory perceptual alterations, as evidenced by hiding from hallucinated dog and wanting nurse to remove hallucinated bugs from her legs.

Answer: 2

Rationale: The physical safety of the client is of highest priority among the diagnoses given. Many opportunities for injury exist when a client misperceives the environment as distorted, threatening, or harmful; when the client exercises poor judgment; and when the client's sensorium is clouded. The other diagnoses, although valid, are of lower priority.

Cognitive level: Analysis
Nursing process: Diagnosis
NCLEX: Safe and Effective Care Environment
See text page: 428

5. An important facet of nursing care for a client with delirium who has fluctuating levels of consciousness, disturbed orientation, and perceptual alterations is
   1. avoidance of physical contact.
   2. application of wrist and ankle restraints.
   3. careful observation and supervision.
   4. a high level of sensory stimulation.

Answer: 3

Rationale: Careful observation and supervision are of ultimate importance because an appropriate outcome would be that the client will remain safe and free from injury while hospitalized. Option 1: Physical contact during caregiving cannot be avoided. Option 2: Restraint is a last resort. Option 4: Sensory stimulation should be reduced.

Cognitive level: Application
Nursing process: Implementation
NCLEX: Safe and Effective Care Environment
See text page: 430

6. What environmental conditions should the nurse arrange for a client with delirium while the client is experiencing perceptual alterations?
   1. Provide a well-lit room without glare or shadows and limit noise
   2. Have the client sit by the nurse's desk while awake and provide rest periods in a room with the television on
   3. Light room brightly around the clock and awaken hourly to check mental status
   4. Keep room shadowy with soft lighting around the clock and keep a radio on continuously

Answer: 1

Rationale: A quiet, shadow-free room offers an environment that produces the fewest sensory perceptual distortions for a client with cognitive impairment associated with delirium. The other options have the potential to produce increased perceptual alterations.

Cognitive level: Application
Nursing process: Implementation
NCLEX: Safe and Effective Care Environment
See text page: 430

7. Which of the following descriptions of client experience and behavior can be assessed as a hallucination? A client
   1. states "I feel bugs crawling on my legs and biting me."
   2. looks at shadows on a wall and tells the nurse "I see scary faces."
   3. becomes anxious whenever the nurse leaves her bedside.

4. tries to hit the nurse when vital signs are being taken.

Answer: 1

Rationale: An illusion is a misinterpreted sensory perception. A hallucination is a false sensory perception occurring without a corresponding sensory stimulus. Feeling bugs on the body when none are present is a tactile hallucination. Option 2: Misinterpreting shadows as faces is an illusion. Options 3 and 4 are examples of behaviors sometimes occurring during delirium that are related to fluctuating levels of awareness and misinterpreted stimuli.

Cognitive level: Application
Nursing process: Assessment
NCLEX: Physiological Integrity
See text page: 426

8. A client whose medical diagnosis is hepatic encephalopathy is admitted to the hospital. The client has abused alcohol for 20 years. The attitude on the part of the nurse assigned to care for the client that would be most detrimental to establishing an effective nurse-client relationship is perceiving that the client
1. has a serious physical condition.
2. did it to himself and is getting what he deserves.
3. will respond best to a calm, caring approach.
4. is challenging, requiring skill in both physical and emotional care.

Answer: 2

Rationale: This attitude is judgmental, whereas the other statements are nonjudgmental. Being judgmental hinders the establishment of a therapeutic relationship.

Cognitive level: Application
Nursing process: Assessment
NCLEX: Safe and Effective Care Environment
See text page: NA

9. A client with Alzheimer's disease requires coaching to bathe and dress, wanders aimlessly throughout the home, displays mood fluctuations from pleasant to irritable, and becomes easily frustrated when performing simple tasks. Which behavior should the nurse assess as an example of cognitive impairment?
1. Inability to bathe and dress independently
2. Wandering
3. Mood lability
4. Ease of frustration

Answer: 1

Rationale: Inability to bathe and dress suggests apraxia, the loss of purposeful movement in the absence of motor or sensory impairment. The other symptoms are less directly attributable to loss of cortical function.

Cognitive level: Application

Nursing process: Assessment
NCLEX: Physiological Integrity
See text page: 426

10. A man, aged 84 years, was stopped for going through a red light in a small town where he has lived all his life. He told the officer "It wasn't there yesterday." He was unable to tell the officer his address and demonstrated labile mood, seeming pleasant one minute and angry the next. The officer took the individual to his home to discuss his condition with the family and found that he lives with his wife, who is legally blind. She stated "He's my eyes and I'm his mind." She also related that her husband wanders around the neighborhood, sometimes taking tools from people's garages, saying they belong to him. She reluctantly agreed that he should go to the emergency department for evaluation. He was diagnosed with Alzheimer's disease. The cardinal sign of Alzheimer's disease demonstrated by the client is
1. aphasia.
2. apraxia.
3. agnosia.
4. memory impairment.

Answer: 4

Rationale: Of the cardinal signs of Alzheimer's disease, the client is presently demonstrating only mnemonic disturbance, or memory loss. Option 1: Aphasia refers to the loss of language ability. Option 2: Apraxia refers to the loss of purposeful movement. Option 3: Agnosia refers to the loss of sensory ability to recognize objects.

Cognitive level: Application
Nursing process: Assessment
NCLEX: Psychosocial Integrity
See text page: 426

11. An elderly man drove from his home to a nearby convenience store and was unable to remember how to get home. He was unable to tell a police officer his address and demonstrated labile mood, seeming pleasant one minute and angry the next. The officer took the individual to his home to discuss his condition with the family. The wife related that her husband often wanders around the neighborhood, sometimes taking tools from people's garages. She reluctantly agreed that he should go to the emergency department for evaluation. He was diagnosed with Alzheimer's disease. On the basis of the client's history, the nurse can make the assessment that the client's Alzheimer's disease has progressed to
1. Stage 1 (mild).
2. Stage 2 (moderate).

Chapter 21 Cognitive Disorders

3. Stage 3 (moderate to severe).
4. Stage 4 (late).

Answer: 2

Rationale: In stage 2, deterioration is evident. Memory loss may include the inability to remember addresses or the date. Mood is labile. Activities such as driving may become hazardous, and frustration by the increasing difficulty of performing ordinary tasks may be experienced. Hygiene may begin to deteriorate. Option 3: Stage 3 finds the individual unable to identify familiar objects or people and needing direction for the simplest of tasks. Option 4: In stage 4 the ability to talk and walk are eventually lost and stupor evolves.
Cognitive level: Analysis
Nursing process: Assessment
NCLEX: Physiological Integrity
See text pages: 434-436

12. As Alzheimer's disease progresses from moderate to severe to late stage, for planning purposes the nurse can anticipate that all but one of the following symptoms will become apparent. The behavior that is *least* likely to affect care planning is
    1. agraphia.
    2. hyperorality.
    3. hypermetamorphosis.
    4. improvement of memory.

Answer: 4

Rationale: The memories of clients with Alzheimer's disease are expected to continue to deteriorate. These clients will demonstrate the inability to read or write (option 1), the need to put everything into the mouth (option 2), and the need to touch everything (option 3).
Cognitive level: Application
Nursing process: Planning
NCLEX: Physiological Integrity
See text page: 436

13. A client with stage 1 Alzheimer's disease is described by her husband as having lost energy and preferring to remain at home rather than attend club meetings and church. The husband has been doing the grocery shopping because his wife cannot remember what to purchase and is unable to find her way around the store unassisted. Which nursing diagnosis commonly used for clients with Alzheimer's disease can be established for the client at this time?
    1. Risk for injury
    2. Impaired memory
    3. Self-care deficit
    4. Caregiver role strain

Answer: 2

Rationale: Memory impairment is present. Data are not present to suggest the other diagnoses.
Cognitive level: Analysis
Nursing process: Diagnosis
NCLEX: Physiological Integrity
See text page: 437

14. A nursing intervention designed to help the client with progressive memory deficit associated with dementia function in his or her environment is
    1. assisting the client to perform simple tasks by giving step-by-step directions.
    2. avoiding frustrating the client by performing routines associated with activities of daily living for the client.
    3. stimulating the client's intellectual functioning by bringing new topics and options to the client's attention.
    4. promoting the use of the client's sense of humor by telling jokes or riddles and discussing cartoons.

Answer: 1

Rationale: Clients with cognitive impairment should perform all tasks of which they are capable. When simple directions are given in a step-by-step fashion, the client is better able to process information and perform simple tasks. Option 3 is likely to prove frustrating for the client. Option 4: Clients with cognitive deficits may lose their sense of humor and find such discussions meaningless.
Cognitive level: Application
Nursing process: Implementation
NCLEX: Psychosocial Integrity
Seem text page: 443

15. B and J both have Alzheimer's disease. B walks up behind J in the hall and shouts "Move along, you're blocking the road. I'll take a stick to you." J turns around, shakes his fist, and shouts "I know what you're up to, you're trying to steal my car." The best action for the nurse to take would be to
    1. reinforce reality by telling B that J can walk in the hall, and telling J that B is not trying to steal his car.
    2. ask the medication nurse to give both clients an as-needed dose of neuroleptic medication.
    3. separate and distract them by directing one to go to the day room and taking the other to the activities area.
    4. step between them, saying "Gentlemen, please quiet down. We do not permit physical violence here."

Answer: 3

Rationale: Separating and distracting prevents escalation from verbal to physical acting out. Neither client loses self-esteem during this intervention, and medication will probably not be necessary. Stepping between two angry, threatening clients is an unsafe action, and trying to reinforce reality during an angry outburst will probably not be successful when the clients are cognitively impaired.

Cognitive level: Application
Nursing process: Implementation
NCLEX: Safe and Effective Care Environment
See text page: 442

16. The elderly client in the intensive care unit who is diagnosed as having disturbed sensory perceptions in the form of visual and auditory illusions will be helped most by
   1. large clocks and calendars on the wall.
   2. personally meaningful objects placed in full view.
   3. wearing her glasses and hearing aids.
   4. keeping the room brightly lit around the clock.

Answer: 3

Rationale: Illusions are sensory misperceptions. Glasses and hearing aids help clarify sensory perceptions. Options 1 and 2: Without glasses, clocks, calendars, and personal objects may not be noticed. Option 4: Round-the-clock lighting promotes sensory overload and sensory perceptual alterations.

Cognitive level: Application
Nursing process: Implementation
NCLEX: Physiological Integrity
See text page: 427

17. A client with stage 2 Alzheimer's disease calls the police, saying an intruder is in her home. The police officer who investigates the call determines the client has seen her own reflection in the mirror and thought an intruder was present. This phenomenon can be assessed as
   1. hyperorality.
   2. aphasia.
   3. apraxia.
   4. agnosia.

Answer: 4

Rationale: Agnosia is the inability to recognize familiar objects, parts of one's body, or one's own reflection in a mirror. Option 1: Hyperorality refers to placing objects in the mouth. Option 2: Aphasia refers to the loss of language ability. Option 3: Apraxia refers to the loss of purposeful movements, such as being unable to dress.

Cognitive level: Application
Nursing process: Assessment
NCLEX: Physiological Integrity
See text page: 426

18. During morning care, the nursing assistant asks a client with dementia "How was your night?" The client replies "It was lovely. My husband and I went out to dinner and to a movie." The nurse who overhears this should make the assessment that the client is
   1. demonstrating a sense of humor.
   2. using confabulation.
   3. perseverating.
   4. delirious.

Answer: 2

Rationale: Confabulation is the making up of stories or answers to questions by a person who does not remember. It is a defensive tactic to protect self-esteem and prevent others from noticing memory loss. Option 1: The client's response was not given facetiously, so it cannot be assessed as an attempt at humor. Option 3: Perseveration refers to repeating a word or phrase over and over. Option 4: Delirium cannot be assessed as present in this scenario.

Cognitive level: Application
Nursing process: Assessment
NCLEX: Psychosocial Integrity
See text page: 426

19. A client with Alzheimer's disease has been determined to have a dressing/grooming self-care deficit. Appropriate interventions to include in the client's nursing care plan are (more than one answer may be correct)
   1. to provide clothing with elastic and hook-and-loop material closures.
   2. to label clothing with the client's name and name of the item.
   3. to provide necessary items and expect the client to proceed independently.
   4. to administer anxiolytic medication before bathing and dressing.
   5. if the client is resistive, use distraction; then try again after a short interval.
   6. if the client moves too slowly to accomplish the task, the staff should perform it.

Answers: 1, 2, 5

Rationale: Option 1 facilitates client independence. Option 2 maintains client identity and dignity (provides information if the client has agnosia). Option 5: Client moods are often labile. The client may be willing to cooperate given a later opportunity.

Chapter 21   Cognitive Disorders

Option 3 is inappropriate. Be prepared to coach by giving step-by-step directions for each task as it occurs. Option 4 is inappropriate. This measure would result in unnecessary overmedication. Option 6: Clients should be allowed to perform all tasks within their capabilities.
Cognitive level: Application
Nursing process: Planning
NCLEX: Psychosocial Integrity
See text page: 443

20. An action the nurse can advise a family to take in the home setting to enhance safety for the client with Alzheimer's disease who wanders at night is
   1. place throw rugs on tile or wooden floors.
   2. elevate bed on 6-inch blocks.
   3. encourage daytime napping.
   4. place locks at the tops of doors.

Answer: 4
Rationale: Placing door locks at the top of the door makes it more difficult for the client with dementia to unlock the door because the ability to look up and reach upward is diminished. Option 1: All throw rugs should be removed to prevent falls. Option 2: Placing a mattress on the floor to prevent falls is a better intervention than raising the height of the bed. Option 3: Day napping should be discouraged with the hope that the client will sleep during the night.
Cognitive level: Application
Nursing process: Planning
NCLEX: Safe and Effective Care Environment
See text page: 445

21. The outcome that should be established for an elderly client with delirium caused by fever and dehydration is that the client will
   1. return to a premorbid level of functioning.
   2. demonstrate motor responses to noxious stimuli.
   3. identify stressors negatively affecting self.
   4. exert control over responses to perceptual distortions.

Answer: 1
Rationale: The desired overall outcome is that the delirious client will return to the level of functioning held before the development of delirium. Option 2 is an indicator appropriate for a client whose arousal is compromised. Option 3 is too nonspecific to be useful for a client with delirium. Option 4 is an unrealistic indicator for a client with sensorium problems related to delirium.
Cognitive level: Application
Nursing process: Planning (Outcome Identification)
NCLEX: Physiological Integrity
See text pages: 428, 429

22. A family states that the father, who has moderate-stage dementia, is incontinent related to forgetting where the bathroom is located. An intervention the nurse should suggest to the family is to
   1. label the bathroom door.
   2. have someone take him to the bathroom hourly.
   3. place the client in disposable diapers.
   4. make sure the client does not eat nonfood items.

Answer: 1
Rationale: The client with moderate Alzheimer's disease has memory loss that begins to interfere with activities. This client may be able to use environmental cues such as labels on doors to compensate for memory loss. Option 2: Regular toileting may be helpful, but a 2-hour schedule is often more reasonable. Option 3: This intervention is more appropriate as a later stage intervention. It is probably unnecessary at this point. Option 4 will be more relevant when the client demonstrates hyperorality.
Cognitive level: Application
Nursing process: Implementation
NCLEX: Safe and Effective Care Environment
See text page: 445

23. A client with dementia no longer recognizes her only daughter. The daughter asks the nurse "How long do you think it will be before my mother will recognize me when I visit her?" The best reply for the nurse would be
   1. "I think that is a question the physician will need to answer."
   2. "Your mother will never again be able to identify you or other family members."
   3. "One never knows; consciousness fluctuates in clients with dementia."
   4. "It is disappointing when someone you love no longer recognizes you."

Answer: 4
Rationale: Therapeutic communication techniques can assist the family to come to terms with the losses and irreversibility dementia imposes on both the loved one and themselves. Options 1 and 2: These responses close communication. The nurse should take the opportunity to foster communication. Option 3 does not present factual information.
Cognitive level: Application
Nursing process: Implementation
NCLEX: Health Promotion and Maintenance
See text pages: 430, 431

24. A client with severe dementia can no longer recognize her only daughter and becomes anxious and agitated when the daughter attempts to reorient her.

An alternative the nurse could suggest to the daughter is to
1. wear a large name tag.
2. visit her mother less often.
3. use validating techniques.
4. place clocks and calendars strategically.

Answer: 3

Rationale: Reorientation may seem like arguing to a client with cognitive deficit and increases the client's anxiety. Validating, talking with the client about familiar, meaningful things and reminiscing, gives meaning to existence both for the client and family members. Option 3 is the only option that addresses an interactional strategy. Options 1 and 4 are reorientation strategies. Option 2 is inadvisable because clients with dementia profit from contacts with interested individuals whether or not they can name the individual.

Cognitive level: Application
Nursing process: Implementation
NCLEX: Health Promotion and Maintenance
See text page: 442

23. A client with marked cognitive impairment is combative and difficult to manage. He has pulled out his nasogastric tube, his intravenous line, and his indwelling urinary catheter. He had climbed out of bed over the side rails while the nurse tried to calm and restrain him. The nurse notifies the doctor on call and can anticipate that the physician will order a
1. small dose of a selective serotonin reuptake inhibitor.
2. large dose of a benzodiazepine.
3. maintenance dose of buspirone.
4. small dose of a high-potency antipsychotic.

Answer: 4

Rationale: Aggressive behavior can be safely managed by antipsychotic medication. Initial dosing should be small and raised cautiously until behavior is controlled. Option 1: Selective serotonin reuptake inhibitors are not indicated for aggressive behavior. Option 2: If a benzodiazepine is used, the initial dose should be low. Option 3: Buspirone is not effective if given on an as-needed basis. It is administered in small divided doses daily to control agitation.

Cognitive level: Application
Nursing process: Planning
NCLEX: Physiological Integrity
See text page: 447

26. The client need that assumes priority when implementing care for a client with late-stage dementia is

1. meaningful verbal communication.
2. promotion of self-care activities.
3. maintenance of nutrition and hydration.
4. prevention of the client from wandering.

Answer: 3

Rationale: In late-stage dementia, the client often seems to have forgotten how to eat, chew, and swallow. Nutrition and hydration needs must be met if the client is to live.

Cognitive level: Analysis
Nursing process: Planning
NCLEX: Physiological Integrity
See text page: 435

27. Which remark by a family member of a client with dementia would allow the nurse to evaluate psychoeducation regarding medications as having been effective? "We understand that medications
1. inhibiting the action of dopamine will restore short-term memory."
2. inhibiting acetylcholine breakdown may slow the progression of the disease."
3. affecting glutamate receptors will provide a cure for late-stage dementia."
4. offer virtually no positive effects on cognitive performance and function of activities of daily living."

Answer: 2

Rationale: Tacrine, donepezil, rivastigmine, and galantamine act by increasing the brain's supply of acetylcholine, a neurotransmitter deficient in people with Alzheimer's disease. These drugs improve functioning and slow the progress of the disease in 20% to 50% of clients. They do not provide a cure. Memantine affects N-methyl-D-aspartate receptors and has also been shown to provide significant benefits when administered with donepezil. Options 1 and 3: Medications affecting dopamine action or glutamate receptors are not indicated in treatment of Alzheimer's disease. Option 4 is untrue.

Cognitive level: Analysis
Nursing process: Evaluation
NCLEX: Health Promotion and Maintenance
See text pages: 444-446

28. Planned assessments of critical importance for a client with delirium include
1. biophysical parameters.
2. the emotional state.
3. speech and language.
4. cognitive symptoms.

Answer: 1

Rationale: Although each area should be assessed initially and systematically thereafter, the biophysical parameters, including vital signs and physical safety needs, are of critical importance to maintenance of biophysical integrity. Delirium is, after all, a physiological disturbance.

Cognitive level: Analysis
Nursing process: Assessment
NCLEX: Safe and Effective Care Environment
See text page: 426

29. The 55-year-old-daughter of a client with late-stage Alzheimer's disease mentions to the nurse that she is concerned that she, too, will have dementia develop. The response that provides accurate information is
   1. "Put aside your worries and make the most of the years you have. You will be symptom free for at least another 20 years."
   2. "Statistics show that relatives of people with Alzheimer's disease are predisposed to the disease, but the risk is not universal."
   3. "You might wish to have genetic testing, because the *APOE* gene analysis can predict development of late-onset symptoms."
   4. "Talk with your doctor. Evidence is conclusive that people who take statin drugs and nonsteroidal antiinflammatory drugs can significantly lower their risk."

Answer: 2
Rationale: Actually, little is known of the genetic and nongenetic risk factors for Alzheimer's disease. Even though relatives of clients with Alzheimer's disease are more likely to develop the disease than the general population, no etiologic hypotheses have been proven. Option 1 may not be a true statement. Option 3 is untrue. Option 4 has not been conclusively proven.

Cognitive level: Comprehension
Nursing process: Implementation
NCLEX: Health Promotion and Maintenance
See text pages: 431, 432

30. When the nurse receives information that a client with delirium is being admitted to the unit, the nurse would expect to document assessment findings that include (more than one answer may be correct)
   1. unimpaired level of consciousness.
   2. disorientation to place and time.
   3. wandering of attention.
   4. perceptual disturbances.
   5. self-care competence.
   6. stable autonomic signs.

Answers: 2, 3, 4
Rationale: Option 2 is an expected finding. Orientation to person (self) usually remains intact. Option 3: Attention span is short, and difficulty focusing or shifting attention as directed is often noted. Option 4: Illusions and hallucinations are commonly experienced by clients with delirium. Option 1: Fluctuating levels of consciousness are expected. Option 5: Self-care deficits are usually noted. Option 6: Autonomic signs, tachycardia, seating, flushing, dilated pupils, and elevated blood pressure are often present.

Cognitive level: Application
Nursing process: Assessment
NCLEX: Physiological Integrity
See text page: 426

31. An intervention appropriate to use for both clients with delirium and clients with dementia is
   1. speaking in a loud, firm voice.
   2. touching the client before speaking.
   3. reorienting the client to the health care worker with each contact.
   4. for aggression, using physical restraint in lieu of medication.

Answer: 3
Rationale: Short-term memory is often impaired in clients with delirium and dementia. Reorientation to staff if often necessary with each contact to minimize misperceptions, reduce anxiety level, and secure cooperation. Option 1: Loud voices may be frightening or sound angry. Option 2: Speaking before touching prevents the client from feeling threatened. Option 4: The least restrictive measure should be used.

Cognitive level: Application
Nursing process: Implementation
NCLEX: Safe and Effective Care Environment
See text page: 430

32. An outcome for the nursing diagnosis of risk for injury that would be appropriate for both a hospitalized client with delirium who misinterprets reality and a client with dementia who wanders about his home is that the client will
   1. remain safe in the present environment.
   2. participate in self-care.
   3. acknowledge reality.
   4. communicate confusion.

Answer: 1
Rationale: Safety maintenance is the desired outcome of the nursing diagnosis. The other outcomes are not

directly related to the stated nursing diagnosis and may or may not be realistic for the clients mentioned because so little is known of their conditions.

Cognitive level: Application
Nursing process: Planning (Outcome Identification)
NCLEX: Safe and Effective Care Environment
See text pages: 428, 429

CHAPTER 22

1. A client, aged 16 years, comes to the crisis clinic with several superficial cuts on her left wrist. She paces around the room and cries with convulsive sobs. She cowers when approached and responds to the nurse's questions with shrugs or monosyllables. The nurse assigned to assess the client should first say
   1. "I can see you are feeling anxious. I am going to stay and talk with you to help you feel better."
   2. "Everything is going to be all right. You are here at the clinic and the staff will keep you safe."
   3. "You need to try to stop crying so I can ask you some very important questions."
   4. "Let's set some guidelines and goals for your visit here."

Answer: 1

Rationale: The two primary thrusts of crisis intervention are to provide for the safety of the individual and use anxiety-reduction techniques so that inner resources can be used. The nurse offers her presence, which provides caring, ongoing observation relative to the client's safety, and gives interpersonal reassurance.

Cognitive level: Application
Nursing process: Implementation
NCLEX: Psychosocial Integrity
See text pages: 463, 464

2. A client, aged 16 years, comes to the crisis clinic with several superficial cuts on her left wrist. She paces around the room and cries with convulsive sobs. She cowers when approached and responds to the nurse's questions with shrugs or monosyllables. After a few minutes spent with the nurse, the client is slightly calmer. To assess the client's perception of the precipitating event, the nurse should ask
   1. "Why are you crying?"
   2. "Why did you injure your wrist?"
   3. "How can I help you feel more comfortable?"
   4. "What was happening just before you started to feel this way?"

Answer: 4

Rationale: A clear definition of the immediate problem provides the best opportunity to find a solution.

Asking about recent upsetting events permits assessment of the precipitating event. Options 1 and 2 use a poor communication technique, asking a "why" question. Option 3 asks the client to make a decision that should be made by the nurse after assessment is completed.

Cognitive level: Application
Nursing process: Assessment
NCLEX: Psychosocial Integrity
See text page: 460

3. A client, aged 16 years, comes to the crisis clinic with several superficial cuts on her left wrist. She paces around the room and cries with convulsive sobs. She cowers when approached and responds to the nurse's questions with shrugs or monosyllables. The nurse states "You are behaving like a very sick person. I wonder why." The client begins to cry and replies "I am at the end of my rope. I need help. My uncle keeps trying to molest me. My mother says I am lying about it. I read about mental illness in a book, and thought I could get help if I behaved that way." The best rationale for identifying this situation as a crisis for the client is that the client
   1. has identified it as a stressful event.
   2. is attempting to cope with an event having a pathological outcome.
   3. is manifesting a state of disequilibrium related to failure of usual coping mechanisms.
   4. is demonstrating a permanent change in coping ability, resulting in a lower level of adaptation.

Answer: 3

Rationale: A crisis occurs when a stressful event over-taxes the individual's usual ability to cope and the individual enters a state of disequilibrium. Option 1 is too simplistic. Not all stressful events result in crises. Option 2 assumes that the outcome will be pathological. Option 4 assumes that the outcome will result in a lower level of adaptation. In fact, an individual in crisis may emerge at a higher level of functioning, the same level of functioning, or a lower level of functioning.

Cognitive level: Application
Nursing process: Assessment
NCLEX: Psychosocial Integrity
See text page: 459

4. A client, aged 16 years, comes to the crisis clinic. The nurse learns she is being molested by her uncle. The client told her mother of the uncle's behavior, but the mother accused the daughter of lying. The client's crisis would be classified as
   1. maturational.

2. situational.

3. adventitious.

4. organic.

Answer: 3

Rationale: An adventitious crisis is a crisis of disaster, that is, not a part of everyday life. It is unplanned or accidental. Adventitious crises include natural disasters, national disasters, and crimes of violence. Sexual molestation falls within this classification. Option 1: Maturational crisis occurs as an individual arrives at a new stage of development, when old coping styles may be ineffective. Option 2: Situational crisis arises from an external source such as a job loss, divorce, or other loss affecting self-concept or self-esteem. Option 4 is not a type of crisis.

Cognitive level: Analysis

Nursing process: Assessment

NCLEX: Psychosocial Integrity

See text page: 459

5. A client, aged 16 years, comes to the crisis clinic. The nurse learns the client is being molested by her uncle. The client told her mother, who accused her of lying. To proceed with crisis intervention, the nurse must assume that

 1. the client has a demonstrated previous ability to cope.

 2. the client will not be open to a therapist's intervention.

 3. the therapist must help the client resolve past and current issues.

 4. the therapist must assume a passive, nondirective role as the client problem solves.

Answer: 1

Rationale: Crisis intervention is aimed at maintaining, at a minimum, the precrisis level of functioning. Crisis intervention is therefore appropriate only for someone who functioned adequately before the crisis. Option 2: This assumption would obstruct crisis intervention. Option 3: The focus of crisis intervention is on only the present problem. Option 4: The therapist must be prepared to assume an active, direct role if necessary.

Cognitive level: Application

Nursing process: Assessment

Client need: Psychosocial Integrity

Text reference: 459

6. A client, aged 16 years, comes to the crisis clinic. The nurse learns she is being molested by her uncle. She has told her mother, who thinks she is lying. In a disjointed fashion, the client tells the nurse the following: (1) "I am all confused. I got desperate and tried to kill myself." (2) "For a few days I just sat in

my room. I told my mother I was sick." (3) "I tried to figure out what to do. First I thought I would live with my friend, but her mother said I couldn't. Then I thought I would go live in a homeless shelter." (4) "I told my mother, hoping she would tell my uncle he couldn't come to the house anymore." The client has actually described the four distinct phases of crisis according to Caplan. Place the statements in the correct order to coincide with Caplan's theory.

 1. 1, 2, 3, 4

 2. 4, 2, 3, 1

 3. 3, 2, 1, 4

 4. 4, 3, 2, 1

Answer: 4

Rationale: Caplan suggests that in stage 1 the individual tries the usual problem-solving methods in an attempt to lower anxiety. In stage 2, trial-and-error attempts at solving the problem are used to restore equilibrium. In stage 3, automatic relief behaviors such as withdrawal and flight are used. In stage 4, the anxiety can be so overwhelming as to lead to serious personality disorganization or suicidal behavior.

Cognitive level: Analysis

Nursing process: Assessment

NCLEX: Psychosocial Integrity

See text page: 459

7. A client, aged 16 years, comes to the crisis clinic. The nurse learns she is being molested by her uncle. The client told her mother of the uncle's behavior, but the mother accused the daughter of lying. The client describes feeling "all confused" and subsequently cutting her wrists. Nursing diagnoses that would be appropriate to consider developing include (more than one choice may be correct)

 1. ineffective coping related to crisis involving attempted sexual abuse by uncle.

 2. disturbed thought processes related to anxiety associated with crisis of sexual abuse.

 3. anxiety related to threat to emotional and physical safety caused by sexual abuse.

 4. compromised family coping related to mother's cooperation with uncle's sexual abuse of client.

Answers: 1, 2, 3

Rationale: Defining characteristics for diagnoses 1, 2, and 3 are present. Option 4: The nurse cannot assume the mother is cooperating with the uncle's attempted sexual abuse of the client. This would require investigation.

Cognitive level: Analysis

Nursing process: Diagnosis

NCLEX: Psychosocial Integrity

See text page: 459

8. A 42-year-old woman seeks crisis intervention. She tells the nurse "I cannot take it anymore! It has to stop. Last year my husband had an affair, and we do not communicate anymore. Three months ago I found a lump in my breast that the doctor is watching closely, and yesterday my 20-year-old daughter told me she is quitting college and moving to another state with her boyfriend." The type of crisis the client is experiencing is
   1. maturational.
   2. situational.
   3. adventitious.
   4. recurring.

Answer: 2

Rationale: A situational crisis arises from an external source and involves a loss of self-concept or self-esteem. Option 3: An adventitious crisis is a crisis of disaster, such as a natural disaster or crime of violence. Option 1: Maturational crisis occurs as an individual arrives at a new stage of development, when old coping styles may be ineffective. Option 4: No classification of recurring crisis exists.

Cognitive level: Analysis
Nursing process: Assessment
NCLEX: Psychosocial Integrity
See text page: 458

9. A client, aged 42 years, seeks crisis intervention. She tells the nurse "I cannot take it anymore! It has to stop. Last year my husband had an affair, and we do not communicate anymore. Three months ago I found a lump in my breast that the doctor is watching closely, and yesterday my 20-year-old daughter told me she is quitting college and moving to another state with her boyfriend." The priority assessment for the nurse is
   1. what measures might be used to help improve the couple's communication.
   2. whether the husband is still engaged in an affair.
   3. how the client feels about the possibility of having a mastectomy.
   4. what the client has in mind when she says she "cannot take it anymore."

Answer: 4

Rationale: During crisis intervention the priority concern is client safety. This question helps assess personal coping skills. The other options are incorrect because the focus of crisis intervention is on the event that occurred immediately before the client seeking help.

Cognitive level: Application
Nursing process: Assessment
NCLEX: Psychosocial Integrity
See text page: 460

10. A client, aged 42 years, seeks crisis intervention. She tells the nurse "I cannot take it anymore! It has to stop. Last year my husband had an affair, and we do not communicate anymore. Three months ago I found a lump in my breast, and yesterday my 20-year-old daughter told me she is quitting college and moving to another state with her boyfriend." After making the assessment that the client's nuclear family is unable to provide the client with sufficient situational support, the nurse should
   1. suggest that the client seek admission to the inpatient crisis unit.
   2. ask what other relatives or friends are available to support her.
   3. tell the client to be emotionally strong and to let her daughter go.
   4. foster insight by relating the present situation to earlier situations involving loss.

Answer: 2

Rationale: The assessment of situational supports should continue. Even though the client's nuclear family may not be supportive, other situational supports may be available. If they are adequate, admission to an inpatient unit will be unnecessary (option 1). Option 3 violates the concept that the therapist can review available options but that the client should actually choose the option. Option 4 describes a traditional psychotherapeutic approach rather than crisis intervention.

Cognitive level: Application
Nursing process: Implementation
NCLEX: Psychosocial Integrity
See text page: 468

11. A client, aged 42 years, seeks crisis intervention. She tells the nurse "I cannot take it anymore! It has to stop. Last year my husband had an affair, and we do not communicate anymore. Three months ago I found a lump in my breast, and yesterday my 20-year-old daughter told me she is quitting college and moving to another state with her boyfriend." The client problem that should be the focus for crisis intervention is
   1. the possible mastectomy.
   2. the impact of her husband's infidelity.
   3. coping with her daughter leaving home.
   4. the disordered family communication.

Answer: 3

Rationale: The focus of crisis intervention is on the most recent problem: "the straw that broke the camel's back." The client had coped with the breast lesion, the husband's infidelity, and the disordered communication; disequilibrium occurred only with the introduction of the daughter leaving college and moving.

12. A client, aged 42 years, seeks crisis intervention. She tells the nurse "I cannot take it anymore! It has to stop. Last year my husband had an affair, and we do not communicate anymore. Three months ago I found a lump in my breast, and yesterday my 20-year-old daughter told me she is quitting college and moving to another state with her boyfriend." The nurse can make the assessment that crisis intervention is likely to be successful for this client because the client.
   1. is experiencing disequilibrium that she finds uncomfortable.
   2. is willing to allow others to make decisions for her.
   3. is experiencing low to moderate levels of anxiety.
   4. has never resorted to seeking help before.

Answer: 1

Rationale: A client in crisis is seeking anxiety reduction and is usually open to the active intervention of the therapist, who may offer possible solutions to the crisis not previously considered by the client. The other options are not predictive of positive outcomes.

Cognitive level: Application
Nursing process: Assessment
NCLEX: Psychosocial Integrity
See text page: 459

13. A client, aged 42 years, seeks crisis intervention. She tells the nurse "I cannot take it anymore! It has to stop. Last year my husband had an affair, and we do not communicate anymore. Three months ago I found a lump in my breast, and yesterday my 20-year-old daughter told me she is quitting college and moving to another state with her boyfriend." The priority nursing diagnosis for the client is
   1. fear related to impending surgery.
   2. deficient knowledge related to breast lesion.
   3. ineffective coping related to daughter moving away.
   4. impaired verbal communication related to spousal estrangement.

Answer: 3

Rationale: This nursing diagnosis is the priority because it reflects the precipitating event associated with the client's crisis. Data are not present to make the other diagnoses of deficient knowledge, fear, or impaired verbal communication.

14. A client who sought crisis intervention agrees after the first interview to return to the clinic daily for two weeks. The nurse offers many suggestions for lifestyle changes the client should make as crisis intervention progresses. After six sessions, which feeling should alert the nurse to the need for supervision?
   1. Caring
   2. Desire to be of assistance
   3. Empathy for the client's recent losses
   4. Wanting the client to be less clingy

Answer: 4

Rationale: The nurse feels unrealistic responsibility to "cure" the client's problems. The nurse must seek supervision and examine the expectations for self and the client. When this has been accomplished, the client's level of functioning can be reevaluated and realistic goals can be established with the client.

Cognitive level: Analysis
Nursing process: Assessment
NCLEX: Safe and Effective Care Environment
See text page: 462

13. The technique used in crisis intervention that is used less often in traditional counseling is
   1. role modeling.
   2. advice giving.
   3. information giving.
   4. empathetic listening.

Answer: 2

Rationale: The nurse working in crisis intervention must be creative and flexible in looking at the client's situation and suggesting possible solutions for the client to consider. Giving advice is part of the active role the crisis intervention therapist takes. The other options are used equally in crisis intervention and traditional counseling roles.

Cognitive level: Application
Nursing process: Implementation
NCLEX: Psychosocial Integrity
See text page: 459

16. Primary crisis intervention is potentially used by the nurse when
   1. teaching a student nurse stress reduction techniques.
   2. assessing the coping strategies used by a client who attempted suicide.

3. providing a postdischarge referral of a client with schizophrenia to a day hospital.
4. obtaining an order for suicide precautions for a depressed client.

Answer: 1

Rationale: Primary crisis intervention promotes mental health and reduces mental illness. Options 2 and 4 are examples of secondary intervention during a crisis, and option 3 is an example of tertiary care.

Cognitive level: Analysis
Nursing process: Implementation
NCLEX: Safe and Effective Care Environment
See text page: 465

---

17. The nurse supervising other staff can correctly assess that the health care worker who will have the most difficulty terminating with a client who has required crisis intervention is
   1. A, who needs to be needed.
   2. B, who has highly developed empathy.
   3. C, who believes clients must participate in goal setting.
   4. D, who identifies highly creative alternatives for clients.

Answer: 1

Rationale: Problems commonly experienced by practitioners of crisis intervention are the need to be needed, the creation of unrealistic goals for clients, difficulty dealing with the issue of suicide, and difficulty terminating. The other options refer to personal qualities that enhance nursing effectiveness.

Cognitive level: Analysis
Nursing process: Assessment
NCLEX: Safe and Effective Care Environment
See text page: 462

---

18. The crisis that occurs as an individual moves from young adulthood to middle age and becomes concerned with loss of his youthful appearance would be assessed by the nurse as
   1. a situational crisis.
   2. a maturational crisis.
   3. a reactive crisis.
   4. an adventitious crisis.

Answer: 2

Rationale: Maturational crises occur when a person arrives at a new stage of development and finds that old coping styles are ineffective but has not yet developed new strategies. Option 1: Situational crises arise from sources external to the individual, such as divorce and job loss. Option 3: No classification called reactive crisis exists. Option 4: Adventitious crises occur when disasters such as natural disasters (e.g., floods, hurricanes), war, or violent crimes disrupt coping.

Cognitive level: Application
Nursing process: Assessment
NCLEX: Health Promotion and Maintenance
See text pages: 457, 458

---

19. The nurse is asked by the spouse of a client seeking crisis intervention to give an example of an adventitious crisis. The nurse should mention
   1. the death of a child from sudden infant death syndrome.
   2. being fired from one's job because of company downsizing.
   3. retirement of a 55-year-old.
   4. a riot at a rock concert.

Answer: 4

Rationale: The rock concert riot is unplanned, accidental, violent, and not a part of everyday life. Options 1 and 2 are examples of situational crises. Option 3 is an example of a maturational crisis.

Cognitive level: Application
Nursing process: Implementation
NCLEX: Psychosocial Integrity
See text page: 459

---

20. The role assumed by the nurse in the crisis intervention clinic would probably never be described by the adjective
   1. active.
   2. supportive.
   3. goal directed.
   4. inflexible.

Answer: 4

Rationale: Flexibility is a personal quality that enhances nursing effectiveness in crisis intervention therapy. Flexibility is required for the nurse to work with the client to identify alternatives compatible with the client's beliefs, personal values, and traditions.

Cognitive level: Application
Nursing process: Implementation
NCLEX: Psychosocial Integrity
See text page: 471

---

21. A client being interviewed on his first visit to the crisis center says he is there because he needs help, but then falters and cannot continue his explanation. Which question would be of value in helping him relate his perception of the precipitating event?
   1. "How can we help you?"
   2. "What led you to seek help today?"

3. "Who is available to help you with your problem?"
4. "What do you usually do to get through difficult times?"

Answer: 2

Rationale: Option 2 will help the client identify the precipitating event. The precipitating event must be identified before planning, goal setting, and intervention can take place. Option 1 is not relevant to identification of the precipitating event. Option 3 focuses on assessment of situational supports. Option 4 focuses on assessing personal coping skills.

Cognitive level: Application
Nursing process: Assessment
NCLEX: Psychosocial Integrity
See text page: 460

22. During the initial interview at the crisis center, a client reveals that his wife asked him for a divorce. He is so anxious that he "cannot think straight." To assess personal coping skills, the nurse could say
   1. "I can see you are upset. You can rely on us to help you feel better."
   2. "What would you like us to do to help you feel more relaxed?"
   3. "In the past, how did you handle difficult or stressful situations?"
   4. "Do you think you deserve to have things like this happen to you?"

Answer: 3

Rationale: Option 3 is the only option that assesses coping skills. Option 1 gives unrealistic reassurance, and option 2 asks the client to decide on his own treatment at a time when, by his own admission, he "cannot think straight." Option 4 is concerned with self-esteem.

Cognitive level: Application
Nursing process: Assessment
NCLEX: Psychosocial Integrity
See text page: 461

23. During his first interview at the crisis center, a client who is having suicidal ideation associated with divorce proceedings tells the nurse he has usually been able to talk over problems with his sister. He also states he finds playing the bagpipes relaxing but had given them up when be became an apartment dweller. He mentions that he took diazepam (Valium) for a short time several years ago but did not like the side effects. The nurse should help the client weigh the consequences of various alternatives, including (more than one answer may be correct)
   1. visiting his sister to talk about his problem.
   2. joining a pipe band at the local YMCA.

3. returning to the clinic in 24 hours.
4. taking diazepam four times daily.

Answers: 1, 2, 3

Rationale: Options 1 and 2 use previously effective coping strategies that could be helpful in this instance. Option 3 is advisable because it provides ongoing support and promotes the feeling that the client is not alone. Option 4 would not be useful because the client disliked the medication's side effects. Furthermore, anxiolytics may not be necessary if other options are successful.

Cognitive level: Application
Nursing process: Implementation
NCLEX: Psychosocial Integrity
See text page: 466

24. The individual whose spouse was killed in a plane crash was noted to cope for the first 24 hours by using denial. Now, reality of the death has set in and the individual is demonstrating severe anxiety. Consistent with phase 2 of crisis, the nurse should expect to assess the client as demonstrating
   1. trial-and-error problem solving.
   2. withdrawal.
   3. suicidal ideation.
   4. violence toward others.

Answer: 1

Rationale: Trial-and-error problem solving is typical of phase 2 of the crisis cycle. Option 2: Withdrawal, an automatic coping behavior, would be seen in phase 3. Options 3 and 4: Suicidal ideation and violence toward others might be seen in phase 4.

Cognitive level: Application
Nursing process: Assessment
NCLEX: Psychosocial Integrity
See text page: 459

25. A client at the crisis clinic has cared for her invalid mother for 10 years. The mother's condition has deteriorated, and placement in a nursing home has been recommended by the mother's physician. The client states she has always seen herself as capable of caring for her mother despite the personal sacrifice it requires. To place the mother in a home threatens her value system. The Nursing Outcomes Classification outcome of highest relevance for this client with the nursing diagnosis of decisional conflict would be
   1. role performance.
   2. decision making.
   3. stress level.
   4. coping.

Answer: 2

Rationale: The Nursing Outcomes Classification outcome of decision making is most closely aligned with the decisional conflict experienced by the client. The relation of the other outcomes to this diagnosis would be more indirect.

Cognitive level: Application

Nursing process: Planning (Outcome Identification)

NCLEX: Psychosocial Integrity

See text page: 463

26. A client at the crisis clinic has cared for her invalid mother for 10 years. The mother's condition has deteriorated, and placement in a nursing home has been suggested by the mother's physician. The client states she has always seen herself as capable of caring for her mother despite the personal sacrifice it requires. To place the mother in a home threatens her value system. Successful resolution of the client's crisis will be most closely related to
   1. resolving the grief associated with the threat to the client's self-concept.
   2. ability of the client to avail herself of situational supports in the community.
   3. reliance on assistance from role models within the client's culture.
   4. mobilization of automatic relief behaviors by the client.

Answer: 1

Rationale: The client's crisis clearly relates to a loss of (or threatened change in) self-concept and self-esteem. Her capacity to care for her mother, regardless of the mother's deteriorating condition, has been challenged. Crisis resolution will involve coming to terms with the grief associated with this loss. Option 2 is relevant, but less so than coming to terms with the loss of self-esteem. Option 3: Reliance on lessons from role models can be helpful but is not the primary factor associated with resolution in this case. Option 4: Automatic relief behaviors will not be helpful. Automatic relief behaviors are part of the fourth phase of crisis.

Cognitive level: Analysis

Nursing process: Planning

Client need: Psychosocial Integrity

See text pages: 458, 459

27. The assumption that will be most useful to the nurse planning crisis intervention for any client who is experiencing a crisis is that the client
   1. is experiencing a type of mental illness.
   2. is experiencing a state of disequilibrium.
   3. has high potential for self-injury.
   4. poses a threat of violence to others.

Answer: 2

Rationale: The only answer universally true for all clients in crisis is option 2. A crisis represents a struggle for equilibrium when problems seem unsolvable. Option 1: Crisis does not reflect mental illness. Options 3 and 4: Potential for self-violence or other-directed violence may or may not be factors in crisis.

Cognitive level: Application

Nursing process: Planning

NCLEX: Psychosocial Integrity

See text pages: 456, 457

28. The priority assessment the nurse must make during the initial crisis intervention interview is the
   1. need for external controls.
   2. adequacy of social supports.
   3. client's perception of the precipitating event.
   4. client's preferred coping mechanism.

Answer: 1

Rationale: Safety needs of clients and others are of high priority; thus assessment of potential for harm to self or others is of greater importance than the other options.

Cognitive level: Application

Nursing process: Assessment

NCLEX: Psychosocial Integrity

See text pages: 460

29. An appropriate question for the nurse to ask to assess situational support is
   1. "Has anything upsetting occurred in the last few days?"
   2. "What led you to seek help at this time?"
   3. "How does this problem affect your life?"
   4. "Who can be helpful to you during this time?"

Answer: 4

Rationale: Only option 4 focuses on situational support. Options 1, 2, and 3 focus on the client's perception of the precipitating event.

Cognitive level: Application

Nursing process: Assessment

NCLEX: Psychosocial Integrity

See text page: 460

30. A 50-year-old man comes to the crisis clinic after being terminated from his job of 15 years. He tells the nurse "I do not know what to do. How will I get another job? Who will pay the bills? How will I get money to feed my three kids? I am not in the driver's seat anymore!" The nursing diagnosis that should be considered is
   1. hopelessness.
   2. powerlessness.

351

3. chronic low self-esteem.

4. disturbed thought processes.

Answer: 2

Rationale: The client describes feelings of lack of control over events in his life. Options 1 and 3: No direct mention is made of hopelessness or chronic low self-esteem. Option 4: The client's thought processes are not shown to be altered at this point.

Cognitive level: Application

Nursing process: Diagnosis

NCLEX: Psychosocial Integrity

See text page: 463

31. The nursing diagnosis of "powerlessness related to lack of a plan to resolve crisis" has been established for a client seeking crisis intervention. An appropriate outcome for this nursing diagnosis would be that the client will

1. sign a no-suicide contract within 30 minutes.

2. meet precrisis role expectations within 36 hours.

3. state he feels less anxious within 4 hours of the interview.

4. state two possible alternative solutions during the first interview.

Answer: 4

Rationale: Determining possible alternative solutions to the problem is the only outcome that addresses the etiology statement of the nursing diagnosis. Option 1 relates to risk for self-directed violence. Option 2 relates to ineffective role performance. Option 3 relates to anxiety.

Cognitive level: Application

Nursing process: Planning (Outcome Identification)

NCLEX: Psychosocial Integrity

See text page: 463

32. The client has completed the contracted number of crisis clinic visits and tells the nurse "I have emerged from this as a stronger person. I realize I am not superwoman; it is OK not to have to do everything for everybody. You supported me as I worked through my feelings of loss and helped me find community resources. My mother is doing well in the nursing home and I am profiting from a support group for the relatives of the residents." From these statements the nurse can evaluate the client's feelings about the psychological care received as

1. not at all satisfied.

2. somewhat satisfied.

3. moderately satisfied.

4. very satisfied.

Answer: 4

Rationale: The client mentions a number of indicators that suggest a high degree of satisfaction with the

Nursing Outcomes Classification outcome of client satisfaction: psychological care. No indicators express low to moderate satisfaction.

Cognitive level: Analysis

Nursing process: Evaluation

NCLEX: Safe and Effective Client Environment

See text pages: 466, 467

33. The client has completed the contracted number of crisis clinic visits and tells the nurse "I have emerged from this as a stronger person. I realize I am not superwoman; it's OK not to have to do everything for everybody. You supported me as I worked through my feelings of loss and helped me find community resources. My mother is doing well in the nursing home and I am profiting from a support group for the relatives of the residents." The nurse responds "I wonder whether you would consider it worthwhile to spend additional time exploring why your feelings about giving up the caregiver role were so intense." When the nurse makes this overture, the assessment can be made that

1. the client is experiencing transference.

2. the client demonstrates need for continuing support.

3. the nurse is having difficulty terminating.

4. the nurse is empathizing client dependency feelings.

Answer: 3

Rationale: The nurse's remark is clearly an invitation to work on other problems and prolong contact with the client. (The focus of crisis intervention is the problem the precipitated the crisis, not other issues.) Option 1: The scenario does not describe transference. Option 2: Client need for continuing support is not demonstrated in the scenario. Option 4: The scenario does not describe client dependency needs the nurse might be empathizing.

Cognitive level: Analysis

Nursing process: Assessment

NCLEX: Psychosocial Integrity

See text page: 462

34. The nurse working with a client with a maturational crisis suggests enhancing the client's stress management skills by learning relaxation techniques. This intervention takes place at the level of care identified as

1. primary.

2. secondary.

3. tertiary.

4. quaternary.

Answer: 1

Rationale: Primary care promotes mental health and reduces mental illness to decrease the incidence of crisis. It includes early recognition of potential problems, teaching an individual specific skills to handle stress, and environmental manipulation to decrease the negative effects of stress. Secondary care provides intervention during an acute crisis. Tertiary care provides support for those recovering from a disabling mental state. Quaternary care does not exist.

Cognitive level: Application
Nursing process: Planning
NCLEX: Psychosocial Integrity
See text pages: 464, 465

35. The health care worker who should be referred to critical incident stress debriefing is
    1. A, who worked 8 hours at the information desk for the intensive care unit answering visitor queries.
    2. B, an emergency medical technician who treated victims of a car bomb attack on a large department store.
    3. C, a nurse who works at an oncology clinic with clients receiving chemotherapy.
    4. D, a case manager whose clientele are the seriously mentally ill being cared for at home.

Answer: 2
Rationale: Although each of the individuals mentioned experiences job-related stress on a daily basis, the person most in need of critical incident stress debriefing is B, who experienced an adventitious crisis event by responding to a bomb attack and providing care to trauma victims.

Cognitive level: Analysis
Nursing process: Planning
NCELX: Psychosocial Integrity
See text pages: 465, 466

36. The nurse assigned to implement a critical incident stress debriefing for a group who responded to a plane crash disaster scene must correctly organize the elements of the debriefing for maximal effectiveness. Put the following elements in the order in which they should occur after an explanation of the purpose and ground rules of the meeting have been given.
    1. Ask each person to tell of his or her involvement in the incident.
    2. Review the material discussed, then ask how closure should proceed.
    3. Ask participants to discuss their first thoughts of the incident.
    4. Ask participants to describe cognitive, physical, and emotional/behavioral symptoms experienced at the scene and symptoms experienced after the initial experience.
    5. Acknowledge and affirm the normality of expressed symptoms; offer anticipatory guidance.

6. Encourage discussion of the worst thing about the incident, what is painful, and what participants would like to forget.

Answers: 1, 3, 6, 4, 5, 2
Rationale: Option 1: The fact phase allows the participants to introduce themselves and tell how each was involved, including what happened from their perspective. Option 3: The thought phase follows, with all participants discussing their first thoughts of the incident. Option 6: First thoughts are followed by a discussion of reactions to the event: the worst thing about the incident, what participants would like to forget, and what was most painful. Option 4: Symptoms are described: what cognitive, physical, emotional, or behavioral experience they encountered at the scene and after the initial experience. Option 5: The normalcy of the symptoms is affirmed and anticipatory guidance is given regarding possible future symptoms. Option 2: What has been discussed is reviewed, how closure should proceed is determined, referrals are provided, and the debriefing experience is summarized.

Cognitive level: Application
Nursing process: Implementation
NCLEX: Health Promotion and Maintenance
See text pages: 465, 466

CHAPTER 23

1. A 20-year-old economics major became severely depressed after failing two examinations in economics. She cried for 2 hours, then called her parents who live in a neighboring state, planning to ask if she could return home. Her parents were in Europe. When her roommate went home for the weekend, the client gave her three expensive sweaters to keep. Later, the dormitory resident assistant returned a book to the client's room and found her unconscious on the floor, with an empty pill bottle nearby. Paramedics took the client to the emergency department, where she was lavaged and a psychiatric assessment was performed. Suicide risk factors present in the scenario include (more than one answer may be correct)
    1. history of earlier suicide attempt.
    2. co-occurring medical illness.
    3. recent lack of social support.
    4. recent stressful life event.
    5. shame or humiliation.
    6. family history of suicide.

Answers: 3, 4, 5
Rationale: Failing examinations in the academic major constitutes a recent stressful life event. Shame and

humiliation related to the failure can be hypothesized. Inability to contact parents can be seen as recent lack of social support, as can the roommate's absence from the dormitory. Options 1, 2, and 6: The scenario does not provide data regarding a history of an earlier suicide attempt, a family history of suicide, or of co-occurring medical illness.

Cognitive level: Comprehension
Nursing process: Assessment
NCLEX: Psychosocial Integrity
See text page: 476

2. The nurse caring for a college student who attempted suicide by overdose believes brain biochemical dysfunction contributes to suicidal behavior. The nurse will be better able to plan necessary health teaching if she identifies the probable neurotransmitter alteration of
   1. acetylcholine excess.
   2. serotonin deficiency.
   3. dopamine excess.
   4. γ-aminobutyric acid deficiency.

Answer: 2
Rationale: Research suggests that low levels of serotonin may play a role in the decision to commit suicide. Knowing this, the nurse would understand the rationale for the use of selective serotonin reuptake inhibitors and plan appropriate health teaching. The other neurotransmitter alterations have not been implicated in suicidal crises.

Cognitive level: Application
Nursing process: Assessment
NCLEX: Health Promotion and Maintenance
See text page: 475

3. A 20-year-old economics major became severely depressed after failing two examinations in economics. She cried for 2 hours, then called her parents who live in a neighboring state, planning to ask if she could return home. Her parents were in Europe. When her roommate went home for the weekend, the client gave her three expensive sweaters to keep. Later, the dormitory resident assistant returned a book to the client's room and found her unconscious on the floor, with an empty pill bottle nearby. The client behavior that provided a clue to the suicide attempt was
   1. calling her parents.
   2. staying in her dorm room.
   3. giving away her sweaters.
   4. excessive crying.

Answer: 3
Rationale: Giving away prized possessions may signal that the individual thinks he or she will have no fur-

ther need for the item, such as when a suicide plan has been formulated. Option 1: Calling her parents would not be a clue in and of itself. Option 2: Remaining in the dorm would be an expected behavior because the client had nowhere else to go. Option 4: Crying does not provide a clue to suicide in and of itself.

Cognitive level: Analysis
Nursing process: Assessment
NCLEX: Psychosocial Integrity
See text page: 477

4. The nurse uses the SAD PERSONS scale as he interviews a client who has expressed suicidal ideation. This tool provides data relevant to
   1. mood disturbance.
   2. suicide potential.
   3. current stress level.
   4. level of anxiety.

Answer: 2
Rationale: The SAD PERSONS tool evaluates 10 major risk factors in suicide potential: sex, age, depression, previous attempt, ethanol use, rational thinking loss, social supports lacking, organized plan, no spouse, and sickness. The tool does not have appropriate categories to provide information on the other options listed.

Cognitive level: Application
Nursing Process: Assessment
NCLEX: Psychosocial Integrity
See text page: 478

5. A college student who attempted suicide by overdose was treated in the emergency department. Because the client lives in the dorm, her roommate is away, and her parents are in Europe, the decision was made to hospitalize her. The nursing diagnosis of highest priority would be
   1. powerlessness.
   2. social isolation.
   3. compromised family coping.
   4. risk for self-directed violence.

Answer: 4
Rationale: This diagnosis is the only one with life-or-death ramifications and is therefore of higher priority than the other options.

Cognitive level: Analysis
Nursing process: Diagnosis
NCLEX: Safe and Effective Care Environment
See text page: 479

6. A college student who attempted suicide by overdose was treated in the emergency department and,

354

because she had no available social supports, was hospitalized. An outcome related to the client's risk for self-directed violence is that the client will

1. exercise suicide self-restraint by refraining from making gestures or attempts to kill self.
2. verbalize a will to live by the end of the second hospital day.
3. describe two new coping mechanisms she can use by the end of the third hospital day.
4. accurately delineate personal strengths by the end of first week of hospitalization.

Answer: 1

Rationale: Suicide self-restraint relates most directly to the priority problem of risk for self-directed violence. The other outcomes are related to hope, coping, and self-esteem.

Cognitive level: Application
Nursing process: Outcome Identification
NCLEX: Psychosocial Integrity
See text page: 480

7. A college student who attempted suicide by overdose was hospitalized until social supports could be put into place. When her parents were contacted, her mother's response was "We cannot understand why our daughter would do this to herself. We have given her everything she ever wanted." The mother's reaction can be assessed as reflecting

1. anxiety.
2. anger.
3. denial.
4. rescue feelings.

Answer: 3

Rationale: Statements such as "I cannot understand why. . ." indicate denial. Denial or minimization of suicidal ideation or attempts is a defense against uncomfortable feelings. Family members are often unable to acknowledge suicidal ideation in someone close to them. The feelings suggested in the other options are not clearly described in the scenario.

Cognitive level: Application
Nursing process: Assessment
NCLEX: Psychosocial Integrity
See text pages: 478, 479

8. A client with suicidal impulses is placed on the most stringent level of suicide precautions. The measures the nurse caring for the client should incorporate into the plan of care include (more than one answer may be correct)

1. maintaining arm-length, one-on-one nursing observation around the clock.
2. allowing no glass or metal on meal trays.
3. keeping client within visual range while he or she

is awake. Check every 15 to 30 minutes while the client is sleeping.
4. checking client whereabouts every 15 minutes and make frequent verbal contacts.
5. checking whereabouts every hour. Make verbal contact at least three times each shift.
6. removing all potentially harmful objects from the client's possession.

Answers: 1, 2, 6

Rationale: One-on-one observation is necessary for anyone who has limited control over suicidal impulses. Plastic dishes on trays and the removal of potentially harmful objects from the client's possession are measures included in any level suicide precautions. The other options are seen in less stringent levels of suicide precautions.

Cognitive level: Application
Nursing process: Planning
NCLEX: Safe and Effective Care Environment
See text page: 481

9. A nurse caring for a client on suicide precautions talks with a new staff nurse about the client's suicide attempt, saying "I have come to understand that I cannot control anyone's suicidal ideas or impulses. Clients are in charge of their own lives." This understanding means the nurse

1. does not assume any responsibility for treatment outcomes.
2. can see herself and the client as partners in planning outcomes.
3. will defer to the client's judgment about outcomes.
4. takes minimal responsibility for instilling hope.

Answer: 2

Rationale: The nurse's statement indicates she has no rescue fantasies and no illusions that she can control outcomes. She recognizes the client as an autonomous individual. In recognizing autonomy, the nurse knows that client can be helped to explore and choose adaptive alternatives. Option 1: Nurses cannot divest themselves of accountability for treatment outcomes. Option 3: Nurses are accountable for using good judgment in helping clients select outcomes. Option 4: Nurses cannot divest themselves of responsibilities such as instilling hope.

Cognitive level: Application
Nursing process: Planning
NCLEX: Safe and Effective Care Environment
See text page: 478

10. The nurse's efforts to assist a suicidal client to examine alternatives to suicide are best supported by

355

1. tricyclic antidepressants.
2. the client's ambivalence.
3. suicide precautions.
4. hospitalization.

Answer: 2

Rationale: Ambivalence is experiencing both the wish to die and the wish to live. The client's ambivalence about dying as a solution to an intolerable life situation is an important asset to the nurse. It provides the nurse with a positive base that can be reinforced. Tricyclic antidepressants take up to 3 weeks to be effective. Hospitals are not 100% suicide proof, and hospitalization may not prompt the client to look for alternatives to suicide. Suicide precautions may not prompt the client to look for alternatives to suicide but rather for ways to evade the precautions.

Cognitive level: Application
Nursing process: Implementation
NCLEX: Safe and Effective Care Environment
See text page: 475

11. When the nurse and client construct a no-suicide contract, the preferable wording would be
    1. "I will not try to harm myself during the next 24 hours."
    2. "In the next 24 hours I will not, for any reason, accidentally or purposely, kill myself."
    3. "I will not kill myself until I call you."
    4. "I will not make a suicide attempt while I am hospitalized."

Answer: 2

Rationale: This statement leaves no loopholes. Option 1: The wording about not harming oneself and not making an attempt can be ignored by the client who thinks "I am not going to harm myself, I am going to kill myself" or "I am not going to attempt suicide, I am going to commit suicide." Option 3: A client may call a therapist and leave the telephone to carry out the suicidal plan. Option 4 leaves a huge loophole.

Cognitive level: Application
Nursing process: Implementation
NCLEX: Safe and Effective Care Environment
See text page: 481

12. A tearful, anxious client comes to the clinic with the chief complaint "I should be dead." The initial task of the nurse conducting the assessment interview is to
    1. assess lethality of suicide plan.
    2. establish rapport with the client.
    3. encourage expression of anger.
    4. determine risk factors for suicide.

Answer: 2

Rationale: Establishing rapport will allow the nurse to obtain relevant assessment data such as the presence of a suicide plan, lethality of plan, and presence of risk factors for suicide. Option 3 is not an identified intervention.

Cognitive level: Application
Nursing process: Implementation
NCLEX: Psychosocial Integrity
See text pages: 477, 478

13. The most helpful response for the nurse to make when a client being treated as an outpatient states "I am considering committing suicide" is
    1. "I am glad you shared this. There is nothing to worry about. We will handle it together."
    2. "We need to talk about the things you have to live for."
    3. "I think you should admit yourself to the hospital to get help with this."
    4. "Bringing this up is a very positive action on your part."

Answer: 4

Rationale: This response gives the client reinforcement and validation for making a positive response rather than acting out the suicidal impulse. It gives neither advice nor false reassurance, and it does not imply stereotypes such as "You have a lot to live for." It uses the client's ambivalence and sets the stage for more realistic problem solving.

Cognitive level: Application
Nursing process: Implementation
NCLEX: Psychosocial Integrity
See text page: 481

14. The tertiary prevention therapy the nurse should recommend for the distressed family and friends of someone who has committed suicide is
    1. psychological postmortem assessment.
    2. attending a self-help group for survivors.
    3. participating in reminiscence therapy.
    4. contracting for two sessions of dynamic group therapy.

Answer: 2

Rationale: Survivors need outlets for their feelings about the loss and the deceased person. Self-help groups provide peer support while survivors work through feelings of loss, anger, and guilt. Option 1 would not provide the support necessary to work through feelings of loss associated with the suicide of a family member. Option 3 is not geared to loss resolution. Option 4 would probably not provide sufficient time to work through the issues associated with a death by suicide.

356

Cognitive level: Application
Nursing process: Planning
NCLEX: Psychosocial Integrity
See text page: 484

15. The statement that provides the best rationale for the nursing intervention of monitoring the severely depressed client closely during antidepressant therapy is
   1. as depression lifts, physical energy becomes available to carry out a plan for suicide.
   2. suicide may be precipitated by a variety of internal and external events.
   3. suicidal clients have difficulty using social supports.
   4. suicide is an impulsive act.

Answer: 1
Rationale: Antidepressant medication has the objective of relieving depression. Risk for suicide is greater as the depression lifts, primarily because the client has more physical energy at a time when he or she may still have suicidal ideation. The other options have little to do with nursing interventions relating to antidepressant medication therapy.
Cognitive level: Application
Nursing process: Planning
NCLEX: Safe and Effective Care Environment
See text page: 485

16. The nurse is taking the history of a client who admits to having been despondent for 2 weeks. He relates that his business is bankrupt and his wife has filed for divorce. The statement the nurse should assess as a covert clue to suicide is
   1. "Life is not worth living."
   2. "I wish I were dead."
   3. "My family will be better off without me."
   4. "I have a plan that will fix everything."

Answer: 4
Rationale: Verbal clues to suicide may be overt or covert. The first three statements are overt references to suicide. The last remark is more veiled. It alludes to the client's suicide as being a way to "fix everything" but does not say it outright.
Cognitive level: Application
Nursing process: Assessment
NCLEX: Psychosocial Integrity
See text page: 477

17. The most appropriate response by the nurse when a despondent client says "nothing matters anymore" would be
   1. "Are you having thoughts of suicide?"
   2. "I am not sure I understand what you are trying to say."

3. "Try to stay hopeful. Things have a way of working out."
4. "Tell me more about the things that interested you before you began to feel depressed."

Answer: 1
Rationale: The nurse must make overt what is covert, that is, the possibility of suicide must be openly addressed. The client often feels relieved to be able to talk about suicidal ideation.
Cognitive level: Application
Nursing process: Implementation
NCLEX: Safe and Effective Care Environment
See page: 477

18. An indicator that the suicidal client is exercising suicide self-restraint is
   1. compliance with antidepressant therapy.
   2. agreeing to sign a no-suicide contract.
   3. disclosing a plan for suicide to staff.
   4. expressing feelings of hopelessness to nurse.

Answer: 3
Rationale: Admitting a plan for suicide to staff is an indicator of suicide self-restraint. By admitting that a plan exists, the client enables staff to take appropriate measures to prevent the client from carrying out the plan. Option 1: Clients may comply with antidepressant therapy and still make suicide attempts. Option 2: Clients may sign no-suicide contracts, knowing they will make a later suicide attempt. Option 4: Expressing hopelessness does not indicate suicide self-restraint.
Cognitive level: Application
Nursing process: Planning (Outcome Identification)
NCLEX: Psychosocial Integrity
See text page: 480

19. When assessing a client's plan for suicide, the priority areas to consider include
   1. client financial and educational status.
   2. client insight into his or her suicidal motivation.
   3. availability of means and lethality of method.
   4. quality and availability of client social support.

Answer: 3
Rationale: If a person has definite plans that include choosing a method of suicide readily available to the person, and if the method is one that is lethal (i.e., will cause the person to die with little probability for intervention), the suicide risk is considered high. These areas provide a better indication of risk than the areas mentioned in the other options.
Cognitive level: Analysis
Nursing process: Assessment
NCLEX: Safe and Effective Care Environment
See text page: 477

357

20. Which understanding about persons who attempt suicide will help the nurse plan care for a suicidal client? Every person who is suicidal should be considered to be
   1. intent on dying.
   2. cognitively impaired.
   3. mentally ill.
   4. experiencing hopelessness.

Answer: 4

Rationale: Hopelessness is the characteristic common among people who attempt suicide. The other options reflect myths about suicide. Option 1: Not all who attempt suicide are intent on dying. Options 2 and 3: Not all are mentally ill and not all are cognitively impaired.

Cognitive level: Comprehension
Nursing process: Planning
NCLEX: Psychosocial Integrity
See text page: 474

21. The statement made by the client during the assessment interview that should alert the nurse to the client's need for immediate, active intervention is
   1. "I am mixed up, but I know I need help."
   2. "I have no one to turn to for help or support."
   3. "It is worse when you are a person of color."
   4. "I tried to get attention before I shot myself."

Answer: 2

Rationale: Lack of social support and social isolation increase the suicide risk. Option 1: Willingness to seek help lowers risk. Option 3: Being a person of color does not suggest higher risk because more whites commit suicide than do individuals of other racial groups. Option 4: Attention seeking is not correlated with higher suicide risk.

Cognitive level: Application
Nursing process: Planning
NCLEX: Safe and Effective Care Environment
See text page: 476

22. The feeling experienced by a client that should be assessed by the nurse as most predictive of elevated suicide risk is
   1. anger.
   2. hopelessness.
   3. elation.
   4. sadness.

Answer: 2

Rationale: Of the feelings listed, hopelessness is most closely associated with increased suicide risk. Depression, aggression, impulsivity, and shame are other feelings noted as risk factors for suicide.

Cognitive level: Application

Nursing process: Assessment
NCLEX: Psychosocial Integrity
See text page: 476

23. Four individuals have given the information about their suicide plans. The plan that should be assessed as indicating the highest suicide risk is
   1. jumping from a 100-foot-high railroad bridge located in a deserted area late at night.
   2. overdosing on aspirin with codeine while the patient's husband is out with friends.
   3. turning on the oven and letting gas escape into the apartment during the night.
   4. cutting the wrists in the bathroom while the patient's husband reads in the living room.

Answer: 1

Rationale: This is a highly lethal method with little opportunity for rescue. The other options are lower lethality methods with higher rescue potential.

Cognitive level: Analysis
Nursing process: Assessment
NCLEX: Psychosocial Integrity
See text page: 477

24. The individual seen in the emergency department who should be considered at highest risk for completing suicide is
   1. A single white man, aged 79 years, with cancer of the prostate.
   2. A single black female church member, aged 38 years, with fibrocystic breast disease.
   3. A 60-year-old married Hispanic man with numerous grandchildren who has type II diabetes.
   4. An adolescent white girl with superior athletic and academic skills who has asthma.

Answer: 1

Rationale: High-risk factors include being elderly, being single, being male, and having a co-occurring medical illness. Cancer is one of the somatic conditions associated with increased suicide risk. Options 2 and 3: Protective factors for African American women and Hispanic individuals include strong religious and family ties. Option 4: Adolescent white girls are at lower risk than adolescent boys.

Cognitive level: Application
Nursing process: Assessment
NCLEX: Psychosocial Integrity
See text pages: 475, 476

23. The nurse working the telephone suicide crisis line receives a call from a man who tells her he lives alone in a home several miles from his nearest neighbors. He has been considering suicide for 2

months. He has had several drinks and has loaded his shotgun, with which he plans to shoot himself in the heart. The nurse should assess the lethality of this plan as having
1. no risk.
2. a low level of lethality.
3. a moderate level of lethality.
4. a high level of lethality.

Answer: 4

Rationale: The client has a highly detailed plan, a highly lethal method, the means to carry it out, lowered impulse control because of alcohol ingestion, and a low potential for rescue.

Cognitive level: Analysis
Nursing process: Assessment
NCLEX: Safe and Effective Care Environment
See text pages: 476, 477

26. A staff nurse tells another nurse "I just used the SAD PERSONS scale to evaluate a new client. His score was 10. I'm wondering if I should send him home after arranging for follow-up." The best reply by the second nurse would be
1. "That would seem appropriate."
2. "Make sure he is followed up closely; he may require hospitalization in the near future."
3. "I think you should strongly consider hospitalization for him."
4. "A score of 7 or higher usually requires immediate hospitalization."

Answer: 4

Rationale: A SAD PERSONS scale score of 0 to 2 suggests home care with follow-up. A score of 3 to 4 calls for close follow-up and possible hospitalization. A score of 5 to 6 requires the nurse to strongly consider hospitalization, and a score of 7 or higher calls for hospitalization.

Cognitive level: Application
Nursing process: Implementation
NCLEX: Safe and Effective Care Environment
See text page: 478

27. When suicidal clients are admitted to a hospital, objects that can easily be used for self-harm are removed from their possession. The rationale for this intervention is that
1. the environment must be made completely safe.
2. psychiatric clients cannot be trusted with dangerous objects.
3. having to depend on staff to meet needs promotes a trusting relationship.
4. removing known harmful objects conveys the staff's concern for client safety.

Answer: 4

Rationale: Promoting client safety is a priority concern. Explaining this to clients reduces anxiety and supports the client's will to live. Option 1: the environment cannot be made completely safe. Option 2: Although some clients can be trusted not to harm themselves or others, some cannot. Thus, to maintain a safe milieu, harmful objects are available for use only under supervision. Option 3 is not an accurate statement.

Cognitive level: Application
Nursing process: Implementation
NCLEX: Safe and Effective Care Environment
See text page: 481

28. A highly suicidal client who has been hospitalized for 2 weeks committed suicide during the night. The measure that will be helpful to staff and clients having to deal with the event is
1. asking the client's roommate not to discuss the event with other clients.
2. allowing only national newspapers on the unit and sending the television "out for repair."
3. holding a staff meeting to express feelings and plan care for other clients.
4. discharging as many clients as possible as quickly as possible to prevent panic.

Answer: 3

Rationale: Interventions should be aimed at helping the staff and clients come to terms with the loss and grow as a result of the incident. A psychological postmortem assessment should be conducted by staff. A community meeting should be scheduled to inform clients. Staff should be prepared to provide additional support and reassurance to clients and should seek opportunities for peer support. Options 1 and 2 will not control information. Option 4 would result in unsafe care.

Cognitive level: Application
Nursing process: Implementation
NCLEX: Safe and Effective Care Environment
See text page: 484

29. The measure that would be considered primary prevention for suicide is
1. hospitalization of a suicidal client.
2. referral of a formerly suicidal client to a support group.
3. advocating laws to require trigger locks on all firearms.
4. suicide precautions for 24 hours for newly admitted clients.

Answer: 3

Rationale: This measure reduces ease of access to a lethal means of suicide. (Firearms are the most common

359

method for suicide for both men and women.) Options 1 and 4 are secondary prevention measures, and option 2 is a tertiary prevention measure.

Cognitive level: Application
Nursing process: Implementation
NCLEX: NA
See test page: 480

30. A new nurse mentions to a peer "My newest client has schizophrenia. At least I will not have to worry about him being suicidal." The most helpful response by the peer would be
    1. "Suicide risk is high in schizophrenic clients, especially early in the course of the illness."
    2. "Command hallucinations often prompt suicide among clients with schizophrenia."
    3. "Suicide is a risk for any client with schizophrenia who uses alcohol or drugs."
    4. "You are correct in saying that schizophrenia does not increase risk for suicide."

Answer: 1
Rationale: Up to 10% of clients with schizophrenia die from suicide, usually related to depressive symptoms occurring in the early years of the illness. Option 2: Depressive symptoms are more related to suicide among clients with schizophrenia than are command hallucinations. Option 3: The scenario does not mention substance use; thus the option has questionable relevance. Option 4 is an incorrect statement.

Cognitive level: Application
Nursing process: Implementation
NCLEX: Safe and Effective Care Environment
See text page: 474

31. The mother of identical twin sons seeks the nurse for advice. She reveals that one son became depressed and made a serious suicide attempt a month ago. Now she is concerned that the other son may also display suicidal tendencies. The nurse can be most helpful if he replies
    1. "Primary prevention can be used to mitigate genetic factors."
    2. "Fortunately for your sons, dizygotic twins are at higher risk than identical twins."
    3. "Your son is most likely to act out suicidal fantasies if he identifies with a suicide victim."
    4. "Because hopelessness underlies suicide, instilling hope is the key to health maintenance."

Answer: 1
Rationale: Twin studies suggest the presence of genetic factors in suicide; however, separating genetic predisposition to suicide from predisposition to depres-

sion or alcoholism is difficult. Primary interventions can be helpful in promoting and maintaining health and possibly counteracting genetic load. Option 2 is an untrue statement. Option 3 is factual but not helpful. Option 4 is an oversimplification.

Cognitive level: Application
Nursing process: Implementation
NCLEX: Psychosocial Integrity
See text page: 475

32. The nurse assessing a client for suicide potential will be most effective if she recognizes that the cognitive style that places a client at increased risk is
    1. being flexible and interested in exploring alternatives.
    2. demonstrating tunnel vision thinking and perfectionism.
    3. demonstrating distractible, scattered thinking.
    4. The presence of strong religious beliefs.

Answer: 2
Rationale: The cognitive style that features rigid all-or-nothing thinking, inability to see different options, and perfectionism contributes to increased suicide risk. Option 1 is associated with mental health. Option 3 is associated with anxiety. Option 4 is a protective factor.

Cognitive level: Comprehension
Nursing process: Assessment
NCLEX: Psychosocial Integrity
See text page: 475

33. A severely depressed client who has been on suicide precautions tells the nurse "I am feeling a lot better, so you can stop watching me. I have taken too much of your time already." The best response for the nurse to make would be
    1. "I wonder what this sudden change is all about. Care to elaborate?"
    2. "I am glad you are feeling better. The team will consider what you have said."
    3. "You should not try to direct your plan for care. Leave that to the team."
    4. "Because we are concerned about your safety, we will continue with our plan."

Answer: 4
Rationale: When a client seeks to have precautions lifted by professing to feel better, the client may be seeking greater freedom in which to attempt suicide. Changing the treatment plan requires careful evaluation of outcome indicators by staff. Option 1 will not cause the client to admit to a suicidal plan. Option 2 does not convey concern for the client. Option 3 remonstrates the client and suggests the client is not a partner in the care process.

Cognitive level: Application
Nursing process: Implementation
NCLEX: Safe and Effective Care Environment
See text page: 479

34. An 80-year-old woman who lives alone has begun calling friends and complaining in an exaggerated fashion about minor aches and pains. He physician found no significant medical problems. Over the course of a month, she obtained a number of prescriptions for pain medication, none of which seemed to be effective. Friends counseled her that aches are a normal part of life for the elderly and tried unsuccessfully to involve her in activities. She often suggested that she would be better off dead, to which one friend responded "Well, perhaps. It would get you out of your misery." As she became increasingly "needy" and demanding of attention, friends agreed that her behavior made them uncomfortable and began to call and visit less. The woman took four pain pills and called a neighbor, saying she had overdosed. The universal reactions toward the type of suicidal client demonstrated in this scenario include (more than one answer may be correct)
   1. denial.
   2. anxiety.
   3. irritation.
   4. avoidance.
   5. fear.
   6. interest.

Answers: 2, 3, 4
Rationale: Anxiety is demonstrated when friends agreed that the client's behavior made them "uncomfortable." Irritation is demonstrated when the friend responded "Perhaps it will get you out of your misery" to the client's statement that she would be better off dead. Avoidance is seen when friends stopped visiting and calling. Option 1: Denial is not reflected in the scenario. Denial would be seen in statements such as "I cannot understand why anyone would want to commit suicide," or "I do not believe she really wants to die." Options 5 and 6 are not considered universal reactions toward suicidal clients and are not demonstrated in the scenario.
Cognitive level: Analysis
Nursing process: Assessment
NCLEX: Psychosocial Integrity
See text pages: 478, 479

35. An 80-year old-woman who lives alone has begun calling friends and complaining in an exaggerated fashion about minor aches and pains. Her physician found no significant medical problems. Over the course of a month, she obtained a number of pre-

scriptions for pain medication, none of which seemed to be effective. Friends counseled her that aches are a normal part of life for the elderly and tried unsuccessfully to involve her in activities. She often suggested that she would be better off dead, to which one friend responded "Well, perhaps. It would get you out of your misery." As she became increasingly "needy" and demanding of attention, friends agreed that her behavior made them uncomfortable and began to call and visit less. The woman took four pain pills and called a neighbor, saying she had overdosed. After medical clearance, the client will be monitored at the mental health clinic. Principles of paramount importance to care planning in this instance include (more than one answer may be correct):
   1. Parasuicide with lethal intent requires emergency hospitalization.
   2. The client should be treated for underlying psychiatric disorder if one exists.
   3. Client perception of isolation is a significant cause for hopelessness.
   4. A nonlethal suicide attempt must be viewed as communication of the client's desperate state of mind.

Answers: 2, 4
Rationale: Option 2: This client should be assessed for depression because 60% to 90% of elderly suicides have at least one psychiatric diagnosis, two thirds of which are single-episode, late-onset depression. The client's somatic symptoms may be depressive equivalents. Option 4: Any suicide attempt communicates the client's inability to find an acceptable solution to the problem. Option 1: The client's suicide attempt would not be considered parasuicide. Parasuicide is defined as a nonfatal self-injury with a clear intent to cause bodily harm or death. Option 3: Data are not present to show that the client perceived self as isolated.
Cognitive level: Analysis
Nursing process: Planning
NCLEX: Safe and Effective Care Environment
See text pages: 479, 480

36. An 80-year-old woman who lives alone has begun calling friends and complaining in an exaggerated fashion about minor aches and pains. Her physician found no significant medical problems. Over the course of a month, she obtained a number of prescriptions for pain medication, none of which seemed to be effective. Friends counseled her that aches are a normal part of life for the elderly and tried unsuccessfully to involve her in activities. She often suggested that she would be better off dead, to which one friend responded "Well, perhaps. It

Chapter 23   Suicide

would get you out of your misery." As she became increasingly "needy" and demanding of attention, friends agreed that her behavior made them uncomfortable and began to call and visit less. The woman took four pain pills and called a neighbor, saying she had overdosed. After medical clearance, the client will be monitored at the mental health clinic. Nursing interventions that have been agreed on for the client include hope instillation, coping enhancement, and support system enhancement. Measures designed to enhance the client's support system include (more than one answer may be correct)
1. providing services in a caring manner.
2. providing a referral to a self-help group.
3. teaching cognitive restructuring.
4. encouraging relationships with friends.
5. identifying areas of hope in life.
6. arranging situations that foster autonomy.

Answers: 1, 2, 4
Rationale: These options are relevant to support system enhancement. Option 3 relates to changing faulty cognitive patterns. Option 5 relates to hope instillation. Option 6 relates to coping enhancement.
Cognitive level: Application
Nursing process: Planning
NCLEX: Psychosocial Integrity
See text pages: 481-485

CHAPTER 24

1. The client who should be assessed as demonstrating aggression is
   1. A, who stomps away from the nurses' station, goes into the day room, and grabs a pool cue from a client standing at the pool table.
   2. B, who bursts into tears, leaves the community meeting, and sits on her bed hugging her pillow and sobbing.
   3. C, who tells her primary nurse "When you told me that I could not have a pass, I felt angry."
   4. D, who tells the medication nurse "I am not going to take that, or any other, medication."

Answer: 1
Rationale: Aggression is harsh physical or verbal action that reflects rage, hostility, and potential for physical or verbal destructiveness. Aggressive behavior violates the rights of others; thus client A would be assessed as displaying aggression. The other options do not feature violation of another's rights.
Cognitive level: Application
Nursing process: Assessment
NCLEX: Psychosocial Integrity
See text page: 490

2. Which statement about aggression would serve as a basis for care planning using behavioral techniques? Aggression
   1. runs in families and is manifested as early as infancy.
   2. results from abnormalities in the temporal lobe of the brain.
   3. results from low levels of the neurotransmitter serotonin.
   4. is motivated by rewards received for previous aggression.

Answer: 4
Rationale: Behavioral theory does not accept aggressive drives as being instinctual or biological. It views aggressive behavior as a learned response that tends to be repeated if reinforced. Lack of reinforcement or reinforcing other, more desirable behavior will help extinguish the aggressive behavior. Option 1 suggests a genetic origin for aggression. Option 2 suggests brain abnormality as the origin for aggression. Option 3 suggests neurotransmitter abnormality as the origin for aggression. Behavioral techniques would not necessarily be chosen for these options.
Cognitive level: Comprehension
Nursing process: Planning
NCLEX: Psychosocial Integrity
See text page: 491

3. A nurse tells a colleague "When the client said 'You have no right to treat me this way!' and hit the nurse, he was responding to the perceived threat of powerlessness when his request for a weekend pass was refused." This comment reflects the clinician's belief that aggression should be assessed in terms of
   1. behavioral theory.
   2. cognitive theory.
   3. biological theory.
   4. genetic theory.

Answer: 2
Rationale: Cognitive theory suggests an event is more likely to lead to anger and aggression if the event is perceived as threatening. Option 1 would require an analysis referring to learned behavior. Option 3 would require an analysis referring to a brain abnormality. Option 4 would require an analysis suggesting an inherited trait.
Cognitive level: Application
Nursing process: Assessment
NCLEX: Safe and Effective Care Environment
See text page: 492

4. The client on the mental health unit who should be assessed as being at highest risk for directing violent behavior toward others is

1. E, who has obsessive-compulsive disorder and performs many rituals.
2. F, who has paranoid delusions that she is being followed by members of the mafia.
3. G, who has severe depression with delusions of worthlessness.
4. H, who has completed alcohol withdrawal and is beginning a rehabilitation program.

Answer: 2

Rationale: F has the greatest disruption of ability to perceive reality accurately. People who feel persecuted may strike out against those believed to be persecutors. The other clients have better reality-testing ability.

Cognitive level: Analysis
Nursing process: Assessment
NCLEX: Safe and Effective Care Environment
See text page: 491

5. The behavior that would be considered inconsistent with the clinical picture of a client who is becoming increasingly aggressive is
   1. pacing.
   2. sobbing inconsolably.
   3. rigid posture with a clenched jaw.
   4. staring with narrowed eyes into the eyes of another.

Answer: 2

Rationale: Crying is not cited by experts as a behavior indicating that the individual has a high potential to behave violently. The other behaviors are consistent with increasing risk for other-directed violence.

Cognitive level: Application
Nursing process: Assessment
NCLEX: Safe and Effective Care Environment
See text page: 493

6. A client is admitted for psychiatric observation after being arrested for breaking windows in the home of his former girlfriend, who had refused to see him. His history reveals abuse as a child by a punitive father, torturing family pets, and one arrest for disorderly conduct. The nursing diagnosis that should be considered for development is
   1. risk for injury.
   2. posttrauma syndrome.
   3. disturbed thought processes.
   4. risk for other-directed violence.

Answer: 4

Rationale: The defining characteristics for risk for violence directed at others include a history of being abused as a child, having committed other violent acts, and demonstrating poor impulse control. The defining characteristics for the other diagnoses are not present in the scenario.

Cognitive level: Analysis
Nursing process: Diagnosis
NCLEX: Psychosocial Integrity
See text page: 494

7. A confused elderly nursing home client is in bed sleeping. When the nurse makes rounds, she enters the room quietly and reaches under the top sheet to feel the bottom sheet to see if it is wet. The client awakens and strikes out, hitting the nurse in the face. The statement best explaining the client's action is
   1. elderly clients often demonstrate exaggerations of behaviors used earlier in life.
   2. the client learned violent behavior by watching excessive television violence.
   3. the client interpreted the health care worker's behavior as potentially harmful.
   4. the crowding that occurs in nursing homes increases individual tendencies toward violence.

Answer: 3

Rationale: Confused clients are not always able to evaluate the actions of others accurately. This client behaved as though provoked by the intrusive actions of the staff.

Cognitive level: Application
Nursing process: Assessment
NCLEX: Safe and Effective Care Environment
See text pages: 501-503

8. A client is pacing the hall near the nurses' station, swearing loudly. An appropriate initial intervention for the nurse would be to address the client by name and say
   1. "Please quiet down."
   2. "Hey, what's up?"
   3. "You seem upset. Tell me about it."
   4. "You need to go to your room to get control of yourself."

Answer: 3

Rationale: Intervention should begin with analysis of the client and the situation. With this response the nurse is attempting to hear the client's feelings and concerns. This leads to the next step of planning an intervention. Options 1 and 4 close off communication. Option 2 is not a concrete request for information and could be misinterpreted.

Cognitive level: Application
Nursing process: Implementation
NCLEX: Safe and Effective Care Environment
See text pages: 495, 496

9. A client who has been seen responding to auditory hallucinations earlier in the morning approaches the nurse and shakes his fist, saying "Back off, bitch!"

363

and then goes into the day room. The nurse follows the client into the day room. The nurse should
1. move to a position that allows the client to be closest to the door.
2. make sure physical space is present between herself and the client.
3. position herself within an arm's length of the client.
4. sit down in a chair near the client.

Answer: 2

Rationale: Making sure space is present between the nurse and the client avoids invading the client's personal space. Personal space needs increase when a client feels anxious and threatened. Option 1: Allowing the client to block the nurse's exit from the room is not wise. Option 3: This closeness may be threatening to the client and provoke aggression. Option 4: Sitting is inadvisable until further assessment suggests the client's aggression is abating.

Cognitive level: Application
Nursing process: Implementation
NCLEX: Safe and Effective Care Environment
See text pages: 495, 496

10. A client who has been seen responding to auditory hallucinations earlier in the morning approaches the nurse and shakes his fist, saying "Back off, bitch!" and then goes into the day room. The nurse goes into the day room. The client continues to mumble and shake his fist. The nursing actions most likely to be effective in achieving the outcome of deescalation would be (more than one answer may be correct)
1. telling the client that he is behaving inappropriately.
2. stating the client cannot be understood when he mumbles.
3. stating the expectation that the client will stay in control.
4. offering to provide the client with as-needed medication.

Answers: 3, 4

Rationale: Stating the expectation that the client will maintain control of his behavior reinforces positive, healthy behavior and avoids challenging the client. Offering as-needed medication provides support for the client trying to maintain control. Option 1: Belittling remarks such as this may lead to aggression. Option 2 will be considered a criticism and probably prompt the client to begin shouting.

Cognitive level: Analysis
Nursing process: Implementation
NCLEX: Safe and Effective Care Environment
See text pages: 495, 496

11. An intramuscular dose of antipsychotic medication needs to be given to a client who is becoming in-

creasingly more aggressive. The client is in the day room. The nurse should
1. enter the day room and say "Would you like to come to your room and take some medication that your doctor has ordered for you?"
2. take three staff members to the day room as a show of solidarity and say "Please come to your room so I can give you some medication that will help you feel more comfortable."
3. take a male nursing assistant to the day room and tell the client "You can come to your room willingly so I can give you this medication, or the aide and I will have to take you there."
4. enter the day room, place the client in a basket hold, and say "I am going to take you to your room to give you an injection of medication to calm you."

Answer: 2

Rationale: A client gains feelings of security if he or she sees others are present to help with control. The nurse gives a simple direction, honestly states what is going to happen, and reassures the client that the intervention will be helpful. This positive approach assumes the client can act responsibly and will maintain control. Physical control measures should be used only as a last resort. Option 1 offers the client a choice, something the nurse does not actually plan to permit. Option 3 threatens the client. Option 4 restrains the client before knowing whether such a measure is necessary.

Cognitive level: Application
Nursing process: Implementation
NCLEX: Safe and Effective Care Environment
See text pages: 495, 496

12. A nurse was battered by an assaultive client. Although no bones were broken, she sustained several facial contusions. Afterward she had difficulty sleeping, startled easily, admitted to being preoccupied with thoughts about the incident, and stated she dreaded having to face intimidating clients. Which response would be considered the most urgent reason to seek supervision?
1. Sleep pattern disturbance
2. Startle reactions
3. Preoccupation with the incident
4. A wish for revenge

Answer: 4

Rationale: The first three symptoms the nurse experienced re considered normal in a client who has been battered. They are similar to the symptoms experienced by clients with posttraumatic stress disorder but are usually are relieved with crisis intervention and follow-up designed to give support, help the individual regain a sense of control, and make sense of the event. The desire for revenge signals an urgent need for professional supervision to work through anger and counteraggressive feelings.

Cognitive level: Analysis
Nursing process: Assessment
NCLEX: Safe and Effective Care Environment
See text page: 498

13. After an incident in which staff intervention was required to control a client's aggressive behavior, a critical incident debriefing will take place. The topic on which minimal time should be spent is
   1. client behavior associated with the incident.
   2. intervention techniques used by staff.
   3. the impact of environmental factors.
   4. review of theories of aggression.

Answer: 4
Rationale: The client's behavior, the intervention techniques used, and the environment in which the incident occurred are important to establish realistic outcomes and effective nursing interventions. Discussing views about the theoretical origins of aggression would be less effective.

Cognitive level: Analysis
Nursing process: Evaluation
NCLEX: Safe and Effective Care Environment
See text page: 498

14. The staff development coordinator planning to teach the use of physical management techniques when clients become assaultive should stress the importance of
   1. spontaneity and surprise.
   2. practice and teamwork.
   3. caution and superior size.
   4. diversion and physical outlets.

Answer: 2
Rationale: Intervention techniques are learned behaviors and must be practiced to be used in a smooth, organized fashion. Every member of the intervention team should be assigned a specific task to carry out before beginning the intervention. The other options are useless if the staff does not know how to use physical techniques and how to apply them in an organized fashion.

Cognitive level: Application
Nursing process: Implementation
NCLEX: Safe and Effective Care Environment
See text pages: 493, 496

15. The limit-setting technique most likely to precipitate violence when intervening with an angry client is

   1. "Your behavior is unacceptable."
   2. "Go to your room for a time out."
   3. "I can see you are angry. Let's talk."
   4. "You are pretty upset just now."

Answer: 1
Rationale: A belittling remark is most likely to escalate anger and precipitate violence because it threatens client self-respect. Option 2 sets limits by offering a solution without providing options. Because it is simple, direct, and does not threaten, clients often comply without becoming increasingly aggressive. Option 3, which uses affect and an option (talk), is not likely to cause escalation. Option 4 uses affect without offering the client an option and is a type of remark well tolerated by most angry clients. It usually leads to discussion of client feelings.

Cognitive level: Application
Nursing process: Implementation
NCLEX: Safe and Effective Care Environment
See text pages: 493, 494

16. An effective nursing intervention for helping angry clients learn to manage anger without violence would be
   1. using cognitive strategies to identify a thought that increases anger, find proof for or against the belief, and substitute reality-based thinking.
   2. providing negative reinforcement such as restraint or seclusion in response to angry outbursts, whether or not violence is present.
   3. administering antipsychotic medications.
   4. administering antianxiety medications.

Answer: 1
Rationale: Anger has a strong cognitive component, so using cognition to manage anger is logical. Option 2 is punitive. Options 3 and 4 may not be necessary and do nothing to help the client learn anger management.

Cognitive level: Application
Nursing process: Implementation
NCLEX: Psychosocial Integrity
See text page: 492

17. The individual who should be assessed as being at greatest risk for demonstrating violent behavior is
   1. A, who has a history of spousal abuse.
   2. B, who is severely agoraphobic.
   3. C, who verbalizes hopelessness and powerlessness.
   4. D, who demonstrates bizarre somatic delusions.

Answer: 1
Rationale: A history of prior aggression or violence is the best predictor of who may become violent. Option 2: Clients with anxiety disorders are not particularly prone to violence unless panic occurs. Option 3:

Clients experiencing hopelessness and powerlessness may have coexisting anger, but violence is not often demonstrated. Option 4: Clients with paranoid delusions are at greater risk for violence than those with bizarre somatic delusions.

Cognitive ability: Analysis
Nursing process: Assessment
NCLEX: Safe and Effective Care Environment
See text pages: 493, 494

18. The unit milieu most likely to have a low incidence of violent behavior is one that has
    1. a rigid and authoritarian structure.
    2. little structure and haphazard unit routines.
    3. unpredictable routines and allows clients to vent anger at staff.
    4. predictable routines and high client autonomy.

Answer: 4
Rationale: The milieu that is predictable and permits clients to behave autonomously as much as possible is less likely to be the scene of violence than units with authoritarian staff, little structure, haphazard routines, or permissive limits about directing anger at staff. Less structured routines create situations in which clients feel slighted, ignored, and insecure, all feelings known to underlie anger. Direct venting of anger at staff often leads to escalation.

Cognitive level: Analysis
Nursing process: Assessment
NCLEX: Safe and Effective Care Environment
See text pages: 492, 497

19. A client has sat in stony silence in the day room for 20 minutes after her appointment with her psychiatrist. She appears tense and vigilant. The nurse sees the client abruptly stand up and pace back and forth across the day room, clenching and unclenching her fists, then stop and stare intently into the face of the psychiatric technician seated at a table. The assessment that can be made is that the client is
    1. working off angry feelings.
    2. attempting to use relaxation strategies.
    3. exhibiting clues to potential aggression.
    4. using withdrawal.

Answer: 3
Rationale: The description of the client's behavior shows the classic signs of someone whose potential for aggression is increasing. Option 1: this assumption cannot be made.

Option 2: No evidence exists that the patient is using relaxation strategies. Option 4: The client's behavior cannot be described as typical of withdrawal.

Cognitive level: Application

Nursing process: Assessment
NCLEX: Safe and Effective Care Environment
See text page: 493

20. The client least likely to become angry and aggressive is the one who has feelings of
    1. fear or physical threat.
    2. rejection.
    3. humiliation.
    4. being valued.

Answer: 4
Rationale: Feelings listed in options 1, 2, and 3 engender anxiety, which is an antecedent to anger. Feeling valued is a positive experience, not one that would engender anger.

Cognitive level: Analysis
Nursing process: Assessment
NCLEX: Psychosocial Integrity
See text page: 497

21. A client with multiinfarct dementia is striking out with her arms and kicking at people who walk past in the hall. Intervention by the nurse should begin by
    1. asking the client what she needs.
    2. saying the client's name to gain contact.
    3. gently touching the client's arm.
    4. approaching from behind and using a bear hug.

Answer: 2
Rationale: Getting the client's attention is fundamental to intervention. The nurse should make eye contact and smile while repeating the client's name until the client focuses on the nurse. Once the nurse has the client's attention, gently touching the client and asking what she needs are appropriate. Striking out usually signals fear or that the client perceives the environment to be out of control. Option 4 would generate greater fear.

Cognitive level: Application
Nursing process: Implementation
NCLEX: Safe and Effective Care Environment
See text page: 498

22. A cognitively impaired client who has been a widow for 30 years is frantically trying to leave the unit, saying "I have to go home to start dinner before my husband comes home from work." To intervene with validation therapy, the nurse should say
    1. "You must come away from the door."
    2. "You have been a widow for many years."
    3. "You want to go home to get your husband's dinner."
    4. "Was your husband abusive when you did not have his dinner ready on time?"

Answer: 3

Rationale: Validation therapy meets the client "where she or he is at the moment" and acknowledges the client's wishes. Validation does not seek to redirect, reorient, or probe.

The other options do not validate client feelings.

Cognitive level: Application
Nursing process: Implementation
NCLEX: Safe and Effective Care Environment
See text page: 499

23. A client who is known to be angry and impulsive is hospitalized after an automobile accident in which he sustained severe orthopedic injuries. When in pain, he loudly berates nursing staff for "not knowing enough to give me my pain medicine when I need it." The nursing diagnosis of "ineffective coping related to inappropriate methods for handling anger associated with delayed pain relief" is recorded. A nursing intervention designed to address this would be
    1. telling the client to notify nursing staff one half-hour before the pain returns so they can prepare his medication.
    2. telling the client his verbal assaults on nurses will do nothing to shorten his wait for as-needed medication.
    3. urging the physician to change the as-needed order for pain medication to every 4 hours.
    4. having the clinical nurse leader request a psychiatric consultation.

Answer: 3

Rationale: Scheduling the medication at specific intervals will help the client anticipate when the medication can be given. Receiving the medication promptly on schedule, rather than expecting nurses to intuitively know his pain level, should reduce anxiety and anger. Option 1 expects the client to predict onset of pain before it occurs. Option 2 is a thinly veiled threat. Option 4 is not necessary at this point.

Cognitive level: Application
Nursing process: Implementation
NCLEX: Physiological Integrity
See text pages: 498, 499

24. A client has, in the past, had a nursing diagnosis of ineffective coping related to impulsively acting out anger as evidenced by striking others. An appropriate plan for forestalling such incidents would be
    1. explaining that restraint and seclusion will be used if violence occurs.
    2. helping a client identify incidents that trigger impulsive acting out.
    3. offer one-on-one supervision to help the client maintain control.

4. request that the client receive lorazepam (Ativan) every 4 hours to reduce anxiety.

Answer: 2

Rationale: Identification of trigger incidents allows the client and nurse to plan interventions to reduce irritation and frustration, which lead to acting out anger, and eventually to put into practice more adaptive coping strategies. Option 1 suggests restraint and seclusion are punitive interventions. Option 3 is too costly. Option 4 provides chemical restraint without cause.

Cognitive level: Application
Nursing process: Planning
NCLEX: Safe and Effective Care Environment
See text pages: 493, 494

25. A client with severe orthopedic injuries after an automobile accident is irritable, angry, and belittles the nurses who provide his care. While the nurse is changing the dressing over a deep laceration, the client screams "Don't touch me! You are so stupid that you will make it worse!" The intervention that uses a cognitive technique is to
    1. wordlessly leave the room.
    2. continue the dressing change, saying "Did you know that the dressing change is necessary so your leg will not become infected?"
    3. stop the dressing change, saying "Since you think you know more than a nurse, perhaps you would like to change your own dressing."
    4. continue the dressing change, saying "Unfortunately, you have no choice in this because your doctor has ordered this dressing change."

Answer: 2

Rationale: Anger is cognitively driven. Option 2 is an intervention that helps the client test his cognitions and may lead to lowering his anger. Option 1 is not possible if the nurse has started the dressing change. Option 3 will escalate the client's anger because it is belittling. Option 4 will escalate the client's anger by increasing his sense of powerlessness.

Cognitive level: Application
Nursing process: Implementation
NCLEX: Safe and Effective Care Environment
See text page: 492

26. The medication protocol the nurse should use to provide immediate intervention for an angry psychotic client whose aggressive behavior continues to escalate despite verbal intervention is
    1. lithium.
    2. trazodone.
    3. valproic acid.
    4. haloperidol.

367

Answer: 4

Rationale: Haloperidol is a short-acting antipsychotic that is useful in calming angry, aggressive clients regardless of diagnosis. The other drugs listed require long-term use to reduce anger. Option 1: Lithium would be used for bipolar clients. Option 2: Trazodone would be used for clients with dementia. Option 3: Valproic acid would be ordered for bipolar or borderline clients.

Cognitive level: Application
Nursing process: Planning
NCLEX: Physiological Integrity
See text page: 497

27. The emergency department nurse realizes that the husband of a client appears increasingly irritable as he waits. Interventions to prevent escalation of anger would include
   1. periodically updating the husband about what is being done for his wife.
   2. explaining that his wife will have to wait because clients are treated in order of need.
   3. asking that he relax, explaining that his wife's condition is not life threatening.
   4. suggesting that he return home and have the physician call with an update in 3 hours.

Answer: 1

Rationale: Periodic updates reduce anxiety and defuse anger. This strategy acknowledges the husband's presence and concern. Options 2, 3, and 4 would be likely to increase anger because they imply that his anxiety is inappropriate.

Cognitive level: Application
Nursing process: Implementation
NCLEX: Psychosocial Integrity
See text page: 499

28. The information noted in a client's history that suggests marginal coping skills and the need for careful assessment of risk for violence is a history of
   1. childhood trauma.
   2. family involvement.
   3. academic problems.
   4. chemical dependence.

Answer: 4

Rationale: The nurse should suspect marginal coping skills in a client with chemical dependence. They are often anxious, may be concerned about inadequate pain relief, and may have personality styles that externalize blame. The other options do not signal as high a degree of risk as chemical dependence.

Cognitive level: Application
Nursing process: Assessment

NCLEX: Safe and Effective Care Environment
See text pages: 499, 500

29. A client being treated for compartment syndrome has been hospitalized for 4 days. He has no history of psychiatric disorder but is described by his family as being "a difficult person who finds fault with others." From the day of admission he has verbally abused the nurses for their inability to provide care that keeps him pain free and comfortable. The most likely explanation lies in
   1. poor child-rearing that did not teach respect for others.
   2. automatic thinking leading to cognitive distortion.
   3. a personality style that externalizes problems.
   4. delusions that others wish to harm him.

Answer: 3

Rationale: Clients whose personality style causes them to externalize blame see the source of their discomfort and anxiety as being outside themselves. They displace anger and are unable to take responsibility for self-soothing. On the basis of family input, the other options are less likely to have a bearing on his behavior.

Cognitive style: Analysis
Nursing process: Assessment
NCLEX: Safe and Effective Care Environment
See text pages: 499, 500

30. A client being treated for compartment syndrome has been hospitalized for 4 days. He has no history of psychiatric disorder but is described by his family as being "a difficult person who finds fault with others." From the day of admission he has verbally abused the nurses for their inability to provide care that keeps him pain free and comfortable. Nursing interventions that should be introduced include (multiple answers may be correct)
   1. providing activities that distract or entertain.
   2. clarifying actions the nurse can take.
   3. providing medication on schedule.
   4. meeting requests only when politely verbalized.
   5. establishing penalties for inappropriate behavior.
   6. encouraging the client to plan with nurse.

Answers: 1, 2, 3, 6

Rationale: Option 1: Helping the client focus on things other than his discomfort can reduce anxiety. Option 2: Clients who externalize discomfort and blame expect relief to come from external sources. They often have unrealistic beliefs about what a nurse can do. Careful explanation that clarifies can reduce unrealistic expectations. Option 6: When the client takes responsibility for planning with staff, the client will have a greater investment in outcomes and will usually agree to modify behaviors in support of having needs met. Option 3: Providing medications and treatment according to a schedule, rather than on an as-needed basis, helps the client establish trust that the staff will meet his needs sooner rather than later. Option 4: The nurse must respond to certain client needs, whether articulated politely or not. Option 5: Establishing penalties would not be an independent nursing intervention.

Cognitive level: Synthesis
Nursing process: Planning
NCLEX: Safe and Effective Care Environment
See text pages: 499, 500

31. A client being treated in the burn injury unit has demonstrated good coping skills for several weeks. Today, a new nurse is assigned to care for him and has proven to be poorly organized. His usual schedule has not been followed and by midafternoon he is angry and raises his voice to complain to the nurse clinician. The best course of action for the nurse clinician would be to
   1. explain the reasons for the disorganization and take over his care for the rest of the shift.
   2. acknowledge and validate his distress and ask what he would like to have happen.
   3. apologize and explain that he will have to live with the situation for the rest of the shift.
   4. ask him to control his anger and tell him allowances must be made for new staff.

Answer: 2
Rationale: When a client with good coping skills is angry and overwhelmed, the goal is to reestablish a means of dealing with the situation. The nurse should problem solve with the client by acknowledging the client's feelings, validating them as understandable, apologizing as necessary, then seeking an acceptable solution. Often clients can tell the nurse what they would like to have happen as a reasonable first step.

Cognitive level: Application
Nursing process: Implementation
NCLEX: Safe and Effective Care Environment
See text pages: 498, 499

32. The principle on which nursing intervention should be predicated when a client's aggression quickly escalates is
   1. staff should match client's affective level, tone of voice, and so forth.
   2. immediately use physical containment measures.
   3. ask the client what will be most helpful to him or her.
   4. begin with the least restrictive measure possible.

Answer: 4
Rationale: Legal constraints require that staff use the least restrictive measure possible. This becomes the guiding principle for intervention. Option 1 would result in greater escalation. Option 2: Physical containment is seldom the least restrictive measure. Option 3: Asking the out-of-control client what to do is rarely helpful. It may be an effective strategy during the preaggressive phase but is less effective during escalation.

Cognitive level: Application
Nursing process: Planning
NCLEX: Safe and Effective Care Environment
See text pages: 496, 497

33. An aggressive client was placed in four-point restraints and given an intramuscular dosage of anxiolytic medication. Systematic assessment to guide interventions during the period of restraint should include (more than one answer may be correct)
   1. hydration.
   2. vital signs.
   3. nutritional status.
   4. elimination needs.
   5. level of awareness.
   6. range of motion and comfort needs.

Answers: 1, 2, 3, 4, 5, 6
Rationale: All the options should be assessed. Each pertains to biological and safety needs of the client. Nurses must follow hospital protocol for care. Generally, clients should be observed for level of consciousness at 15-minute intervals, given food at normal meal times or more often if they are hyperactive, given fluids hourly, have vital signs taken at 4-hour intervals or less if medication administration has caused hypotension, taken to the bathroom every 2 hours, and released from restraint and given range of motion every 2 hours.

Cognitive level: Application
Nursing process: Assessment
NCLEX: Safe and Effective Care Environment
See text pages: 496, 497

34. The nurse directs the intervention team who must take an aggressive client to seclusion. Other clients have been removed from the area. Before approaching the client, the nurse should ensure that staff (more than one answer may be correct)
   1. remove jewelry, glasses, and harmful items from their persons.
   2. select the person who will communicate with the client.
   3. quickly approach the client and take hold of the closest arm or leg.

Chapter 24   Anger and Aggression

4. move behind the client to use the element of surprise.
5. appoint a person to clear a path and open, close, or lock doors.

Answers: 1, 2, 5

Rationale: Option 1 prevents injury to staff and the client. Option 2: Only one person should explain what will happen and direct the client. This may be the nurse or a staff member with a good relationship with the client. Option 5 is essential because those restraining a limb cannot use keys, move furniture, or open doors. The nurse is usually responsible for administering medication once the client has been restrained. Option 3: Each staff member should have an assigned limb rather than just grabbing the closest. This system could leave one or two limbs unrestrained. Option 4: Approaching in full view of the client reduces suspicion.

Cognitive level: Application
Nursing process: Planning
NCLEX: Safe and Effective Care Environment
See text page: 498

35. Six hours after a client lost control and required seclusion and as-needed medication, she is out of seclusion, calm, and sitting in her room reading. Postassaultive stage care measures that should be taken by the nurse include (more than one option may be chosen)
1. avoiding mention of the incident.
2. suggesting that the client may wish to apologize.
3. helping the client identify the precipitating event.
4. reviewing possible alternative coping strategies with client.

Answers: 3, 4

Rationale: Postincident processing should be attempted when the client is calm. This processing helps the client and staff understand what happened and how further incidents of violence can be avoided. Identification of the precipitating event is critical. Once this is accomplished, the client and nurse can discuss possible alternative coping strategies and role play those chosen. Options 1 and 2 do nothing to help the client learn more effective coping strategies.

Cognitive level: Application
Nursing process: Implementation
NCLEX: Safe and Effective Care Environment
See text page: 498

36. A newly admitted client required seclusion immediately on entering the inpatient unit. Assessment had not been completed and no medical orders had been written. Immediately after secluding the client the priority action of the nurse should be to

1. provide an opportunity for the client to go to the bathroom.
2. notify the physician and obtain a seclusion order.
3. notify the hospital risk manager.
4. debrief staff.

Answer: 2

Rationale: Emergency seclusion can be effected by a credentialed nurse but must be followed by securing a medical order within a period of time specified by the state and the agency. The other options are not immediately necessary from a legal standpoint.

Cognitive level: Application
Nursing process: Implementation
NCLEX: Safe and Effective Care Environment
See text pages: 496, 497

37. A client being admitted to the inpatient unit suddenly removes a knife from his coat pocket and threatens to kill himself or anyone who tries to take him into a room. A psychiatric emergency code is called and the client is safely disarmed and placed in seclusion. The rationale for use of seclusion was that the client
1. clearly evidenced a thought disorder, rendering him incapable of rational decision.
2. presented a clear and present danger to self and others.
3. presented a clear escape risk.
4. was psychotic.

Answer: 2

Rationale: The client's threat to kill himself or others with the knife he possessed constituted a clear and present danger to self and others. The other three options are not considered sufficient reasons for seclusion.

Cognitive level: Analysis
Nursing process: Planning
NCLEX: Safe and Effective Care Environment
See text pages: 496, 497

CHAPTER 25

1. A community mental health nurse is assigned to visit the home of a child, aged 11 years, to investigate his frequent school absences. The nurse finds the child caring for his siblings, aged 4 months, 11/2 years, and 3-year-old twins. Both parents are at work. The house is cluttered and dirty. The child tells the nurse he would like to attend school regularly, but whenever his mother is called to work at her part-time job, he must watch the kids because the family cannot afford to pay a babysitter. He mentions that it does not make a difference anyway, be-

370

cause he is "too dumb to learn much." He adds "I don't have any friends at school, probably because I don't deserve any." Based on the information obtained thus far, what preliminary assessment can be made?

1. Insufficient data are present to make an assessment.
2. The child and his siblings are experiencing neglect.
3. The children are at high risk for sexual abuse.
4. The children are experiencing physical abuse.

Answer: 2

Rationale: The child is experiencing educational neglect when his parents deprive him of the opportunity to attend school. It is possible that the other children may be experiencing physical neglect, but more data should be gathered before making the actual assessment. Options 3 and 4: The information presented does not indicate high risk for sexual abuse, and no hard evidence of physical abuse is present.

Cognitive level: Analysis
Nursing process: Assessment
NCLEX: Psychosocial Integrity
See text page: 514

2. A child, aged 11 years, stays home from school to care for his siblings while his mother works because the family cannot afford a babysitter. The home is cluttered and dirty. When asked about his parents, the child reluctantly reveals that he thinks his father does not like him very much because he calls him "stupid" and says he can never do anything right. This should be assessed as
   1. physical abuse.
   2. sexual abuse.
   3. emotional abuse.
   4. economic abuse.

Answer: 3

Rationale: Examples of emotional abuse include having an adult demean a child's worth or frequently criticize or belittle the child. No data support physical battering or endangerment, sexual abuse, or economic abuse.

Cognitive level: Analysis
Nursing process: Assessment
NCLEX: Psychosocial Integrity
See text page: 514

3. A child, aged 11 years, stays home from school to care for his siblings while his mother works because the family cannot afford a babysitter. The home is cluttered and dirty when the community mental health nurse visits to investigate the child's school

absences. The nurse learns that the parents are due home in half an hour and decides to wait and interview them. While waiting, the nurse does a mental review of personal feelings. The feelings most commonly experienced by a nurse working with abusive families include
   1. sympathy for the victim and anger toward the abuser.
   2. outrage toward the victim and sympathy for the abuser.
   3. unconcern for the victim and dislike for the abuser.
   4. vulnerability for self and empathy with the abuser.

Answer: 1

Rationale: Intense protective feelings, sympathy for the victim, and anger and outrage toward the abuser are common emotions of a nurse working with an abusive family.

Cognitive level: Application
Nursing process: Assessment
Client need: Safe and Effective Care Environment
See text pages: 512, 513

4. The rationale for the nurse needing to be aware of feelings while working with a family experiencing family violence is best explained as
   1. awareness protects one's own mental health.
   2. strong negative feelings interfere with assessment and judgment.
   3. strong positive feelings lead to underinvolvement with the victim.
   4. positive feelings promote the development of sympathy for clients.

Answer: 2

Rationale: Strong negative feelings cloud the nurse's judgment and interfere with assessment and intervention, no matter how well the nurse tries to cover or deny feelings. Option 3: Strong positive feelings lead to overinvolvement with victims. Options 1 and 4 are neither wholly true nor entirely relevant.

Cognitive level: Application
Nursing process: Assessment
NCLEX: Psychosocial Integrity
See text pages: 513, 514

5. A child, aged 11 years, stays home from school to care for his siblings while his mother works because the family cannot afford a babysitter. The home is cluttered and dirty when the community mental health nurse visits to investigate the child's school absences. When the parents arrive home from work, the nurse sees that the parents are young, aged 25

and 26 years. They married after the woman became pregnant. What in the oldest child's life might indicate that he is vulnerable to abuse?
1. He is a male.
2. He is the oldest child.
3. His birth was unplanned.
4. Both parents work outside the home.

Answer: 3
Rationale: An unwanted child is at risk for abuse. The other factors do not place him at high risk for abuse.
Cognitive level: Application
Nursing process: Assessment
NCLEX: Psychosocial Integrity
See text pages: 509, 510

6. A child, aged 11 years, stays home from school to care for his siblings while his mother works because the family cannot afford a babysitter. The home is cluttered and dirty when the community mental health nurse visits to investigate the child's school absences. When the parents arrive home from work the child's father behaves angrily. He orders his wife and son about. He finds fault with the son, asking him twice "Why are you such a stupid kid?" The wife tells the nurse she has difficulty disciplining the children and gets frustrated easily. The nurse's goal is to continue to gather assessment data. The remark or question that would create a block is
   1. "Tell me how you punish your children."
   2. "When your baby cries, how do you get him to stop?"
   3. "Caring for five small children must be difficult."
   4. "Do you or your husband ever beat the children?"

Answer: 4
Rationale: An interview with possible abusing individuals should be built on concern and carried out in a nonthreatening, nonjudgmental way. This question would be threatening. Option 3: Empathetic remarks are helpful in creating rapport. Options 1 and 2: Questions requiring a descriptive response are less threatening and elicit more relevant information than questions that can be answered by yes or no.
Cognitive level: Analysis
Nursing process: Assessment
NCLEX: Safe and Effective Care Environment
See text page: 512

7. A child, aged 11 years, stays home from school to care for his siblings while his mother works because the family cannot afford a babysitter. The home is cluttered and dirty when the community mental health nurse visits to investigate the child's school absences. The nurse's legal responsibility if child abuse or neglect is suspected is to

1. discuss the family in a team meeting with the child's teacher, principal, and school psychologist.
2. document the observations and speculations in the family health record.
3. report the suspected abuse or neglect according to state regulations.
4. schedule a return visit for reassessment in 1 week.

Answer: 3
Rationale: Each state has specific regulations for reporting child abuse that must be observed. The nurse is usually a mandated reporter. The reporter does not need to be absolutely sure that abuse or neglect is occurring, only that it is suspected.
Cognitive level: Application
Nursing process: Implementation
NCLEX: Safe and Effective Care Environment
See text pages: 519, 520

8. A child, aged 11 years, has to stay home from school to care for his siblings while his mother works because the family cannot afford a babysitter. The home is cluttered and dirty when the community mental health nurse visits to investigate the child's school absences. When asked about his parents, he reluctantly reveals that he thinks his father does not like him very much. The level of prevention for work with this family will be
   1. primary.
   2. secondary.
   3. tertiary.
   4. prevention is not possible.

Answer: 2
Rationale: Secondary prevention involves intervention in abusive situations to minimize their disabling or long-term effects. Community resources are mobilized to help find alternative ways to deal with stress. Option 1: Primary prevention refers to measures to prevent or reduce the occurrence of abusive situations. Option 3: Tertiary prevention refers to interventions aimed at reducing the severity of mental illness or handicaps resulting from long-term, abusive trauma.
Cognitive level: Application
Nursing process: Assessment
NCLEX: Safe and Effective Care Environment
See text pages: 520, 521

9. A child, aged 11 years, stays home from school to care for his siblings while his mother works because the family cannot afford a babysitter. The home is cluttered and dirty when the community mental health nurse visits to investigate the child's school absences. During the visit the child reveals that he thinks his father does not like him very much be-

cause he calls him "stupid" all the time. Furthermore, the child states he thinks he is too dumb to learn much. The child states he has no friends at school and suggests the reason for this is because he does not deserve them. On the basis of the assessment data, the nursing diagnosis that should be considered for the child is
1. chronic low self-esteem related to negative feedback about self from father.
2. deficient knowledge related to missing school.
3. noncompliance: school attendance related to parental rules.
4. disturbed personal identity related to negative self-evaluation.

Answer: 1

Rationale: The child has indicated he believes he may be too dumb to learn and does not deserve to have friends. He receives frequent negative and demeaning feedback from his father. Option 2: Deficient knowledge is a nursing diagnosis that refers to knowledge of health care measures. Option 3: Noncompliance refers to an individual's informed decision not to adhere to a therapeutic recommendation. Option 4: Disturbed personal identity refers to an alteration in the ability to distinguish between self and nonself.

Cognitive level: Analysis
Nursing process: Diagnosis
NCLEX: Psychosocial Integrity
See text page: 518

10. A child, aged 11 years, stays home from school to care for his siblings while his mother works because the family cannot afford a babysitter. The home is cluttered and dirty when the community mental health nurse visits to investigate the child's school absences. During the visit the child reveals that he thinks his father does not like him very much because he calls him "stupid" all the time. The child states he has no friends at school and suggests the reason for this is because he does not deserve them. The desired outcome for the child is
1. abuse cessation.
2. abuse recovery: sexual.
3. abuse recovery: physical.
4. abusive behavior: self-restraint.

Answer: 1

Rationale: Abuse cessation is a desirable outcome. Indicators to be monitored are cessation of emotional abuse, such as calling the child "stupid." Options 2 and 3: Data are not present to suggest sexual or physical abuse. Option 4: Abusive behavior: self restraint has relevance to the perpetrator rather than the victim.

Cognitive level: Application
Nursing process: Planning (Outcome Identification)
NCLEX: Safe and Effective Care Environment
See text pages: 518, 519

11. A child, aged 11 years, stays home from school to care for his siblings while his mother works because the family cannot afford a babysitter. The home is cluttered and dirty when the community mental health nurse visits to investigate the child's school absences. During the visit the child reveals that he thinks his father does not like him very much because he calls him "stupid" all the time. The wife mentions that the father is easily frustrated and has trouble disciplining the children. In planning interventions to stabilize the home situation and maintain a violence-free atmosphere, the nurse should consider suggesting
1. anger management counseling for the father.
2. placing the children in a children's shelter.
3. continuing home visits to give support.
4. group sessions to teach child-rearing practices.
5. a safety plan for the wife and children.

Answers: 1, 3, 4

Rationale: Option 1 would be appropriate. Option 3: Support for this family will be an important component of treatment. Option 4: By the wife's admission the family has deficient knowledge of parenting practices. Option 2: Whenever possible, the goal of intervention should be to keep the family together; thus removing the children from the home should be considered a last resort. Option 5: Physical abuse is not suspected, so this would not be a priority at this time.

Cognitive level: Analysis
Nursing process: Planning
NCLEX: Safe and Effective Care Environment
See text pages: 519-524

12. A community mental health nurse working with a family demonstrating emotional abuse of a child by the father has put several interventions in place designed to stabilize the home and maintain a violence-free atmosphere. Several weeks later the child tells the nurse that his parents and all the children go to a clinic and talk to a man about how to get along. He says the man asked him how he felt when his dad called him "stupid," and that his dad cried when the child described feeling "awful." The child is describing the type of therapy called
1. Parents Anonymous.
2. group therapy.
3. family therapy.
4. individual therapy.

Chapter 25   Family Violence

Answer: 3

Rationale: Family therapy involves the entire family meeting with a family therapist to learn to listen to each other and ultimately decrease the frequency and intensity of abuse. Option 1: Parents Anonymous is a self-help group for abusing parents. Option 2: Group therapy would involve having the abuser meet with other clients in a supportive atmosphere. Option 4: Individual therapy would involve meetings of a single client with a therapist.

Cognitive level: Application
Nursing process: Assessment
NCLEX: Psychosocial Integrity
See text page: 524

13. A 35-year-old married woman who works full time in a factory has recently been absent for 3-day periods on several occasions. Each time she returned to work wearing dark glasses. Facial and body bruises were apparent. Her supervisor became suspicious that she was a victim of battering and referred her to the occupational health nurse. The assessment priority when the nurse interviews the client is
   1. leisure skills.
   2. work habits.
   3. physical injuries.
   4. socialization skills.

Answer: 3

Rationale: The woman has been referred to be assessed for possible battering. Physical injuries are abuse indicators and are the primary focus for assessment. No data support the other options.

Cognitive level: Application
Nursing process: Assessment
NCLEX: Safe and Effective Care Environment
See text page: 512

14. A 35-year-old married woman who works full time in a factory has recently been absent for 3-day periods on several occasions. Each time she returned to work wearing dark glasses. Facial and body bruises were apparent. Her supervisor became suspicious that she was a victim of battering and referred her to the occupational health nurse. The priority question for the nurse to ask is
   1. "How did this happen to you?"
   2. "Do you drink excessively?"
   3. "Did your husband beat you?"
   4. "What did you do to deserve this?"

Answer: 1

Rationale: Obtaining the victim's explanation is necessary. If the explanation does not match the injuries or if the victim minimizes the injury, abuse should be suspected. Option 2 suggests the victim is to blame. Option 3 is too direct. Option 4 is judgmental.

Cognitive level: Application
Nursing process: Implementation
NCLEX: Safe and Effective Care Environment
See text page: 512

15. A 35-year-old married woman who works full time in a factory has recently been absent for 3-day periods on several occasions. Each time she returned to work wearing dark glasses. Facial and body bruises were apparent. Her supervisor became suspicious that she was a victim of battering and referred her to the occupational health nurse. When the nurse interviews her, the worker admitted her husband beat her. She stated he was "upset" because he lost his job. The next step for the nurse to take would be to
   1. call the police.
   2. call the adult protective agency.
   3. have her admitted to the hospital.
   4. document injuries with a body map and photographs.

Answer: 4

Rationale: Documentation of injuries provides a basis for possible legal intervention. Options 1 and 2 are not appropriate for the nurse to take. The woman would need to make the decision to involve the police. Because the worker is not an elder and is competent, the adult protective agency is unable to assist her. Option 3: Admission to the hospital is not necessary.

Cognitive level: Application
Nursing process: Implementation
Client need: Safe and Effective Care Environment
Text reference: 514

16. A woman who is a victim of severe emotional violence tells the nurse that her husband abuses her most often when he is intoxicated, just as his father had beaten him and his mother. The woman is aware of the location of a safe house and has considered leaving home with her two children, but she cites being brought up to believe "you keep quiet and stay together, no matter what happens." She states the husband is always apologetic and remorseful after an incident. What evidence exists that the husband is at risk of becoming a perpetrator of physical abuse? He
   1. is unable to make lasting behavioral changes.
   2. was an abused child.
   3. is without a job.
   4. experiences remorse.

Answer: 2

Rationale: An abuse-prone individual is an individual who has experienced family violence and has usually been abused as a child. The other options are not relevant in this scenario.

Cognitive level: Application
Nursing process: Assessment
NCLEX: Psychosocial Integrity
See text pages: 508, 509

17. A woman who is a victim of severe emotional violence tells the nurse that her husband abuses her most often when he is intoxicated, just as his father had beaten him and his mother. She states he is always apologetic and remorseful after an incident. She has considered leaving home with her two children but has not been able to bring herself to actually leave. The stage in the cycle of violence that prevents her from leaving her husband is the
   1. tension-building stage.
   2. acute battering stage.
   3. honeymoon stage.
   4. recovery stage.

Answer: 3
Rationale: The honeymoon stage is characterized by kindly, loving behaviors toward the abused spouse when the perpetrator feels remorseful. The victim believes the promises and drops plans to leave or seek legal help. Option 1: The tension-building stage is characterized by minor violence in the form of abusive verbalization or pushing. Option 2: The acute battering stage involves the abuser beating the victim. Option 4: The violence cycle does not include a recovery stage.

Cognitive level: Application
Nursing process: Assessment
NCLEX: Safe and Effective Care Environment
See text page: 510

18. A battered wife tells the nurse she was brought up to believe "you stay together, no matter what happens." She also states her husband is always apologetic and remorseful after an incident. The myth that can be identified is
   1. a family life is private and sacred.
   2. women who are abused are mentally ill.
   3. men have a right to keep their wives in line.
   4. battered women like to be beaten.

Answer: 1
Rationale: The only myth verbalized by the victim relates to the confidentiality of what occurs within the family. The other statements are commonly held myths, but no evidence exists that the victim holds any of them.

Cognitive level: Application
Nursing process: Assessment
NCLEX: Psychosocial Integrity
See text page: 515

19. A victim of physical abuse by her domestic partner is being treated for a broken humerus. She tells the nurse her partner abuses her most often when he is intoxicated. She has considered going to a safe house. She cites being brought up to believe "you stay together, no matter what happens." She also states her partner is always apologetic and remorseful after an incident. The nursing diagnosis that can be established for this client is
   1. impaired social interaction related to husband's unemployment.
   2. risk for injury related to husband's physical abuse when intoxicated.
   3. deficient knowledge: community supports related to unreadiness to learn.
   4. disturbed sleep pattern related to problems in the home, as evidenced by behavior of husband and children.

Answer: 2
Rationale: Risk for injury is a viable diagnosis because the partner has already inflicted physical injury during violent episodes. Options 1 and 4: Data have not been obtained showing that the client's social interactions are impaired or that she has disturbed sleep patterns, although both are common among victims of violence. Option 3: Deficient knowledge cannot be substantiated because she is aware of a safe house.

Cognitive level: Analysis
Nursing process: Diagnosis
NCLEX: Safe and Effective Care Environment
See text page: 518

20. A victim of physical abuse by her domestic partner is being treated for a broken humerus. She tells the nurse her partner abuses her most often when he is intoxicated. She has considered going to a safe house. She cites being brought up to believe "you stay together, no matter what happens." She also states her partner is always apologetic and remorseful after an incident. Which indicator for the outcome of abuse protection can be met before the client leaves the emergency department? The client will
   1. name two community resources she can contact.
   2. demonstrate insight into the abusive relationship.
   3. limit contact with the perpetrator by a restraining order.
   4. facilitate counseling for the perpetrator.

Answer: 1
Rationale: The only outcome indicator clearly attainable within this time is for staff to provide the victim with information about community resources she can contact. Option 2: Development of insight into the abusive relationship will require time. Option 3:

375

Securing a restraining order can be accomplished quickly but not while the client is in the emergency department. Option 4: Facilitating the perpetrator's counseling may require weeks or months.
Cognitive level: Analysis
Nursing process: Planning (Outcome Identification)
NCLEX: Safe and Effective Care Environment
See text pages: 518, 519

21. A victim of spousal abuse comes to the emergency department for treatment of a broken nose. She appears hypervigilant and anxious and admits to sleep disturbance when the nurse questions the dark circles under her eyes. She reluctantly tells the nurse the abuse usually occurs when the husband has been drinking, although she concedes he is always jealous and controlling. She is a stay-at-home mother of two preschool children. The family has lived in this town for 1 month. The client states she has fleetingly considered suicide but must stay alive to care for her children. She denies having had the desire to kill her husband. The assessments the nurse should document in the medical record include noting that (more than one option may be correct)
    1. signs of high anxiety and chronic stress are present.
    2. the client relies on the perpetrator for basic needs.
    3. the client is isolated from individual and community support.
    4. suicide risk is high.
    5. homicide potential is low.
    6. a safety plan should be constructed.

Answers: 1, 2, 3, 5, 6
Rationale: Option 1: Client and family coping is impaired as evidenced by client symptoms, recently sustained physical abuse, and perpetrator substance abuse and overcontrolling aspects of family life. Option 2: Powerlessness is evident. Option 3: The client does not have support systems available. Option 5: The scenario supports this assessment. Option 6: Because the client has already sustained physical injury, and the perpetrator abuses alcohol and is both jealous and obsessive about the relationship, risk for further injury is high. The client should have a plan for going to a safe site in the event this becomes necessary. Option 4: Data do not support the assessment that the client's suicide risk is *high*.
Cognitive level: Analysis
Nursing process: Assessment
NCLEX: Safe and Effective Care Environment
See text page: 512

22. A mother of one, who is the victim of partner abuse, describes her partner as someone who is easily frus-

trated and more likely to abuse her after a experiencing an event in which self-esteem is challenged. The most recent episodes of violence were related to feeling "upset" over job loss. The type of therapy that would provide the greatest help to the client's partner is
    1. individual therapy focusing on decision making.
    2. group therapy focusing on anger management.
    3. couples therapy focusing on assertiveness.
    4. family therapy focusing on parenting.

Answer: 2
Rationale: Group therapy provides assurance that the abuser is not alone and that positive change is possible. By learning to recognize signs of escalating anger and ways to channel anger nonviolently, the cycle of abuse may be broken. Option 1 is inappropriate because decision making is not an identified problem. Option 3: Therapy focusing on assertiveness might be premature. The partner needs to work with the problem of anger first, or the abuse may intensify as the client becomes more assertive. Option 4: Family therapy focusing on parenting would not focus on the priority problem.
Cognitive level: Application
Nursing process: Planning
NCLEX: Safe and Effective Care Environment
See text pages: 524, 525

23. An 82-year-old widow with Alzheimer's disease lives with her daughter's family, which owns a catering business. During the week, the client attends a day care center for clients with Alzheimer's disease. During the evenings, members of the family care for the client. One day the nurse at the day care center notices the client's appearance is disheveled. She has a strong odor of urine and her hair is uncombed. When the nurse took the client to the bathroom, she noticed bruises on her limbs and back. From the nurse's observations, what type of abuse might be occurring?
    1. Psychological abuse
    2. Physical abuse
    3. Financial abuse
    4. Sexual abuse

Answer: 2
Rationale: The assessment of physical abuse would be supported by the nurse's observation of bruises. Physical abuse includes evidence of improper care as well as physical endangerment behaviors such as reckless behavior toward a vulnerable person that could lead to serious injury. No data substantiate the other options.
Cognitive level: Application
Nursing process: Assessment
NCLEX: Safe and Effective Care Environment
See text page: 510

376

24. An 82-year-old widow with Alzheimer's disease lives with her daughter's family. The daughter runs a catering business. During the week, the client attends a day care center for clients with Alzheimer's disease. During the evenings, members of the family care for her. The characteristic that makes the client vulnerable to abuse is
1. confused behaviors.
2. blaming the caregiver for abuse.
3. being home only in the evening.
4. being part of a busy family.

Answer: 1

Rationale: Elders at high risk for violence include those with cognitive impairments. The other characteristics are not identified as placing an individual at high risk.

Cognitive level: Application
Nursing process: Assessment
NCLEX: Safe and Effective Care Environment
See text pages: 509, 510

25. A client, aged 82 years, has Alzheimer's disease. She lives with her daughter's family and goes to a day care facility on weekdays. The nurse at the day care center noticed the client was unkempt and had multiple bruises. When the daughter arrived to pick her up, the nurse discussed her observations. The daughter became defensive and said that her mother was very difficult to manage. She stated "My mother is not my mother anymore. She is confused and she wanders all night. When I have to be out in the evening on business, one of my teenagers has to watch her. Then I have to watch her all night. Last night I fell asleep and she fell down the stairs. Sometimes I just cannot bear to care for her." The nursing diagnosis that can be established for the client is
1. risk for injury related to poor judgment associated with cognitive impairment and lack of family caregiver supervision.
2. noncompliance related to confusion and disorientation, as evidenced by lack of cooperation.
3. anxiety related to confused state, as evidenced by the client wandering at night.
4. impaired verbal communication related to brain impairment, as evidenced by the client's confusion.

Answer: 1

Rationale: The client is at high risk for injury because of her confusion. The risk increases when caregivers are unable to give constant supervision. No assessment data support the diagnoses of anxiety, impaired verbal communication, or noncompliance.

Cognitive level: Analysis
Nursing process: Diagnosis
NCLEX: Safe and Effective Care Environment
See text page: 518

26. A client, aged 82 years, has Alzheimer's disease. She lives with her daughter's family and goes to a day care facility on weekdays. The nurse at the day care center noticed the client was unkempt and had multiple bruises. The nurse discussed her observations with the daughter, who became defensive and said that her mother was very difficult to manage. She stated "My mother is not my mother anymore. She is confused and she wanders all night. When I have to be out in the evening on business, one of my teenagers has to watch her. Then I have to watch her all night. Last night I fell asleep and she fell down stairs. Sometimes I just cannot bear to care for her." What nursing diagnosis can be established for the client's family?
1. Deficient knowledge related to effects of aging
2. Grieving related to mother's aging
3. Interrupted family processes related to elderly mother in home
4. Impaired parenting related to lack of time to spend with teenage children

Answer: 3

Rationale: Interrupted family processes can be diagnosed on the basis of the defining characteristic: inability of the family to meet the physical needs of a member. No data support the diagnoses of deficient knowledge, grieving, or impaired parenting.

Cognitive level: Application
Nursing process: Diagnosis
NCLEX: Safe and Effective Care Environment
See text page: 518

27. A client, aged 82 years, has Alzheimer's disease. She lives with her daughter's family and goes to a day care facility on weekdays. The family cares for her during the evening and at night. Noting the client had several bruises, the nurse discussed her observations with the daughter, who became defensive and said that her mother was very difficult to manage because she is confused and wanders all night. The bruises resulted from a fall down stairs. The daughter states "I have lost my mother." The nursing intervention that should take priority is
1. teaching the daughter more about the effects of Alzheimer's disease.
2. identifying two resources that can be used for the mother's evening and night care.
3. supporting the daughter to grieve the loss of her mother's ability to function.
4. teaching the family how to give physical care more effectively and efficiently.

Answer: 2

Rationale: The client's daughter and her family were coping with care until the client began to wander more

Chapter 25   Family Violence

at night. The family needs assistance with evening and night care to resume their precrisis state of functioning. Secondary prevention calls for the nurse to mobilize community resources to relieve overwhelming stress. The other interventions may then be accomplished.

Cognitive level: Analysis
Nursing process: Planning
NCLEX: Safe and Effective Care Environment
See text pages: 519, 520

28. A client, aged 82 years, has Alzheimer's disease. She lives with her daughter's family and goes to a day care facility on weekdays. The family cares for her during the evening and at night. Noting the client had several bruises, the nurse discussed her observations with the daughter, who became defensive and said that her mother was very difficult to manage because she is confused and wanders all night. The bruises resulted from a fall down stairs. The daughter states "I have lost my mother." The nurse plans to talk with the daughter in 1 week. In the meantime, the client's physical condition will be monitored by day care staff. If new bruises are noted the nurse should plan to
   1. notify the adult protective agency.
   2. phone the client's physician.
   3. have the client admitted to the hospital.
   4. press criminal charges against the daughter.

Answer: 1
Rationale: Investigating suspected elder abuse is within the scope of the adult protective services agency. The agency is responsible for reporting any suspected abusive situation. Suspicion is all that is required. The adult protective agency is responsible for further investigation. The other options are beyond the scope of the day care facility.

Cognitive level: Application
Nursing process: Planning
NCLEX: Safe and Effective Care Environment
See text page: 519, 520

29. The emotional reaction to family violence that is desirable for a nurse to experience is
   1. anger.
   2. empathy.
   3. shock.
   4. revulsion.

Answer: 2
Rationale: Strong negative feelings get in the way of being able to be objective and therapeutic. Empathy, a positive feeling, would not hamper objectivity and the ability to be therapeutic.

Cognitive level: Application
Nursing process: Implementation
NCLEX: Safe and Effective Care Environment
See text pages: 512, 513

30. A nurse is working with a perpetrator of family violence who has a long history of violent outbursts of temper when frustrated and periods of remorse after each outburst. The nurse is most likely to establish the nursing diagnosis of
   1. risk for injury related to victim reprisal.
   2. risk for other-directed violence related to stress.
   3. ineffective coping related to poor anger management.
   4. caretaker role strain related to feelings of being overwhelmed.

Answer: 3
Rationale: Ineffective coping considers the long-term nature of the problem. Option 1: Risk for injury is more relevant for the victim. Options 2 and 4 suggest a recent problem.

Cognitive level: Analysis
Nursing process: Diagnosis
NCLEX: Psychosocial Integrity
See text page: 518

31. The plan of care for a client who has demonstrated outbursts of physical violence against his family when frustrated and periods of remorse after each outburst would be considered successful when the client
   1. expresses frustration verbally instead of physically.
   2. agrees to seek counseling at a future time.
   3. explains the rationale for his behavior to the victim.
   4. identifies three personal strengths.

Answer: 1
Rationale: Option 1 indicates that the client has developed a healthier way of coping with frustration. The other options do not confirm the success of the interventions.

Cognitive level: Analysis
Nursing process: Evaluation
NCLEX: Psychosocial Integrity
See text page: 525

32. The referral essential for the nurse to make for a wife who has been severely beaten by her husband, has no relatives or friends in the community, is afraid to return home, has no financial resources of her own, and has no job skills is
   1. community food cupboard.
   2. vocational counseling.

3. law enforcement.
4. a women's shelter.

Answer: 4
Rationale: Because the wife wishes to leave the home and has no safe place to go, referral to a shelter is necessary. The shelter will provide other referrals as necessary.
Cognitive level: Application
Nursing process: Implementation
NCLEX: Safe and Effective Care Environment
See text page: 521

33. The family scenario that presents the greatest risk for family violence is
   1. a husband who is unemployed and has low self-esteem associated with lack of employability, a wife who loses her job, and a developmentally delayed 3-year-old son.
   2. a husband who finds employment 2 weeks after a layoff from his previous job, a wife who has stable employment, and a child doing well in school.
   3. a single mother with an executive position, a 10-year-old precocious daughter, and a widowed grandmother living in the household to provide child care for the 10-year-old child.
   4. a single gay male parent, an adolescent son who has just begun dating girls, and the father's unmarried sister who has come to visit for 2 weeks.

Answer: 1
Rationale: The family in option 1 has the greatest number of stressors. The other families described have fewer negative events occurring.
Cognitive level: Analysis
Nursing process: Assessment
NCLEX: Psychosocial Integrity
See text page: 512

34. The nurse in the emergency department explains to a client who is the victim of domestic violence that the client's psychosocial history, statements about the battering, a body map detailing injuries, and the photos taken will be placed in the medical record. The nurse also asks the client to return in 2 days for additional photos. The victim begs the nurse not to save the information for fear the perpetrator will find out. The information the nurse can give to the client that will be of greatest relevance in helping her accept the plan includes the facts that the medical record (more than one option may be correct)
   1. is not available to the perpetrator or his legal counsel.
   2. will be valuable to the client if she takes legal action later.

3. makes pertinent information available to other care providers.
   4. will provide evidence to law enforcement if another incident occurs.
   5. can be a resource to providers of treatment to the perpetrator or the victim.

Answers: 1, 2, 3
Rationale: Options 1, 2, and 3 are important facts for the client to know. The medical record is a powerful tool if legal action is initiated. Even if legal action is not taken at the time, the record is begun and the next provider will not have to stumble across the problem and will be in a better position to offer support. Options 4 and 5 are of lesser relevance.
Cognitive level: Application
Nursing process: Implementation
NCLEX: Safe and Effective Care Environment
See text pages: 517, 518

35. The nurse is assisting a victim of spousal abuse to create a plan for escape if it becomes necessary. Components of the plan should include (more than one option may be correct)
   1. determining a code word to signal children that it is time to leave.
   2. having the phone number for the nearest shelter.
   3. hiding money with which to buy new clothes.
   4. assembling birth certificates, Social Security cards, and licenses to take.
   5. bringing change with which to make phone calls.
   6. securing a supply of current medications.
   7. taking enough toys to amuse the children for 2 days.

Answers: 1, 2, 4, 5, 6
Rationale: All the options except 3 and 7 should be considered. Accumulating enough money to purchase clothing may be difficult. The woman should be advised to hide a small suitcase containing a change of clothing for herself and each child. Taking a large supply of toys would be cumbersome and might compromise the plan. Women are advised to take one favorite small toy or security object for each child.
Cognitive level: Application
Nursing process: Planning
NCLEX: Safe and Effective Care Environment
See text page: 521

36. Several children are seen in the emergency department for treatment of illnesses and injuries daily. The situation that would create a high index of suspicion of child abuse is a child
   1. who has repeated middle ear infections.
   2. who has severe colic.

Chapter 25   Family Violence

3. who has bite marks.

4. who has croup.

Answer: 3

Rationale: Injuries such as immersion or cigarette burns, facial fractures, whiplash, bite marks, traumatic injuries, bruises, and fractures in various stages of healing suggest the possibility of abuse. In older children, vague complaints such as back pain may also be suspicious. Ear infections, colic, and croup are not problems that have been induced by violence.

Cognitive level: Application
Nursing process: Assessment
NCLEX: Safe and Effective Care Environment
See text page: 514

37. The nurse at the clinic is interviewing a client who offers a number of vague somatic complaints that might not ordinarily prompt a visit to a caregiver, such as fatigue, back pain, headaches, and sleep disturbance. The client seems tense, and after having spoken of her symptoms seems reluctant to provide more information and is in a hurry to leave. The nurse can best serve the client by

1. asking if the client has ever had psychiatric counseling.

2. having the client fill out an abuse assessment screen.

3. exploring the possibility of client social isolation.

4. asking the client to disrobe so the nurse can look for signs of physical abuse.

Answer: 2

Rationale: In this situation the nurse should consider the possibility that the client is a victim of domestic violence. Although the client is reluctant to discuss issues, she may be willing to fill out an abuse assessment screen, which would then open the door to discussion. Option 1 is prejudicial. Option 3 is only one area for assessment and may be seen by the client as irrelevant and increase her reluctance to disclose. Option 4 will be threatening to the client and probably be met with refusal.

Cognitive level: Analysis
Nursing process: Assessment
NCLEX: Psychosocial Integrity
See text page: 517

CHAPTER 26

1. A single woman who works from 3 to 11 PM as an aide in a nursing home was grabbed from behind by a man who put a gun to her head as she walked home. The attacker warned her not to scream or he would

"blow [her] head off." He put tape over her mouth, tied her hands, forced her into his car, took her to an isolated spot, and raped her. When found, she was confused and disoriented. A rescue unit was called and she was taken to the hospital emergency department, where rape evidence was collected and she received treatment. During the emergency room stay the client sobbed incoherently for the first 30 minutes and intermittently thereafter. She appeared tense, restless, and agitated throughout the stay. The nurse correctly assessed the client's style of coping as

1. controlled.

2. expressed.

3. suicidal.

4. somatic.

Answer: 2

Rationale: The expressed style includes such overt behaviors as crying, smiling, laughing, joking, restlessness, agitation, hysteria, volatility, anger, confusion, incoherence, disorientation, and tenseness. Option 1: The controlled style involves confusion, incoherence, expressionless face, calm, subdued appearance, shock, numbness, and difficulty making decisions. Option 3: There is no suicidal rape-trauma coping style. Option 4: Somatic reactions involve physical symptoms such as headaches, sleep disturbances, and gastrointestinal symptoms.

Cognitive level: Application
Nursing process: Assessment
NCLEX: Psychosocial Integrity
See text page: 533

2. A woman who works from 3 to 11 PM was grabbed from behind by a man who put a gun to her head as she walked home. The attacker warned her not to scream or he would "blow [her] head off." He put tape over her mouth, tied her hands, forced her into his car, took her to an isolated spot, and raped her. When found, she was confused and disoriented. A rescue unit was called and she was taken to the hospital emergency department, where rape evidence was collected and she received treatment. The nurse correctly assessed the aspect of the client's crisis that produced the greatest amount psychological trauma as

1. the threat to her life.

2. the memory of the event.

3. the physical pain experienced.

4. the need for collecting evidence.

Answer: 1

Rationale: Psychological trauma associated with rape is produced by a number of factors. Of the options given, the threat to life is by far the most traumatic aspect of the crisis. The other options may, however, add significantly to the trauma.

Cognitive level: Application
Nursing process: Assessment
NCLEX: Safe and Effective Care Environment
See text page: 535

3. A woman was abducted and raped at gunpoint by an unknown assailant. When found she was confused and disoriented. The nurse makes the following observations about the client. She is talking rapidly in disjointed phrases, is unable to concentrate, and is indecisive when asked to make simple decisions. The client's level of anxiety can be assessed as
    1. severe.
    2. moderate.
    3. mild.
    4. nonexistent.

Answer: 1
Rationale: Acute anxiety results from the personal threat to the victim's safety and security. In this case, the client's symptoms of rapid, dissociated speech, inability to concentrate, and indecisiveness indicate severe anxiety. Options 2 and 3: Mild and moderate levels of anxiety would allow the client to function at a higher level.
Cognitive level: Analysis
Nursing process: Assessment
NCLEX: Physiological Integrity
See text page: 534

4. A client was abducted and raped at gunpoint by an unknown assailant. When found she was confused and disoriented. What behaviors would indicate that the client is in the acute phase of the rape-trauma syndrome?
    1. Confusion and disbelief
    2. Flashbacks and dreams
    3. Decreased motor activity
    4. Fears and phobias

Answer: 1
Rationale: Impact reactions of the acute phase of the rape-trauma syndrome include shock, emotional numbness, confusion, disbelief, restless, and agitated motor activity. Options 2 and 4: Flashbacks, dreams, fears, and phobias are seen in the long-term reorganization phase of the rape-trauma syndrome. Option 3: Decreased motor activity, by itself, is not indicative of any particular phase.
Cognitive level: Application
Nursing process: Assessment
NCLEX: Psychosocial Integrity
See text pages: 532, 533

5. A client was abducted and raped at gunpoint by an unknown assailant. When found she was confused and

disoriented. The client tells the nurse "I cannot talk about it! Nothing happened. I have to forget!" The client's present coping strategy can be assessed as
    1. use of a somatic reaction.
    2. use of denial.
    3. phobia development.
    4. desire for revenge.

Answer: 2
Rationale: The patient's statements reflect use of the ego defense mechanism denial. This mechanism may be unconsciously used to protect the person from the emotionally overwhelming reality of the rape. The client's statements do not reflect somatic symptoms, phobias, or desire for revenge.
Cognitive level: Application
Nursing process: Assessment
NCLEX: Psychosocial Integrity
See text page: 534

6. A client was abducted and raped at gunpoint by an unknown assailant. When found she was confused and disoriented. The intervention that would be appropriate for the nurse to implement while caring for the client in the emergency department is
    1. placing her in a private room and reassuring her that someone will be with her as soon as possible.
    2. putting an arm around her and reassuring her that a nurse will be there to help her at all times.
    3. posing questions in nonjudgmental, empathetic ways and allowing her to talk at a comfortable pace.
    4. allowing her family to be in the room and involving them in the history-taking process.

Answer: 3
Rationale: Neutral, nonjudgmental care and emotional support are critical to crisis management for the rape victim. Option 1: The rape victim should not be left alone. Option 2: The rape victim's anxiety may escalate when touched by a stranger, even when the stranger is a nurse. Option 3 is not universally appropriate. Some rape victims prefer not to have family involved.
Cognitive level: Application
Nursing process: Implementation
NCLEX: Psychosocial Integrity
See text pages: 534, 538, 541

7. An 11-year-old was abducted and raped by an unknown assailant. In the emergency department, the victim is confused and crying. The personal reaction experienced by the nurse that could interfere with the victim's care would be
    1. empathy.
    2. concern.

381

3. anger.

4. understanding.

Answer: 3

Rationale: Feelings of empathy, concern, and understanding are helpful. Anger, on the other hand, may make objectivity impossible.

Cognitive level: Application

Nursing process: Assessment

NCLEX: Safe and Effective Care Environment

See text page: 536

8. The assessment that should be given priority when the nurse interviews a rape victim in the emergency department is
   1. coping mechanisms the client is using.
   2. the client's previous sexual experience.
   3. adequacy of interpersonal relationships.
   4. whether the client has ever had a venereal disease.

Answer: 1

Rationale: Of the options listed, the priority assessment should be the victim's coping mechanisms. The other options have little relevance.

Cognitive level: Application

Nursing process: Assessment

NCLEX: Safe and Effective Care Environment

See text page: 534

9. A client who is a rape victim perplexedly asks the emergency department nurse "How can I determine if I was at fault for what happened to me?" The therapeutic intervention the nurse should use is to
   1. reassure that the outcome of the situation will be positive.
   2. support the client as she separates issues of vulnerability from blame.
   3. pose questions about the rape, using the adverb "why" whenever possible.
   4. make decisions for the client because she is perplexed and confused.

Answer: 2

Rationale: Although the victim may have made choices that made her vulnerable, she is not to blame for the rape. This thinking allows the victim to begin to restore a sense of control. This is a positive response to victimization. Option 1 does not permit the victim to begin to restore a sense of control. Option 3 suggests the use of a nontherapeutic communication technique. Option 4 does not permit the victim to restore control.

Cognitive level: Application

Nursing process: Implementation

NCLEX: Psychosocial Integrity

See text page: 538

10. When a rape victim tells the emergency department nurse "I should have never been out on the street alone," the most helpful response by the nurse would be
    1. "Your actions had nothing to do with what happened."
    2. "Blaming yourself only increases your anxiety and discomfort."
    3. "You believe this would not have happened if you had not been alone."
    4. "You are right. You should not have been alone on the street at night."

Answer: 3

Rationale: A reflective communication technique is more helpful than discounting the victim's role. Looking at one's role in the event serves to explain events that the victim would otherwise find incomprehensible.

Cognitive level: Application

Nursing process: Implementation

NCLEX: Psychosocial Integrity

See text page: 538

11. The nursing diagnosis of rape-trauma syndrome has been selected for a rape victim being cared for in the emergency department. What short-term outcome could be achieved by the time the client leaves the emergency department? The client will state that
    1. she feels safe and is entirely relaxed.
    2. the memory of the rape is less vivid and less frightening.
    3. her physical symptoms of pain and discomfort are no longer present.
    4. she will keep a follow-up appointment with the rape victim advocate.

Answer: 4

Rationale: Outcomes 1, 2, and 3 are unlikely to be met during the limited time the victim is in the emergency department. Agreeing to keep a follow-up appointment is a realistic short-term outcome.

Cognitive level: Application

Nursing process: Planning (Outcome Identification)

NCLEX: Psychosocial Integrity

See text page: 537

12. When the emergency department nurse helps a rape-trauma victim prepare for reactions that may be experienced during the long-term reorganization phase, which reaction can be omitted from the teaching?
    1. Flashbacks and dreams
    2. Decreased motor activity
    3. Development of fears and phobias
    4. Anxiety and mood swings

382

Answer: 2

Rationale: Victims of rape frequently have a period of increased motor activity rather than decreased motor activity during the long-term reorganization phase. The other reactions listed are common to the long-term reorganization phase.

Cognitive level: Application
Nursing process: Planning
NCLEX: Health Promotion and Maintenance
See text page: 533

13. A rape victim whose nursing diagnosis was rape-trauma syndrome received initial treatment in the emergency department and has visited a rape crisis counselor weekly for 8 weeks. The client report that would support nursing evaluation that the long-term process of reorganization has been successfully completed is
   1. absence of signs or symptoms of posttraumatic stress disorder.
   2. presence of mild somatic reaction.
   3. occasional episodic nightmares.
   4. moderate doubts about self-worth.

Answer: 1

Rationale: Rape-trauma syndrome is a variant of posttraumatic stress disorder. Reporting the absence of signs and symptoms of posttraumatic stress disorder suggests that the long-term reorganization phase has been successfully completed. The other options suggest that the process is ongoing.

Cognitive level: Analysis
Nursing process: Evaluation
NCLEX: Psychosocial Integrity
See text page: 539

14. A victim of rape visits the rape crisis counselor weekly. She reports to the counselor that her family is "not very supportive." The belief that contributes to a negative family response is
   1. rape is an act of aggression.
   2. no women ask to be raped.
   3. nice girls do not get raped.
   4. any woman is a potential rape victim.

Answer: 3

Rationale: The myth that nice girls do not get raped may contribute to the family's withdrawal and lack of support. Believing this myth allows the family to attribute blame to the victim. The other statements are facts, rather than myths, about rape and if understood by the family would prompt support.

Cognitive level: Application
Nursing process: Assessment
NCLEX: Psychosocial Integrity
See text page: 536

15. The nurse working a rape telephone hotline should focus the call so as to
   1. provide the caller with a sympathetic listener.
   2. provide the immediate steps the victim may take.
   3. arrange long-term client counseling.
   4. obtain information to relay to the local police.

Answer: 2

Rationale: The telephone counselor establishes where the victim is and what has happened and provides the necessary information to enable the victim to decide what steps to take immediately. Option 1 is incorrect because counselors are trained to be empathetic rather than sympathetic. Option 3 is inappropriate. Long-term aftercare is not the focus until immediate problems are resolved. Option 4: The victim remains anonymous.

Cognitive level: Application
Nursing process: Implementation
NCLEX: Psychosocial Integrity
See text page: 538

16. A rape victim tells the emergency room nurse "I feel so dirty. Please let me take a shower before the doctor examines me. I just cannot stand being so filthy." The nurse should
   1. arrange for the client to shower.
   2. give the client a basin of hot water and towels.
   3. explain that washing would destroy evidence.
   4. explain that bathing facilities are not available in the emergency department.

Answer: 3

Rationale: As uncomfortable as the client may be, she should not bathe until the physician's examination is completed. The collection of evidence is critical if she is to be successful in court. Options 1 and 2 will result in destruction of evidence. Option 4 is not true.

Cognitive level: Application
Nursing process: Implementation
NCLEX: Psychosocial Integrity
See text page: 537

17. Which of the following would be considered consensual sex rather than rape?
   1. S's husband forces vaginal sex when he comes home intoxicated from a party. S objects.
   2. J, aged 22 years, has a date with her boyfriend, aged 24 years, during which he pleads with her to have oral sex. She capitulates, then regrets the action.
   3. K is beaten, robbed, and forced to have anal intercourse by his assailant, who threatens to kill him if he shouts.
   4. N's dentist gives her intravenous anesthesia for a dental procedure, then has intercourse with her while she is unconscious.

Answer: 2

Rationale: Only option 2 describes a scenario in which the sexual contact is consensual. Consensual sex is not considered rape if the participants are at least the age of majority.

Cognitive level: Analysis
Nursing process: Assessment
NCLEX: Psychosocial Integrity
See text page: 530

18. The sexual assault nurse examiner at the hospital is an advanced practice nurse with prescription privileges. The activity that would be outside the scope of practice of this nurse is
   1. collecting and preserving evidence.
   2. obtaining signed consents for photographs and examinations.
   3. providing pregnancy and sexually transmitted disease prophylaxis if the client wishes.
   4. requiring HIV testing of a victim.

Answer: 4

Rationale: HIV testing is not mandatory for a victim of sexual assault. The other activities would be included within the advanced practice role.

Cognitive level: Application
Nursing process: Implementation
NCLEX: Physiological Integrity
See text page: 539

19. When a victim of sexual assault is discharged from the emergency department, the nurse should
   1. notify the client's family of the problem to seek client support.
   2. give referral information verbally and in writing.
   3. offer to stay with the client until she regains stability.
   4. advise the client to try not to think about the assault.

Answer: 2

Rationale: Immediately after the assault, rape victims are often disorganized and unable to think well or remember what they have been told. Written information acknowledges this fact and provides a solution. Option 1 violates the client's right to privacy. Option 3 is part of a rescue fantasy. Option 4 offers a platitude that is neither therapeutic nor effective.

Cognitive level: Application
Nursing process: Implementation
NCLEX: Psychosocial Integrity
See text pages: 537

20. A victim of a sexual assault occurring approximately 1 hour ago is sitting in the emergency department cubicle, rocking back and forth and repeat-ing over and over "I cannot believe he raped me." This behavior should be assessed as characteristic of
   1. the controlled impact reaction to rape-trauma syndrome.
   2. the angry stage of rape-trauma syndrome.
   3. the delayed reaction to rape-trauma syndrome.
   4. phobic reaction to rape-trauma syndrome.

Answer: 1

Rationale: The victim's response is controlled rather than uncontrolled. Her response is immediate and does not include a display of anger or the development of a phobia.

Cognitive level: Application
Nursing process: Implementation
NCLEX: Psychosocial Integrity
See text page: 533

21. An outcome for a client in the delayed reaction stage of rape-trauma syndrome is that the client will
   1. resume optimal level of functioning.
   2. identify situations that generate anxiety.
   3. develop feelings of being in control.
   4. make decisions about life activities.

Answer: 1

Rationale: Resuming optimal functioning is an achievable, comprehensive, long-term outcome; the other statements are short-term indicators.

Cognitive level: Application
Nursing process: Planning (Outcome Identification)
NCLEX: Psychosocial Integrity
See text page: 537

22. A rape victim has been diagnosed as having rape-trauma syndrome: silent reaction. The nurse who will be her counselor should carefully assess for the presence of (more than one option may be correct)
   1. the desire to repeatedly describe the rape.
   2. the onset of phobic behaviors.
   3. a reliance on alcohol or illegal drugs.
   4. increased anxiety during the interview.
   5. a pattern of sound sleep nightly.
   6. a changed relationship with sexual partner.

Answers: 2, 4, 6

Rationale: Option 2: Onset of phobias is common. Option 4: Increased anxiety during interviews is evidenced by blocking, long periods of silence, stuttering, or evidence of physical distress. Option 6: Abrupt changes in relationships with sexual partners is common. Option 1: The usual reaction is the inability to describe or discuss the rape. Option 3: Reliance on alcohol or illegal drugs is more often seen in rape-trauma syndrome: compound reaction. Option 5: Nightmares commonly disturb sleep.

384

Cognitive level: Application
Nursing process: Assessment
NCLEX: Psychosocial Integrity
See text page: 537

23. The outcome universally applicable to consider for rape victims is
    1. knowledge: personal safety.
    2. client satisfaction: safety.
    3. risk detection.
    4. grief resolution.

Answer: 4

Knowledge: Rape victims must work through grief caused by the various losses perceived as associated with rape, such as emotional, physical, and sexual well-being and self-esteem. Option 1: Personal safety focuses on prevention of unintentional injuries rather than victimization associated with rape. Option 2: Client satisfaction: safety focuses on the client's perception of procedures, information, and nursing care to prevent harm or injury. Option 3: Risk detection focuses on personal actions to identify personal health threats. These latter three outcomes have limited relevance for rape victims.

Cognitive level: Analysis
Nursing process: Planning (Outcome Identification)
NCLEX: Psychosocial Integrity
See text page: 537

24. A client in the long-term reorganization phase of the rape-trauma syndrome is experiencing intrusive thoughts of the rape and over the past week has developed a fear of being alone. Indicators for the outcome of fear self-control that should be monitored by the nurse include the client
    1. planning coping strategies for fearful situations.
    2. using increased activity to reduce fear.
    3. temporarily withdrawing from social situations.
    4. expressing willingness to be sexual.

Answer: 1

Rationale: This indicator shows willingness and ability to take personal action to reduce disabling fear. Options 2 and 3 are not desirable. Option 4 is an indicator related to the outcome of sexual functioning rather than fear self-control.

Cognitive level: Application
Nursing process: Evaluation
NCLEX: Psychosocial Integrity
See text page: 537

25. The nurse enters the emergency department cubicle of a rape victim and hears the client scream "What are you doing to me?" The nurse notes a technician standing with a comb who is about to begin comb-ing the client's pubic hair. The client right that has been violated is
    1. advocacy.
    2. confidentiality.
    3. informed consent.
    4. crisis intervention counseling.

Answer: 3

Rationale: The client has a right to have rape protocol explained and to give consent to proceed through the protocol. Options 1 and 2: Data are not conclusive that the rights to advocacy or confidentiality have been violated. Option 4: Crisis intervention counseling is not a specific right, although the client does have a right to be treated.

Cognitive level: Application
Nursing process: Implementation
NCLEX: Safe and Effective Care Environment
See text page: 537

26. A client who has come to the hospital for treatment of injuries sustained when he was raped abruptly decides to refuse treatment and return home. Before the client leaves, the nurse should
    1. provide written information about physical and emotional reactions that he may experience.
    2. tell him he cannot leave until given prophylactic sexually transmitted disease treatment.
    3. give verbal information about legal resources.
    4. mention the need for HIV testing.

Answer: 1

Rationale: All information given to a client before he or she leaves the emergency department should be in writing. Clients who are anxious are unable to concentrate and therefore cannot retain much of what is verbally imparted. Written information can be read and referred to at later times. Options 3 and 4 ignore the need for written information. Option 2 is inappropriate. Clients cannot be kept against their will or coerced into receiving medication as a condition of being allowed to leave. This constitutes false imprisonment.

Cognitive level: Application
Nursing process: Implementation
NCLEX: Safe and Effective Care Environment
See text page: 537

27. A teenager is brought to the emergency department by a girlfriend who accompanied her to a party. The friend found the client unconscious in a bedroom. Emergency department staff note semen on her underclothes. The priority actions of staff should be focused on
    1. preserving rape evidence.
    2. obtaining a description of the rape.

385

Chapter 26   Sexual Assault

3. determining what drug was ingested.
4. maintaining the client's airway.

Answer: 4

Rationale: Because the client is unconscious, the risk for airway obstruction is present. Options 2 and 3 are probably not possible to accomplish and take lower priority than preserving physiological integrity. Option 1 is also of lower priority than preserving physiological functioning.

Cognitive level: Analysis
Nursing process: Planning
NCLEX: Safe and Effective Care Environment
See text page: 532

28. A victim of a violent rape perpetrated by a stranger has been in the emergency department for 3 hours. The collection of evidence is completed and the sexual assault nurse examiner reenters the room to begin discharge counseling. The client says softly "I will never be the same again. I will never be able to face my friends. There is no sense of trying to go on." The most astute response by the nurse would be
1. "Are you thinking of committing suicide?"
2. "It will take time, but you will feel the same."
3. "Your friends will understand when you tell them."
4. "You will be able to find meaning in this experience as time goes on."

Answer: 1

Rationale: The client's words suggest hopelessness. Whenever hopelessness is present, so is suicide risk. The nurse should directly address the possibility of suicidal ideation with the client. The other options attempt to offer reassurance before making an assessment.

Cognitive level: Analysis
Nursing process: Intervention
NCLEX: Safe and Effective Care Environment
See text page: 535

CHAPTER 27

1. A client has been admitted for treatment of a compound fracture of the femur sustained when she fell while intoxicated. The nurse has cared for the client on previous admissions for similar problems. The nurse admits to feeling angry and frustrated at seeing the client in this condition. The action by the nurse that would be most beneficial for the client is to
1. ask to be reassigned because he cannot help the client.
2. cover his feelings by being particularly pleasant to the client.

3. ask how he can help the client find a better solution to her problems.
4. seek supervision to get help with negative feelings about the client.

Answer: 4

Rationale: The nurse who uses the approach of honestly acknowledging feelings is able to maintain congruence between nonverbal and verbal communication. This approach shows the nurse's concern for the client's well-being. Option 1, an avoidant approach by the nurse, would confirm for the client her lack of worth and the hopelessness of her situation. Option 2 is not an honest approach. The nurse's true feelings would probably be conveyed nonverbally. Option 3: This approach reveals the nurse's feelings of helplessness.

Cognitive level: Application
Nursing process: Implementation
NCLEX: Safe and Effective Care Environment
See text page: 559

2. The blood alcohol level of a client admitted last night with a compound fracture of the femur sustained in a fall while intoxicated was not assessed at the time of admission. The nurse should
1. request that the blood be drawn stat for this test.
2. do nothing because the time for the assessment has passed.
3. obtain a Breathalyzer from the emergency department to assess blood alcohol level.
4. ask the client about quantity and frequency of recent drinking and when she had her last drink.

Answer: 4

Rationale: These questions allow the nurse to gain vital information about the likelihood of withdrawal symptoms occurring and the general time of their onset. The blood alcohol level at the time of admission is useful for assessment purposes but is not a necessity. Options 1 and 3: Information relevant for planning can be obtained with option 4. Option 2 is not the best solution. Ascertaining if and when withdrawal symptoms may appear is important.

Cognitive level: Analysis
Nursing process: Assessment
NCLEX: Safe and Effective Care Environment
See text page: 554

3. If an intoxicated client admitted for trauma treatment last night at 2 AM is going to have withdrawal symptoms, nurses should be alert for the symptoms to begin
1. between 8 and 10 AM today (6 to 8 hours after drinking stopped).

2. about 2 AM tomorrow (24 hours after drinking stopped).
3. about 2 AM of hospital day 2 (48 hours after drinking stopped).
4. about 2 AM of hospital day 3 (72 hours after drinking stopped).

Answer: 1

Rationale: Alcohol withdrawal usually begins 6 to 8 hours after cessation or marked reduction of alcohol intake.

Cognitive level: Application
Nursing process: Assessment
NCLEX: Physiological Integrity
See text page: 554

4. The blood pressure and pulse rates for a client admitted last night with a compound fracture of the femur sustained in a fall while intoxicated, are recorded as follows:
admission 2 AM, 122/80 mm Hg and 72 beats/min
4 AM, 126/78 mm Hg and 76 beats/min
6 AM, 124/80 mm Hg and 72 beats/min
8 AM, 132/88 mm Hg and 80 beats/min
10 AM, 148/88 mm Hg and 96 beats/min
The priority action for the nurse to take is to
1. encourage the client to drink plenty of liquids.
2. obtain a clean-catch urine sample.
3. place the client in a vest-type restraint.
4. notify the physician.

Answer: 4

Rationale: Elevated pulse and blood pressure may indicate that the client is going into withdrawal delirium and that additional sedation is warranted. None of the other options takes into account the possible need for sedation. Options 2 and 3: No indication is present that the client may have a urinary tract infection or is presently in need of restraint. Option 1 is too nonspecific. Overhydration may bring on its own set of problems.

Cognitive level: Analysis
Nursing process: Implementation
NCLEX: Physiological Integrity
See text pages: 554, 555

5. A client admitted last night with a compound fracture of femur, sustained in a fall while intoxicated, points to the traction apparatus and screams that she sees a hangman's noose. The assessment that can be made is that the client is experiencing
1. an illusion.
2. a delusion.
3. hallucinations.
4. hypnagogic phenomenon.

Answer: 1

Rationale: The client is misinterpreting a sensory perception when she sees a noose instead of traction. Illusions are common in early withdrawal from alcohol. Option 2: A delusion is a fixed, false belief. Option 3: Hallucinations are sensory perceptions occurring in the absence of a stimulus. Option 4: Hypnagogic phenomena are sensory disturbances that occur between waking and sleeping.

Cognitive level: Application
Nursing process: Assessment
NCLEX: Physiological Integrity
See text pages: 554, 555

6. A client admitted for trauma sustained while intoxicated has been hospitalized for 48 hours. He is shaky, irritable, and anxious and tells of having vivid nightmares for 2 nights. An hour later, the nurse finds the client restless and perspiring. His pulse is 130 beats/min. He shouts "There are bugs crawling on my bed. I have got to get out of here," and begins to thrash about. The most accurate assessment of the situation would be the client
1. is attempting to obtain attention by manipulating staff.
2. may have sustained a head injury before admission.
3. is having a recurrence of an acute psychosis.
4. is demonstrating symptoms consistent with withdrawal delirium.

Answer: 4

Rationale: Symptoms of agitation, elevated pulse, and perceptual distortions point to alcohol withdrawal delirium, a medical emergency. Option 1: His behaviors are inconsistent with manipulative attempts. Options 2 and 3: The physical symptoms are inconsistent with both head injury and functional psychosis.

Cognitive level: Analysis
Nursing process: Assessment
NCLEX: Physiological Integrity
See text pages: 554, 555

7. A client admitted for treatment of trauma sustained in a fall while intoxicated believes bugs are crawling on the bed. The client is anxious, agitated, and diaphoretic. A nursing diagnosis of high priority that should be developed is
1. ineffective health maintenance.
2. ineffective coping.
3. ineffective denial.
4. risk for injury.

Answer: 4

Rationale: The client's clouded sensorium, sensory perceptual distortions, and poor judgment put him at

Chapter 27   Care of the Chemically Impaired

risk for injury. The scenario does not provide data to support the other diagnoses.
Cognitive level: Analysis
Nursing process: Diagnosis
NCLEX: Physiological Integrity
See text page: 561

8. A client admitted for treatment of trauma sustained in a fall while intoxicated believes bugs are crawling on the bed. The client is anxious, agitated, and diaphoretic. The nurse can anticipate that the physician will order a
   1. benzodiazepine such as diazepam (Valium) or chlordiazepoxide (Librium).
   2. phenothiazine such as chlorpromazine (Thorazine) or thioridazine (Mellaril).
   3. monoamine oxidase inhibitor such as phenelzine (Nardil).
   4. narcotic such as codeine.

Answer: 1
Rationale: Sedation allows for safe withdrawal from alcohol. Benzodiazepines are the drugs of choice in most regions because of their high therapeutic safety index and anticonvulsant properties.
Cognitive level: Application
Nursing process: Planning
NCLEX: Physiological Integrity
See text page: 568

9. A client admitted for treatment of trauma sustained in a fall while intoxicated believes bugs are crawling on the bed. The client is anxious, agitated, and diaphoretic. While the client is experiencing sensory perceptual disturbances and clouded sensorium, the nursing intervention that should be instituted is
   1. checking the client every 15 minutes.
   2. providing one-on-one supervision.
   3. keeping the room dimly lit.
   4. rigorously encouraging fluid intake.

Answer: 2
Rationale: One-on-one supervision will be necessary to promote physical safety until sedation reduces the client's feelings of terror. Option 1: Checks every 15 minutes would not be sufficient to provide for safety. Option 3: A dimly lit room promotes illusions. Option 4: Excessive fluid intake can cause overhydration because fluid retention normally occurs when blood alcohol levels fall.
Cognitive level: Application
Nursing process: Planning
NCLEX: Safe and Effective Care Environment
See text page: NA

10. A client admitted with trauma sustained while intoxicated has withdrawal delirium. The client's sensorium cleared after 5 days. A few days later, the client tells the nurse that drinking helps her cope with being a single parent and working mother. Which response by the nurse would help the client view her drinking more objectively?
    1. "Sooner or later your drinking will kill you. Then what will happen to your child?"
    2. "I hear a lot of defensiveness in your voice. Do you really believe this?"
    3. "If you were coping so well, what are you doing here again?"
    4. "Tell me what happened the last time you drank."

Answer: 4
Rationale: This response will help the client see alcohol as a cause of her problems, not a solution. This approach can help the client become receptive to the possibility of change. The other responses directly confront and attack defenses against anxiety that the client still needs. They reflect the nurse's frustration with the client.
Cognitive level: Application
Nursing process: Implementation
NCLEX: Psychosocial Integrity
See text pages: 562, 563

11. A client asks the nurse "What is Alcoholics Anonymous all about?" The best response for the nurse would be
    1. "It is a group that learns about drinking from a group leader."
    2. "It is a form of group therapy led by a psychiatrist."
    3. "It is a self-help group for which the norm is sobriety."
    4. "It is a group that advocates strong punishment for drunk drivers."

Answer: 3
Rationale: Alcoholics Anonymous (AA) is a peer support group for recovering alcoholics. Neither professional nor peer leaders are appointed. Option 4 describes organizations such as Mothers Against Drunk Driving.
Cognitive level: Application
Nursing process: Implementation
NCLEX: Psychosocial Integrity
See text page: 566

12. The police bring a client to the emergency department to be examined after an automobile accident. He is ataxic, has slurred speech, and seems mildly confused. His blood alcohol level is 400 mg/dL (0.40 mg%). From the relation between his behavior

388

and his blood alcohol level, the nurse can make the assessment that the client
1. rarely drinks alcohol.
2. has a high tolerance to alcohol.
3. has been treated with disulfiram (Antabuse).
4. has ingested both alcohol and sedative drugs recently.

Answer: 2

Rationale: A nontolerant drinker would be in coma with a blood alcohol level of 400 mg/dL (0.40 mg%). The fact that the client is walking and talking shows a discrepancy between blood alcohol level and expected behavior and strongly suggests that the client's body has become tolerant to the drug. Option 3: If disulfiram and alcohol are ingested together, an entirely different clinical picture would result. Option 4: The blood alcohol level gives no information about ingestion of other drugs.
Cognitive level: Analysis
Nursing process: Assessment
NCLEX: Physiological Integrity
See text page: 554

13. A client who admits himself to an alcoholism rehabilitation program tells the nurse that he is a social drinker, usually having a drink or two at brunch and a few cocktails during the afternoon, wine at dinner, and several drinks throughout the evening. The client can be assessed as demonstrating
1. projection.
2. rationalization.
3. denial.
4. introjection.

Answer: 3

Rationale: Minimizing one's drinking is a form of denial of alcoholism. By his own description, he is more than a social drinker. Option 1: Projection involves blaming another for one's faults or problems. Option 2: Rationalization involves making excuses. Option 4: Introjection involves taking a quality into one's self system.
Cognitive level: Application
Nursing process: Assessment
NCLEX: Psychosocial Integrity
See text pages: 552, 553

14. A client who admits himself to an alcoholism rehabilitation program tells the nurse that he is a social drinker, usually having a drink or two at brunch and a few cocktails during the afternoon, wine at dinner, and several drinks throughout the evening. A response designed to help the client view his drinking more honestly would be

1. "I see," and use interested silence.
2. "I think you may be drinking even more than you report."
3. "To me, being a social drinker involves having a drink or two once or twice a week."
4. "You describe drinking rather steadily throughout the day and evening. Am I correct?"

Answer: 4

Rationale: Option 4 summarizes and validates what the client reported, but is acceptant rather than strongly confrontational, as are options 2 and 3. Defenses cannot be removed until healthier coping strategies are in place. Strong confrontation does not usually take place so early in the program. Option 1 would not assist the client to begin to explore the problem.
Cognitive level: Application
Nursing process: Implementation
NCLEX: Psychosocial Integrity
See text pages: 562, 563

15. A client admits himself to an alcoholism rehabilitation program. During the third week of treatment, his wife tells the nurse that once her husband is discharged from the alcoholism rehabilitation program, she is sure everything will be "just fine." Which remark by the nurse will be most helpful to the client's wife?
1. "It is good that you are supportive of your husband's sobriety and want to help him maintain it."
2. "While your husband's sobriety solves some problems, new ones may come to light as he adjusts to living without alcohol."
3. "It will be important for you to structure his life to avoid as much stress as you can. You will need to protect him."
4. "Remember, your husband is basically a self-destructive person. You will need to observe his behavior carefully."

Answer: 2

Rationale: During recovery, clients identify and use alternative coping mechanisms to reduce reliance on alcohol. Physical adaptations must occur. Emotional responses, formerly dulled by alcohol, are now fully experienced and may cause considerable anxiety. These changes inevitably have an effect on the spouse and children, who should be given anticipatory guidance. Option 1 does not provide anticipatory guidance. Option 3 provides inaccurate information. Option 4 provides inappropriate instruction.
Cognitive level: Application
Nursing process: Implementation
NCLEX: Health Promotion and Maintenance
See text page: 564

16. A client undergoing alcohol rehabilitation decides he will take disulfiram to help him avoid impulsively responding to drinking cues. Discharge teaching for the client should include the need to (more than one answer may be correct)
  1. read labels of all liquid medications.
  2. avoid aged cheeses.
  3. avoid alcohol-based skin products.
  4. wear sunscreen and avoid bright sunlight.
  5. maintain and adequate dietary intake of sodium.
  6. refrain from eating foods prepared with alcohol.
  7. avoid breathing fumes of paints, stains, and stripping compounds.

Answers: 1, 3 ,6, 7
Rationale: The client must avoid hidden sources of alcohol. Many liquid medications, such as cough syrups, contain small amounts of alcohol that could trigger an alcohol-disulfiram reaction. Using alcohol-based skin products such as aftershave or cologne; smelling alcohol-laden fumes; and eating foods prepared with wine, brandy, beer, or spirits of any sort may also trigger reactions. The other options do not relate to hidden sources of alcohol.
Cognitive level: Application
Nursing process: Planning
NCLEX: Physiological Integrity
See text page: 569

17. The wife of a client attending an alcoholism rehabilitation program goes to an Al-Anon meeting. The fundamental Al-Anon teaching that will help the client's wife cope with her husband's drinking is
  1. the drinker's abstinence must be supervised.
  2. the client is responsible for his or her own drinking.
  3. maintenance of sobriety cannot be expected.
  4. significant others need her to meet client dependency needs.

Answer: 2
Rationale: Al-Anon teaches family members that they did not cause the disease, that they cannot control it, and they cannot cure it. They advocate making the alcoholic responsible for his or her own behavior. None of the other options is a basic teaching in Al-Anon.
Cognitive level: Application
Nursing process: Implementation
NCLEX: Psychosocial Integrity
See text page: 566

18. The most therapeutic approach for the nurse to take when working with a client entering treatment for alcohol abuse is

  1. strongly confrontive.
  2. empathetic, supportive.
  3. cool and somewhat distant.
  4. skeptical and wary.

Answer: 2
Rationale: Support and empathy assist the client to feel safe enough to start looking at problems. Counseling during the early stage of treatment needs to be direct, open, and honest. The other approaches will increase client anxiety and cause the client to cling to defenses.
Cognitive level: Application
Nursing process: Implementation
NCLEX: Psychosocial Integrity
See text pages: 562, 563

19. A client comes to her outpatient therapy appointment obviously intoxicated. Her husband tells the nurse "There was nothing I could do to stop her when she started drinking this morning." The nurse should
  1. talk with him about strategies to limit his wife's drinking.
  2. have the client admitted to the inpatient psychiatric unit.
  3. arrange for emergency admission to a detoxification unit.
  4. tell the client that therapy cannot take place while she is intoxicated.

Answer: 4
Rationale: One cannot conduct meaningful therapy with an intoxicated client. The client should be taken home to recover, then make another appointment.
Cognitive level: Application
Nursing process: Implementation
NCLEX: Physiological Integrity
See text page: 564

20. A client who came to her previous outpatient therapy appointment obviously intoxicated tells the nurse "I could not help what happened last week. I am an alcoholic and cannot control my drinking." The client is using
  1. denial.
  2. projection.
  3. rationalization.
  4. selective attention.

Answer: 3
Rationale: The client is making excuses for her behavior, saying she is not responsible because she is an alcoholic. Option 1: Denial would call for her to say she has no problem. Option 2: Projection would have

her using blaming behavior. Option 4: Selective attention would involve only attending to what can be coped with to minimize anxiety.

Cognitive level: Application
Nursing process: Assessment
NCLEX: Psychosocial Integrity
See text pages: 552, 553

21. An individual uses alcohol to relieve tension. When he first began self-medicating with alcohol, two drinks made him relaxed and drowsy. Now, after 1 year, he needs four drinks to bring himself to the same relaxed, drowsy state. The reason for this is
   1. the alcohol is less potent.
   2. he is developing tolerance.
   3. hypomagnesemia.
   4. antagonistic effects.

Answer: 2
Rationale: Tolerance refers to needing higher and higher doses of a drug to produce the desired effect. Option 1: The potency of the alcohol is stable. Options 3 and 4: Neither hypomagnesemia nor antagonistic effects would account for this change.

Cognitive level: Application
Nursing process: Assessment
NCLEX: Physiological Integrity
See text page: 549

22. A client's blood alcohol level is 100 mg/dL (0.10 mg%). He is clumsy and slightly off balance as he performs the roadside sobriety tests. A second client's blood alcohol level is 300 mg/dL (0.30 mg%). He is clumsy and slightly off balance as he performs the roadside sobriety tests, but not appreciably more affected than the other client. How can this be accounted for?
   1. The second client is an alcohol-tolerant person.
   2. The first client is an alcohol-tolerant person.
   3. The second client takes disulfiram.
   4. The first client takes naltrexone.

Answer: 1
Rationale: An individual who has developed a tolerance for a drug will show fewer signs of intoxication than a nontolerant person who has used the same amount of the drug. Options 3 and 4: Neither disulfiram nor naltrexone use would account for the similarity in behaviors.

Cognitive level: Application
Nursing process: Assessment
NCLEX: Physiological Integrity
See text page: 554

23. A student who is assigned to observe in the chemical dependency center asks "What is the difference between drug abuse and drug dependence?" The nurse replies "Abuse implies maladaptive, consistent use of the drug despite having problems related to the drug." Which statement should be used to describe dependency?
   1. Dependence involves the lack of control of drug use, tolerance, and withdrawal symptoms when intake is reduced or stopped.
   2. Dependence occurs when psychoactive drug use interferes with the work of neurotransmitters.
   3. Dependence refers to symptoms that occur when two or more drugs affecting the central nervous system (CNS) are used for their additive effects.
   4. Dependence refers to taking a combination of drugs to weaken or inhibit the effect of another drug.

Answer: 1
Rationale: According to the *DSM-IV-TR,* option 1 defines psychoactive substance dependence. Option 2 does not explain dependence. Option 3 describes synergistic effect, and option 4 describes antagonistic effect.

Cognitive level: Application
Nursing process: Implementation
NCLEX: Safe and Effective Care Environment
See text page: 550

24. An unconscious client is brought to the emergency department, accompanied by a friend who is in an obviously intoxicated state. The friend is unable to give any information regarding what caused the client to lapse into unconsciousness. The nurse can anticipate that the physician will order a toxicological screening. This will require the nurse to
   1. assist with passing a nasogastric tube to collect a sample of gastric contents.
   2. obtain urine and blood samples in the presence of a witness.
   3. conduct a complete neurological and psychological assessment.
   4. prepare and administer a dose of naloxone and observe the client for 2 hours after administration.

Answer: 2
Rationale: Toxicological screening usually requires 100 mL of urine and 20 mL of blood. The specimens are obtained and labeled with a witness at hand to ensure correct identification and handling of the specimen in the event the results become legal evidence. The drug screening provides vital information needed for emergency treatment and possibly for long-term care planning. Option 1: Gastric contents are not tested. Option 3: Neurological and psychological assess-

Chapter 27   Care of the Chemically Impaired

ment will be performed but are not specifically part of a toxicological screening. Option 4: Naloxone would be administered as an opiate antagonist, not as a routine part of a toxicological screen.

Cognitive level: Application
Nursing process: Planning
NCLEX: Safe and Effective Care Environment
See text page: NA

25. In the emergency department, a client's blood pressure is 66/40 mm Hg, pulse is 140 beats/min, and respirations are 8 breaths/min and shallow. He receives naloxone (Narcan). The nursing diagnosis established is ineffective breathing pattern: depression of respiratory center secondary to narcotic overdose. The outcome indicator for which the nurse will evaluate is that the client will
    1. be stable within 8 hours, as evidenced by vital signs within normal values.
    2. be able to describe a plan for home care before release from the emergency department.
    3. demonstrate effective coping skills within 1 week of admission.
    4. identify two community resources for treatment of substance abuse by discharge.

Answer: 1
Rationale: This short-term outcome is the only one relating to the client's physical condition. It is expected that vital signs will return to normal when the CNS depression is alleviated.
Cognitive level: Application
Nursing process: Evaluation
NCLEX: Physiological Integrity
See text pages: 560, 561

26. The nursing intervention necessary after the administration of naloxone is to
    1. monitor the airway and take vital signs every 15 minutes.
    2. insert an indwelling urinary catheter.
    3. insert a nasogastric tube.
    4. treat hyperpyrexia with cooling measures.

Answer: 1
Rationale: Narcotic antagonists such as naloxone quickly reverse CNS depression, but because the narcotics have a longer span of action than antagonists, the client may lapse into unconsciousness or require respiratory support again. Options 2, 3, 4 are measures unrelated to naloxone use.
Cognitive level: Application
Nursing process: Planning
NCLEX: Physiological Integrity
See text pages: 549, 551

27. A nurse worked at Community Hospital for several months, then resigned and took a position at General Hospital. At General he was seen as a "super nurse" and given increasing responsibility. He often volunteered or arranged with others to be assigned as medication nurse. After a year, he began to call in sick frequently and was noticed to be more irritable and unsociable. Then he made several serious medication errors in rapid succession. As these were investigated, it was learned that he had been allowed to resign from Community Hospital when he was found diverting client narcotics for his own use. One evening shortly after the investigation began, the nurse was found unconscious in the locker room. The nurse manager retrospectively identified an early indicator of the nurse's drug use as
    1. assuming responsibility for errors.
    2. high sociability with peers during the shift.
    3. seeking to be in possession of the narcotic keys.
    4. presenting a neat physical appearance.

Answer: 3
Rationale: The nurse who is intent on diverting drugs for personal use or who uses drugs while on duty usually attempts to isolate himself or herself from peers and may manipulate others to gain access to the keys to the narcotics. Appearance often deteriorates and errors are blamed on others.
Cognitive level: Application
Nursing process: Assessment
NCLEX: Psychosocial Integrity
See text pages: 559, 560

28. A nurse with a history of narcotic abuse was found unconscious in the hospital locker room after overdosing. The nurse is transferred from the emergency department to the inpatient psychiatric unit. Attitudes or behaviors on the part of nursing staff that may be assessed as enabling behaviors include
    1. conveying understanding that pressures experienced in nursing underlie substance use.
    2. pointing out that work problems are the result, not the cause, of substance abuse.
    3. empathizing when the nurse discusses fear of disciplinary action by the state board.
    4. providing health teaching about stress management.

Answer: 1
Rationale: Enabling denies the seriousness of the client's problem or supports the client as he or she shifts responsibility from self to circumstances. The other options are therapeutic and appropriate.
Cognitive level: Analysis
Nursing process: Assessment
NCLEX: Safe and Effective Care Environment
See text page: 551

29. The treatment most appropriate for a client with antisocial tendencies who has been treated several times for substance addiction and has relapsed is
1. a 12-step self-help program.
2. a 1-week detoxification program.
3. long-term outpatient therapy.
4. a residential program.

Answer: 4

Rationale: Residential programs and therapeutic communities have as goals complete change in lifestyle, abstinence from drugs, elimination of criminal behaviors, development of employable skills, self-reliance, and honesty. Residential programs have been found to be more effective for clients with antisocial tendencies than outpatient programs.

Cognitive level: Application
Nursing process: Planning
NCLEX: Safe and Effective Care Environment
See text page: 566

30. A nursing diagnosis commonly applied to both paranoid schizophrenic clients and clients with amphetamine-induced psychosis is
1. disturbed thought processes.
2. powerlessness.
3. ineffective thermoregulation.
4. deficient knowledge.

Answer: 1

Rationale: Paranoid delusions are commonly experienced by both types of clients; thus the nursing diagnosis of disturbed thought processes is appropriate for both. The other options are not specifically applicable to both.

Cognitive level: Analysis
Nursing process: Diagnosis
NCLEX: Psychosocial Integrity
See text page: 560

31. An important nursing intervention when giving care to a client withdrawing from a CNS stimulant is to
1. make physical contact by frequently touching the client.
2. offer intellectual activities requiring concentration.
3. observe for depression and suicidal ideation.
4. avoid manipulation by denying all client requests.

Answer: 3

Rationale: Rebound depression occurs with withdrawal from CNS stimulants, probably related to neurotransmitter depletion. Option 1: Touch may be misinterpreted if the client is experiencing paranoid tendencies. Option 2: Concentration is impaired during

withdrawal. Option 4: Denying all requests is inappropriate; maintaining established limits will suffice.

Cognitive level: Application
Nursing process: Planning
NCLEX: Safe and Effective Care Environment
See text pages: 552, 553

32. The head nurse tells a new staff nurse "We anticipate this client will have symptoms of withdrawal from sedative-hypnotics. Watch her closely." For which symptoms should the staff nurse assess the client?
1. Dilated pupils, tachycardia, elevated blood pressure, elation
2. Mood lability, incoordination, fever, drowsiness
3. Nausea, vomiting, diaphoresis, anxiety, tremors
4. Excessive eating, constipation, headache

Answer: 3

Rationale: The symptoms of withdrawal from sedative-hypnotic or anxiolytic drugs are similar to those of alcohol withdrawal. Grand mal seizures are possible. Option 1 might be seen in CNS stimulant use. Options 2 and 4 are merely collections of symptoms with no relation to sedative-hypnotic withdrawal.

Cognitive level: Application
Nursing process: Assessment
NCLEX: Safe and Effective Care Environment
See text page: 553

33. A client has smoked two packs of cigarettes daily for many years. When she does not smoke or tries to "cut back," she becomes anxious, craves a cigarette, cannot concentrate, and gets a headache. This scenario would be assessed as
1. substance abuse.
2. substance intoxication.
3. substance dependence.
4. recreational use of a social drug.

Answer: 3

Rationale: Nicotine meets the criteria for "substance," the criterion for dependence (tolerance) is present, and withdrawal symptoms are noted with abstinence or reduction of dose. The scenario does not meet criteria for substance abuse, intoxication, or recreational use of a social drug.

Cognitive level: Application
Nursing process: Assessment
NCLEX: Physiological Integrity
See text page: 550

34. Symptoms the nurse should expect to confirm for an individual who has just "shot up" with heroin are
1. anxiety, restlessness, and paranoid delusions.
2. muscle aching, dilated pupils, and tachycardia.

Chapter 27   Care of the Chemically Impaired

3. heightened sexuality, insomnia, and euphoria.
4. drowsiness, constricted pupils, and slurred speech.

Answer: 4

Rationale: Heroin, an opiate, is a CNS depressant. Blood pressure, pulse, and respirations will be decreased and attention will be impaired. Option 1 describes behaviors consistent with amphetamine use. Option 2 describes symptoms of narcotic withdrawal. Option 3 describes cocaine use.

Cognitive level: Application
Nursing process: Assessment
NCLEX: Psychosocial Integrity
See text page: 556

35. A client newly admitted to the medical unit has needle tracks on both arms. A friend has stated that the client uses heroin. The nurse should assess the client for
    1. slurred speech, excessive drowsiness, and bradycardia.
    2. runny nose, yawning, insomnia, and chills.
    3. anxiety, agitation, and aggression.
    4. paranoid delusions, tactile hallucinations, and panic.

Answer: 2

Rationale: Early signs and symptoms of narcotic withdrawal resemble symptoms of onset of a flulike illness, minus the temperature elevation. Option 1 reflects signs of intoxication or CNS depressant overdose. Option 3 might be noted with CNS stimulant or hallucinogen use. Option 4 is consistent with CNS stimulant (amphetamine, cocaine) use.

Cognitive level: Application
Nursing process: Assessment
NCLEX: Physiological Integrity
See text page: 556

36. A nurse is called to the home of a neighbor and finds an unconscious woman still holding a medication bottle labeled pentobarbital sodium. The nurse's first action should be to
    1. test reflexes.
    2. check pupils.
    3. initiate vomiting.
    4. establish a patent airway.

Answer: 4

Rationale: Maintaining a patent airway is the priority when the client is unconscious. Options 1 and 2: Assessing neurological function can wait. Option 3: Vomiting should not be induced when a client is unconscious because of the danger of aspiration.

Cognitive level: Analysis
Nursing process: Implementation

NCLEX: Safe and Effective Care Environment
See text page: 553

37. A 24-year-old woman comes to the emergency department, stating "I feel restless. Everything I look at wavers. Sometimes I am outside my body looking at myself. I can hear colors. I think I am losing my mind." Vital signs are slightly elevated. The nurse should suspect
    1. a schizophrenic episode.
    2. cocaine overdose.
    3. PCP intoxication.
    4. LSD ingestion.

Answer: 4

Rationale: The client who is high on lysergic acid diethylamide (LSD) often experiences synesthesia (visions in sound), depersonalization, and concerns about going "crazy." Option 1: Synesthesia is not common in schizophrenia. Option 2: CNS stimulant overdose more commonly involves elevated vital signs and assaultive, grandiose behaviors. Option 3: Phencyclidine (PCP) use commonly causes bizarre or violent behavior, nystagmus, elevated vital signs, and repetitive jerking movements.

Cognitive level: Application
Nursing process: Assessment
NCLEX: Psychosocial Integrity
See text page: 557

38. In what significant way should the therapeutic environment differ for a client who has ingested LSD from that of a client who has ingested PCP?
    1. For LSD ingestion, have one person stay with the client and provide verbal support. For PCP ingestion, maintain a regimen of limited contact with one staff member accompanied by two or more staff.
    2. For PCP ingestion, place client on one-on-one intensive supervision. For LSD ingestion, maintain a regimen of limited interaction and minimal verbal stimulation.
    3. For LSD ingestion, provide continual midlevel stimulation involving as many senses as possible. For PCP ingestion, provide continual high-level stimulation.
    4. For LSD ingestion, place the client in restraints. For PCP ingestion, place the client on seizure precautions.

Answer: 1

Rationale: Clients who have ingested LSD respond well to being "talked down" by a supportive person. Clients who have ingested PCP are very stimulation sensitive and display frequent, unpredictable, violent behavior. While one person should perform care

and talk gently to the client, no one should be alone in the room with the client. Take adequate staff to manage violent behavior if it occurs.
Cognitive level: Analysis
Nursing process: Planning
NCLEX: Safe and Effective Care Environment
See text page: 557

39. A 16-year-old client was brought to the 24-hour drug clinic after taking her first dose of LSD and having a bad trip. The drug effects wore off after 8 hours. What health teaching should be performed before the client's release from the drug clinic?
    1. Provide a list of untoward effects of narcotic use.
    2. Explain the dangers of cocaine use.
    3. Discuss the carcinogenic effects of marijuana on the lungs.
    4. Describe flashbacks and what to do if one occurs.

Answer: 4
Rationale: Flashbacks are a common effect of hallucinogenic drugs. They can be terrifying to experience. Information about their possible occurrence can be helpful. The other options deal with information about drugs other than LSD.
Cognitive level: Application
Nursing process: Planning
NCLEX: Health Promotion and Maintenance
See text page: 557

40. A client is seen in the 24-hour drug clinic. She's thin, tense, jittery, and has dilated pupils and bad breath. She tells the nurse "I have been speeding, and now I am burning up and need help." She permits an oral temperature to be taken (it is 104° F), but then becomes suspicious and moves away from staff, refusing to allow further examination. She states, "You could be trying to kill me." The assessment that can be made is the client is most likely under the influence of
    1. PCP.
    2. heroin.
    3. barbiturates.
    4. amphetamines.

Answer: 4
Rationale: The physical symptoms are consistent with CNS stimulation. Suspicion and paranoid ideation are also present. Amphetamine use should be suspected. Option 1: PCP use would probably result in bizarre, violent behavior. Options 2 and 3 would result in symptoms of CNS depression.
Cognitive level: Application
Nursing process: Assessment
NCLEX: Psychosocial Integrity
See text page: 555

41. Which nursing diagnosis would be appropriate for most clients who are chemically impaired?
    1. Constipation
    2. Hyperthermia
    3. Risk for injury
    4. Disturbed personal identity

Answer: 3
Rationale: Substance abuse, regardless of the drug used, offers a variety of ways an individual might sustain injury: falls, skin infection, aspiration, etc. The defining characteristics for the other nursing diagnoses are not universally present among substance abusers.
Cognitive level: Application
Nursing process: Diagnosis
NCLEX: Physiological Integrity
See text pages: 554, 555

42. For care planning purposes the nurse should understand that the drug that normally produces the least complicated withdrawal syndrome is
    1. cocaine.
    2. heroin.
    3. amphetamine.
    4. diazepam.

Answer: 2
Rationale: The withdrawal syndrome for narcotics produces flulike symptoms, including severe aching, but has fewer profound effects on the cardiovascular, respiratory, and nervous systems than the other options.
Cognitive level: Analysis
Nursing process: Planning
NCLEX: Physiological Integrity
See text pages: 554, 555

43. A short-term outcome that can be identified for a client completing his fourth alcohol detoxification program in 1 year is: that the client will
    1. use denial and rationalization in a healthier way.
    2. identify constructive outlets for anger.
    3. state that he sees the need for ongoing treatment.
    4. develop a dependent relationship with one staff member.

Answer: 3
Rationale: Option 3 refers to the need for ongoing treatment after detoxification and is a reasonable goal related to controlling recidivism. Options 1 and 4 are undesirable. Option 2: The scenario does not give enough information to allow the learner to know whether anger has been identified as a problem.
Cognitive level: Analysis
Nursing process: Planning (Outcome Identification)
NCLEX: Psychosocial Integrity
See text pages: 560, 561

Chapter 27   Care of the Chemically Impaired

44. The question of highest priority a nurse should ask a newly admitted client with a history of alcohol abuse is
1. "Has drinking caused you any problems?"
2. "Have you ever had blackouts?"
3. "When did you take your last drink?"
4. "When did you decide to seek treatment?"

Answer: 3
Rationale: Learning when the client had the last drink is essential to knowing when to begin to observe for symptoms of withdrawal. The other questions are relevant but of lower priority.
Cognitive level: Analysis
Nursing process: Assessment
NCLEX: Physiological Integrity
See text page: 554

45. A client in an alcohol rehabilitation program tells the nurse "I have been such a loser all my life! I feel so ashamed of what I put my family through! Now, here I am in a program and I am not even sure I can succeed at staying sober." The nurse should consider the nursing diagnosis of
1. chronic low self-esteem.
2. powerlessness.
3. ineffective health maintenance.
4. risk for violence.

Answer: 1
Rationale: Low self-esteem is present when a client sees the self as inadequate. Data are not present to support the other options.
Cognitive level: Analysis
Nursing process: Diagnosis
NCLEX: Psychosocial Integrity
See text page: 560

46. A client brought to the emergency department after an automobile accident tells the nurse that she attended a cocktail party and consumed four drinks over the last hour. Her blood alcohol level is 150 mg/dL (0.15 mg%) and she describes herself as "tipsy." What conclusion can the nurse draw?
1. The client is intoxicated.
2. The client has a problem of alcohol dependence.
3. The client's blood alcohol is in the dangerous-to-life range.
4. Insufficient data are present to draw any conclusion.

Answer: 1
Rationale: The client's blood alcohol level indicates she is intoxicated. Because her behavior and the blood alcohol level correspond, one can assume the client does not have a high tolerance to alcohol. Option 2 is not a conclusion that can be drawn. Option 3 is

not a true statement. The blood alcohol level for coma and death is 0.40 to 0.50 mg%. Option 4 is incorrect. A conclusion can be drawn.
Cognitive level: Analysis
Nursing process: Assessment
NCLEX: Physiological Integrity
See text page: 554

47. What behaviors would indicate that the treatment plan for a client in alcohol rehabilitation can be evaluated as effective?
1. Abstinent 10 days; states she can maintain sobriety for 1 day at a time; has spoken with employer, who is willing to have her start work in 3 weeks.
2. Abstinent 15 days; states she has her problems licked; plans to seek a new job where she will not have to face peers who know her history.
3. Attends AA daily; states many of the members are real alcoholics; thinks she may be able to help some of them find jobs in her company.
4. Abstinent 21 days; states in future she will never drink during the day or on the job; plans to stop by the bar after work occasionally to show her friends her newly found health.

Answer: 1
Rationale: Option 1 reflects the AA beliefs. Options 2, 3, and 4 each contain a statement that suggests early relapse.
Cognitive level: Evaluation
Nursing process: Evaluation
NCLEX: Psychosocial Integrity
See text pages: 564, 565

48. A client admitted for a heroin overdose received naloxone, which relieved his altered breathing pattern. Two hours later he reported muscle aching and abdominal cramps. He sniffs and points to the gooseflesh on his arms. He says he feels "terrible." Which assessment can be made?
1. An idiosyncratic reaction to naloxone is occurring.
2. The client should be monitored closely for seizures.
3. The client is experiencing a relapse.
4. Symptoms of narcotic abstinence are present.

Answer: 4
Rationale: The symptoms given in the question are consistent with narcotic withdrawal. Early symptoms of narcotic withdrawal are flulike in nature. Option 1: This is an expected reaction. Naloxone has caused withdrawal symptoms to appear. Option 2: Seizures are more commonly seen in alcohol withdrawal syndrome. Option 3: The client is experiencing withdrawal symptoms.

396

Cognitive level: Analysis
Nursing process: Assessment
NCLEX: Physiological Integrity
See text page: 556

49. The wife of a heroin addict asks the nurse "What is methadone maintenance all about?" The nurse's explanation should be based on the information that methadone
   1. replaces a more potent drug.
   2. is safe even in large doses.
   3. is a deterrent to use of both hard and soft drugs.
   4. blocks the craving for and the action of opiates.

Answer: 4
Rationale: The only true statement is that methadone administration, in sufficient dosage, blocks the craving for and action of opiates.
Cognitive level: Application
Nursing process: Implementation
NCLEX: Health Promotion and Maintenance
See text page: 569

50. A client is admitted in a comatose state after ingestion of 30 capsules of pentobarbital sodium. As she responds to emergency care, her husband tells staff that she often takes more of the drug than is ordered and frequently drinks alcohol concurrently. The nurse assesses that the use of alcohol with this drug
   1. diminishes the effect.
   2. stimulates metabolism of the drug.
   3. causes no effect.
   4. has a synergistic effect.

Answer: 4
Rationale: Both pentobarbital and alcohol are CNS depressants and have synergistic effects. Taken together, the action of each would potentiates the other. Option 1: The effects are enhanced. Option 2 is untrue. Option 3: The effect is synergistic.
Cognitive level: Application
Nursing process: Assessment
NCLEX: Safe and Effective Care Environment
See text page: 549

51. A client is admitted in a comatose state after ingesting a lethal dose of diazepam. The intern tells the nurse "Give him 30 mL of ipecac stat, then help me start this IV." The nurse should
   1. do as ordered.
   2. ask if the IV should be the first priority.
   3. question the dose of ipecac to be given.
   4. refuse to give the ipecac.

Answer: 4

Rationale: A comatose client should receive nothing by mouth because of the lack of ability to swallow and an absent gag reflex.
Cognitive level: Analysis
Nursing process: Implementation
NCLEX: Safe and Effective Care Environment
See text page: NA

52. Three days after admission to a drug treatment program, a client is found crying. She describes seeing her arm floating in space and feeling as though if she moves she will be swallowed by the bed on which she is lying. These symptoms suggest that the client is experiencing
   1. withdrawal delirium.
   2. a flashback.
   3. crashing.
   4. sedative withdrawal.

Answer: 2
Rationale: Loss of ego boundaries and synesthesia are common experiences during flashbacks. Synesthesia is not experienced in the other options. The symptoms described are not characteristic of withdrawal delirium, crashing, or sedative withdrawal.
Cognitive level: Application
Nursing process: Assessment
NCLEX: Psychosocial Integrity
See text page: 549

53. After a methamphetamine overdose, priority nursing and medical measures will center around
   1. repeated lavage.
   2. acidification of urine.
   3. maintenance of nutrition and elimination.
   4. reduction of fever and prevention of seizures.

Answer: 4
Rationale: Hyperpyrexia and convulsions are common when a client has overdosed on a CNS stimulant. These problems are life threatening and take priority. Option 1: Lavage is not needed when the drug was injected. Option 2: Acidification of urine will not enhance drug clearance. Option 3: Problems of nutrition and elimination are not priorities in an overdose situation.
Cognitive level: Application
Nursing process: Planning
NCLEX: Physiological Integrity
See text page: 555

54. Which medication is the nurse most likely to see ordered as part of the treatment plan for both a client who is in an alcoholism treatment program and a

Chapter 27   Care of the Chemically Impaired

client who is in a program for treatment of opioid addiction?
1. Methadone
2. Disulfiram
3. Naltrexone
4. Bromocriptine

Answer: 3

Rationale: Naltrexone (ReVia) is useful for treating both opioid and alcohol addiction. An opioid antagonist, it blocks the action of opioids and because it blocks the mechanism of reinforcement; it also reduces or eliminates alcohol preference.

Cognitive level: Application
Nursing process: Planning
NCLEX: Physiological Integrity
See text page: 569

55. When assessing a client who has been given fluni-trazepam (Rohypnol), the nurse would expect to find that the client demonstrated
1. hypothermia.
2. hallucinations.
3. acrophobia.
4. anterograde amnesia.

Answer: 4

Rationale: Flunitrazepam is also known as the "date rape drug" because it produces disinhibition and relaxation of voluntary muscles as well as anterograde amnesia for events that occur. The other options do not reflect symptoms commonly seen after use of this drug.

Cognitive level: Application
Nursing process: Assessment
NCLEX: Physiological Integrity
See text pages: 558, 559

56. A client seeking detoxification after a family intervention session tells the nurse "My husband told me I am no companion to him because I am always drunk. My daughter told me she cannot bring friends home because my behavior embarrasses her. They say I do not care about anyone and that they have to be responsible for all the things I once did." The nurse should consider the nursing diagnosis of
1. self-care deficit.
2. activity intolerance.
3. ineffective health maintenance.
4. interrupted family processes.

Answer: 4

Rationale: The client describes a change in family relationships and functioning associated with family tasks, mutual support, and availability for intimacy, each of which is a defining characteristic for this nursing diagnosis. Defining characteristics for the other options are not present in the scenario.

Cognitive level: Analysis
Nursing process: Diagnosis
NCLEX: Psychosocial Integrity
See text page: 561

57. Aspects of substance abuse relapse prevention in which the nurse can assist the client and family include (more than one answer may be correct)
1. advising the client to accept residential treatment if relapse occurs.
2. assisting the client to identify life skills needed for effective coping.
3. rehearsing techniques to handle anticipated stressful situations.
4. educating regarding physical changes to expect as the body adapts to functioning without substances.

Answers: 2, 3, 4

Rationale: Option 2: Nurses can be helpful as a client assesses needed life skills and in providing appropriate referrals. Option 3: Anticipatory problem solving and role playing are good ways of rehearsing effective strategies for handling stressful situations. The nurse can participate in role playing and can help the client evaluate the usefulness of new strategies. Option 4: The nurse can provide valuable information about physiological changes that can be expected and ways in which to cope with these changes. Option 1: Residential treatment is not usually necessary after relapse.

Cognitive level: Application
Nursing process: Planning
NCLEX: Psychosocial Integrity
See text page: 565

58. The nurse discussing substance abuse relapse prevention with a client will be most effective if he or she instills the idea that relapse is best viewed as
1. an opportunity to define the client change effort.
2. a failure of the treatment program.
3. a learning experience.
4. a personal failure.

Answer: 3

Rationale: Relapses can be seen as learning experiences rather than all-or-nothing events associated with failure. Relapse prevention is aimed at recognizing and learning how to avoid threats to recovery. Lifestyle changes do not happen all at once; they are learned and applied a few at a time over an extended period of time.

Cognitive level: Application

59. A substance-abusing client tells the nurse he has been disowned by his parents. He has two siblings who have told him to "stay out of our lives." He has not had a stable relationship with a significant other for several years and has lost touch with co-workers since being fired from his job. The client states he feels anxious about his ability to maintain a drug-free state. The nurse should give highest consideration to referring the client for treatment using
1. an inpatient program.
2. outpatient therapy.
3. family therapy.
4. AA.

Answer: 1

Rationale: People with little support often do best in inpatient programs that provide structure and support. Option 2: Outpatient programs work best for employed substance abusers who have good social support systems. Option 3: The client has no family with which to participate in such a program. Option 4: AA meetings account for only a few hours daily. A client with little or no other social supports may do better with an inpatient program.

Cognitive level: Application
Nursing process: Planning
NCLEX: Psychosocial Integrity
See text page: 562

60. The nurse notes that the appearance of a client being treated in the clinic for bronchitis suggests heavy alcohol use. The nurse wishes to use the FRAMES acronym. The only intervention listed below that is consistent with FRAMES is to
1. arrange to have a blood alcohol level drawn.
2. suggest the use of disulfiram or naltrexone.
3. assist in developing a relapse prevention plan.
4. counsel regarding risks of heavy alcohol use.

Answer: 4

Rationale: FRAMES makes use of brief interventions that allow the nurse to take advantage of brief interactions with substance-abusing clients. Option 4 is consistent with FRAMES because the F of the acronym stands for feedback of personal risk. R refers to responsibility to the patient (personal control). A refers to advice to change. M refers to a menu of ways to reduce drinking (options). E stands for empathic counseling and S for self-efficacy or optimism of the patient. None of the other options listed fits the FRAMES framework.

Cognitive level: Application
Nursing process: Implementation
NCLEX: Physiological Integrity
See text page: 564

61. The treatment team discusses the fact that a client diagnosed with paranoid schizophrenia and cannabis abuse is experiencing increased hallucinations and delusions and has recently used cannabis on a daily basis. To plan effective treatment the team must
1. consider each diagnosis primary and provide simultaneous treatment.
2. first treat the schizophrenia, then establish goals for substance use treatment.
3. withdraw the client from cannabis, then treat the symptoms of schizophrenia.
4. hospitalize the client for the longest possible stay permitted by insurance.

Answer: 1

Rationale: Dual diagnoses clinical practice guidelines for both outpatient and inpatient settings suggest that the substance disorder and the psychiatric disorder should both be considered primary and receive simultaneous treatment. In addition, outcomes should be individualized to support progress in small steps over a long period of time. Thus options 2 and 3 are ruled out as correct answers. Option 4: In today's health care climate, long hospitalizations are rarely allowed by insurers.

Cognitive level: Application
Nursing process: Planning
NCLEX: Safe and Effective Care Environment
See text page: 564

62. The spouse of a client who abuses crack cocaine tells the nurse that she has been in the habit of calling her husband's employer to cover for his job absences and has even written reports for him "to keep him out of trouble." She peevishly states "He promises to change but never follows through." The nurse should make the assessment that the spouse demonstrates
1. synergism.
2. petulance.
3. codependence.
4. manipulative tendencies.

Answer: 3

Rationale: Codependent behaviors permit the substance abuser to continue unhealthy behaviors without having to become accountable for them. Making excuses and covering for the client are ways of condoning the substance abuse. Option 1 has no

Chapter 27   Care of the Chemically Impaired

relevance to the spouse's actions. Option 2: Petulance does not explain what is described in the scenario. Option 4: The spouse's behaviors are codependent rather than manipulative.

Cognitive level: Analysis
Nursing process: Assessment
NCLEX: Psychosocial Integrity
See text page: 551

63. An appropriate outcome to select for the initial treatment phase for a client who has abused cocaine is
   1. psychosocial adjustment: life change.
   2. abusive behavior: self-restraint.
   3. risk control: drug use.
   4. compliance behavior.

Answer: 3
Rationale: Risk control: drug use is defined as actions to prevent, eliminate, or reduce drug use that poses a threat to health. This outcome is most pertinent to treatment for cocaine abuse. Option 1 refers to adaptive psychosocial response of an individual to a significant life change. It is less specific than option 3. Option 2 refers to self-restraint of abusive behaviors toward others. Option 4 refers to personal actions to promote wellness, recovery, and rehabilitation based on professional advice. It is less specific than option 3.

Cognitive level: Analysis
Nursing process: Planning (Outcome Identification)
NCLEX: Psychosocial Integrity
See text pages: 560, 561

64. To effectively teach the client about cross tolerance and alcohol, benzodiazepines, and barbiturates, the nurse must understand that these drugs act on the
   1. dopamine system.
   2. γ-aminobutyric acid system.
   3. opioid system.
   4. serotonin system.

Answer: 2
Rationale: The nurse must be able to explain that alcohol and other CNS depressants act on γ-aminobutyric acid receptors. Because the receptor sites are the same for each of these classes of drugs, cross tolerance and cross addiction readily occur. Clients need this information to avoid the pitfalls of inappropriate medication usage. Option 1: This system is affected by neuroleptics. Option 2: This system is affected by opioids and synthetic opioids. Option 4: This system is affected by selected antidepressant medication.

Cognitive level: Application
Nursing process: Planning
NCLEX: Health Promotion and Maintenance
See text page: 548

65. The nurse performing a client assessment will identify the following data as consistent with psychodynamic factors associated with chemical addictions (more than one answer may be correct):
   1. High tolerance for frustration and pain
   2. Lack of success in life
   3. Stable mature relationships
   4. Low self-esteem
   5. Propensity for risk taking

Answers: 2, 4, 5
Rationale: These characteristics commonly coexist with substance dependence and abuse. Other characteristics include low tolerance for frustration and pain and immature, troubled interpersonal relationships.

Cognitive level: Application
Nursing process: Assessment
NCLEX: Psychosocial Integrity
See text page: 548

CHAPTER 28

1. When asked by a client's wife what characterizes severe mental illness, the nurse should reply, "It is
   1. mental illness of more than 2 weeks' duration."
   2. mental illness accompanied by physical impairment and severe social problems."
   3. a major mental illness that is chronic and is marked by pervasive functional impairment."
   4. a major mental illness that cannot be treated to prevent deterioration of cognitive and social abilities."

Answer: 3
Rationale: "Severe mental illness" has replaced the term "chronic mental illness." Thus option 3 is the best explanation. Neither option 1 nor option 2 considers the long-term aspect of severe mental illness. Option 4: Severe mental illness can, in fact, be treated, but remissions and exacerbations are part of the course of the illness.

Cognitive level: Application
Nursing process: Implementation
NCLEX: Health Promotion and Maintenance
See text page: 579

2. A client with residual schizophrenia, aged 60 years, spent 5 years in a state hospital before being discharged to a community residence. The client, who is now monitored by the community mental health nurse, requires much encouragement to voice her needs and take independent action to get her needs met. The nurse assesses this passive behavior as being the probable result of
   1. dependency caused by institutionalization.

400

2. cognitive deterioration from schizophrenia.
3. brain damage from recreational drug use.
4. neuroleptic drug side effects.

Answer: 1

Rationale: Institutionalization brought about a decreased sense of self, resulting in lack of autonomy in many clients. Clients became dependent on the hospital and its staff to meet their needs. When these clients were discharged into the community many continued to demonstrate passive behaviors despite efforts to rehabilitate them. Option 2: Although the long-term effects of the disease process may contribute to passivity, institutionalization was probably a greater determinant of the behavior. Option 3: The scenario does not suggest recreational drug use. Option 4: Neuroleptic drug side effects would result in different behaviors.

Cognitive level: Analysis
Nursing process: Assessment
NCLEX: Psychosocial Integrity
See text page: 576

3. A client, aged 30 years, tells his case manager "I do not have bipolar disorder anymore, so I do not need the medicine and the blood tests. I was in the hospital twice for a few days a year or so ago. Then you got into the act to get me a place to live and SSI checks. All that is wrong now is I am bored and I do not have any friends." The nurse assesses the client as demonstrating
   1. denial.
   2. projection.
   3. rationalization.
   4. identification.

Answer: 1

Rationale: The client scenario describes denial. Many young clients with severe mental illness have limited experience with hospital-based formal treatment programs. Short-term hospitalizations and community follow-up contribute to these clients failing to see that they have a problem. Option 2: The client is not blaming another for a personal weakness. Option 3: The client is not making socially acceptable excuses. Option 4: The client is not identifying with another.

Cognitive level: Analysis
Nursing process: Assessment
NCLEX: Psychosocial Integrity
See text page: 576

4. A client, aged 30 years, tells his case manager "I do not have bipolar disorder anymore, so I do not need the medicine and the blood tests. I was in the hospi-

tal twice for a few days a year or so ago. Then you got into the act to get me a place to live and SSI checks. All that is wrong now is I am bored and I do not have any friends." The nurse should plan to refer the client to (more than one answer may be correct)
   1. psychoeducation classes.
   2. crisis intervention.
   3. social skills training.
   4. a homeless shelter.

Answers: 1, 3

Rationale: The client does not understand his illness and the need for adherence to the medication regimen. Psychoeducation for the client (and family) can address this lack of knowledge. The client, who considers himself friendless, could also profit from social skills training to improve the quality of interpersonal relationships. Many clients with severe mental illness have such poor communication skills that others are uncomfortable interacting with them. Interactional skills can be effectively taught by breaking the skill down into smaller verbal and nonverbal components. Option 2: The nurse case manager will function in the role of crisis stabilizer. Option 4: The client presently has a home and does not require the services of a homeless shelter.

Cognitive level: Analysis
Nursing process: Planning
NCLEX: Psychosocial Integrity
See text pages: 582, 583

5. Economic factors that are highly critical to the success of discharge planning for a client with severe and persistent mental illness include (more than one answer may be correct)
   1. access to housing.
   2. income adequate to meet basic needs.
   3. availability of health insurance.
   4. ongoing interdisciplinary evaluation.

Answers: 1, 2, 3

Rationale: The success of discharge planning requires careful attention to the client's economic status. Access to housing is the first priority of the seriously mentally ill, and lack of income and health insurance are barriers to effective treatment and rehabilitation.

Option 4: Although an important aspect of ongoing care of the seriously mentally ill client, this option is not classified as an economic factor.

Cognitive level: Comprehension
Nursing process: Planning
NCLEX: Psychosocial Integrity
See text pages: 576-578

6. A nursing diagnosis that should be considered for individuals who are severely mentally ill and homeless is
1. substance abuse.
2. chronic low self-esteem.
3. disturbed sleep pattern.
4. impaired environmental interpretation syndrome.

Answer: 2

Rationale: Of the 40% to 70% of individuals with severe mental illness who do not live with their families, many become homeless. Life on the street or in a shelter has a negative influence on the individual's self-esteem, making this nursing diagnosis one that should be considered. Option 1: Substance abuse is not an approved North American Nursing Diagnosis Association diagnosis. Option 3: Disturbed sleep pattern may be noted in some clients but is not a universal problem. Option 4 refers to persistent disorientation, which is not seen in a majority of the homeless.

Cognitive level: Analysis
Nursing process: Diagnosis
NCLEX: Psychosocial Integrity
See text pages: 577-578

7. A client with severe and persistent schizophrenia is seen at the adult outpatient clinic. He is delusional and experiencing auditory hallucinations. He tells the nurse "I am here to save the world. I threw away the pills because they interfere with hearing God's voice." The nurse identifies the client's reason for medication nonadherence as
1. poor therapeutic alliance with clinicians.
2. inadequate discharge planning.
3. dislike of side effects.
4. poor insight.

Answer: 4

Rationale: The client's noncompliance is most closely related to lack of insight into his illness. The client believes he is an exalted personage who hears God's voice, rather than an individual with a serious mental disorder who needs medication to control his symptoms. Data do not suggest any of the other factors often related to medication nonadherence.

Cognitive level: Analysis
Nursing process: Assessment
NCLEX: Physiological Integrity
See text page: 578

8. The nurse at the adult outpatient clinic plans to use the Abnormal Involuntary Movement Scale to examine a client who has taken typical antipsychotic medication (chlorpromazine, haloperidol) over a period of several years. The purpose of this examination is to detect
1. neuroleptic malignant syndrome.
2. anticholinergic side effects.
3. tardive dyskinesia.
4. akathisia.

Answer: 3

Rationale: The Abnormal Involuntary Movement Scale is a tool used to detect symptoms of tardive dyskinesia, a serious, often irreversible side effect of typical antipsychotic medication use. Early detection and changing to an atypical antipsychotic medication can prevent worsening of the symptoms. Clients with severe mental illness should be monitored regularly for signs of medication side effects. This scale is not useful for detecting neuroleptic malignant syndrome, anticholinergic side effects, or akathisia.

Cognitive level: Application
Nursing process: Assessment
NCLEX: Physiological Integrity
See text page: 578

9. Health maintenance and promotion efforts for clients with severe and persistent schizophrenia should include education about the importance of regular
1. home safety inspections.
2. monitoring of self-care ability.
3. screening for cancer, hypertension, and diabetes.
4. determination of adequacy of client support system.

Answer: 3

Rationale: Individuals with severe mental illness have an increased prevalence of several disorders, including those mentioned in option 3. Clients should be taught the importance of regular visits to a primary care physician for screening for these illnesses.

Option 1: Home safety inspections are more often suggested for clients with physical impairments. Option 2: Evaluating self-care ability is usually accomplished by caregivers and family rather than the client. Option 4: Assessment of client support system is not usually considered part of health promotion and maintenance.

Cognitive level: Application
Nursing process: Planning
NCLEX: Health Maintenance and Promotion
See text page: 578

10. The nurse planning care for a client with the dual diagnoses of bipolar disorder and substance abuse disorder, cocaine, should consider the fact that the client has increased risk for (more than one answer may be correct)
1. injury.
2. suicide.

3. homelessness.
4. HIV infection.

Answers: 1, 2, 3, 4

Rationale: Clinical consequences of substance abuse among the severely mentally ill include all the options listed, along with medication nonadherence, increased rates of violence, relapse of psychosis, and increased use of institutional services.

Cognitive level: Comprehension
Nursing process: Planning
NCLEX: Psychosocial Integrity
See text pages: 578, 579

11. A client with severe mental illness had been living independently in an apartment but was evicted when the landlord became aware that the client was causing disturbances in the neighborhood as the result of responding to auditory hallucinations commanding her to report terrorists to the FBI. After a short hospitalization with discharge to a group home, the client regained her state of adjustment before relapse and attempted to rent her old apartment. The landlord told her he was not willing to risk "more trouble" if her "craziness" returned. The problem the client is experiencing is
   1. grief.
   2. stigma.
   3. homelessness.
   4. lack of parity in insurance coverage.

Answer: 2

Rationale: The inability to obtain shelter because of negative attitudes about mental illness is an example of stigma. Stigma is defined as damage to reputation, the covert and sometimes overt shame and ridicule our society places on mental illness. Option 1: Data are not present to identify grief as a client problem. Option 3: Data do not suggest that the client is actually homeless. Option 4: Insurance parity is not relevant to the scenario.

Cognitive level: Application
Nursing process: Assessment
NCLEX: Psychosocial Integrity
See text page: 579

12. A client who is severely and persistently mentally ill with bipolar disorder also abuses alcohol. He comes to the mental health clinic for his lithium level to be tested. The results suggest the client has not been medication compliant. The nurse ascertains that the client's lithium was stolen from his pocket while he was intoxicated and sleeping. This is the third time this has happened. The nursing diagnosis of highest priority that should be formulated is

1. risk for injury related to frequent intoxication.
2. noncompliance with medication regimen related to denial of illness.
3. ineffective therapeutic regimen management related to situational obstacles (theft of medication).
4. decisional conflict related to unpleasant side effects of medication.

Answer: 3

Rationale: Ineffective therapeutic regimen management related to situational obstacles is a viable diagnosis. It recognizes the client's inability to regulate and integrate the medication program as a result of the theft of the medication. Options 1 and 2: The client has not made an informed decision not to adhere to the therapeutic recommendation, and the client is not denying illness. Option 4: Risk for injury is not the priority at this time, and no data support decisional conflict.

Cognitive level: Analysis
Nursing process: Diagnosis
NCLEX: Physiological Integrity
See text page: 578

13. A client with severe mental illness has been homeless for 3 years. He states he is a loner. He lost contact with his family and is suspicious of anyone who approaches him. He has had several psychiatric admissions when his behaviors have been highly bizarre. When hospitalized he takes medication, but after discharge he is medication nonadherent and does not keep aftercare appointments. The client's lifestyle can be assessed as
   1. stable.
   2. compliant.
   3. socially isolated.
   4. interdependent.

Answer: 3

Rationale: Social isolation is characterized by being cut off from family, community, and peer support and involvement. Data are not present to support any of the other options.

Cognitive level: Analysis
Nursing process: Assessment
NCLEX: Psychosocial Integrity
See text page: 576

14. A client who has been homeless for the last 3 years states he is a loner. He lost contact with his family and is suspicious of anyone who approaches him. He has had several psychiatric admissions, but after discharge stops taking medication and does not keep aftercare appointments. The illness symptom that

may actually contribute to his ability to survive on the streets is his
1. suspiciousness.
2. ability to relate.
3. self-confidence.
4. assertiveness.

Answer: 1

Rationale: Affable, eager-to-please individuals are easily manipulated and vulnerable on the streets. Individuals who are suspicious of the motives of others are not as vulnerable to harm on the street. The scenario does not suggest that the client relates well to others, has self-confidence, or is assertive.

Cognitive level: Analysis
Nursing process: Assessment
NCLEX: Psychosocial Integrity
See text page: 576

15. A client with severe mental illness who lived on the streets before his most recent hospitalization will be discharged to a shelter until other housing can be arranged. The advantage of placement in the shelter is the provision of
1. privacy.
2. a safe environment.
3. freedom to do as he pleases.
4. supplemental Social Security income.

Answer: 2

Rationale: The shelter will provide a safer environment than living on the street. Options 1, 3, and 4: Shelters do not provide a great deal of privacy or autonomy, and they do not secure SSI for clients.

Cognitive level: Application
Nursing process: Planning
NCLEX: Safe and Effective Care Environment
See text page: 580

16. An individual with severe mental illness is persuaded to enter a shelter for the homeless. The shelter has an interdisciplinary team of health care workers available to assist residents. What initial activity will the team undertake with the client?
1. Development of a treatment plan
2. A behavioral and needs assessment
3. Intervention with his suspiciousness
4. Evaluation of his reaction to the shelter

Answer: 2

Rationale: Assessment must be performed before treatment planning, intervention, or evaluative processes can be successful.

Cognitive level: Application
Nursing process: Assessment
NCLEX: Psychosocial Integrity
See text pages: 579, 580

17. An individual with severe mental illness is persuaded to enter a shelter for the homeless. The shelter has an interdisciplinary team of health care workers available to assist residents. The intervention that should be the nurse's initial priority is
1. developing a relationship.
2. finding him employment.
3. administering prescribed medication.
4. teaching appropriate health care practices.

Answer: 1

Rationale: Basic psychosocial needs do not change because a person is homeless. The first step in caring for health care needs is establishing rapport. Once a trusting relationship is established, options 3 and 4 become possible. Eventually, employment may be considered.

Cognitive level: Application
Nursing process: Planning
NCLEX: Psychosocial Integrity
See text pages: 579, 580

18. An individual with severe mental illness who has been living on the street is persuaded to enter a shelter for the homeless, where there is an interdisciplinary team of health care workers available to assist residents. After 2 days in the shelter the client tells the nurse that he feels confused in his new surroundings and feels a need to be on his guard. The nursing diagnosis that should be considered is
1. risk for injury.
2. ineffective denial.
3. relocation stress syndrome.
4. noncompliance with medication regimen.

Answer: 3

Rationale: Relocation stress syndrome is defined as physiological or psychosocial disturbance after transfer from one environment to another. Data are not present to support options 1, 2, or 4.

Cognitive level: Analysis
Nursing process: Diagnosis
NCLEX: Psychosocial Integrity
See text page: 577

19. A client with severe and persistent paranoid schizophrenia has had several hospitalizations. He responds quickly to antipsychotic medication but stops taking the medication soon after discharge. Discharge planning after this hospitalization will include follow-up at the adult mental health clinic, placement in a group home, and daily attendance at a psychosocial rehabilitation program. Evidence-based pharmacologic guidelines recommend prescribing
1. chlorpromazine (Thorazine).
2. thioridazine (Mellaril).

404

3. fluphenazine decanoate (Prolixin decanoate).
4. long-acting risperidone (Risperdal).

Answer: 4

Rationale: First-line treatment with atypical antipsychotics such as risperidone, olanzapine, or quetiapine is recommended in evidence-based pharmacological guidelines. A long-acting form of risperidone is available and appropriate given the client's propensity for medication nonadherence. The other options are typical antipsychotics that are less effective in treating secondary symptoms of schizophrenia.
Cognitive level: Analysis
Nursing process: Planning
NCLEX: Physiological Integrity
See text page: 578

20. A client with severe and persistent mental illness who has just moved into a homeless shelter tells the nurse that his "life just got out of control." He stated that he could not depend on others, so he kept to himself. Then he added "I am like a leaf at the mercy of the wind." The nurse adds the nursing diagnosis of powerlessness to his care plan. The outcome that should be identified as most relevant is
1. hope.
2. self-esteem.
3. personal autonomy.
4. anxiety self-control.

Answer: 3

Rationale: On the basis of information in the scenario, the most relevant outcome is personal autonomy. The client speaks of loss of control over his life and of being like a leaf blown about. Data are not present to suggest hopelessness, low self-esteem, or increased anxiety.
Cognitive level: Analysis
Nursing process: Planning (Outcome Identification)
NCLEX: Psychosocial Integrity
See text page: 581

21. A client with severe and persistent mental illness who has just moved into a homeless shelter tells the nurse that his "life just got out of control." Then he added "I am like a leaf at the mercy of the wind." The nurse formulates the nursing diagnosis of powerlessness. An appropriate outcome indicator to monitor is that the client will
1. participate in health care decisions.
2. demonstrate low anxiety levels.
3. express satisfaction with stress level.
4. process information accurately.

Answer: 1

Rationale: Personal autonomy is a desired outcome for powerlessness. An indicator of personal autonomy is participation in decision making. The other options, although desirable, are not as clearly related to the nursing diagnosis of powerlessness.
Cognitive level: Analysis
Nursing process: Planning (Outcome Identification)
NCLEX: Psychosocial Integrity
See text: 581

22. A severely and persistently mentally ill client who lives in a homeless shelter has a nursing diagnosis of powerlessness. An intervention related to this nursing diagnosis is
1. reinforcing participation in activity.
2. encouraging mutual goal setting.
3. verbally communicating empathy.
4. demonstrating an accepting attitude.

Answer: 2

Rationale: Mutual goal setting is an intervention designed to promote feelings of personal autonomy and dispel feelings of powerlessness. The health care provider's available resources of time and talent are frequently strained by the severe psychosocial and physical needs of homeless and severely and persistently mentally ill clients. Although it might be easier and faster for the nurse to establish a plan and outcomes, this action would contribute to the client's sense of powerlessness. Involving the client in decision making empowers the client and reduces feelings of powerlessness. Option 1 is an intervention associated with activity therapy. Options 3 and 4 are interventions related to presence.
Cognitive level: Application
Nursing process: Planning
NCLEX: Psychosocial Integrity
See text page: 581

23. A seriously mentally ill client who was highly suspicious and delusional entered the shelter and was given depot antipsychotic medication. After 4 weeks in residence the outreach team holds a case conference to evaluate client progress. The client statement that would indicate the client had significantly improved is
1. "I am feeling pretty comfortable here. Nobody hassles me."
2. "They will not let me drink wine in here, so I am going back to the street."
3. "Those guys are always watching me. I think they are going to steal my shoes."
4. "That shot you gave me made my arm sore. I am not going to have any more of them."

405

Answer: 1

Rationale: Final evaluation of a client's progress is made on the basis of client satisfaction with the new health status and the health care team's estimation of improvement. For a formerly delusional client to admit to feeling comfortable and free of "hassles" denotes improvement in the client's condition. The other options suggest that the client is in danger of relapse.

Cognitive level: Evaluation
Nursing process: Evaluation
NCLEX: Psychosocial Integrity
See text page: 581

24. The nurse in the emergency department is caring for a client with a long history of schizophrenia whose chief complaint is sores on her legs. As the nurse takes the history, the client gives vague answers to questions about eating and sleeping habits and activities of daily living. The nurse notes that the client's personal hygiene is poor and that she has a large canvas duffle bag with her. The nurse wonders if the client is a homeless person. The nurse should
   1. ask if the client has someone with her that the nurse might speak to.
   2. ask the client during the mental status examination to state her address.
   3. avoid mentioning the topic because it is not relevant to treatment of a physical problem.
   4. ask the client directly about her living arrangements.

Answer: 4

Rationale: The topic of homelessness should be approached directly. Homelessness affects planning for aftercare because the client's ability to carry out prescribed measures may be severely compromised. The individual living on the street will find it difficult to obtain even minimal resources for the care of the leg ulcers.

Cognitive level: Application
Nursing process: Assessment
NCLEX: Physiological Integrity
See text pages: 577, 578

25. The brother of a client who is severely and persistently mentally ill with bipolar disorder asks why the client has been assigned a case manager. The nurse's reply should cite the major advantage of the use of case management as
   1. "The case manager can modify traditional psychotherapy for homeless clients."
   2. "With one coordinator of services, resources can be more efficiently used."
   3. "The case manager can focus on social skills training and esteem building."
   4. "The case manager can adjust medication dosage to manage side effects."

Answer: 2

Rationale: The case manager not only provides entrance into the system of care, he or she can coordinate the multiple referrals that so often confuse the severely and persistently mentally ill client and the client's family. Case management promotes efficient use of services. The other options are lesser advantages or may be irrelevant.

Cognitive level: Application
Nursing process: Implementation
NCLEX: Safe and Effective Care Environment
See text page: 580

26. A family is talking with the nurse about the impact a schizophrenic son has had on the family. The father mentions that his health insurance provides limited coverage for psychiatric hospitalization and even less coverage for outpatient treatment. Consequently, the family savings have been depleted over the past 2 years. The mother relates that she has had to quit her job to provide supervision for the son, who, if left to his own devices, brings drugs into the home, becomes violent, and destroys furniture. The client's younger sister mentions she feels lost because her parents are so focused on her brother that it seems as though they have no time for her. The topics discussed are called
   1. life cycle stressors.
   2. psychobiological issues.
   3. the family burden of mental illness.
   4. stigma associated with mental illness.

Answer: 3

Rationale: Family burden refers to the meaning that the experience of living with a mentally ill person has for families. Option 1: The stressors mentioned are not related to live cycle issues. Option 2: The stressors described are psychosocial in nature. Option 4: *Stigma* refers to shame and ridicule associated with mental illness.

Cognitive level: Application
Nursing process: Assessment
NCLEX: Psychosocial Integrity
See text page: NA

27. A responsibility of a basic level nurse case manager for severely and persistently mentally ill clients is
   1. coordinating referrals.
   2. prescribing medications.
   3. making medical diagnoses.
   4. budgeting for community outreach programs.

Answer: 1

Rationale: Coordinating referrals is within the responsibility of a case manager. Medications can be pre-

406

scribed by physicians or by nurse practitioners in selected states. Making medical diagnoses is the purview of the physician or advanced practice nurse, not the basic level nurse. Budgeting is the responsibility of facility managers, not basic level staff.

Cognitive level: Application
Nursing process: Implementation
NCLEX: Safe and Effective Care Environment
See text page: 580

28. The mother of a severely and persistently mentally ill client says to the nurse "Why are you getting my daughter involved in that vocational rehabilitation program? She is too sick to ever be able to hold a job." The best reply for the psychiatric rehabilitation nurse would be
   1. "We do this to be eligible for federal funding for our programs."
   2. "Are you concerned that we are trying to make Anna too independent?"
   3. "If you think the program is detrimental to Anna, we can postpone it for a time."
   4. "Most clients are capable of employment at some level, competitive or sheltered."

Answer: 4
Rationale: Studies have shown that most clients who complete vocational rehabilitation programs are capable of some level of employment and, in addition, demonstrate significant improvement in assertiveness and work behaviors as well as decreased feelings of depression.

Cognitive level: Application
Nursing process: Implementation
NCLEX: Psychosocial Integrity
See text pages: 583, 584

29. Illness management is an agreed-on outcome for a client with severe mental illness receiving outpatient therapy for exacerbation of hallucinations and delusions associated with paranoid schizophrenia. Nursing interventions appropriate to include in the client's care plan include (more than one answer may be correct)
   1. teaching the client respect for mental health professionals.
   2. planning strategies to reduce susceptibility to relapse.
   3. assisting the client in identifying personal goals.
   4. practicing techniques to dismiss hallucinations.

Answers: 2, 4
Rationale: Illness management refers to helping the client gain control over symptoms. Planning strategies to reduce susceptibility to relapse is a means of retaining control over symptoms of the disorder.

Practicing techniques to cope more effectively with symptoms, such as hallucinations, is another means of managing illness. Option 1: A more appropriate intervention is to teach the client how to work in collaboration with mental health treatment members for the client to gain maximal benefit from the expertise of the treatment team professionals. Option 3: Identification of personal goals is a focus during recovery, the stage after relief of symptoms.

Cognitive level: Application
Nursing process: Planning
NCLEX: Psychosocial Integrity
See text page: 581

30. An appropriate focus for nursing intervention for a client who is in the sixth month of recovery from a bipolar episode would be
   1. promoting client awareness of personal identity, time, and environment.
   2. assisting the client in performing instrumental activities of daily living.
   3. assisting the client in developing a self-concept beyond illness.
   4. teaching the use of appropriate eye contact.

Answer: 3
Rationale: Recovery refers to the period of time after the relief of symptoms. The focus is on developing and accomplishing personal goals. Clients are assisted in developing self-confidence, a sense of well-being and hope, and a self-concept beyond illness. Options 1 and 2 would be addressed during the early stage of treatment, when the focus is illness management. Option 4 would be addressed for a client with schizophrenia during social skills training. Clients with bipolar disorder usually make appropriate eye contact.

Cognitive level: Application
Nursing process: Implementation
NCLEX: Psychosocial Integrity
See text page: 581

31. A client with severe mental illness who lived independently in an apartment and attended a psychosocial rehabilitation program 5 days a week appears at the emergency department seeking admission to the inpatient unit. The mental status examination reveals no acute symptoms of psychiatric disorder. Her chief complaint is that she has no money to pay her rent or refill her antipsychotic medication prescription. The best action for the emergency department nurse would be to
   1. arrange for a short in-patient admission and begin discharge planning.
   2. send the client to a homeless shelter until housing can be arranged.

407

3. involve the client's case manager to provide crisis intervention.
4. explain that one must have psychiatric symptoms to be admitted.

Answer: 3

Rationale: The client is experiencing a crisis. Crisis stabilization, undertaken by the case manager who knows the client, can undoubtedly avert an unnecessary hospitalization.

Options 1 and 2 carelessly uses scarce resources. Option 4 may prompt the client to feign symptoms.

Cognitive level: Analysis
Nursing process: Implementation
NCLEX: Safe and Effective Care Environment
See text pages: 581, 582

32. The case manager providing crisis stabilization for a client with severe mental illness who states his wallet was stolen and who is left without means of paying the rent will use several principles. Put the interventions in the order in which they should be implemented.
    1. Actively engage in problem solving to find new resources, as needed
    2. Determine availability of additional social support
    3. Clarify the reality of the situation
    4. Identify realistic goals

Answer: 3, 4, 2, 1

Rationale: The case manager, using principles of crisis stabilization, would first clarify the situation, then identify realistic goals considering the client's strengths. The case manager would then assess availability of additional help from the client's social support system. If additional help from the support system is not possible, the case manager must actively engage in problem solving to find new resources to assist the client.

Cognitive level: Application
Nursing process: Implementation
NCLEX: Safe and Effective Care Environment
See text pages: 581, 582

33. A nurse working at an adult outpatient clinic for clients with severe mental illness is given the task of determining topics appropriate for the psychoeducation program.

    Select four basic topics supported by evidence-based practice that the nurse should incorporate as part of the program.
    1. The instillation of hope and a sense of well-being in clients
    2. Improvement of client self-esteem

3. Information about the illness
4. Principles of illness management and treatment
5. Information about medication and methods to improve adherence
6. Stress management for family members

Answers: 3, 4, 5, 6

Rationale: These topics, along with a focus on improved functioning in all family members, are recommended as topics for education for both the family and the client.

The other two topics are not as fundamental.

Cognitive level: Application
Nursing process: Planning
NCLEX: Health Promotion and Maintenance
See text pages: 582, 583

34. The nurse wishes to enroll a client with poor social skills in a training program for clients with severe and persistent schizophrenia. The basis for such a program is evidence that
    1. complex interpersonal skills can be taught by breaking them into simple behaviors.
    2. improved functioning reduces relapses and the need for hospitalization.
    3. group teaching is superior to work with individual clients.
    4. learned skills must be repeatedly reinforced if they are to persist.

Answer: 1

Rationale: Research studies have shown that complex interpersonal skills can be taught by breaking them down into simpler behaviors, including verbal and nonverbal parts. Clients observe and role play new behaviors until they can perform the skill in and outside class. Option 2: This statement reflects a goal of social skills classes rather than explains the basis on which the programs work. Option 3 is not proven. Social skills can be taught in groups or to individual clients. Option 4: Follow-up has shown that learned skills persist over time and may be transferred to new settings for some clients.

Cognitive level: Comprehension
Nursing process: Planning
NCLEX: Psychosocial Integrity
See text page: 583

35. The case manager has the option to refer a client with severe mental illness to a vocational rehabilitation program. Which model, supported by evidence, should the nurse choose for the client?
    1. Referral to a state vocational rehabilitation agency for prevocational training
    2. Referral to a sheltered workshop with later placement in a competitive job

3. Job placement followed by individualized, on-the-job training
4. Cognitive interventions alternating with job skill training

Answer: 3

Rationale: Placing the client in the job first, then giving individualized training in the field describes the supported employment model that is now an evidence-based practice.

Options 1 and 2 are not supported by evidence as superior models. Option 4 is not a vocational rehabilitation model.

Cognitive level: Comprehension
Nursing process: Planning
NCLEX: Psychosocial Integrity
See text pages: 583, 584

CHAPTER 29

1. A diabetic client is to have a mid-thigh amputation of his left leg. He tells the nurse "I guess I will be called 'Gimpy' after the surgery. My life is really going to change when I cannot carry out my exercise program any more." The nurse assesses that the client is at risk for the nursing diagnosis of
   1. spiritual distress.
   2. ineffective denial.
   3. disturbed body image.
   4. impaired social interaction.

Answer: 3

Rationale: The nature of the surgery, which involves an actual change in body structure, places the client at greater risk for developing disturbed body image than any of the other diagnoses listed. The client's statements about what he is expecting also suggest risk for this diagnosis.

Cognitive level: Analysis
Nursing process: Diagnosis
NCLEX: Psychosocial Integrity
See text page: 596

2. A client's breast cancer was diagnosed after a mammogram. Her doctor advised a lumpectomy, followed by radiation and chemotherapy. The client schedules consultations with the surgeon, the radiation oncologist, and the medical oncologist so that she may ask questions regarding her treatment. The coping strategy being used can be identified as
   1. keeping busy and distracting oneself.
   2. conforming and complying.
   3. sharing concern and finding consolation.
   4. seeking information and obtaining guidance.

Answer: 4

Rationale: The client is coping by gathering information that will help her understand her treatment goals and the effects of treatment. Most clients who use this strategy believe knowledge reduces anxiety. Option 1: Keeping busy and distracting oneself has as its goal postponing dealing with the problem. Option 2: Conforming and complying would involve simply accepting the physician's treatment plan. Option 3: Sharing concern and finding consolation are usually carried out with family and friends and would not necessitate medical appointments.

Cognitive level: Analysis
Nursing process: Assessment
NCLEX: Psychosocial Integrity
See text page: 596

3. Of the common client problems listed below, the one taking priority for nursing assessment and intervention is the client's
   1. fear of the unknown.
   2. future plans.
   3. present level of pain.
   4. reaction to the illness.

Answer: 3

Rationale: Pain is considered a physiological warning of tissue damage, and as such would take priority over the other client problems listed. Pain management begins with assessment. Once the level of pain has been assessed, appropriate intervention can occur. Intervention may be necessary before further psychosocial assessment can take place.

Cognitive level: Analysis
Nursing process: Assessment
NCLEX: Physiological Integrity
See text pages: 594, 595

4. Which situation indicates use of a negative coping strategy by a client?
   1. A client states "That heart attack was no fun, but at least it woke me up to my need for a better diet and more exercise."
   2. A client tells the nurse "I am going to do whatever my doctor advises; after all, he knows more about things than I do."
   3. The client muses "I definitely have cancer. Now I need to look at the effects of treatment and decide whether I will be able to work daily."
   4. A client states "I would not be in this position if the company had a better safety program. I blame them for not explaining the hazards of that machine."

Answer: 4

409

Rationale: Blaming someone else is not usually considered a highly adaptive coping strategy. Options 1 (redefinition), 2 (conforming), and 3 (confronting) are seen as more effective.
Cognitive level: Analysis
Nursing process: Assessment
NCLEX: Psychosocial Integrity
See text page: 596

5. A staff nurse tells the clinical nurse leader "I feel as though I am at a total loss as to how to cope with this client. He has so many physical needs as a result of his head and neck surgery! Those needs have to be my primary focus, but sometimes it seems he must have emotional pain, too. I don not know how to help with that." The staff nurse should be referred to
   1. the psychiatric liaison nurse.
   2. the psychiatrist in the crisis clinic.
   3. the unit social worker.
   4. the hospital chaplain.

Answer: 1
Rationale: The psychiatric liaison nurse is a resource for the nursing staff who feel unable to intervene therapeutically with a client. The other professionals might be helpful, but problems such as these are the specialty of the liaison nurse.
Cognitive level: Application
Nursing process: Implementation
NCLEX: Psychosocial Integrity
See text page: 598

6. Which modality would be least helpful to include in the plan of care for a client who is being treated for severe chronic low back pain?
   1. Biofeedback, to promote relaxation of muscle groups and relief of tension that aggravates pain
   2. Guided imagery, as a way of deepening relaxation and desensitizing the client to pain
   3. Hypnosis, to achieve a state of resting alertness and the ability to block out painful sensations
   4. Psychoanalytic psychotherapy, to develop insight about the underlying psychological reasons for the symptom

Answer: 4
Rationale: Analytic therapy has been found to be largely ineffective in helping clients cope with chronic pain. Supportive therapy, behavior therapy, cognitive therapy, and antidepressants have proved helpful, as have the modalities listed in options 1, 2, and 3.
Cognitive level: Application
Nursing process: Planning
NCLEX: Physiological Integrity
See text pages: 596, 597

7. A client, who is recovering from a severe myocardial infarction, was moved from the cardiac intensive care unit to the cardiac step-down unit. He tells the new nurse "I will be fine once I get home. None of that 'watch your cholesterol, watch your calories, watch your stress' stuff is for me. Nobody has mentioned it, so it will be business as usual." Which nursing diagnosis should the nurse consider adding to the client's care plan?
   1. Fear related to unknown aspects of hospitalization
   2. Deficient knowledge related to new diagnosis of myocardial infarction
   3. Health-seeking behaviors related to desire to seek a higher level of wellness
   4. Powerlessness related to unmet need to remain in control

Answer: 2
Rationale: The client may be denying the seriousness of his condition or he may simply not know about risk factors and posthospital treatment plans. By receiving health teaching regarding risk factors related to his condition and his treatment plan, denial can be diminished and knowledge can be increased. The defining characteristics are not present for any of the other diagnoses listed as options.
Cognitive level: Analysis
Nursing process: Diagnosis
NCLEX: Psychosocial Integrity
See text page: 592

8. A client has had a total knee replacement and will need assistance for several weeks after discharge. She tells the nurse caring for her "I do not intend to assume the 'sick role.'" The nurse knows the client is objecting to
   1. coordinating various aspects of medical and nursing care.
   2. giving up financial responsibility for hospital and medical care.
   3. giving up independent functioning to assume a dependent role.
   4. using a variety of defense mechanisms to reduce anxiety associated with hospitalization.

Answer: 3
Rationale: Hospitalized clients give up a certain amount of independent functioning. They give up clothing, customary roles, and occasionally a name, such as when they are referred to as "the client with pneumonia in room 213." The "sick role" usually refers to being dependent on others. Orthopedic surgery often requires the client to assume a more dependent role because of the inability to ambulate indepen-

410

dently. The other options are not associated with the "sick role."
Cognitive level: Application
Nursing process: Assessment
NCLEX: Psychosocial Integrity
See text page: 593

9. A client hospitalized after a myocardial infarction is restlessly moving about in bed. Her pulse, blood pressure, and respiratory rate are elevated. In a shaky voice, she tells the nurse "I think I am going to die. The pain is gone, but it could come back anytime. Where is the doctor? Why isn't the doctor here with me?" The nurse should analyze this behavior as suggesting the nursing diagnosis of
   1. spiritual distress.
   2. ineffective breathing pattern.
   3. noncompliance.
   4. anxiety.

Answer: 4
Rationale: The clinical picture is typical of anxiety. The client is experiencing uneasy feelings arising from a nonspecific source. Anxiety typically produces elevated vital signs. Data are not present for the other nursing diagnoses.
Cognitive level: Analysis
Nursing process: Diagnosis
NCLEX: Psychosocial Integrity
See text pages: 590, 592

10. A client is to have a nephrostomy. A concern the nurse might anticipate relates to the client's
    1. reproductive ability.
    2. ability to think rationally.
    3. body image.
    4. friends.

Answer: 3
Rationale: A nephrostomy, like a colostomy, has serious implications for body image. Options 1 and 4: Concerns with reproductive ability and acceptance by friends are less certain to occur than body image changes. Option 2: The ability to think rationally should not be affected.
Cognitive level: Application
Nursing process: Assessment
NCLEX: Psychosocial Integrity
See text page: 596

11. An elderly client's children had always assumed they would be able to care for her until she died. However, the client had diabetes develop, had a below-the-knee amputation that is healing poorly, and recently had a cerebrovascular accident that left her paralyzed on the right side. The family has been told the client can be cared for at home if sufficient help can be obtained, or she can be placed in a nursing home. The siblings cannot make up their minds. The nursing diagnosis most appropriate would be
    1. compromised family coping.
    2. anticipatory grieving.
    3. decisional conflict.
    4. impaired verbal communication.

Answer: 3
Rationale: Decisional conflict occurs when a state of uncertainty about a course of action exists and when the action to be taken involves a challenge to personal values. The siblings had assumed they would be competent to care for their mother and now question this assumption.
Cognitive level: Analysis
Nursing process: Diagnosis
NCLEX: Psychosocial Integrity
See text page: 596

12. An elderly client's children had always assumed they would be able to care for her until she died. However, the client had diabetes develop, had a below-the-knee amputation that is healing poorly, and recently had a cerebrovascular accident that left her paralyzed on the right side. The family has been told the client can be cared for at home if sufficient help can be obtained, or she can be placed in a nursing home. The siblings cannot make up their minds. The nurse could be helpful by
    1. making the decision for the family.
    2. encouraging the client to make the decision.
    3. reporting the situation to the elder abuse hotline.
    4. helping the family clarify the advantages and disadvantages of each option.

Answer: 4
Rationale: Decision making requires accurate information and understanding of choices. The other options are inappropriate.
Cognitive level: Application
Nursing process: Implementation
NCLEX: Psychosocial Integrity
See text page: 596

13. Which client would the nurse assess as being at greatest risk for becoming noncompliant with his or her treatment recommendations?
    1. G, who has diabetic neuropathy and depression
    2. H, who has had a mild stroke and arteriosclerosis
    3. I, who has chronic obstructive pulmonary disease and altered role performance
    4. J, who has unstable angina and type 2 diabetes

Chapter 29   Psychological Needs of the Medically Ill

Answer: 1

Rationale: Evidence tells us that comorbid depression creates increased risk for noncompliance with the medical regimen. The other comorbidities have not been investigated for increased risk of noncompliance.

Cognitive level: Analysis
Nursing process: Assessment
NCLEX: Psychosocial Integrity
See text page: 590

14. A client with amyotropic lateral sclerosis is becoming increasingly debilitated. Recently, he told the nurse "It bothers me that I cannot get to church anymore. Since I have not been able to get to services, I feel out of touch with God. I pray but I wonder if my prayers are heard." The nurse should consider the nursing diagnosis of
   1. powerlessness.
   2. death anxiety.
   3. spiritual distress.
   4. disturbed thought processes.

Answer: 3

Rationale: The client is verbalizing his concern about his relationship with God and his inability to participate in religious services. Both are defining characteristics for the nursing diagnosis of spiritual distress. Data are not present to suggest the other nursing diagnoses.

Cognitive level: Analysis
Nursing process: Diagnosis
NCLEX: Psychosocial Integrity
See text pages: 593, 594

15. A client has spastic lower limbs and bouts of severe pain. A nursing intervention useful for helping the client learn to manage the pain would be
   1. teaching relaxation techniques.
   2. using cognitive behavior therapy.
   3. performing a holistic lifestyle assessment.
   4. obtaining an overall quality-of-life assessment.

Answer: 1

Rationale: Relaxation techniques can be helpful in diminishing pain perception and reactions to pain. Option 2: Cognitive behavior therapy may be useful to the client but would not be a nursing intervention that can be independently initiated by a basic level nurse. Options 3 and 4 refer to assessments rather than intervention.

Cognitive level: Application
Nursing process: Planning
NCLEX: Physiological Integrity
See text page: 597

16. The client who would probably require long-term intervention to promote adaptation to his or her medical condition is
   1. M, who has had a negative scalene node biopsy.
   2. N, who has bacterial pneumonia.
   3. O, who has Crohn's disease.
   4. P, who has gout.

Answer: 3

Rationale: O has a chronic debilitating disease that may, at some point, require surgical treatment that will cause body image change. Option 1: M's surgery has provided good news. Option 2: N's illness is considered a short-term acute infection. Option 4: P's illness is chronic but is neither threatening to life nor causative of major lifestyle change.

Cognitive level: Analysis
Nursing process: Assessment
NCLEX: Psychosocial Integrity
See text page: 588

17. Which client, waiting to be seen in the emergency department, is at greatest risk for stigmatization by health care personnel?
   1. Q, a student who is a victim of date rape
   2. R, a street addict who has cellulitis caused by dirty needles
   3. S, a visitor from Canada who has acute abdominal pain of unknown origin
   4. T, a housewife whose husband beat her during a domestic dispute

Answer: 2

Rationale: The greater the client's disenfranchisement, the greater the possibility for stigmatization. The lifestyle of street addicts is seen by medical staff as undesirable, hence they are often stigmatized as "bad." At best, they are labeled as psychiatric clients, misfits, or losers. The are apt to be avoided and receive less-than-optimal care. The other clients described in the options would receive adequate responses from the health care team.

Cognitive level: Analysis
Nursing process: Assessment
NCLEX: Psychosocial Integrity
See text pages: 597, 598

18. An unconscious client is brought to the emergency department by ambulance for trauma treatment. The client is wearing a cocktail dress, high heels, and a wig, but on close inspection has facial and body hair consistent with being male. Further inspection determines that the client is male. Several staff laugh and make remarks about transvestism as they stabilize the client. The most appropriate action for the nurse is to say

1. "Your focus should be treatment, not ridicule."
2. "Each client deserves our respect."
3. "Your behavior constitutes client abuse."
4. "Grow up, you have seen this before."

Answer: 2

Rationale: The scenario is an example of a stigmatization of a medically ill client. The nurse should advocate for the client in this situation. Option 2 is a simple, straightforward reminder of the need to respect the dignity of each individual. Remembering that clients who are unconscious may still be able to hear should cause the nurse to attempt to immediately put an end to the negative comments being made without being argumentative or accusative.

Cognitive level: Application
Nursing process: Implementation
NCLEX: Psychosocial Integrity
See text pages: 597, 598

19. During the psychosocial assessment the nurse determines that a client who is HIV positive believes his family is "burned out" and has little energy left to provide care for him as his condition worsens. He mentions that they maintain communication with him and express concern for him but find it difficult to listen as he speaks of his anxieties and concerns regarding dying. The nurse should assess family support as
   1. rarely demonstrated.
   2. sometimes demonstrated.
   3. often demonstrated.
   4. consistently demonstrated.

Answer: 2

Rationale: Maintaining communication and expressing concern suggest that the support is sometimes demonstrated. Other needs such as providing physical care and bearing painful feelings are not met; thus options 3 and 4 are not appropriate choices.

Cognitive level: Analysis
Nursing process: Assessment
NCLEX: Psychosocial Integrity
See text pages: 594, 595

20. A client who has been diagnosed with polymyalgia rheumatica has muscle pain and weakness and has curtailed physical and social activities to accommodate her condition. She tells the nurse "I cannot do anything. I have to depend on other people to help me. I do not enjoy much of anything any more; even food does not taste good. I cannot see that my situation will change, so I feel pretty hopeless." The priority action the nurse should take is to
   1. point out positive aspects of the client's situation.
   2. discuss the importance of physical exercise.

3. inquire about her social support system.
4. assess for depression.

Answer: 4

Rationale: The client has given several indications that she may be depressed. A thorough assessment for depression should be completed. Depression that goes unrecognized and untreated is often responsible for worsening the medical condition and diminishing functional abilities. Depression also presents a risk factor for nonadherence to the treatment plan. The other options do not address the leads the client has given.

Cognitive level: Analysis
Nursing process: Implementation
NCLEX: Psychosocial Integrity
See text page: 590

21. A client who has been diagnosed with breast cancer has many questions related to surgery, radiation therapy, and chemotherapy. The nurse provides education about the disease and treatments but perceives that the client has further questions about coping with day-to-day situations. The action of greatest benefit to the client would be
   1. suggesting cognitive-behavioral therapy.
   2. teaching her to monitor her stress level.
   3. suggesting she enroll in a pain management program.
   4. referring her to a support group for individuals with breast cancer.

Answer: 4

Rationale: Clients with breast cancer are often helped by the support and knowledge shared in support group meetings. Techniques for coping can be learned from women who have had similar experiences. Option 1: There is no indication that the client is demonstrating negative cognitions. Option 2: Monitoring stress level is insufficient. The client would also need to be taught stress management techniques. Option 3: Pain management is not currently indicated.

Cognitive level: Analysis
Nursing process: Implementation
NCLEX: Psychosocial Integrity
See text page: 596

22. A client being treated for a myocardial infarction has been transferred to a step-down unit from the intensive care unit. She uses the call bell as often as every 15 minutes. She makes a seemingly small request or complains each time a staff member is summoned. Several staff tell the primary nurse that the client is "obnoxious" and that they feel inadequate

413

because they can never seem to satisfy her needs. The primary nurse can be most helpful by
1. explaining that the client's anxiety is being demonstrated by demanding behaviors.
2. "laying down the law" to the client and saying she may use the call light once hourly.
3. rotating caregivers each day to give staff a much-needed respite from her complaints.
4. offering to co-assign an agency temporary nurse to the client to share the burden.

Answer: 1

Rationale: Teaching staff the probable basis for the behavior will change their perspective. They will realize the problem is anxiety expressed as self-centeredness, rather than perversity, and that they are not inadequate to the task of lowering the client's anxiety. They must address the anxiety rather than the complaints. Option 2 will only increase the client's anxiety. Options 3 and 4 do not address the client's real need for anxiety reduction.

Cognitive level: Analysis
Nursing process: Implementation
NCLEX: Physiological Integrity
See text pages: 590, 592

23. A client being treated for a myocardial infarction has been transferred from the intensive care unit to a step-down unit. She uses the call bell as often as every 15 minutes. She makes a seemingly small request or complains each time a staff member is summoned. Several staff tell the primary nurse that the client is "obnoxious" and that they feel inadequate because they can never seem to satisfy her needs. The primary nurse decides to intervene directly with the client. The most appropriate way to begin problem solving would be to say
1. "I am wondering if you are feeling anxious about your condition and being left alone."
2. "The staff are concerned that you are not satisfied with the care you are receiving."
3. "Let's talk about why you use your call light so frequently."
4. "I think you are giving staff a negative message."

Answer: 1

Rationale: This opening conveys the nurse's willingness to listen to the client's feelings and an understanding of the commonly seen concern about not having a nurse always nearby as in the intensive care unit. Verbalization is an effective outlet for anxiety. Also, knowing that staff understand her anxiety and will meet her needs without being summoned so frequently can reduce the client's anxiety level from severe to moderate or lower.

Cognitive level: Analysis

Nursing process: Implementation
NCLEX: Psychosocial Integrity
See text pages: 590, 592

24. A client being treated for a myocardial infarction has been transferred from the intensive care unit to a step-down unit. She uses the call bell as often as every 15 minutes and makes a seemingly small request or complains each time the staff member enters the room. Several staff tell the primary nurse that the client is "obnoxious" and that they feel inadequate because they can never seem to satisfy her needs. The best indicator to monitor for the outcome of anxiety self-control is that the client will
1. monitor duration of episodes of anxiety.
2. maintain adequate sleep of 7 hours nightly.
3. maintain social relationships and role performance.
4. control anxiety response by using call bell appropriately.

Answer: 4

Rationale: This indicator is directly related to the behavior described in the scenario. The other indicators are not as indicative of improvement in self-control in the area identified in the scenario.

Cognitive level: Analysis
Nursing process: Planning (Outcome Identification)
NCLEX: Psychosocial Integrity
See text pages: 590, 592

25. A client with diabetes and coronary artery disease asks health care staff and family what they think she should do each time a decision is to be made. She often fails to follow therapeutic advice after seeking professional opinions. On the basis of this information, the information that would be found on axis III of the *DSM-IV-TR* would be
1. diabetes and coronary artery disease.
2. dependent personality.
3. maladaptive health behaviors: high-fat diet, lack of exercise.
4. persistent failure to follow professional advice of health care staff.

Answer: 3

Rationale: This option identifies maladaptive health behaviors in which the client engages that have an impact on the medical conditions identified on axis I. Option 1: This information would be found on axis I. Option 2: This information would be found on axis II. Option 4 is not an appropriate statement for axis III.

Cognitive level: Application
Nursing process: Assessment
NCLEX: Safe and Effective Care Environment
See text page: 588

26. In planning client education relating to coping with stents inserted to treat coronary disease, the nurse should include (more than one answer may be correct)
  1. specific information about the client's condition.
  2. caution to keep a tight rein on expression of emotions.
  3. the need to self-monitor for anxiety and depression.
  4. the need to adhere to good general health practices.

Answers: 1, 3, 4
Rationale: Option 1: Knowledge reduces anxiety and allows the client to understand options and make appropriate decisions. Option 3: Self-assessment of mood and emotions allows the client to seek help if depression or anxiety occur. Option 4: Good health practices promote general health, a sense of well-being, and a healthy immune system. Option 2: Expressing feelings by sharing them with a supportive person or writing a journal should be encouraged in the teaching sessions.
Cognitive level: Application
Nursing process: Planning
NCLEX: Health Promotion and Maintenance
See text page: 597

27. The nurse sees a client with coronary artery disease 3 months after stenting. The client states he is doing "great." He indicates he has read of the benefits of alcohol on coronary artery disease and has incorporated this theory into his lifestyle. When asked describe his lifestyle, he mentions he arises at 9 AM, has a bloody Mary, works at his computer until lunch and again after lunch, enjoys "a couple of Manhattans" before dinner, has a good dinner with some red wine and then finishes the bottle of wine during the evening. The nurse can make the assessment that the client is
  1. at risk for substance abuse disorder.
  2. grieving for lost abilities.
  3. self-medicating for anxiety.
  4. using protective denial.

Answer: 1
Rationale: The client is drinking excessively and is at risk for developing alcoholism. The scenario does not provide data to suggest that any of the other options is correct.
Cognitive level: Analysis
Nursing process: Assessment
NCLEX: Physiological Integrity
See text page: 592

CHAPTER 30

1. A client, aged 54 years, confides to a nurse "I found a lump in my neck and now they tell me I have an incurable disease. I cannot believe it. I am too young to die." The client's reaction shows the pattern of response called
  1. restitution.
  2. shock and denial.
  3. somatic distress.
  4. reorganization.

Answer: 2
Rationale: The reaction described is shock and disbelief, in which denial acts as a buffer against the pain of acknowledgment. Options 1 and 4: Restitution and reorganization both imply healing or wellness. Option 3: Somatic distress would involve client display of bodily symptoms.
Cognitive level: Analysis
Nursing process: Assessment
NCLEX: Psychosocial Integrity
See text page: 614

2. A client's fiancée died in an auto accident several days ago. She finds herself crying and experiencing feelings of guilt and anger. The nurse can assess this behavior as characteristic of the stage of acute grief called
  1. reorganization.
  2. denial.
  3. developing awareness.
  4. preoccupation with the lost object.

Answer: 3
Rationale: As denial fades, awareness of the finality of loss develops and is accompanied by painful feelings of loss, anger with others, and guilt for taking or not taking specific actions. Reorganization implies movement toward healing. Denial is manifested by the inability to believe the reality of an event. Preoccupation with the lost object would involve the client dwelling on thoughts of the deceased.
Cognitive level: Application
Nursing process: Assessment
NCLEX: Psychosocial Integrity
See text page: 614

3. For several days after her husband's death, a client repeats over and over "I should have made him go to the doctor when he said he did not feel good." It can be assessed that the individual is experiencing
  1. preoccupation with the image of the deceased.
  2. sensations of somatic distress.

415

3. anger.
4. guilt.

Answer: 4

Rationale: Guilt is expressed by the bereaved person's self-reproach. Option 1: Preoccupation refers to dwelling on images of the deceased. Option 2: Somatic distress would involve bodily symptoms. Option 3: Anger cannot be assessed from data given in the scenario.

Cognitive level: Application
Nursing process: Assessment
NCLEX: Psychosocial Integrity
See text page: 615

4. A widower for a year and a half tells his friends "I think I will begin to go out socially, maybe even take someone out to dinner. I am beginning to feel more like being with other people." This phenomenon suggests that the individual is
1. accepting the reality of his loss.
2. working through his grief.
3. adjusting to being alone.
4. ready to reinvest in new relationships.

Answer: 4

Rationale: Toward the end of the grief process, the person renews interest in people and activities. At the same time, the person is released from the relationship with the deceased. Option 1: The client has progressed beyond this point. Option 2: The client has progressed beyond grief. Option 3: The client is seeking to move into new relationships so that he is not alone.

Cognitive level: Application
Nursing process: Assessment
NCLEX: Psychosocial Integrity
See text page: 615

5. After the death of his wife, a man tells the nurse "I can never live without her. She was my whole life." The most therapeutic reply for the nurse to make is
1. "Remember, she is no longer suffering."
2. "Her death is a terrible loss for you."
3. "Each day will get a little better."
4. "Your friends will help you cope with this."

Answer: 2

Rationale: A statement that validates the bereaved person's loss is more helpful than banalities and clichés. It signifies understanding. The other options are clichés.

Cognitive level: Application
Nursing process: Implementation
NCLEX: Psychosocial Integrity
See text page: 617

6. A woman has just received the news that her husband died. She approaches the nurse who cared for him during his last hours and says angrily "If you had given him your undivided attention instead of running off to care for others, he would still be alive." The nurse's response should consider that
1. the client is warning staff of a malpractice suit.
2. anger is a phenomenon that is experienced during grieving.
3. the client had ambivalent feelings about her husband.
4. in some cultures, grief is expressed solely through anger.

Answer: 2

Rationale: Anger may protect the bereaved from facing the devastating reality of loss. Anger expressed during mourning is not directed toward the nurse personally, even though accusations and blame may make her feel as though it is. Option 1 is somewhat unlikely because the angry feelings are likely to subside. Option 3: Data are not present to warrant this conclusion. Option 4: This is not a true statement.

Cognitive level: Application
Nursing process: Implementation
NCLEX: Psychosocial Integrity
See text page: 615

7. A wife has just received the news that her husband died of heart failure. She has called her family to come to the hospital. She approaches the nurse who cared for her husband during his last hours and, in the middle of the corridor, shouts angrily "If you had given him your undivided attention instead of running off to care for others, he would still be alive." The best response for the nurse to make would be
1. "You are mistaken. Your husband's heart was so severely damaged that it could no longer pump."
2. "I will call my supervisor to discuss this matter with you."
3. "I understand you are feeling very upset. Let's go into this room and I will stay with you until your family comes."
4. "It will be all right if you give in and cry."

Answer: 3

Rationale: When bereaved family behaves in a disturbed manner, the nurse should show patience and tact while offering sympathy and warmth. Option 1 is defensive. Option 2 is evasive. Option 4 is placating.

Cognitive level: Application
Nursing process: Implementation
NCLEX: Psychosocial Integrity
See text page: 604

8. A client who was widowed 18 months ago tells the nurse "I have gotten to the point that I can remember the good times my wife and I shared without getting a lump in my throat. Sometimes I even think about the disappointments, like not having children. I have gotten used to being without her by my side." The nurse can make the evaluation that the work of mourning
  1. is beginning.
  2. is progressing abnormally.
  3. is at or near completion.
  4. has not begun.

Answer: 3
Rationale: The work of mourning has been successfully completed when the bereaved can remember both positive and the negative memories about the deceased and when the task of restructuring the relationship with the deceased is completed.
Cognitive level: Evaluation
Nursing process: Evaluation
NCLEX: Psychosocial Integrity
See text page: 616

9. The nurse can anticipate that the mourning process will be more difficult when the bereaved
  1. was relatively independent of the deceased.
  2. had few unresolved conflicts in the relationship with the deceased.
  3. has a good support system with meaningful relationships evident.
  4. has experienced a number of previous losses.

Answer: 4
Rationale: The following factors have negative effects on the mourning process: high dependency on the deceased, ambivalence toward the deceased, a poor or absent support system, a high number of past losses or other recent losses, poor physical or mental health, and young age of the deceased. Data do not support the other options.
Cognitive level: Application
Nursing process: Planning
NCLEX: Psychosocial Integrity
See text pages: 617, 618

10. For planning purposes nurses should understand task-based models of mourning because such models
  1. provide guidelines to help those who are coping with mourning.
  2. explain cultural variations in the expression of grief.
  3. identify factors that affect the successful completion of mourning.
  4. identify the role played by delayed grief and unresolved grief in mental health.

Answer: 1
Rationale: Having a task-based model offers a framework that incorporates diverse coping skills that can be identified and taught. A task-based theory does not explain cultural variations or the origins of unresolved or delayed grief, and it does not cite factors that interfere with successful mourning.
Cognitive level: Application
Nursing process: Planning
NCLEX: Psychosocial Integrity
See text pages: 613, 614

11. A 60-year-old retiree was awakened early one morning by a police officer who informed her that her husband had died while jogging. The next 3 days the widow went through the funeral ritual in a state of numbness. Several of her friends tried to get her to vent her feelings by crying. Which statements offer plausible explanations for the widow's inability to cry? (More than one answer may be correct.)
  1. The acute stage of grief involves shock and disbelief that may last for several days.
  2. Culture is a determinant of grief responses. Some groups view emotional displays negatively.
  3. Psychologically unhealthy individuals are likely to have atypical grief reactions.
  4. The unconscious use of denial is considered normal for several days after a loss. It protects the individual from the intolerable pain of loss.

Answers: 1, 2, 4
Rationale: Options 1, 2, and 4 are true statements with relevance to the scenario. Option 3: This statement is not based on fact. It has no relevance to the individual's inability to cry during the initial stage of grieving, which is marked by shock, disbelief, and denial.
Cognitive level: Analysis
Nursing process: Assessment
NCLEX: Psychosocial Integrity
See text page: 614

12. A woman learned that her husband had died while jogging in the early morning. Two weeks later, the widow went to visit her late husband's doctor. While waiting to see the doctor, the nurse converses with her. An appropriate statement for the nurse to make would be
  1. "At least your husband did not suffer."
  2. "It is better to go quickly as your husband did."
  3. "Your husband's loss must be very painful for you."
  4. "You'll begin to feel better after you get over the shock."

Answer: 3
Rationale: The most helpful responses by others validate the bereaved's experience of loss. Banalities should

417

be avoided because they increase the individual's sense of isolation.
Cognitive level: Application
Nursing process: Implementation
NCLEX: Psychosocial Integrity
See text page: 617

13. A recently widowed client tells the doctor that she has a great deal of discomfort in the epigastric region. She adds "I wonder if I have an ulcer." The diagnostic tests are negative. The nurse assesses the symptom as
   1. preoccupation with the deceased.
   2. disorganization and depression.
   3. early reorganization behavior.
   4. a normal phenomenon of mourning.

Answer: 4
Rationale: Sensations of somatic distress are often experienced during the acute stage of grieving. They include tightness in the throat, shortness of breath, exhaustion, and pain or sensations such as those experienced by the dead person.
Cognitive level: Application
Nursing process: Assessment
NCLEX: Psychosocial Integrity
See text page: 615

14. Which behavior would the nurse evaluate as indicating successful completion of a bereaved individual's grieving process?
   1. After 15 months, the widow realistically remembers both the pleasures and disappointments of her relationship with her husband.
   2. Three years after her husband's death, the widow talks about her husband as if he were alive, then weeps when others mention his name.
   3. For 2 years after her husband's death, the widow has kept his belongings in their usual places.
   4. Eighteen months after her husband's death, the widow states she has never cried or experienced feelings of loss even though they were very close.

Answer: 1
Rationale: The work of grieving is over when the bereaved can remember the individual realistically and acknowledge both the pleasure and disappointments associated with the loved one. The individual is then free to enter into new relationships and activities. The other options suggest unresolved grief.
Cognitive level: Evaluation
Nursing process: Evaluation
NCLEX: Psychosocial Integrity
See text page: 616

15. Which actions by the nurse would contribute to protecting the rights of a client who is terminally ill with lymphoma? (More than one answer may be correct.)
   1. Providing interventions that convey respect
   2. Giving choices and fostering personal control
   3. Supporting the client's quest for spiritual growth
   4. Maintaining the pose that his prognosis is positive

Answers: 1, 2, 3
Rationale: Options 1, 2, and 3 support the rights of the dying individual. Option 4: Acting on false information robs a client of the opportunity for honest dialogue and places barriers to achieving end-of-life developmental opportunities.
Cognitive level: Analysis
Nursing process: Implementation
NCLEX: Psychosocial Integrity
See text pages: 601, 602

16. A hospice nurse is asked by another nurse "Who should be referred for hospice care?" The best reply would be
   1. "Clients in the end stage of any disease are eligible."
   2. "Hospice is primarily for terminally ill cancer sufferers."
   3. "We are best equipped to care for clients with end-stage renal disease."
   4. "Clients with progressive neurological disease can be admitted once respiration is affected."

Answer: 1
Rationale: A hospice cares for terminally ill clients regardless of diagnosis.
Cognitive level: Application
Nursing process: Implementation
NCLEX: Safe and Effective Care Environment
See text pages: 602, 603

17. A newly admitted hospice client tells the nurse "I am dying, but I am still living. I want to be in control as long as I possibly can be." A reply that indicates the nurse was actively listening is
   1. "Our staff will do the best they can to make you feel comfortable."
   2. "Most people do not know what to do to help. Try not to be hard on them."
   3. "You want people to stop focusing exclusively on your weaknesses."
   4. "Your mind and spirit are healthy, although your body is weak."

Answer: 4
Rationale: The client is asking for acknowledgment that he is not totally sick, that even in his terminal state

418

he has strengths and capabilities. Option 4 provides that acknowledgment. The other responses are tangential.
Cognitive level: Application
Nursing process: Implementation
NCLEX: Psychosocial Integrity
See text pages: 616-618

18. A terminally ill client receiving palliative care tells the nurse "I know I am not going to get well... but still..." His voice trails off. A therapeutic response would be
   1. "What are you hoping for?"
   2. "No, you are not going to get well."
   3. "Do you have questions about what is happening?"
   4. "When you have questions, it is best to talk to the doctor."

Answer: 1
Rationale: This open-ended response is an example of following the client's lead. It provides an opportunity for the client to speak about whatever is on his mind. Option 2 may block further communication. Option 3 refocuses the conversation. Option 4 gives advice and suggests the nurse is uncomfortable with the topic.
Cognitive level: Application
Nursing process: Implementation
NCLEX: Psychosocial Integrity
See text page: 604

19. A wife whose husband is terminally ill tells the nurse "I do not want to cry in front of my husband. I do not want him to know how close he is to death or how sad I am." A therapeutic response would be
   1. "You are right to protect him at a time when he is so vulnerable."
   2. "You need to consider the fact that time is running out."
   3. "He might be more reassured than disturbed by your tears."
   4. "You definitely need to be honest about your feelings."

Answer: 3
Rationale: Many people try to protect the dying person from experiencing emotions; however, emotional honesty is important to both the client and the family. The client may be reassured knowing that the family is facing the inevitable. Giving advice and making judgmental statements are not helpful.
Cognitive level: Application
Nursing process: Implementation
NCLEX: Psychosocial Integrity
See text pages: 604, 607, 608

20. A husband asks the nurse what he can say or do when his terminally ill wife mentions that she will soon die. The nurse could suggest that he say
   1. "I think you will be around for a long time yet."
   2. "I do not want you to give up trying to get well."
   3. "I do not think I am ready to talk about this yet."
   4. "I feel so sad when I think of life without you."

Answer: 4
Rationale: This response is emotionally honest. It will allow both husband and wife the opportunity to express emotions and further resolve issues in the relationship and explore end-of-life developmental opportunities for the wife. The other options are evasive.
Cognitive level: Application
Nursing process: Implementation
NCLEX: Psychosocial Integrity
See text pages: 604, 608-610

21. As death approaches, a client terminally ill with AIDS tells the nurse "I really do not want to see a lot of visitors anymore. Just my parents and Jim can come in for a while each day." What action should the nurse take?
   1. Discuss this with the parents and Jim and suggest that they explain the client's decision to his friends.
   2. Ask the client to reconsider his decision because he has many interested friends.
   3. Suggest that the client discuss his wishes with his physician.
   4. Place a "no visitors" sign on his door.

Answer: 1
Rationale: As many clients approach death, they begin to withdraw. In the stage of acceptance, many clients are exhausted and tired, and interactions of a social nature are a burden. Many prefer to have someone present at the bedside who will sit without talking constantly. Options 2 and 3 imply the client should revise his position. Option 4 could keep out the visitors the client actually wants to see.
Cognitive level: Application
Nursing process: Implementation
NCLEX: Safe and Effective Care Environment
See text pages: 607, 608

22. The clinical nurse leader notices that staff spend minimal time with a client who is terminally ill with AIDS. The client confides in the nurse leader that he is having intense emotional reactions to his illness, sometimes feeling angry, sometimes afraid, sometimes feeling abandoned. As the nurse leader considers how to approach the problem of client avoid-

419

Chapter 30   Care for the Dying and for Those Who Grieve

ance with staff, he can hypothesize that the most likely reason for the staff's avoidance is
1. the need to use extra infection control precautions.
2. feelings of inadequacy in dealing with complex emotional needs.
3. knowledge that the client needs time alone with family and friends.
4. disapproval of the client's former high-risk lifestyle.

Answer: 2

Rationale: Many nurses tend to be more comfortable with meeting physical needs than in focusing on emotional needs. Option 1 is not an acceptable answer because universal precautions are necessary for all clients. Option 3 assumes friends and family are available to the client, which might not be true. Option 4 assumes the client led a high-risk lifestyle, which might not be accurate.

Cognitive level: Application
Nursing process: Assessment
NCLEX: Safe and Effective Care Environment
See text pages: 612, 613

23. The statements by a client that would give the nurse information that pertains to spiritual assessment include (more than one answer may be correct)
    1. "I think I can trust the doctor to prescribe enough medication to keep me comfortable in the days to come."
    2. "I have prepared advance directives to spare my children the need to make difficult decisions."
    3. "I plan to use these last weeks to experience the process of dying as fully as I experienced the richness of living."
    4. "I find that listening to hymns helps deepen my relaxation and the relief I get from my pain medication."

Answers: 3, 4

Rationale: Option 3 suggests the individual will find meaning in the process of dying as he or she has found growth potential in all life's events. This equates to the motif identified as "quest." Option 4 identifies an activity that connects the client to his or her beliefs and is helpful in calming anxieties. The other options are not as directly related to spiritual aspects.

Cognitive level: Analysis
Nursing process: Assessment
NCLEX: Psychosocial Integrity
See text page: 605

24. A terminally ill client is described by her family as "strong." The client tells the nurse that her life has been good. She is proud of being self-educated and rising to the top of her profession. She states she has overcome many adversities by the sheer force of willpower and that her philosophy of giving the best and expecting things to turn out well has been effective. She adds "I intend to die as I lived: optimistic." From this, the nurse planning care for the client would assess a critical need to
1. provide aggressive pain and symptom management.
2. help the client reassess and explore existing conflicts.
3. assist the client to focus on the meaning in life and death.
4. support the client's use of her own resources to meet challenges.

Answer: 4

Rationale: The client whose intrinsic strength and endurance have been a hallmark often wishes to approach dying by staying optimistic and in control. Helping the client use her own resources to meet challenges would be appropriate. Option 1 is important for all clients, but less of a factor than supporting use of the client's own strengths. Options 2 and 3: This client would not find these activities particularly meaningful.

Cognitive level: Analysis
Nursing process: Planning
NCLEX: Psychosocial Integrity
See text pages: 611, 612

25. The wife of a client being cared for in hospice has begun to "micromanage" the client's care, seeing to each and every detail herself. She angrily tells the hospice nurse the care the hospice aide and other family members provide leaves the client uncomfortable, so she must do everything herself. She asks "Why is this happening? Why can't someone help before I go crazy?" The hospice nurse should
1. provide teaching about anticipatory grieving.
2. refer the client for crisis intervention.
3. assign new hospice personnel to the case.
4. arrange for hospitalization for the client.

Answer: 1

Rationale: The behaviors described in the scenario are consistent with anticipatory grieving. The client needs to receive education about the process of anticipatory grieving and counseling to validate what she is experiencing and enhance coping with the physical, emotional, and cognitive symptoms she is experiencing. The other options are not appropriate to the situation.

Cognitive level: Analysis
Nursing process: Implementation
NCLEX: Health Promotion and Maintenance
See text pages: 607, 608

26. As the hospice nurse begins work with a terminally ill client and his family, an important self-care action for her to take during the first encounters is to
    1. provide the family with her home phone number to facilitate after-hours contact.
    2. clearly state both what she can do and what her professional limitations are.
    3. resolve not to become emotionally involved with the client or the family.
    4. encourage the family to consent to the dying of their loved one.

Answer: 2

Rationale: This action protects both the client and the nurse. The client can formulate appropriate expectations and the nurse is helped to avoid overinvolvement. The action facilitates self-care by the health professional. Option 1 promotes unrealistic expectations that the nurse is available at all hours. Option 3 is easier said than done. Emotional involvement is inevitable in hospice nursing. Option 4: This measure is not a self-care action, and the first meeting is too early to accomplish the task.

Options do not facilitate self care.

Cognitive level: Application
Nursing process: Implementation
NCLEX: Safe and Effective Care Environment
See text page: 610

27. The children of a widow confer with the bereavement nurse because their mother persists in repeatedly telling people the details of finding her husband not breathing, performing CPR, and going to the emergency department with him by ambulance and seeing him pronounced dead. The family are concerned that this is traumatic to those who have to hear the story and ask what they can do. The nurse should counsel the family that
    1. they can interpret their feelings to their mother and ask for a change in behavior.
    2. the retelling should be limited to once daily to avoid unnecessary stimulation.
    3. repeating the story and her feelings is a helpful and necessary part of grieving.
    4. retelling of memories is to be expected as part of the aging process.

Answer: 3

Rationale: Nurses are encouraged to tell bereaved clients that telling the personal story of loss as many times as needed is acceptable and healthy because repetition is a helpful and necessary part of grieving. Options 1 and 2 would not be helpful because they limit the expression of feelings. Option 4 is not a true or relevant statement.

Cognitive level: Application
Nursing process: Implementation
NCLEX: Health Promotion and Maintenance
See text page: 618

28. A client grieving her husband's sudden death tells the bereavement nurse "I am not feeling very well. Yesterday, I was sitting in my kitchen and a saw my husband walk through the door and stop and smile at me. Then he just faded away. I think I must be going crazy." The most appropriate action for the nurse to take is to
    1. assess for recent substance use.
    2. suggest a referral to the mental health clinic.
    3. arrange for a prescription for risperidone.
    4. counsel that visualizations are a normal part of grieving.

Answer: 4

Rationale: Grieving clients often dream about, visualize, think about, or search for the lost loved one. The client should be told that this is considered a normal phenomenon and not a sign of mental illness. Option 1: Visualization does not suggest substance use in this case. Option 2: This is premature because visualization is normal. Option 3: This is inappropriate because the client is not mentally ill.

Cognitive level: Analysis
Nursing process: Implementation
NCLEX: Health Promotion and Maintenance
See text page: 618

29. A grieving client tells the nurse "It has been 8 months since my husband died. I thought I would be feeling better by this time, but lately I have felt worse. I have no energy. I feel lonely, but I do not want to be around people. What should I do?" The best counsel would be to
    1. attend a bereavement group.
    2. become active in a church.
    3. seek psychotherapy.
    4. understand this is normal.

Answer: 4

Rationale: The client needs understanding and support that her feelings are normal. Although feelings of depression generally decline over the period of a year after the death of a loved one, the decline is not linear. Loneliness and aimlessness are most pronounced 6 to 9 months after the death. The client should be given this and other information about phenomena experienced during bereavement if she has not already received it. If it has been previously given, the information should be reinforced and the

client given understanding and support. The other options are not clearly indicated.
Cognitive level: Analysis
Nursing process: Implementation
NCLEX: Health Promotion and Maintenance
See text page: 615

30. Soon after leaving nursing school a nurse cared for a terminally ill client over a period of a month. The nurse found that she looked forward to spending time with this client. When the client died, the nurse realized that she experienced feelings of sadness. As time went on, the nurse found herself sleeping poorly, lacking energy, and feeling mildly depressed. Eventually the nurse explained her feelings to her mentor. The mentor should counsel the nurse
   1. about stress reduction strategies.
   2. to seek therapy for dysfunctional grief.
   3. about the experience of disenfranchised grief.
   4. to consider taking a leave of absence to pursue healing.

Answer: 3
Rationale: The nurse is experiencing disenfranchised grief. Nurses often incur loss that is not openly acknowledged or publicly mourned. Loss of a client may not be recognized or acknowledged by others, so the grief is solitary and uncomforted and may be difficult to resolve. Option 1 does not address the actual problem. Option 2: The grief is not dysfunctional. Option 4 is inappropriate.
Cognitive level: Application
Nursing process: Implementation
NCLEX: Health Promotion and Maintenance
See text page: 613

CHAPTER 31

1. An individual with severe and persistent paranoid schizophrenia killed a homeless man when his auditory hallucinations commanded him to do so. He was found not guilty by reason of insanity. The forensic nurse understands that the best placement for the individual would be to be
   1. released into the community without supervision.
   2. sent to a forensic unit in the state prison system.
   3. admitted to the inpatient unit at a community mental health center.
   4. incarcerated in a state prison.

Answer: 2
Rationale: The individual who responds to command hallucinations is too dangerous to be released into the community but too ill to be held within the general population of the state prison system. A forensic unit would provide the needed treatment and confinement.
Cognitive level: Application
Nursing process: Planning
NCLEX: Safe and Effective Care Environment
See text pages: 625, 626

2. A prison inmate has paranoid schizophrenia, for which he is given fluphenazine. He meets with a small group of inmates and the correctional mental health nurse to talk about problems with returning to the community. This inmate and several others speak openly of abusing alcohol when they are living in the community. The nurse should plan to
   1. continue to focus on problems anticipated by the group when released.
   2. advocate in the prison system for treatment for prisoners with dual diagnosis.
   3. suggest the prisoners keep in mind joining AA on release.
   4. recognize the probability of reincarceration for the inmate.

Answer: 2
Rationale: The need for treatment for prisoners with dual diagnosis is great. Currently only a few such programs exist. A poor outcome can be anticipated unless both diagnoses are addressed. Option 1: This is not optimal. Option 3: Dual diagnosis treatment would be a better solution. Option 4: Planning an intervention would be more helpful.
Cognitive level: Application
Nursing process: Planning
NCLEX: Psychosocial Integrity
See text pages: 625, 626

3. The correctional mental health nurse learns that an inmate with bipolar II disorder ran out of lithium and did not seek an additional supply, leading to a relapse. When the individual was psychotic she assaulted several people in a convenience store. She was arrested, tried, convicted, and sentenced. An outcome the nurse and the inmate might establish is that by release the inmate will
   1. be agreeable to taking lithium.
   2. identify community resources for obtaining medication.
   3. understand that physical assault violates the rights of others.
   4. agree to maintain contact with the nurse after discharge.

Answer: 2
Rationale: The individual should become aware of community resources that can be accessed for ongoing

treatment, medication refills, and crisis intervention once she is released from the correctional facility. Option 1 is insufficient in scope because the individual has no objection to taking lithium when it is available. Option 3 is not directly related to the problem of medication availability. Option 4 is not appropriate.
Cognitive level: Analysis
Nursing process: Planning (Outcome Identification)
NCLEX: Health Promotion and Maintenance
See text pages: 625, 626

4. The correctional mental health nurse assesses a new prisoner who is beginning his incarceration for committing a sex crime. The prisoner speaks in a low voice, is tearful, and tells the nurse that his life may as well be over as there is no hope that he will ever be able to fit into society after he is released from prison. He states his family has disowned him and that wherever he goes his reputation will follow him. The priority intervention would be to
   1. arrange to meet with him weekly to discuss feelings.
   2. offer to contact his family to speak of his remorse.
   3. advise the guards to place him in solitary confinement.
   4. arrange to implement suicide precautions.

Answer: 4
Rationale: Suicide attempts are often made in prison. The inmate shows evidence of hopelessness, an important predictor of suicide. Options 1, 2, 3: Safety is the primary issue. None of these options is appropriate relative to suicide prevention.
Cognitive level: Application
Nursing process: Implementation
NCLEX: Safe and Effective Care Environment
See text pages: 625, 626

5. A correctional mental health nurse working in the jail of a large city assesses new inmates with symptoms of psychiatric disorder and those who report that they currently take psychotropic medication. Because of the high number of newly incarcerated individuals the nurse sees, a priority skill for the nurse to have is the ability to
   1. establish chain-of-custody of evidence.
   2. make an assessment of suicide risk.
   3. access community resources.
   4. provide spiritual support.

Answer: 2
Rationale: Newly incarcerated prisoners are often in crisis and may be suicidal. Being able to perform an as-

sessment of suicide risk is an essential skill for the forensic nurse.
   Option 1: This is not a skill needed in the scenario mentioned. Option 3: Community resource identification is not a priority until the end of the sentence. Option 4: This would not be a priority need.
Cognitive level: Application
Nursing process: Implementation
NCLEX: Safe and Effective Care Environment
See text pages: 625, 626

6. A psychiatric forensic nurse is speaking to a group of student nurses about his responsibilities. He should point out that the distinct elements combined in forensic nursing include (more than one option may be chosen)
   1. nursing science.
   2. forensic science.
   3. the criminal justice system.
   4. the body of tort law.
   5. formal report writing.
   6. parole/probation follow-up.

Answers: 1, 2, 3
Rationale: This specialty area of nursing combines elements of nursing science, forensic science, and the criminal justice system. Option 4: Knowledge of tort law is not a requirement for psychiatric forensic nursing. Option 5: Formal report writing is an element subsumed under nursing science and forensic science. Option 6: Knowledge of parole/probation follow-up is an element subsumed under the criminal justice system.
Cognitive level: Comprehension
Nursing process: Implementation
NCLEX: NA
See text pages: 623, 624

7. A forensic nurse educating graduate students in nursing about the specialty area of psychiatric forensic nursing would state the specialty is most clearly defined by (more than one option may be correct)
   1. its practice setting, such as a correctional facility.
   2. the clients served, such as incarcerated individuals.
   3. the nature of the nurse-client relationship, such as working with an alleged victim or an alleged perpetrator.
   4. the nursing role function being performed, such as meeting needs of the court or the alleged perpetrator.

Answers: 3, 4
Rationale: The nurse-client relationship in the subspecialty areas within forensic nursing practice have in

423

common that the nurse is engaged in working with either an alleged victim or an alleged perpetrator. In addition, the specialty is further defined by the nursing role functions being performed, functions that center on the identification, collection, documentation, and preservation of potential evidence; and assessment of competence, risk, and dangerousness. Options 1 and 2 are not related to the definition of forensic nursing.

Cognitive level: Comprehension
Nursing process: Implementation
NCLEX: NA
See text pages: 623, 624

8. The nurse-client relationship in forensic nursing is predicated on
   1. preservation of potential evidence.
   2. assessment of risk of dangerousness.
   3. the possibility a crime has been committed.
   4. treatment of symptoms of psychiatric disorder.

Answer: 3
Rationale: The possibility of a crime having been committed is the actual basis on which the nurse-client relationship is predicated. The other options are elements of forensic nursing practice.

Cognitive level: Knowledge
Nursing process: Implementation
Client need: Psychosocial Integrity
See text pages: 623, 624

9. Which statements can be used to explain forensic nursing to the prison staff? (More than one option may be correct.)
   1. Forensic nurses work exclusively with alleged perpetrators of crimes.
   2. The needs of the court or attorney dictate the focus of psychiatric forensic nurse-client interactions.
   3. Psychiatric forensic nurses make specialized assessments related to competence, sanity, risk, and dangerousness.
   4. Psychiatric forensic nurses become advocates for defendants in all legal proceedings.

Answers: 2, 3
Rationale: Option 2: When the client is the court, the focus of the nurse's interactions with the client is dictated by the needs of the court. Option 3: Assessments of competence, risk, and dangerousness are the special focus of psychiatric forensic nurses, psychiatrists, and psychologists. Other specialty groups of nurses are not concerned with these assessments. Option 1: Physiological forensic nurses focus on the alleged victim. Psychiatric forensic

nurses work with alleged perpetrators. Option 4: Forensic nurses remain neutral and objective, advocating for the legal process rather than for the client.

Cognitive level: Analysis
Nursing process: Implementation
NCLEX: NA
See text page: 624

10. A staff member at the mental hospital asks the psychiatric forensic nurse who is working with a defendant as a competency therapist "Why are you spending so much time with that guy? You spend one-to-one time with him and even go to activities with him. And I have seen you writing volumes. Usually we just give these people medication for a while, then return them to the court." The best reply for the nurse would be
    1. "My role is to become an advocate for the defendant, so I have to know him well."
    2. "The specialized assessments I make on behalf of the court require lengthy interviews."
    3. "My focus is providing intensive psychotherapy to ensure the defendant's competency when he returns to court."
    4. "I spend time observing, assessing, and documenting to determine the defendant's competency, write a report, and provide expert witness testimony in court."

Answer: 4
Rationale: Option 4 best explains the need for the competency therapist to spend large amounts of time with the defendant. The competency therapist collects evidence by spending many hours with a defendant and carefully documenting the dialogue. A complete formal report is prepared for the court and, in addition, the competency therapist may provide expert witness testimony. Option 2: This response is more nonspecific than option 4. Option 1: The role of the competency therapist is to advocate for the judicial process, not the defendant. Option 3: The psychiatric forensic nurse working as a competency therapist does not provide psychotherapy for the defendant.

Cognitive level: Application
Nursing process: Implementation
NCLEX: NA
See text page: 627

11. When a defendant is arraigned, she demonstrates bizarre behavior, talking to unseen people, failing to respond to questions asked by the judge, and shouting obscenities during the proceedings. The judge orders an evaluation by a forensic examiner. The in-

formation of highest priority the examiner will be asked to provide for the court is
1. the defendant's competence to proceed.
2. the cause of the defendant's courtroom behavior.
3. a reconstruction of the defendant's mental state at the time of the alleged crime.
4. a synopsis of the defendant's history, past diagnoses, personality traits, and cognitive abilities.

Answer: 1

Rationale: Competence to proceed is defined as the capacity to assist one's attorney and to understand legal proceedings. In the United States no one is tried unless deemed to be competent. An incompetent individual is remanded to a locked facility for treatment to regain competency. Option 2: This information may or may not be ascertainable. It may be associated with competence to proceed but is not the priority. Option 3: Legal sanity is not the priority concern in this instance. Option 4: These data are of interest but are not the priority concern.

Cognitive level: Analysis
Nursing process: Assessment
NCLEX: Psychosocial Integrity
See text page: 627

12. The psychiatric forensic nurse has been asked by the defendant's lawyer to determine the client's legal sanity. The priority task of the nurse will be to
1. determine whether the defendant understands the legal charges and is capable of assisting in his own defense.
2. reconstruct the defendant's mental state at the time of the crime.
3. presents a danger to self or others in the immediate future.
4. determine whether a crime has been committed.

Answer: 2

Rationale: Legal sanity is determined for the specific time of the alleged crime; thus reconstructing the defendant's mental state at the time of the alleged crime is essential to making the determination. Option 1: This refers to competence to proceed. Option 3 is an assessment dealing with the future and is separate from determination of legal sanity. Option 4 is not associated with determination of legal sanity.

Cognitive level: Analysis
Nursing process: Assessment
NCLEX: Psychosocial Integrity
See text pages: 626, 627

13. A question the psychiatric forensic nurse would ask to provide data with which to assess legal sanity is
1. "On the day of the shooting, were you having any unusual experiences, such as hearing voices or thinking someone wanted to harm you?"
2. "If you found a letter with a stamp lying near a postal box, what would you do?"
3. "At this time, are you experiencing any phenomena others might think strange?"
4. "Do you feel as though you would like to harm anyone at the present time?"

Answer: 1

Rationale: Legal sanity refers to the individual's ability to know right from wrong with reference to the act charged, the capacity to know the nature and quality of the act charged, and the capacity to form the intent to commit the crime. It is determined for the specific time of the act. Only option 1 refers to the client's state at the time of the alleged crime.

Cognitive level: Analysis
Nursing process: Assessment
NCLEX: Psychosocial Integrity
See text pages: 626, 627

14. In which instance would a psychiatric forensic nurse determine that the legal insanity defense could be used by a defendant? The defendant
1. experienced persistent auditory hallucinations commanding her to drown her newborn.
2. admitted to being angry with his wife for committing adultery and tampered with the brakes of her car, leading to her death in a traffic accident.
3. shot the drug dealer who refused to give her cocaine when she had no money to purchase the drug.
4. poisoned his wife with warfarin after she refused to agree to a divorce.

Answer: 1

Rationale: The defendant, demonstrating symptoms of paranoid schizophrenia and acting on the direction of command hallucinations, could use the defense of legal insanity because she could not control her behavior because of a psychiatric illness. The other options suggest the defendant knew right from wrong, had the capacity to know the nature and quality of the act, and had the capacity to form intent to commit the crime.

Cognitive level: Analysis
Nursing process: Assessment
NCLEX: Psychosocial Integrity
See text pages: 626, 627

15. A correctional nurse testified about care received by a specific client in the 8 hours before his successful suicide. The nurse responds to questions about what

he saw and heard and the interventions he performed and documented during the work shift. The nurse was acting as a(n)

1. forensic nurse examiner.
2 physiological forensic nurse.
3. expert witness.
4. fact witness.

Answer: 4

Rationale: A fact witness testifies regarding first-hand experience only. Option 1: Forensic nurse examiners conduct court-ordered examinations and provide written reports and court testimony regarding the findings of the examinations. Option 2: Physiological forensic nurses work with the alleged victim rather than the alleged perpetrator. Option 3: An expert witness testifies regarding involvement with the client and any documentation made by the expert witness and provides a professional opinion based on professional expertise.

Cognitive level: Application
Nursing process: Assessment
NCLEX: Psychosocial Integrity
See text page: 627

16. The highest degree of credibility is required by a nurse who provides testimony before the court as a(n)

1. expert witness.
2. fact witness.
3. correctional nurse.
4. emergency department trauma nurse.

Answer: 1

Rationale: An expert witness is recognized by the court as having a higher level of skill or expertise in a specific area. In addition to testifying about involvement with the individual and documentation of the interactions, the court permits the expert witness to give a professional opinion. Option 2: A fact witness may testify only regarding what was seen, heard, performed, or documented regarding first-hand nursing care. Option 3: A correctional nurse would testify as a fact witness. Option 4: An emergency department trauma nurse would testify as a fact witness.

Cognitive level: Comprehension
Nursing process: Implementation
NCLEX: NA
See text page: 627

17. The psychiatric forensic nurse assigned to a tactical team is deployed along with the team. The nurse's role within the team would include

1. directing personnel deployment.

2. suggesting negotiation techniques to a negotiator.
3. determining the competency of the perpetrator.
4. describing the type of person holding the hostages.

Answer: 2

Rationale: The forensic nurse assigned to a tactical team may suggest negotiation techniques to the negotiator based on assessments the nurse makes regarding behaviors of the perpetrator, understanding of principles of effective communication, understanding of cultural factors, and the ability to think clearly under stress. Option 1: The nurse has no authority to direct the operation, only to advise. Option 3: This assessment is more relevant to the determination of the client's ability to assist with his own court defense. Option 4: Criminal profiling would not be a priority role.

Cognitive level: Application
Nursing process: Implementation
NCLEX: Safe and Effective Care Environment
See text page: 628

18. The difference between the role of the community mental health nurse and the psychiatric forensic nurse advising a hostage negotiating team is the that community mental health nurse

1. is prepared at the master's level; the psychiatric forensic nurse has a PhD.
2. works best on a one-to-one basis; the psychiatric forensic nurse works best with a team.
3. has responsibility but no authority; the psychiatric forensic nurse has responsibility and authority.
4. is an advocate for the client; the psychiatric forensic nurse is concerned with the process of hostage negotiation.

Answer: 4

Rationale: A psychiatric forensic nurse assisting with hostage negotiation remains objective. His or her allegiance is to the process of hostage negotiation, rather than the individual. The community mental health nurse role calls for the nurse to be a client advocate. Option 1: In all probability, each would be prepared at the master's level. Option 2: This is not a valid distinction. Option 3: The opposite is true.

Cognitive level: Comprehension
Nursing process: NA
NCLEX: Safe and Effective Care Environment
See text page: 628

19. The characteristics most important for a psychiatric forensic nurse to possess include (more than one option may be correct)

1. empathy.

2. neutrality.
3. detachment.
4. assertiveness.
5. supportiveness.
6. acceptance.

Answers: 2, 3, 4
Rationale: Forensic nurses need objectivity/neutrality and detachment to perform the duties required by their clients (the court, attorneys, etc.). Positions such as competency therapist, forensic examiner, advisor to hostage negotiator, and criminal profiler require the ability to exercise objectivity rather than become subjectively involved with the alleged perpetrator. Assertiveness is a requisite because the nurse is often breaking new ground. Empathy, supportiveness, and acceptance impede the work of the forensic nurse.
Cognitive level: Comprehension
Nursing process: Implementation
NCLEX: Psychosocial Integrity
See text pages: 626-629

20. The psychiatric forensic nurse describes her work as follows: "I apply my knowledge of psychopathology as I investigate and reconstruct the crime and attempt to understand the criminal's reasoning process. This allows me to compile information on the type of individual who would have committed the crime." The work the nurse describes is
   1. forensic examiner.
   2. competency therapist.
   3. hostage negotiator.
   4. criminal profiler.

Answer: 4
Rationale: Criminal profilers attempt to provide law enforcement with specific information and the type of individual who would have committed a certain crime. Profilers use behavioral and psychological indicators left at violent crime scenes and apply their understanding of psychopathology, attempt to reconstruct the crime, formulate hypotheses, and develop a profile, which is then tested against known data. The other options refer to roles the psychiatric forensic nurse may fill, but none of these roles fits the description given in the scenario.
Cognitive level: Application
Nursing process: Implementation
NCLEX: NA
See text page: 628

21. A physiological forensic nurse would be most likely to be involved with
   1. assessing the victim of sexual assault.

2. determining legal sanity of an alleged perpetrator.
3. acting as a competency therapist.
4. establishing a profile of a suspected serial rapist.

Answer: 1
Rationale: Physiological forensic nurses focus on the application of forensic aspects of health care in the investigation and treatment of trauma and medicolegal issues. They often work as abuse specialists, coroners, or death investigators. Psychiatric forensic nurses assume the roles listed in options 2, 3, and 4.
Cognitive level: Application
Nursing process: Implementation
NCLEX: Safe and Effective Care Environment
See text page: 629

22. In which case would the psychiatric forensic nurse assess the alleged perpetrator as competent to proceed? The individual
   1. believes the FBI has paid assassins to kill him.
   2. hears voices commanding him to kill the president of the United States.
   3. is developmentally disabled with a mental age of 5 years.
   4. is able to understand the legal proceedings and assist in his defense.

Answer: 4
Rationale: Competence to proceed is determined by the defendant's thinking in the future, that is, at the time of trial, and is determined by the defendant's capacity to assist the attorney and understand the legal proceedings. The other options suggest mental incapacity.
Cognitive level: Analysis
Nursing process: Assessment
NCLEX: Psychosocial Integrity
See text page: 627

23. When asked by nurses wishing to learn about correctional nursing, the correctional nurse would characterize the health problems of inmates as
   1. simple, subacute health disorders.
   2. chronic, long-term, and infectious diseases.
   3. acute, short-term problems similar to the nonincarcerated population.
   4. mostly preventable or correctable with diet, exercise, and violence prevention.

Answer: 2
Rationale: Correctional nurses provide care for inmates who have disproportionately high rates of tuberculosis, AIDS, hepatitis, diabetes, and other chronic illnesses. Option 1: The health problems of inmates are more complex. Option 3: Inmates have higher

Chapter 31   Psychiatric Forensic Nursing

rates of sexually transmitted diseases, diabetes, and HIV than the nonincarcerated population. Option 4: Most health problems of inmates are more complex than this description implies.
Cognitive level: Analysis
Nursing process: Implementation
NCLEX: Physiological Integrity
See text page: 625

24. A role function assumed by correctional nurses not appropriate for psychiatric forensic nurses is
    1. teacher.
    2. examiner.
    3. investigator.
    4. advocate for the defendant/inmate.

Answer: 4
Rationale: Correctional nurses advocate for inmates regarding needed care. The psychiatric forensic nurse remains objective, neutral, and detached in his or her relationship with the defendant, advocating instead for the judicial process. Option 1: Both correctional nurses and psychiatric forensic nurses may engage in teaching. Option 2: The forensic nurse may function as examiner and or investigator, roles not usually assumed by the correctional nurse.
Cognitive level: Application
Nursing process: Implementation
NCLEX: Psychosocial Integrity
See text page: 625

25. The psychiatric forensic nurse role functions include making assessments to determine (more than one answer may be correct)
    1. perpetrator ability to formulate intent.
    2. risk for future violent acts.
    3. evidence of sexual assault.
    4. legal sanity.
    5. ability to understand legal proceedings.
    6. patterns of injury in abuse.

Answers: 1, 2, 4, 5
Rationale: Options 1, 2, 4, and 5 are assessments the psychiatric forensic nurse makes. Options 3 and 6 are assessments made by the physiological forensic nurse. The physiological forensic nurse focuses on the victim of the alleged crime, whereas the psychiatric forensic nurse focuses on the perpetrator of the alleged crime.
Cognitive level: Application
Nursing process: Assessment
NCLEX: Psychosocial Integrity
See text pages: 625, 629

CHAPTER 32

1. The mother of a 4-year-old tells the nurse that her son spends his day in constant motion. The mother tries to get him interested in playing with his toys, but he is easily distracted and does not seem to listen. He talks appropriately but excessively. He gets out of bed in the morning before his mother. She reports that one morning he broke the screen on the TV. She enrolled him in preschool, but the teacher was unable to handle him. The suggestion was made that he should be evaluated at the mental health clinic. The nurse can assess that the child's problem is most consistent with the *DSM-IV-TR* criteria for
   1. pervasive developmental disorder.
   2. mental retardation.
   3. oppositional defiant disorder.
   4. attention deficit hyperactivity disorder.

Answer: 4
Rationale: The excessive motion, distractibility, and excessive talkativeness are seen in attention deficit hyperactivity disorder (ADHD). The behaviors presented in the scenario do not suggest the other possible choices. Developmental delays would be seen if pervasive developmental disorder or mental retardation were present. Oppositional defiant disorder would include serious violations of the rights of others.
Cognitive level: Analysis
Nursing process: Assessment
NCLEX: Psychosocial Integrity
See text page: 643

2. A child, aged 4 years, who was removed from preschool when the teacher was unable to handle his excessive motor activity and talking, is to be treated by a psychiatric clinical nurse specialist. What aspect of the child's care can be performed by a clinical nurse specialist but would not be performed by a nurse generalist?
   1. Formulating nursing diagnoses
   2. Planning nursing interventions
   3. Participating in child psychotherapy
   4. Evaluating responses to nursing actions

Answer: 3
Rationale: The clinical nurse specialist roles include individual, group, and family psychotherapist; educator of nurses, other professions, and the community; clinical supervisor; consultant to professional and nonprofessional groups; and researcher.
Cognitive level: Analysis
Nursing process: Planning
NCLEX: Psychosocial Integrity
See text page: NA

3. A child, aged 4 years, has been referred to the mental health clinic for evaluation of hyperactive, impulsive behaviors. At the first visit nursing staff begin observing and assessing his behavior in the play area. What developmental task should the child have achieved?
   1. Forming satisfactory relationships with peers
   2. Separation from parents and ability to socialize outside the family
   3. Ability to establish goals
   4. A sense of autonomy

Answer: 4
Rationale: A 4-year-old should have attained the developmental tasks of children aged 11/2 to 3 years: autonomy. Options 1, 2, and 3 are goals of children aged 3 to 6 years and 6 to 9 years.
Cognitive level: Application
Nursing process: Assessment
NCLEX: Psychosocial Integrity
See text page: 639

4. The tool the clinical nurse specialist uses to organize data about three-generational relationships within a client's family system is
   1. play.
   2. genogram.
   3. word association.
   4. projective story-telling cards.

Answer: 2
Rationale: A genogram displays family information over at least three generations and provides data for hypothesizing about the child's problem in relation to the family. The other options would not be useful to organizing data.
Cognitive level: Knowledge
Nursing process: Assessment
NCLEX: Psychosocial Integrity
See text page: 639

5. A 7-year-old with ADHD is being evaluated at the mental health clinic. The nurse establishes the nursing diagnosis of delayed growth and development related to neurological status, as evidenced by hyperactivity and distractibility preventing participation in play. The plan for care includes administration of methylphenidate (Concerta). The outcome indicator the nurse should monitor is
   1. child socialization skills.
   2. expressive communication.
   3. participation in play activities.
   4. anxiety self-control.

Answer: 3
Rationale: This outcome indicator is directly related to improvement in the child's hyperactivity and dis-

tractibility. Options 1 and 3 are more relevant for a child with pervasive developmental disorder. Option 4 is more relevant for a child with anxiety disorder.
Cognitive level: Analysis
Nursing process: Planning (Outcome Identification)
NCLEX: Psychosocial Integrity
See text page: 645

6. A 5-year-old boy with ADHD bounces out of his chair in the clinic waiting room and runs over to another child and begins to slap her. The best action for the nurse to take is to
   1. tell the boy's mother to take him home immediately.
   2. direct him to stop, then comfort the other child.
   3. call for emergency assistance from other staff.
   4. take him to a room with toys to act out feelings.

Answer: 4
Rationale: Use of play to express feelings is appropriate because the cognitive and language abilities of the child may require acting out of feelings if verbal expression is limited. Option 1 would not be advantageous to the child. Option 2 provides no outlet for feelings or opportunity to develop coping skills. Option 3 would be unnecessary.
Cognitive level: Application
Nursing process: Implementation
NCLEX: Safe and Effective Care Environment
See text page: 646

7. Which statement by the nurse who has been working with a child with ADHD might indicate overinvolvement with the child and a need for supervision?
   1. "There are times I want to spank him, like when he throws things."
   2. "He is beginning to concentrate more when he plays."
   3. "He responds best when I stay calm and neutral."
   4. "Decreasing environmental stimuli helps him concentrate."

Answer: 1
Rationale: Negative feelings may indicate the presence of countertransference, signaling an unresolved conflict. The other comments are appropriate and suggest no overinvolvement.
Cognitive level: Application
Nursing process: Assessment
NCLEX: Psychosocial Integrity
See text pages: 644, 645

8. The physician mentions to the nurse that a child with ADHD will begin medication therapy. The nurse should prepare a plan to teach the family about

429

1. methylphenidate (Ritalin).
2. fluphenazine (Prolixin).
3. diazepam (Valium).
4. haloperidol (Haldol).

Answer: 1

Rationale: Central nervous system stimulants such as methylphenidate and pemoline (Cylert) increase blood flow to the brain and have proved helpful in reducing hyperactivity in children and adolescents with attention deficit hyperactivity disorder. The other medications listed would not be appropriate.

Cognitive level: Application
Nursing process: Planning
NCLEX: Physiological Integrity
See text page: 644

9. Shortly after her parents announced that they were divorcing, a 15-year-old high-school junior stopped participating in cheerleading and began to sit alone at lunch and avoid former friends. At home she spends most of her time in her room. She tells the nurse "All the kids at school have families. Now that my parents are divorcing, I am an outsider. If my parents loved me, they would work out their problems." What nursing diagnosis should be considered based on the assembled data?
   1. Decisional conflict
   2. Social isolation
   3. Disturbed thought processes
   4. Disturbed personal identity

Answer: 2

Rationale: This diagnosis refers to aloneness that the client perceives negatively, even when self-imposed. Defining characteristics that the teen displays include expressing feelings of being different from others and self-imposed isolation from peers and family. The other options are not supported by data in the scenario.

Cognitive level: Analysis
Nursing process: Diagnosis
NCLEX: Psychosocial Integrity
See text page: 648

10. Shortly after her parents announced that they were divorcing, a 15-year-old high-school junior stopped participating in cheerleading and began to sit alone at lunch and avoid former friends. At home she spends most of her time in her room. She tells the nurse "All the kids at school have families. Now that my parents are divorcing, I am an outsider. If my parents loved me, they would work out their problems." The nursing intervention that would be appropriate to consider for her is to

1. communicate disbelief relative to the client's feelings.
2. develop a plan for activities of daily living.
3. assist the client to distinguish reality from perceptions.
4. assess and document the client's level of fatigue twice daily.

Answer: 3

Rationale: The client's perception that all the other kids are from two-parent households and that she is different is not based on reality. Helping her test the accuracy of her perception will be helpful. Option 1 is nontherapeutic. Options 2 and 4 are not appropriate on the basis of the available information.

Cognitive level: Analysis
Nursing process: Planning
NCLEX: Psychosocial Integrity
See text page: 651

11. The nurse working with a teen client who has become moody and withdrawn because her parents are divorcing will make the establishment of a therapeutic alliance a priority because
   1. focusing on the strengths of an individual increases the individual's self-esteem.
   2. the client should express feelings and not keep them inside.
   3. acceptance and trust convey feelings of security to the client.
   4. therapeutic activities provide an outlet for tension.

Answer: 3

Rationale: Trust is frequently an issue because the child or adolescent may never have had a trusting relationship with an adult. In this client's situation, the trust she once had in her parents has been shattered, robbing her of feelings of security. Only option 3 relates to the therapeutic alliance.

Cognitive level: Application
Nursing process: Planning
NCLEX: Safe and Effective Care Environment
See text page: NA

12. Which therapeutic intervention could the nurse generalist use to help a child gain insight into feelings and learn new ways to cope with difficult situations?
   1. Bibliotherapy
   2. Family therapy
   3. Psychodrama
   4. Insight-oriented individual therapy

Answer: 1

Rationale: Bibliotherapy involves reading stories about children in situations similar to the client's. Books can help children deal with divorce, death, fears, and separation. The other modalities are reserved for advanced practice nurses and other therapists with additional training.

Cognitive level: Application
Nursing process: Implementation
NCLEX: Psychosocial Integrity
See text page: 653

13. When assessing a 2-year-old child with suspected autistic disorder, the nurse should be particularly alert for
1. failure to develop interpersonal skills.
2. hyperactivity and attention deficits.
3. high levels of anxiety when separated from the mother.
4. a history of disobedience and destructive acts.

Answer: 1

Rationale: Autistic disorder involves distortions in development of social skills and language that include perception, motor movement, attention, and reality testing. Caretakers nearly always mention the child's failure to develop interpersonal skills. Option 2 is more relevant for assessment of ADHD. Option 3 is more relevant to children with separation anxiety. Option 4 becomes more important in the assessment of children with conduct disorder.

Cognitive level: Application
Nursing process: Assessment
NCLEX: Psychosocial Integrity
See text page: 640

14. A 3-year-old cries and screams from the time his mother drops him off at kindergarten until she picks him up 4 hours later. He is calm and relaxed when he is with his mother. His mother asks their neighbor, a nurse, what she should do. The best advice would be
1. "Talk with the school about withdrawing him until he is more mature."
2. "Arrange with the teacher to let him call home at play time."
3. "Send a picture of yourself to school to keep with him."
4. "Talk with your doctor about referring him to a mental health clinic."

Answer: 4

Rationale: Separation anxiety disorder becomes apparent when the child is separated from the attachment figure. Often, the first time separation occurs is when the child goes to kindergarten or nursery school. Separation anxiety may be based on the child's fear that something will happen to the at-

tachment figure. The other options are "short-term" fixes." The child needs professional help.

Cognitive level: Application
Nursing process: Implementation
NCLEX: Psychosocial Integrity
See text page: 646

15. A 15-year-old has been referred to the adolescent mental health clinic by the juvenile court after being arrested for prostitution. She has run away from home several times and has lived in homeless shelters. Her parents told the court they could not manage her, that she was physically abusive to her mother and defiant and hostile to her father. From the history, the nurse might anticipate that the psychiatrist will consider the diagnosis of
1. attention-deficit hyperactivity disorder.
2. autistic disorder.
3. conduct disorder.
4. childhood depression.

Answer: 3

Rationale: Conduct disorders are manifested by a persistent pattern of behavior in which the rights of others and age-appropriate societal norms are violated. *DSM-IV-TR* identifies this type of conduct disorder as conduct disorder: serious violations of rules. The client's clinical manifestations do not coincide with *DSM-IV-TR* descriptions of the other disorders.

Cognitive level: Analysis
Nursing process: Assessment
NCLEX: Psychosocial Integrity
See text pages: 643, 644

16. A client, aged 15 years, has been referred to the mental health center by the juvenile court after being arrested for prostitution. Her parents told the court they could not manage her, that she was physically abusive to her mother and defiant and hostile to her father. At the mental health center she refused to participate in scheduled activities. She also pushed an elderly client, causing her to fall. The approach by nursing staff that would be most therapeutic is
1. neutrally permitting refusals.
2. coaxing to gain compliance.
3. offering rewards in advance.
4. establishing firm limits.

Answer: 4

Rationale: Firm limits are necessary to ensure physical safety and emotional security. Limit setting will also protect other clients from the teen's thoughtless or aggressive behavior. Permitting refusals to participate in the treatment plan, coaxing, and bargaining are strategies that do not help the client learn to abide by rules or structure.

431

Cognitive level: Application
Nursing process: Planning
NCLEX: Psychosocial Integrity
See text page: 646

17. A client, aged 15 years, has been referred to the adolescent mental health clinic by the juvenile court after being arrested for prostitution. She has run away from home several times and has lived in homeless shelters. Her parents told the court they could not manage her, that she was physically abusive to her mother and defiant and hostile to her father. The client tells the nurse she hates her parents because they focus attention on her older brother "who is simply perfect in their eyes." Based on the accumulated data, the therapy that might promote the greatest change in the client's behavior is
   1. bibliotherapy.
   2. play therapy.
   3. family therapy.
   4. art therapy.

Answer: 3
Rationale: Family therapy would focus on problematic family relationships and interactions. The client had already identified problems within the family. Options 1 and 4 could be useful to a lesser extent. Option 2 would be more useful with a younger child. Option
Cognitive level: Application
Nursing process: Planning
NCLEX: Psychosocial Integrity
See text page: 649

18. A client, aged 15 years, has been referred to the adolescent mental health clinic by the juvenile court after being arrested for prostitution. She has run away from home several times and has lived in homeless shelters. Her parents told the court they could not manage her, that she was physically abusive to her mother and defiant and hostile to her father. The client tells the nurse she hates her parents because they focus attention on her older brother "who is simply perfect in their eyes." A nursing diagnosis that can be identified for the client is
   1. ineffective coping related to seeking parental attention, as evidenced by acting out.
   2. chronic low self-esteem related to knowing her brother is the parental favorite.
   3. hopelessness related to feeling unloved by parents.
   4. disturbed personal identity related to living on the streets.

Answer: 1

Rationale: The client demonstrates an inability to problem solve by using adaptive behaviors to meet life's demands and roles. The defining characteristics are not present for the other nursing diagnoses listed. The client has never mentioned hopelessness, low self-esteem, or disturbed personal identity.
Cognitive level: Analysis
Nursing process: Diagnosis
NCLEX: Psychosocial Integrity
See text page: 644

19. Which fact obtained during nursing assessment would cause the nurse to consider a child to be at risk for the development of a psychiatric disorder?
   1. Being raised by a depressed mother
   2. Regular prenatal care for the mother
   3. Developmental milestones achieved on schedule
   4. Marital harmony in the household

Answer: 1
Rationale: Statistics tell us that children raised by a depressed mother have a 30% to 50% chance of developing an emotional disorder. The other factors are not risk enhancing.
Cognitive level: Application
Nursing process: Assessment
NCLEX: Psychosocial Integrity
See text page: 637

20. The child the nurse would assess as showing behaviors indicative of psychopathology is
   1. A, aged 3 months, who cries after feeding until burped and sucks her thumb.
   2. B, aged 6 months, who does not eat vegetables well and likes to be rocked.
   3. C, aged 3 years, who is mute, impassive toward adults, and twirls and flaps while walking.
   4. D, aged 4 years, who lisps and became enuretic after the birth of a sibling.

Answer: 3
Rationale: C's symptoms are consistent with symptoms of pervasive developmental disorder. The behaviors of the other children are within normal ranges.
Cognitive level: Analysis
Nursing process: Assessment
NCLEX: Psychosocial Integrity
See text page: 640

21. The child most likely to receive haloperidol to control symptoms is
   1. E, with attention deficit hyperactivity disorder.
   2. F, with Rett syndrome.

432

3. G, with separation anxiety.
4. H, with autistic disorder.

Answer: 4

Rationale: Haloperidol is useful for relieving irritability and labile affect of some autistic children. It is not indicated in any of the other disorders.

Cognitive level: Application
Nursing process: Assessment
NCLEX: Physiological Integrity
See text page: 642

22. A 12-year-old boy has been the neighborhood bully for several years. His peers avoid him. His mother says she cannot believe a thing he tells her. Recently he was observed shooting at several dogs with a pellet gun. Yesterday he was caught setting fire to a dumpster outside a supermarket. A nurse could assess his behaviors as being most consistent with
1. conduct disorder.
2. attention deficit.
3. anxiety over separation from parent.
4. defiance of authority.

Answer: 1

Rationale: The behaviors mentioned are most consistent with *DSM-IV-TR* criteria for conduct disorder, for example, aggression against people and animals; destruction of property; deceitfulness; rule violations; and impairment in social, academic, or occupational functioning. The behaviors are not consistent with attention deficit and separation anxiety and are more pervasive than defiance of authority.

Cognitive level: Application
Nursing process: Assessment
Client need: Psychosocial Integrity
See text pages: 643, 644

23. An autistic child engages in head banging and biting his fist. The nurse can evaluate the plan of care as effective when the child
1. seeks help from staff to avoid engaging in these behaviors.
2. has to be placed in a basket hold to stop these behaviors.
3. wears padded mittens to prevent injury to his hands.
4. hits other children instead of self-mutilating.

Answer: 1

Rationale: Seeking intervention to prevent self-mutilation signifies understanding of the relation between feelings and behaviors, a mark of progress for an autistic individual. Options 2 and 3 do not suggest client self-control of the behaviors. Option 4 is not a desirable substitution.

Cognitive level: Evaluation
Nursing process: Evaluation
NCLEX: Psychosocial Integrity
See text pages: 643, 644

24. A child of 11 years, diagnosed with oppositional defiant disorder, becomes angry and defiant over the rules of the day treatment program. The nurse at whom the child is shouting might defuse the situation by
1. suggesting that B go to the gym and shoot baskets.
2. placing B in a basket hold.
3. calling staff to seclude B.
4. providing as-needed anxiolytic medication.

Answer: 1

Rationale: Redirecting the expression of feelings into nondestructive, age-appropriate behaviors such as a physical activity helps the child learn how to modulate the expression of feelings and exert self-control. This is the least restrictive alternative of those listed and should be tried before resorting to more restrictive measures.

Cognitive level: Application
Nursing process: Implementation
NCLEX: Safe and Effective Care Environment
See text page: 646

25. A teen client acts out in disruptive ways. When he threatens to throw a pool ball at another adolescent, which intervention would set limits and give permission?
1. "You will be taken to seclusion if you throw that ball."
2. "Do not throw the ball. Put it back on the pool table."
3. "Attention, everyone. We are all going to the crafts room."
4. "Please, do not lose control of your emotions."

Answer: 2

Rationale: Setting limits and giving permission uses clear, sharp statements about which behavior is not allowed and gives permission for performing the behavior that is expected. Option 1 is a threat. Option 3 uses restructuring, which would be inappropriate in this instance. Option 4 is a direct appeal to the child's developing self-control that may be ineffective.

Cognitive level: Application
Nursing process: Implementation
NCLEX: Safe and Effective Care Environment
See text page: 646

26. When a client, aged 5 years, is disruptive the nurse tells her "You must take a time-out." The expectation for the child is that she will
1. go to her room until called for the next meal.
2. slowly count to 20 before returning to the milieu.
3. sit quietly on the lap of one of the staff members.
4. sit on the periphery of the activity until able to regain self-control and review the episode.

Answer: 4

Rationale: Time-out is designed so that staff can be consistent in their interventions. Time-out may require going to a designated room or sitting on the periphery of an activity until the child gains self-control and reviews the episode with a staff member. Time-out may not require going to a designated room and does not involve special attention such as holding. Counting to 10 or 20 is not sufficient.

Cognitive level: Application
Nursing process: Implementation
NCLEX: Safe and Effective Care Environment
See text page: 646

27. The parents of a child with ADHD tell the nurse clinician "We try to teach him how to behave, but he does not listen. He just rushes in and does things his way. We feel as though we are terrible parents." The most helpful reply would provide information about
1. children with difficult temperaments.
2. ADHD risk as it relates to marital discord.
3. traumatic life events as precipitating factors in ADHD.
4. the relationship of ADHD and dopamine system abnormalities.

Answer: 4

Rationale: Recent findings suggest that abnormalities in dopamine receptors and transporters are implicated in ADHD. Parents who understand the possible biochemical causation may be less likely to blame their parenting methods for the child's behavior.
The other options have no relevance to ADHD.

Cognitive level: Application
Nursing process: Implementation
NCLEX: Health Promotion and Maintenance
See text page: 637

28. A 12-year-old client has been diagnosed with dissociative identity disorder. Nurses gathering assessment data should be particularly alert to references that may relate to
1. low socioeconomic status.
2. lack of cultural role models.
3. physical or sexual abuse.
4. parental marital discord.

Answer: 3

Rationale: Physical or sexual abuse of children puts them at risk for developing dissociative identity disorder as a defense against anxiety associated with the abuse. Although the other options cause increased social and environmental stress for children, these stressors do not seem to predispose to dissociative identity disorder.

Cognitive level: Application
Nursing process: Assessment
NCLEX: Psychosocial Integrity
See text page: 637

29. An adult client with paranoid schizophrenia lives in a homeless shelter with her 13-year-old daughter. The nurse establishes a relationship with the daughter and determines that the child has adapted to shelter life, having formed a relationship with one of the shelter volunteers who encourages her to attend school. The teen relates that she has a friendship with a classmate. When she describes this relationship, the nurse determines that the teen is able to exercise both social skills and problem-solving skills. The nurse can make the assessment that the teen
1. displays resiliency.
2. has a difficult temperament.
3. is at risk for developing posttraumatic stress disorder.
4. manifests neuroendocrine problems.

Answer: 1

Rationale: Resiliency enables a child to handle the stresses of a difficult childhood. Resilient children can adapt to changes in the environment, take advantage of nurturing relationships with adults other than parents, distance themselves from emotional chaos occurring within the family, learn and use problem-solving skills, and develop good social intelligence. The other options are not supported by data given in the scenario.

Cognitive level: Analysis
Nursing process: Assessment
NCLEX: Psychosocial Integrity
See text page: 637

30. An adult client with paranoid schizophrenia lives in a homeless shelter with her 13-year old-daughter. The mother is fragile but not psychotic most of the time. The nurse establishes a relationship with the daughter and determines that the child has adapted to shelter life, having formed a relationship with one of the shelter volunteers who encourages her to attend school. The teen relates that she has a friendship with a classmate. When she describes this relationship, the nurse determines that the teen is able to

exercise both social skills and problem-solving skills. The mobile treatment team asks the nurse to make a recommendation regarding what should be done to assist the teenage daughter. The best recommendation would be to
1. suggest foster home placement.
2. seek assistance from the domestic violence program.
3. make referrals for existing and emerging developmental problems.
4. foster healthy characteristics and existing environmental supports.

Answer: 4

Rationale: Because the teenage daughter shows no evidence of poor mental health, the best action would be to foster existing healthy characteristics and environmental supports. No other option is necessary or appropriate under the current circumstances.

Cognitive level: Analysis
Nursing process: Planning
NCLEX: Safe and Effective Care Environment
See text page: 637

31. A child, aged 10 years, is referred to the mental health clinic by the school psychologist. The child tells the advanced practice nurse that she wants to die "because no one likes me." She adds that "the other girls laugh at me." She is unable to pinpoint a cause for the behavior of the other girls and does not think she can ever change their feelings about her. When she is asked if she has decided on a plan for taking her life, she states she will jump from the bridge over the river near her home some night after the family is asleep. She believes this will accomplish her goal because she saw her father throw kittens off the bridge and knows they died in the water because, like her, they couldn't swim. The nurse should make the assessment that suicide risk is
1. nonexistent.
2. low.
3. moderate.
4. high.

Answer: 4

Rationale: The suicide risk is high. The child is experiencing feelings of hopelessness and helplessness. The method she has chosen is lethal and the means to carry out the plan are available.

Cognitive level: Analysis
Nursing process: Assessment
NCLEX: Safe and Effective Care Environment
See text page: 648

32. The intake data for an 11-year-old child notes the probability of Asperger syndrome. The nurse will expect to assess
1. absence of verbal language.
2. presence of tics and twitching.
3. severe developmental delays.
4. limited social skills and empathy.

Answer: 4

Rationale: Most children with Asperger's syndrome manifest poor social skills and problems empathizing with others as their major behavioral symptoms. Option 1: Verbal skills are rarely impaired. Option 2: Tics and twitching are more often a part of the clinical picture of Tourette's syndrome. Option 3: Severe developmental delays are part of the clinical picture of autism rather than Asperger's syndrome.

Cognitive level: Application
Nursing process: Assessment
NCLEX: Psychosocial Integrity
See text page: 641

33. The assessment data for a child aged 9 years reveals that she blurts out answers to questions before the question is completed, is unable to wait her turn, and persistently interrupts and intrudes in the conversations of others. The nurse would assess these behaviors as relating primarily to
1. hyperactivity.
2. impulsivity.
3. inattention.
4. defiance.

Answer: 2

Rationale: These behaviors are most directly related to impulsivity. Option 1: Hyperactive behaviors are more physical in nature, such as running, pushing, and the inability to sit. Option 3: Inattention is demonstrated by failure to listen. Option 4: Defiance is demonstrated by willfully doing what an authority figure has said not to do.

Cognitive level: Comprehension
Nursing process: Assessment
NCLEX: Psychosocial Integrity
See text page: 643

34. A psychiatric technician asks the nurse "What is the primary distinguishing factor between the behavior of children with oppositional defiant disorder and those with conduct disorder (CD)?" The facts that should be used by the nurse to formulate a reply include the child with (more than one response may be correct)
1. ODD tests limits and disobeys authority figures.
2. CD often violates the rights of others.

435

3. ODD relives traumatic events by acting them out.
4. CD uses stereotypical or repetitive language.
5. ODD has difficulty separating from the parents.
6. CD engages in eating nonnutritive substances.

Answers: 1, 2

Rationale: Children with ODD are negativistic, disobedient, and defiant toward authority figures without seriously violating the basic rights of others, whereas children with conduct disorder frequently behave in ways that violate the rights of others and age-appropriate societal norms. Option 3: Reliving traumatic events occurs with posttraumatic stress disorder. Option 4: Stereotypical language behaviors are seen in autistic children. Option 5: Separation problems with resultant anxiety occur with separation anxiety disorder. Option 6 describes a child with pica.

Cognitive level: Application
Nursing process: Planning
NCLEX: Safe and Effective Care Environment
See text pages: 643, 644

35. When group therapy is to be used as a treatment modality, the nurse would suggest placement of a child aged 9 years in a therapy group that used
1. play activities exclusively.
2. group discussion exclusively.
3. talk focused on a specific issue.
4. play and talk about the play activity.

Answer: 4

Rationale: Group therapy for young children takes the form of play. For elementary school children therapy combines play and talk about the activity. For adolescents, group therapy involves more talking.

Cognitive level: Application
Nursing process: Implementation
NCLEX: Psychosocial Integrity
See text pages: 649, 650

CHAPTER 33

1. A client who has degenerative arthritis of the knees and hips for which she takes nonsteroidal antiinflammatory drugs tells the nurse "For the past month I have been having a lot of trouble sleeping. I cannot seem to fall asleep, and then when I finally do get to sleep, I find I wake up a number of times during the night." Which information should the nurse seek initially?
1. "Are you snoring a lot?"
2. "Do you have pain at night?"
3. "Do you sleep better with the radio on?"
4. "Can you define 'good sleep' for me?"

Answer: 2

Rationale: Clients with diseases such as arthritis may have sleep disturbance related to nightly pain. Because the pain is chronic the client may fail to realize it is the reason for the inability to sleep. The other options do not follow the client's lead.

Cognitive level: Analysis
Nursing process: Assessment
NCLEX: Physiological Integrity
See text pages: 659, 660

2. A nurse who works the night shift tells the nurse practitioner who is her primary caregiver "I am exhausted most of the time. I sleep through my alarm and have to have a friend phone me to make sure I get up to go to work. Sometimes while I am on duty, my brain does not seem to work right. I am beginning to be concerned that I might make a practice error." What question will the nurse need to ask before problem solving?
1. "How much sleep to you get in a 24-hour period?"
2. "Do you exercise just before going to bed?"
3. "What stress are you experiencing in your life?"
4. "Have you ever used a hypnotic to help you sleep?"

Answer: 1

Rationale: Total sleep hours need to be ascertained before giving advice to correct a sleep disorder. In this case the client describes sleep deprivation symptoms rather than a sleep disorder. Option 1 is the only option that addresses total sleep hours.

Cognitive level: Application
Nursing process: Assessment
NCLEX: Physiological Integrity
See text page: 659

3. A factory night shift worker tells the industrial nurse that he is having trouble getting to sleep when he goes home after a night's work. He mentions that he has a hearty breakfast and a few cups of coffee, reads the paper, does his exercises, and then goes to bed and lies awake until it is nearly time to get up to be with his family at dinner. What change should the nurse suggest? (More than one answer may be correct.)
1. Drink decaffeinated coffee after 3 AM.
2. Do not read the paper.
3. Exercise after awakening.
4. Eat a light breakfast.

Answers: 1, 3, 4

Rationale: Sleep can be disrupted by caffeine, a central nervous system stimulant, exercise performed just before trying to sleep, and eating a heavy meal before retiring. Option 2: Reading the newspaper is not

likely to be so stimulating that it disrupts the client's ability to sleep.
Cognitive level: Analysis
Nursing process: Implementation
NCLEX: Health Promotion and Maintenance
See text page: 670

4. A client goes to the clinic to report that the medication prescribed to help her get to sleep worked well when she took it each night for 1 month. However, now that the medication is gone, her insomnia is worse than ever and she has had nightmares the last two nights. The nurse can hypothesize that the physician had prescribed a
   1. hypnotic.
   2. neuroleptic.
   3. central nervous system stimulant.
   4. tricyclic antidepressant.

Answer: 1
Rationale: Hypnotics can worsen existing sleep disturbances when they induce drug-dependency insomnia. Once the drug is discontinued the individual may have rebound insomnia and nightmares. Neuroleptics rarely worsen insomnia. CNS stimulants worsen insomnia while they are in use. Tricyclic antidepressants may help insomnia.
Cognitive level: Application
Nursing process: Assessment
NCLEX: Physiological Integrity
See text pages: 662-665

5. A client with primary insomnia asks the nurse why day naps do not really compensate for a lost night's sleep. The best reply for the nurse is
   1. "Circadian cycles give daytime naps a structure different from nighttime sleep."
   2. "The body clock operates on a 25-hour cycle, making nap effectiveness unpredictable."
   3. " It is a matter of habit and expectation. We expect to be more refreshed from a
      night's sleep."
   4. "Sleep restores homeostasis but works more efficiently when aided by melatonin secreted at night."

Answer: 1
Rationale: A regular 90- to 100-minute sleep cycle occurs with nighttime sleep, with progression through two distinct physiological states: four stages of non—rapid eye movement (REM) sleep and a period of REM sleep. Naps often contain different amounts of REM sleep, thus changing the physiology of sleep as well as the psychological and behavioral effects of sleep. Options 2 and 4 are not true statements.

Option 3 has little bearing on the reason for lack of refreshment.
Cognitive level: Analysis
Nursing process: Implementation
NCLEX: Health Promotion and Maintenance
See text pages: 661, 662

6. A client mentions to the nurse "Everyone says we should sleep 8 hours a night. I can only sleep 6 hours, no matter how hard I try. Am I doing harm to my body?" The best response for the nurse to make is
   1. "Tell me the things you have done to try to increase your total sleep hours."
   2. "If you have really tried it all, perhaps you should consult with your physician."
   3. "Lack of sleep does act as a stressor on the body and can cause physical changes."
   4. "If you function well with 6 hours sleep, you are what is called a 'short sleeper.'"

Answer: 4
Rationale: Some individuals require less sleep than others. Those who need less are called "short sleepers," compared with "long sleepers," who require more than 8 hours. Options 1 and 2 do not provide information the client is seeking. Option 3 is not strictly true in all cases.
Cognitive level: Analysis
Nursing process: Implementation
NCLEX: Health Promotion and Maintenance
See text pages: 661, 662

7. A client tells the advanced practice nurse that she has trouble falling asleep at night and might lie awake until 3 or 4 AM before falling sleep. The appropriate pharmacological treatment would be
   1. zolpidem (Ambien).
   2. methylphenidate (Ritalin).
   3. flurazepam (Dalmane).
   4. risperidone (Risperdal).

Answer: 1
Rationale: Zolpidem is a short-acting hypnotic that will help the client initiate sleep and allow her to awaken without untoward symptoms of drowsiness. Option 2: This medication is a central nervous system stimulant. Option 3 is a long-acting hypnotic that will produce hangover drowsiness during the day. Option 4: This medication is an antipsychotic and is not useful in promoting sleep.
Cognitive level: Application
Nursing process: Implementation
NCLEX: Physiological Integrity
See text pages: 663, 665

437

8. The sleep record of a client with major depression shows the client waking at 3 AM and being unable to resume sleep. The physician decides to prescribe the client a serotonin-reuptake inhibitor and additionally orders a sleep-deprivation protocol. The outcome expected is
   1. self-control of suicidal ideation.
   2. rapid response to the antidepressant.
   3. self-control of auditory hallucinations.
   4. increased anxiety self-control.

Answer: 2

Rationale: Recent studies have shown that sleep deprivation has proven effective in speeding response to antidepressant medication and to improving sleep pattern. Sleep deprivation has not shown effectiveness in providing direct control of suicidal ideation, auditory hallucinations, or symptoms of anxiety.

Cognitive level: Application
Nursing process: Planning (Outcome Identification)
NCLEX: Physiological Integrity
See text pages: 666, 667

9. The sleep disturbance the nurse caring for a client with bipolar I disorder would consider when planning client care is
   1. early morning awakening.
   2. fragmentation of sleep.
   3. decreased REM sleep.
   4. hypersomnia.

Answer: 4

Rationale: Hypersomnia is often part of the depressed phase of bipolar I disorder and is also frequently seen in mild depressive disorder. Careful scheduling of therapy times and activities can take advantage of periods when the client is most able to benefit from therapy. Option 1: Early morning awakening is seen in major depression. Options 2 and 3: Fragmentation of sleep and decreased REM sleep are associated with a number of other medical and psychiatric conditions.

Cognitive level: Application
Nursing process: Planning
NCLEX: Physiological Integrity
See text pages: 666, 667

10. A client at the sleep disorders clinic tells the nurse "I have not slept well in years. As a result, I never feel good. After all these years, I do not expect things will ever improve or be any different." A nursing diagnosis the nurse should consider developing is
    1. disturbed body image.
    2. health-seeking behaviors.
    3. adult failure to thrive.
    4. hopelessness.

Answer: 4

Rationale: The client sees limited alternatives and provides verbal clues to hopelessness; thus defining characteristics are present for this nursing diagnosis. Defining characteristics are not present for the other options.

Cognitive level: Analysis
Nursing process: Diagnosis
NCLEX: Psychosocial Integrity
See text page: 668

11. A client at the sleep disorders clinic tells the nurse, "I have not slept well in years. As a result, I never feel good. After all these years, I do not expect things will ever improve or be any different." Nursing interventions the nurse should consider implementing include (more than one answer may be correct)
    1. providing instruction in relaxation techniques.
    2. advising to use alcohol as a sedative.
    3. health teaching regarding factors that influence sleep.
    4. counseling to address cognitive distortions.
    5. advising to engage in fatigue-producing activities to become overtired.
    6. promoting lengthy daytime sleep periods.

Answers: 1, 3, 4

Rationale: Interventions that could be helpful include teaching relaxation techniques, such as meditation or progressive relaxation to relieve the tension that sometimes prevents initiation of sleep. Option 3: Reviewing factors that influence sleep can assist the client to diagnose and remove barriers to sleep. Option 4: Cognitive therapy could be helpful in combating the hopelessness verbalized by the client. Option 2: Alcohol consumption actually disrupts sleep. Option 5: Becoming overtired may be a barrier to nighttime sleep. Option 6: Naps may help replace lost sleep, but lengthy daytime sleep will prevent the client from sleeping well at night.

Cognitive level: Application
Nursing process: Planning
NCLEX: Psychosocial Integrity
See text pages: 668, 669

12. The indicators the nurse would find useful for evaluation of outcomes relating to sleep improvement include (more than one answer may be correct)
    1. fewer than 5 hours of sleep.
    2. decreased time falling asleep.
    3. fewer awakenings.
    4. dependence on sleep aids.
    5. ability to resume sleep after awakening.
    6. client perception of improvement.

438

Answers: 2, 3, 5, 6

Rationale: Options 2, 3, 5, and 6 suggest normalization of sleep. Option 1 refers to an amount of sleep generally thought to be insufficient. Option 4: Normalization of sleep should not depend on use of sleep aids.

Cognitive level: Application
Nursing process: Planning (Outcome Identification)
NCLEX: Physiological Integrity
See text page: 670

13. A client reports that nearly every night she awakens feeling frightened after a bad dream. The dream usually involves being hunted by individuals who wish to harm her. She tells the nurse that the awakening consistently takes place between 4 and 5 AM. The nurse assesses this disorder as being most consistent with *DSM-IV-TR* criteria for
  1. sleep talking.
  2. nightmare disorder.
  3. night terror disorder.
  4. REM sleep behavior disorder.

Answer: 2

Rationale: Nightmares are long, frightening dreams from which people awaken in a frightened state. They occur during REM sleep late in the night. Sleep talking occurs without fright and often without awakening the sleeper. Night terror disorder occurs as arousal in the first third of the night during non-REM sleep and is accompanied by feelings of panic. REM sleep behavior disorder involves acting out a violent dream during REM sleep.

Cognitive level: Analysis
Nursing process: Assessment
NCLEX: Physiological Integrity
See text page: 666

14. A 32-year-old man tells the nurse at the sleep disorders clinic that he awakens almost nightly in the midst of acting out a violent dream in which he is defending himself against multiple attackers. When he awakens, he finds he has been hitting and kicking his wife to the point of bruising her face, arms, body, and legs. His wife insists that he must get help if she is to sleep in the same bed with him. The nurse assesses this disorder as being most consistent with criteria for
  1. sleep paralysis.
  2. sleep-related bruxism.
  3. night terror disorder.
  4. REM sleep behavior disorder.

Answer: 4

Rationale: The scenario describes REM sleep behavior disorder in which the client engages in violent and complex behaviors during REM sleep as though acting out his dreams. Option 1: Sleep paralysis refers to the sudden inability to perform voluntary movement either at sleep onset or awakening from sleep. Option 2: Bruxism refers to grinding teeth during stage 2 sleep. Option 3: Night terror disorder occurs as arousal in the first third of the night during non-REM sleep and is accompanied by feelings of panic.

Cognitive level: Analysis
Nursing process: Assessment
NCLEX: Physiological Integrity
See text page: 666

15. A client tells the nurse that he was considered "hyper" as a child and took some sort of medication for a few years while he was in grade school. The medication was discontinued when he was 13 years old. He remembers being an underachiever in high school and just barely graduating. He describes himself now as being disorganized and having problems in occupational functioning. The nurse should recognize this description as being consistent with the clinical picture of
  1. borderline personality disorder.
  2. generalized anxiety disorder.
  3. stress intolerance disorder.
  4. adult attention deficit hyperactivity disorder (ADHD).

Answer: 4

Rationale: ADHD is usually diagnosed in early life and treated until adolescence. Treatment is often stopped because professionals think the disorder resolves itself because the hyperactive impulsive behaviors may diminish. The inattentive and disorganized behaviors tend to persist, however. Options 1 and 2: The scenario description is inconsistent with borderline personality disorder and generalized anxiety disorder. Option 3: Stress intolerance disorder is not found in the *DSM-IV-TR*.

Cognitive level: Analysis
Nursing process: Assessment
NCLEX: Psychosocial Integrity
See text page: 671

16. A client tells the nurse "I make a lot of careless mistakes at work and I have a lot of trouble staying 'on task.' Sometimes I know I should be listening to what a speaker is saying, but I cannot seem to tune in. When it comes to organizing, I have a bad time putting things in the right order and I often lose the tools and things I need to complete a task." The nurse correctly assesses these concerns as problems with
  1. inattention.
  2. impulsivity.

3. hyperactivity.
4. social impairment.

Answer: 1

Rationale: Inattention refers to failure to pay attention as described by the client's inability to "tune in." A number of the other problems are the result of failure to pay attention. Option 2: Impulsivity refers to acting without thinking through consequences. Option 3: Hyperactivity refers to excessive motor activity. Option 4: Social impairment refers to failure to use appropriate social skills.

Cognitive level: Analysis
Nursing process: Assessment
NCLEX: Psychosocial Integrity
See text page: 671

17. The nurse about to interview a client with suspected adult ADHD should prepare assessment questions to elicit information about the ADHD symptom that predominates in adults with this disorder. The focus of such a question would be on
    1. social impairment.
    2. inattention.
    3. hyperactivity.
    4. impulsivity.

Answer: 2

Rationale: Although hyperactivity, impulsivity, and social impairment usually diminish as troublesome symptoms during adolescence and early adulthood, inattention usually persists from childhood into adult ADHD.

Cognitive level: Application
Nursing process: Assessment
NCLEX: Psychosocial Integrity
See text page: 671

18. Basic premises the nurse should include in health teaching for adults with ADHD and significant others are (more than one premise may be correct)
    1. ADHD is a genetically transmitted biological condition.
    2. clients with ADHD respond best to negative reinforcement to modify behavior.
    3. psychostimulants effective for children with ADHD are rarely helpful for adults.
    4. cognitive therapy is useful to challenge internalized negative beliefs about self.

Answers: 1, 4

Rationale: Evidence suggests that ADHD has a biological basis. This fact can help adults with the disorder cope with lowered self-esteem that is often the result of negative treatment and lack of acceptance in childhood. Cognitive therapy is helpful in reframing negative beliefs about self. The other options are untrue statements.

Cognitive level: Analysis
Nursing process: Planning
NCLEX: Health Promotion and Maintenance
See text pages: 670, 672, 673

19. The nurse case manager has agreed to become a coach for a client with ADHD. Responsibilities of the coach should include
    1. reminding the client of priorities and deadlines.
    2. teaching work-related skills such as basic math.
    3. establishing penalties for failure to organize tasks.
    4. giving encouragement and strategies for managing and organizing.

Answer: 4

Rationale: The coach's major responsibilities lie with encouraging the client to learn and use necessary skills, assisting the client to stay on task. The coach is not an ever-present taskmaster or penalizer, however. Neither does the coach teach work-related skills. That task would be assumed by vocational staff.

Cognitive level: Application
Nursing process: Implementation
NCLEX: Psychosocial Integrity
See text page: 676

20. A client with adult ADHD reflects "I make a lot of careless mistakes at work and I have a lot of trouble staying 'on task.' Sometimes I cannot seem to tune in to what others are telling me. My thoughts seem to drift and I do not connect facts. When it comes to organizing, I have a bad time putting things in the right order." The physician tells the nurse that she believes medication will help the client. The nurse should expect to provide health teaching about a class of drugs known as
    1. benzodiazepines.
    2. psychostimulants.
    3. neuroleptics.
    4. anxiolytics.

Answer: 2

Rationale: Psychostimulants such as methylphenidate and amphetamines provide the basis for treatment of both adult and childhood ADHD. They are the most commonly used medications, so the nurse could expect the physician would order a drug in this class. None of the other drugs given as options have proven useful in the treatment of ADHD.

Cognitive level: Application

Nursing process: Implementation
NCLEX: Health Promotion and Maintenance
See text page: 673

21. A 22-year-old beginning treatment with methyl-phenidate (Concerta) for adult ADHD tells the nurse "I have been stupid ever since I was a kid. I was wild and never sat still. I drove the teachers nuts. My parents could not do anything with me. I hung out with the losers when I was a teen because they were the only ones who would accept me. Now, I cannot please my wife or keep a decent job. Everyone gets all bent out of shape because I cannot remember dates and times and I cannot seem to concentrate to get jobs done." The nurse planning care for the client should initially consider
   1. cognitive therapy to help address internalized beliefs.
   2. group therapy to allow comparison of feelings with others.
   3. marriage counseling to sustain interpersonal relationships.
   4. vocational counseling to identify needed occupational skills.

Answer: 1
Rationale: Cognitive therapy and knowledge of ADHD will make it possible for the client to reframe the past and the present in a more positive and realistic light and to challenge internalized false beliefs about himself. Option 2: Group therapy may be valuable at a later time to allow testing new coping behaviors in a safe environment. Option 3: Marriage counseling can be used to strengthen newly reframed thinking and help replace blaming, anger, and frustration with commitment to change. Option 4: Vocational counseling can help the client explore suitable career options as he pursues treatment.
Cognitive level: Analysis
Nursing process: Planning
NCLEX: Psychosocial Integrity
See text pages: 673, 674

22. A new staff nurse tells the clinical nurse specialist "I am unsure about my role when clients bring up sexual problems." The clinical nurse specialist should give clarification by saying "All nurses
   1. qualify as sexual counselors. Each has knowledge about the biopsychosocial aspects of sexuality throughout the life cycle."
   2. should be able to screen for sexual dysfunction and give basic information about sexual feelings, behaviors, and myths."
   3. should defer questions about sex to other health

care professionals because of their limited knowledge of sexuality."
   4. who are interested in sexual dysfunction can provide sex therapy for individuals and couples."

Answer: 2
Rationale: The basic education of nurses provides information sufficient to qualify the generalist to assess for sexual dysfunction and perform health teaching. Taking a detailed sexual history and providing sex therapy requires additional training in sex education and counseling. Options 1 and 4: Nurses with basic education are not qualified to be sexual counselors. Additional education is necessary. Option 3: Basic information about sexual function may be provided by the registered nurse. Complex questions may require referral.
Cognitive level: Application
Nursing process: Implementation
NCLEX: Safe and Effective Care Environment
See text page: 677

23. A nurse is performing a nursing assessment for a 59-year-old man who is hypertensive. What is the rationale for including questions about prescribed medications and their effects on sexual function in the assessment?
   1. Sexual dysfunction may result from use of prescription and nonprescription drugs.
   2. Such questions are a indirect way of learning about the client's drug intake.
   3. These questions ease the transition to questions about sexual practices.
   4. A variety of medical conditions alter sexual functioning.

Answer: 1
Rationale: The side effects of several groups of drugs include impotence or delayed ejaculation in men and decreased responsiveness in women. This rationale relates directly to the question, whereas the other options are tangential.
Cognitive level: Application
Nursing process: Assessment
NCLEX: Physiological Integrity
See text page: 685

24. A middle-aged client tells the nurse that he has delayed ejaculation. Which of the drugs currently prescribed for the client is most likely to be at fault for this condition?
   1. Warfarin
   2. Doxycycline
   3. Lovastatin
   4. Fosinopril

441

Answer: 4

Rationale: Antihypertensive agents often cause or contribute to sexual dysfunction. The other options do not usually cause this problem.

Cognitive level: Analysis
Nursing process: Assessment
NCLEX: Physiological Integrity
See text page: NA

25. A 55-year-old client is recuperating from a myocardial infarction. At a follow-up visit to his physician's office, he tells the nurse practitioner "I have not had much interest in sex since my heart attack. My wife is wondering if something's wrong with me. The truth is, I know having sex puts a strain on my heart and I do not know if my heart is strong enough." The nursing diagnosis for this client should be written as
   1. sexual dysfunction related to self-esteem disturbance.
   2. sexual dysfunction related to knowledge deficit resulting in fear.
   3. disturbed body image related to lifestyle changes resulting in anxiety.
   4. disturbed body image related to treatment side effects.

Answer: 2

Rationale: Clients who have had a myocardial infarction often believe sexual intercourse will cause another heart attack. These clients should receive information about when sexual activity may begin, positions that conserve energy, and so forth. Option 1: The scenario does not suggest self-esteem disturbance. Options 3 and 4: The scenario pinpoints sexual dysfunction rather than suggests disturbed body image.

Cognitive level: Analysis
Nursing process: Diagnosis
NCLEX: Physiological Integrity
See text page: 687

26. The nursing diagnosis the nurse can most easily rule out when analyzing possible diagnoses for clients with problems of sexual functioning such as orgasmic disorders or sexual pain disorders is
   1. sexual dysfunction.
   2. ineffective sexuality patterns.
   3. disturbed body image.
   4. ineffective coping.

Answer: 4

Rationale: Ineffective coping is least likely to have relevance when sexual functioning is the problem. This diagnosis is more related to the general ability of the individual to function effectively than to sexual functioning.

Cognitive level: Analysis
Nursing process: Diagnosis
NCLEX: Psychosocial Integrity
See text page: 687

27. The nursing action that takes priority when working with a client who has a problem of sexual functioning is
   1. acquiring knowledge of client's sexual roles.
   2. developing an understanding of human sexual response.
   3. clarifying the nurse's personal values.
   4. assessing the client's sexual functioning.

Answer: 3

Rationale: Before a nurse can be helpful to clients with sexual dysfunction, each must be aware of and comfortable with his or her own feelings about sex and sexuality. As a corollary, nurses must be comfortable with the idea that clients have a right to their own values and must avoid criticism and censure.

Cognitive level: Application
Nursing process: Implementation
NCLEX: Psychosocial Integrity
See text page: 677

28. The question that would be best to ask when the nurse wishes to introduce the topic of the client's sexual functioning is
   1. "Have you recently experienced a change in your self-esteem?"
   2. "Has anything, such as illness, pregnancy, or a health problem, interfered with your role as a wife (or husband)?"
   3. "Has anything, such as a heart attack or surgery, changed the way you feel about yourself as a man (or woman)?"
   4. "Has anything, such as surgery or disease, changed your body's ability to function sexually?"

Answer: 4

Rationale: Although each of the questions has relevance to the client's sexual history, option 4 directly relates to sexual function.

Cognitive level: Application
Nursing process: Assessment
NCLEX: Physiological Integrity
See text pages: 684, 685

29. A client tells the nurse that his sexual functioning is normal when his wife wears short red nightgowns. He states, "Without the red nighties, I am not interested in sex." The nurse can assess this as consistent with
   1. pedophilia.
   2. exhibitionism.

3. fetishism.

4. voyeurism.

Answer: 3

Rationale: A person with a sexual fetish finds it necessary to have some external object present, in fantasy or in reality, to be sexually satisfied. Option 1: Pedophilia refers to the preference for having sexual relations with a child. Option 2: Exhibitionism refers to exposing ones genitalia publicly. Option 4: Voyeurism refers to viewing others in intimate situations.

Cognitive level: Application

Nursing process: Assessment

NCLEX: Psychosocial Integrity

See text page: 681

30. While performing a nursing assessment the nurse says to a client, "While growing up, most of us have heard some half-truths about sexual matters that continue to puzzle us as adults. Do any come to your mind now?" The purpose of this question is to

1. determine possible homosexuality.

2. identify sexual misinformation.

3. identify areas of sexual dysfunction for treatment.

4. introduce the topic of masturbation.

Answer: 2

Rationale: Misinformation about normal sex and sexuality is common. Lack of knowledge may affect the individual's sexual adjustment. Once myths have been identified, the nurse can give information to dispel the myth.

Cognitive level: Application

Nursing process: Implementation

NCLEX: Psychosocial Integrity

See text page: 686

31. A client, aged 25 years, tells the nurse he is living a miserable existence. All his life, he states, he has thought, felt, and acted like a woman while living in the body of a man. He has lived as a female and dressed in feminine attire for more than a year. He has decided to change jobs so as not to compromise a new identity. The request the client is most likely to make of the physician is

1. "Will you order estrogen therapy?"

2. "Can you refer me for psychological testing?"

3. "Will you alter my medical records?"

4. "What should I tell my parents?"

Answer: 1

Rationale: Before sexual reassignment surgery, the step that follows living as a member of the other sex is hormone therapy. The client's decision to live as a woman makes this a natural request. Option 1: Psychological testing would be undertaken before

sexual reassignment surgery, often after hormone therapy has begun. Option 3 would be an inappropriate request. Option 4: The client has likely told his parents by this point.

Cognitive level: Analysis

Nursing process: Assessment

NCLEX: Psychosocial Integrity

See text pages: 680, 681

32. The manager of a health club has been discovered to have placed a hidden video camera in the women's locker room and has taped several women as they showered and dressed. The nurse who reads this in the paper can assess that the club manager probably is a

1. homosexual.

2. exhibitionist.

3. pedophile.

4. voyeur.

Answer: 4

Rationale: Voyeurism is the viewing of others in intimate situations such as undressing, bathing, or having sexual relations. Voyeurs are often called "peeping Toms." Option 1: A homosexual individual would be interested in watching members of the same sex. Option 2: Exhibitionists are interested in exposing their genitals to others. Option 3: Pedophiles seek sexual contact with prepubescent children.

Cognitive level: Application

Nursing process: Assessment

NCLEX: Psychosexual Integrity

See text page: 681

CHAPTER 34

1. A student nurse visiting a nutrition center for the elderly tells the nursing instructor "It is so depressing to see all these old people. They seem so weak and frail. I doubt if I will be able to do my assessment paper because they are probably all senile." The student is expressing

1. reality.

2. ageism.

3. vulnerability.

4. empathy.

Answer: 2

Rationale: Ageism is defined as a bias against older people because of their age. None of the other options can be identified from the ideas expressed by the student.

Cognitive level: Application

Nursing process: Assessment

NCLEX: Psychosocial Integrity

See text pages: 693, 694

443

2. A community mental health nurse has the task of planning an educational program for staff of a home health agency specializing in care of the elderly. A topic of high priority should be
1. identifying clinical depression in older adults.
2. providing cost-effective foot care for the elderly.
3. identifying dietary deficiencies in the elderly.
4. psychosocial stimulation for those who live alone.

Answer: 1

Rationale: The topic of greatest immediacy is the identification of clinical depression in older adults. Home health staff are better versed in the physical aspects of care and are less knowledgeable about mental health topics. Statistics show that elderly clients with mental health problems are less likely than young adults to be accurately diagnosed. This is especially true for depression and anxiety, both of which are likely to be misinterpreted as normal aging. Undiagnosed and untreated depression and anxiety result in unnecessary suffering. The other options are of lesser importance.

Cognitive level: Analysis
Nursing process: Planning
NCLEX: Psychosocial Integrity
See text page: 693

3. A nurse is asked by staff to explain the reasons ageism is a problem among health care workers. The outcomes the nurse should cite include the facts that ageism results in (more than one option may be correct)
1. staff shortages because caregivers prefer working with younger adults.
2. failure of the elderly to receive necessary medical information.
3. development of public policy that favors programs for the elderly.
4. the perception that elderly consume less than their share of medical resources.

Answers: 1, 2

Rationale: Because of society's negative stereotyping of the elderly as having little to offer, some staff avoid working with older clients. Staff shortages in long-term care are often greater than those for acute care. Elderly clients are often given less information about their conditions and are given fewer treatment options than younger clients because some health care staff perceive them as less able to understand. Option 3: Public policy discriminates against programs for the elderly. Option 4: Anger exists because the elderly are perceived to consume a disproportionately large share of medical resources.

Cognitive level: Analysis

Nursing process: Implementation
NCLEX: Psychosocial Integrity
See text pages: 692, 693

4. Factors that will affect the provision of safe, effective care for elderly clients include the fact(s) that (more than one option may be correct)
1. sexual interest declines with aging.
2. the elderly are prone to become crime victims.
3. aging results in a 50% decline in restorative sleep.
4. older adults are unable to learn new tasks.

Answers: 2, 3

Rationale: Older individuals are more prone to become crime victims. A decline in restorative sleep does occur as one ages. These factors affect care delivery by nurses. The other two options reflect myths about aging.

Cognitive level: Comprehension
Nursing process: Planning
NCLEX: Safe and Effective Care Environment
See text page: 695

5. The optimal way for a nurse to begin an interview with an elderly client is
1. "Hello, _____ [call client by first name]. I am going to be asking you a number of questions to get to know you better."
2. "Hello. My name is _____. I am a nurse here. Please tell me how you would like to addressed by staff."
3. "I am going to be asking you a number of questions about yourself. I would like to call you by your first name if you do not mind."
4. "Hi. You look as though you are comfortable and ready to participate in an admission interview. Shall we get started?"

Answer: 2

Rationale: This opening identifies the nurse's role and politely seeks direction for addressing the client in a way that will make him or her comfortable. This is particularly important when a considerable age difference exists between the nurse and the client. Option 1: The nurse has assumed the client wants to be called by a first name but has not introduced self. Option 3: Again, the nurse seeks to use the client's first name and fails to introduce self. Option 4: The nurse fails to introduce self and does not identify the client.

Cognitive level: Analysis
Nursing process: Implementation
NCLEX: Psychosocial Integrity
See text pages: 694, 695

6. A client, aged 75 years, has come to the clinic with a report of frequent headaches. Immediately after introducing herself to the client at the outset of the interview, the nurse should
   1. ask if the client if can hear clearly as she speaks.
   2. initiate a neurological assessment to determine risk for stroke.
   3. obtain a medication order for the client's headache.
   4. suggest that the client lie down in a darkened room for a few minutes.

Answer: 1

Rationale: Before proceeding with any further assessment, the nurse should assess the client's ability to hear questions. Impaired hearing could lead to inaccurate answers.

Cognitive level: Application
Nursing process: Assessment
NCLEX: Safe and Effective Care Environment
See text pages: 694, 695

7. The statement about aging that provides a rationale for focused assessment for elderly clients is that
   1. the majority of elderly are demented.
   2. the elderly are often socially isolated and lonely.
   3. the senses of vision, hearing, touch, taste, and smell decline with age.
   4. as people age, they become more rigid in their thinking and more set in their ways.

Answer: 3

Rationale: Only option 3 is a true statement. It cues the nurse to assess carefully elderly client sensory function. Correcting vision and hearing are critical to providing safe care. Options 1, 2, and 4 are myths about aging.

Cognitive level: Application
Nursing process: Planning
NCLEX: Safe and Effective Care Environment
See text pages: 694, 695

8. To which question should the answer "yes" from an elderly client prompt the nurse to include the Geriatric Depression Scale as part of the assessment?
   1. "Would you say your mood is often low?"
   2. "Do you often experience moderate to severe pain?"
   3. "Have you noticed an increase in your alcohol use?"
   4. "Are you having any trouble with your memory?"

Answer: 1

Rationale: Feeling low may be a symptom of depression. Low moods occurring with regularity should signal the need to further assess for other symptoms of depression. The other options do not focus on mood.

Cognitive level: Application
Nursing process: Assessment
NCLEX: Psychosocial Integrity
See text pages: 694, 695

9. A nursing home resident, aged 78 years, who is being treated for hypertension and cardiac disease is usually alert and well oriented. This morning she tells the nurse that her granddaughter came to visit her during the night and stood at the foot of the bed talking to her. In reality, the client's granddaughter is a nurse who lives 50 miles away. The client does consider this night visit a bit strange but shrugs the strangeness off. The nurse should suspect that the resident may
   1. have cognitive impairment because of a high blood level of a medication.
   2. have had a ministroke and developed sensory perceptual alteration.
   3. be developing Alzheimer's disease associated with advanced age.
   4. have alcohol-related cognitive impairment.

Answer: 1

Rationale: A resident taking medications is at high risk for becoming confused because of medication side effects, drug interactions, and delayed excretion. The nurse should report the event and continue to assess for cognitive impairment. Option 2: Residual impairment would probably continue to be present in the event of a vascular event. Option 3: Symptoms of dementia tend to develop slowly but persist over time. Option 4: The history would alert the nurse to alcohol-related cognitive impairment.

Cognitive level: Analysis
Nursing process: Assessment
NCLEX: Safe and Effective Care Environment
See text pages: 694, 695, 704, 706

10. The physician visits and writes new orders for a nursing home resident. In addition to antihypertensive medication orders, the nurse finds the following: (1) 2-g sodium diet, (2) restraint as needed, (3) fluids to 2000 mL daily, (4) milk of magnesia 30 mL orally once if no bowel movement for 3 days. The nurse should
   1. transcribe the orders as written.
   2. question the order for restraint.
   3. question the fluid order.
   4. question the milk of magnesia order.

Answer: 2

Rationale: Restraints may be imposed only on the written order of the physician that specifies the duration during which the restraints can be used. Joint Commission on Accreditation of Healthcare

445

Organizations guidelines and Omnibus Budget Reconciliation Act regulations also mandate a number of other conditions that must be considered and documented before restraints are used. The other orders would be considered appropriate for implementation.

Cognitive level: Analysis
Nursing process: Implementation
NCLEX: Safe and Effective Care Environment
See text pages: 701, 702

11. If an elderly client must be physically restrained, who is responsible for the safety of the client during the duration of restraint use? The
    1. physician who ordered the application of restraint.
    2. nurse assigned to care for the client.
    3. nursing assistant who applies the restraint.
    4. family member who agrees to the application of the restraint.

Answer: 2
Rationale: Although restraint is ordered by a physician, the restraint is a measure carried out by nursing staff. The nurse assigned to care for the client is ultimately responsible for safe application of restraining devices and for providing safe care while the client is restrained. Nurses may delegate the application of restraining devices and the care of the client in restraint but, as delegators, remain responsible for outcomes. Option 4: Even when family agree to restraint, nurses are responsible for providing safe outcomes.

Cognitive level: Analysis
Nursing process: Implementation
NCLEX: Safe and Effective Care Environment
See text pages: 701, 702

12. The treatment team has decided that the emotional distress of an elderly client who experiences threatening auditory hallucinations warrants the use of haloperidol (Haldol). As a result, the nursing staff must take action to reduce the risk of
    1. falls.
    2. seizures.
    3. dehydration.
    4. fecal impaction.

Answer: 1
Rationale: The incidence of falls increases when chemical restraint with neuroleptics or anxiolytics is used to reduce emotional distress. Medication does not place the client at great risk for the other options.

Cognitive level: Application
Nursing process: Planning
NCLEX: Safe and Effective Care Environment
See text page: 702

13. A new nurse mentions "I think Mrs. Z. is in pain, but her dementia prevents me from using the tools I usually use to assess pain. What can I do?" The nurse's mentor should recommend using the
    1. Baker-Wong Faces Pain Rating Scale.
    2. Visual Analog Scale.
    3. McGill Pain Questionnaire.
    4. Pain Assessment in Advanced Dementia Scale.

Answer: 4
Rationale: This scale is used to evaluate the presence and severity of pain in clients with advanced dementia. It evaluates breathing, negative vocalizations, body language, and consolability. The other scales are more useful when clients have the cognitive ability to respond to the scale.

Cognitive level: Application
Nursing process: Assessment
NCLEX: Safe and Effective Care Environment
See text pages: 702, 703

14. The nurse caring for a client with severe dementia has assessed the client's level of pain as moderate and has provided pain relief medication. An hour after the medication is administered, reassessment suggests that the client is still in pain. The best action for the nurse to take would be to
    1. seek an order for additional analgesia.
    2. reposition the client.
    3. offer oral intake.
    4. give adjuvant medication.

Answer: 2
Rationale: Repositioning the client offers an opportunity to provide a simple, yet often effective, comfort measure. Another tip is to ensure the patency of the indwelling catheter if the client has one. Blocked urine flow can create pain associated with a distended bladder. Options 1 and 4: Seeking additional or adjuvant medication an hour after analgesic administration is not advised. Option 3: Oral intake may not be feasible because many clients with severe dementia have difficulty swallowing.

Cognitive level: Analysis
Nursing process: Implementation
NCLEX: Physiological Integrity
See text page: 704

15. The nurse will derive plans for a client knowing that the client's living will gives valid direction to health care givers when the client has
    1. Alzheimer's disease.
    2. Parkinson's disease.
    3. multiple sclerosis and is unable to speak.
    4. terminal carcinoma and is incapacitated.

Answer: 4
Rationale: Living wills are invoked only in cases of terminal illness.
Cognitive level: Application
Nursing process: Planning
NCLEX: Psychosocial Integrity
See text page: 706

16. A client with whom the nurse is discussing advance directives asks "What advantage does a durable power of attorney for health care have over a living will?" The nurse should reply
   1. "A durable power of attorney for health care gives your agent the ability to speak for you during any illness if you become incapacitated."
   2. "A durable power of attorney for health care can be used only if you have a terminal illness and become incapacitated."
   3. "A durable power of attorney for health care cannot go into effect for 30 days so you have time to rethink your decision."
   4. "A durable power of attorney can be given only to a relative who would have your best interests at heart."

Answer: 1
Rationale: A durable power of attorney for health care is an instrument that appoints a person other than a physician to act as an individual's agent in the event that he or she is unable to make medical decisions. No waiting period is required for it to become effective, and the individual does not have to be terminally ill or incompetent for the person appointed to act on the individual's behalf.
Cognitive level: Application
Nursing process: Implementation
NCLEX: Psychosocial Integrity
See text page: 707

17. Relative to risk for AIDS among the elderly, nurses should consider providing health teaching aimed at
   1. supporting unprotected sex.
   2. encouraging condom use.
   3. explaining AIDS dementia.
   4. avoiding blood transfusions.

Answer: 2
Rationale: Because the risk for pregnancy is nonexistent in postmenopausal women, condom use is diminished. This puts elderly women at risk for AIDS and other sexually transmitted diseases. Safe sex continues to be important and should be taught to the elderly population. Option 3: AIDS dementia presents clinically with many of the same symptoms as Alzheimer's disease. This topic is of much less im-

portance than educating about the use of condoms. Option 4: Little to no danger exists from blood transfusions.
Cognitive level: Analysis
Nursing process: Planning
NCLEX: Health Promotion and Maintenance
See text pages: 707, 708

18. A single male client, aged 79 years, tells the visiting nurse "I have been feeling down for the last few days. I do not have much to live for. My family and friends are all dead. My money is running out, and my health is failing." The nurse should assess this as
   1. normal pessimism of the elderly.
   2. a cry for sympathy.
   3. normal grieving.
   4. evidence of suicide risk.

Answer: 4
Rationale: The client describes loss of significant others, loss of economic security, and loss of health. He describes mood alteration and voices the thought that he has little to live for. Combined with his age, sex, and single status, each is a risk factor for suicide.
Cognitive level: Application
Nursing process: Assessment
NCLEX: Safe and Effective Care Environment
See text page: 708

19. A client appears sad and speaks slowly and haltingly. She tells the nurse of the death of her husband of 50 years and the death of her daughter in a recent automobile accident. The client has no other family but has a circle of close friends who offer support. What nursing diagnosis should be considered for this client?
   1. Spiritual distress related to being angry with God for taking her family
   2. Anxiety related to sudden and abrupt lifestyle change
   3. Social isolation related to loss of existing family
   4. No nursing diagnosis listed is warranted at this time

Answer: 4
Rationale: The client is experiencing normal grief related to the loss of her family. No defining characteristics exist for the diagnoses listed in options 1, 2, and 3, and no defining characteristics exist for the diagnosis of dysfunctional grieving.
Cognitive level: Analysis
Nursing process: Assessment
NCLEX: Psychosocial Integrity
See text pages: 708, 709

Chapter 34   Psychosocial Needs of the Older Adult

20. When a distinction must be made as to whether a client is demonstrating confusion related to depression or dementia, what nursing assessment would be of particular value?
    1. The client with dementia is pervasively angry and hostile.
    2. Early morning agitation and hyperactivity are present in dementia.
    3. The depressed client is preoccupied with leaving the facility to return home.
    4. Confusion seems to worsen at night when dementia is present.

Answer: 4
Rationale: Both dementia and depression in the elderly may produce symptoms of confusion. To help distinguish whether depression or dementia is producing the confused behavior, note whether the confusion seems to increase at night. This occurs more often with dementia than with depression. The other options are not necessarily true.
Cognitive level: Application
Nursing process: Assessment
NCLEX: Psychosocial Integrity
See text page: 709

21. To thoroughly evaluate an elderly client's memory, reminiscence strategies are helpful because they
    1. reduce the client's anxiety.
    2. produce a positive mood.
    3. stimulate memory chains through associations.
    4. allow evaluation of the client's judgment and general fund of knowledge.

Answer: 3
Rationale: Reminiscence can be used to stimulate memory chains by attempting to recall patterns of association that will improve the client's recollection. The statements made in the other options are not necessarily true.
Cognitive level: Application
Nursing process: Implementation
NCLEX: Physiological Integrity
See text page: 699

22. A client who is 80 years old and has difficulty walking because of arthritis tells the nurse "It is awful to be old. It seems as though every day is a struggle. No one cares about an old person." The best response from the nurse would be
    1. "Oh, let's not focus on the negative. Tell me something good."
    2. "It is a hard truth. We are a youth-oriented society."
    3. "It sounds as though you are having a difficult time. Tell me about it."

4. "You are still able to get around, and your mind is as sharp as a tack."

Answer: 3
Rationale: The nurse uses empathetic understanding to permit the client to express her frustration and clarify her "struggle" for the nurse. The other options block communication.
Cognitive level: Application
Nursing process: Implementation
NCLEX: Psychosocial Integrity
See text page: 698

23. A client, aged 74 years, is regressed and apathetic. Left to his own devices he would sit in a chair near the nurses' station and interact with others only when they initiate the interaction. What form of therapy would be most useful to promote resocialization?
    1. Life review
    2. Individual psychotherapy
    3. Remotivation
    4. Group psychotherapy

Answer: 3
Rationale: Remotivation therapy is designed to resocialize regressed and apathetic clients by focusing on a single topic, creating a bridge to reality as group members talk about the world in which they live and work and hobbies related to the topic. Group members are given acceptance and appreciation by group leaders.
Cognitive level: Application
Nursing process: Planning
NCLEX: Psychosocial Integrity
See text page: 699

24. The clinic nurse saw four clients this morning. Which client would the nurse assess as being a geriatric problem drinker?
    1. X, who had intermittent problems with alcohol misuse early in life, then abused alcohol constantly from age 45 years onward
    2. Y, who had no history of alcohol-related problems until age 65 years, when she retired and began to drink large amounts of alcohol daily "to keep her mind off her arthritis"
    3. S, who drank socially all his adult life and continues this pattern, maintaining he has earned the right to do as he pleases
    4. T, who abused alcohol between the ages of 25 and 40 years, and now at age 70 years abstains and occasionally attends AA

Answer: 2

Rationale: A geriatric problem drinker is defined as someone who has no history of alcohol-related problems but develops an alcohol abuse pattern in response to the stresses of aging. Aging alcoholics, on the other hand, have had alcohol problems earlier in life that continue into old age.

Cognitive level: Analysis
Nursing process: Assessment
NCLEX: Psychosocial Integrity
See text pages: 710-713

25. An elderly client with depression who is being treated with a tricyclic antidepressant should be carefully observed for
   1. orthostatic hypotension and urinary retention.
   2. photosensitivity and skin rashes.
   3. pseudo-Parkinsonism and tardive dyskinesia.
   4. diarrhea and electrolyte imbalance.

Answer: 1
Rationale: Both orthostatic hypotension and urinary retention are side effects of tricyclic antidepressants. The elderly often have circulatory problems predisposing them to orthostatic hypotension and often are particularly sensitive to the anticholinergic side effects of these drugs, which may cause urinary retention.

Cognitive level: Application
Nursing process: Assessment
NCLEX: Physiological Integrity
See text page: 710

26. An elderly client with depression is to be treated with the selective serotonin reuptake inhibitor sertraline. This drug is often chosen for elderly clients because it
   1. is effective when given in smaller doses.
   2. has relatively few side effects.
   3. has few adverse interactions with other drugs.
   4. has a high degree of sedation.

Answer: 2
Rationale: The elderly are particularly susceptible to side effects, so choosing a drug with a low side-effect profile is desirable. Options 1, 3, and 4 are either incorrect or of lesser relevance.

Cognitive level: Application
Nursing process: Planning
NCLEX: Physiological Integrity
See text page: 710

27. When admitting an elderly client to the long-term care unit, the nurse must take measures based on the knowledge that at the time of admission, health care agencies receiving federal funds must provide clients written information about

   1. the financial status of the institution.
   2. their rights to have advance health care directives.
   3. how to sign out against medical advice.
   4. the institution's policy on "coding" individuals.

Answer: 2
Rationale: The Patient Self-Determination Act of 1990 requires that clients have the opportunity to prepare advance directives.

Cognitive level: Application
Nursing process: Implementation
NCLEX: Psychosocial Integrity
See text page: 706

28. Discharge planning is underway for an elderly client who has been hospitalized for 2 weeks for treatment of major depression with selective serotonin reuptake inhibitors. The client has been determined to need ongoing mental status assessment, socialization opportunities, health education regarding medication, and relapse prevention. The client lives with her daughter, who works during the week. The best referral for the client would be
   1. partial hospitalization.
   2. home care.
   3. a nursing home.
   4. a halfway house.

Answer: 1
Rationale: Partial hospitalization would provide the services the client needs and would give supervision and meals to the client while her daughter is at work. Home care would not provide socialization. The nursing home could not as easily provide the necessary teaching. A halfway house provides 24-hour care and usually expects involvement in off-campus programs.

Cognitive level: Analysis
Nursing process: Planning
NCLEX: Safe and Effective Care Environment
See text pages: 698-701

29. A physically frail, cognitively impaired elderly client is being referred to a facility that can provide supervision and safety as well as recreation and social interaction during the day. The client will be cared for by family during the evening and night. The type of community-based facility that would meet the client's needs is
   1. social day care.
   2. adult day health care treatment.
   3. maintenance day care.
   4. partial hospitalization.

Answer: 1
Rationale: Social day care provides recreation and social interaction. Nursing, medical, and rehabilitative care

449

are usually not provided. Option 2: Adult day health care goes beyond meeting recreational and social needs by providing medical interventions and nursing and rehabilitation services. Option 3: Maintenance day care provides services for clients at high risk for institutionalization. Option 4: Partial hospitalization provides acute psychiatric hospital programs in a day care setting.

Cognitive level: Analysis
Nursing process: Planning
NCLEX: Safe and Effective Care Environment
See text pages: 698-701

30. When the nurse wishes to pursue assessment of suicidal ideation in an elderly client, a question that would provide valuable data is
   1. "What thoughts do you have about a person's right to take his or her life?"
   2. "Do you have any risk factors that potentially contribute to suicide?"
   3. "Do you think you are vulnerable to developing depressed mood?"
   4. "If you felt suicidal, would you communicate your feelings to anyone?"

Answer: 1
Rationale: This question is clear, direct, and respectful. It will produce information relative to the acceptability of suicide as an option to the client. If the client deems suicide unacceptable, no further assessment is necessary. If the client deems suicide as acceptable, the nurse can continue to assess intent, plan, means to carry out the plan, lethality of the chosen method, and so forth. The other options are less direct and will produce responses that may be unclear.

Cognitive level: Analysis
Nursing process: Assessment
NCLEX: Safe and Effective Care Environment
See text page: 708

31. The nurse assessing an elderly client for suicide potential should include questions about mood as well as seek information about (more than one option may be correct)
   1. sleep pattern changes.
   2. increased appetite.
   3. increased concern with bodily functions.
   4. enhanced self-esteem.
   5. anhedonia and anergia.

Answers: 1, 3, 5
Rationale: These symptoms are often noted in elderly clients with depression. Somatic symptoms are often present but are missed by nurses as being related to depression. Option 2: Anorexia, rather than hy-

perphagia, is seen in major depression. Option 4: Low self-esteem is more often associated with major depression.

Cognitive level: Application
Nursing process: Assessment
NCLEX: Safe and Effective Care Environment
See text page: 709

32. When the nurse assembles assessment data for an elderly client seeking mental health care, which risk factors should be identified as predisposing the client to development of geriatric problem drinking? (More than one option may be correct.)
   1. History of alcohol abuse starting in young adulthood
   2. Retirement
   3. Loss of spouse
   4. Mild recent memory impairment

Answers: 2, 3
Rationale: The geriatric problem drinker begins drinking in later life, often in response to stressors such as retirement, loss of spouse, and loneliness. Once the demands of job, career, and care of a family and household are gone, the structure of daily life is disrupted and little impetus remains to stay sober. Option 4: Mild cognitive impairment is not a predisposing factor in the development of geriatric problem drinking.

Cognitive level: Application
Nursing process: Assessment
NCLEX: Psychosocial Integrity
See text page: 710

33. A home care client who has been identified as drinking a six-pack of beer daily tells the community mental health nurse that his arthritis has been "acting up" recently and he is taking acetaminophen arthritis formula four times daily for pain. The priority interventions the nurse should take include (more than one option may be correct)
   1. determining the safety of the dose the client is ingesting daily.
   2. advising the client of the harmful effect of alcohol and acetaminophen on the liver.
   3. suggesting increasing the acetaminophen dose because alcohol causes faster excretion.
   4. inquiring about sleep disturbance caused by mixing alcohol and analgesics.
   5. assessing for declining functional status associated with medication-induced dementia.

Answers: 1, 2
Rationale: The nurse should be concerned with the client's use of alcohol and acetaminophen because the toxicity of acetaminophen is enhanced by alco-

hol and by the age-related decrease in clearance. The nurse must determine whether the acetaminophen dose is within safe limits or is excessive and provide this information to the client. Next, the nurse must provide health education regarding the danger of combined use of acetaminophen and alcohol. The client will likely need to discontinue alcohol or consult the physician about another analgesic that is less hepatotoxic. Option 3: This would cause greater liver damage. Option 4: This is not a current priority. Option 5: This is not a priority.

Cognitive level: Analysis
Nursing process: Planning
NCLEX: Physiological Integrity
See text page: 711

CHAPTER 35

1. A client tells the members of the inpatient therapy group that he hears voices saying his doctor is going to poison him. He continues "I look around to see who is talking to me, and I cannot see anybody." Another client replies "I used to hear voices, too. I found out they were my imagination. The voices you hear are not real, either." Which phenomenon common to groups is exemplified in this interchange?
   1. Ventilation
   2. Universality
   3. Catharsis
   4. Symptom management

Answer: 4
Rationale: Symptom management can be taught by peers by helping the individual validate his or her perception of reality. Additionally, group members can help each other manage symptoms by monitoring each member's reactions and behaviors and providing feedback in an open and nonthreatening manner. Option 1: Ventilation refers to expressing feelings. Option 2: Universality refers to members realizing they are not alone with their problems and feelings. Option 3: Catharsis refers to sharing intense feelings.

Cognitive level: Application
Nursing process: Assessment
NCLEX: Psychosocial Integrity
See text page: 724

2. The inpatient group is meeting in the solarium. The group is discussing aftercare. A client tells the group about the activities of a psychosocial club for former inpatients. She explains the club's purpose, the referral process, and the club's location. In this interaction the client has taken the role of

1. Harmonizer
2. Evaluator
3. Information giver
4. Procedural technician

Answer: 3
Rationale: Group roles refer to the parts various members play within the group. The client was acting as an information giver as she explained facts about a psychosocial club to the group as part of a discussion of aftercare. Harmonizers mediate conflicts. Evaluators measure group work against a standard. The procedural technician role is to assist by taking on tasks such as arranging chairs or passing out papers.

Cognitive level: Application
Nursing process: Assessment
NCLEX: Psychosocial Integrity
See text page: 720

3. The nurse psychotherapist looks at the records of the clients admitted over the weekend to determine whom to include in the inpatient symptom management group focusing on self-esteem issues. Which client will the nurse consider inappropriate to bring into the group?
   1. A, aged 32 years, a client with chronic paranoid schizophrenia
   2. B, aged 59 years, a client with depression
   3. C, aged 22 years, a client with panic disorder
   4. D, aged 30 years, a client with antisocial personality disorder

Answer: 4
Rationale: Clients with antisocial personality disorders frequently do not conform to social norms regarding lawful behavior. They tend to be impulsive, have little regard for the truth, and use others for their own ends. They do not benefit from group therapy, and they do not contribute to group cohesion or goal attainment. The other clients could profit from the group experience.

Cognitive level: Analysis
Nursing process: Assessment
NCLEX: Psychosocial Integrity
See text pages: 724, 725

4. During the morning community meeting on the inpatient psychiatric unit, a 40-year-old hypomanic client threatens to strike another client. The nurse therapist should intervene by
   1. immediately sending the other clients out of the room.
   2. telling the client he must leave the meeting.
   3. summoning the assistance of several other staff.
   4. firmly telling the client he can talk about being angry in group, but he cannot act out.

451

Answer: 4

Rationale: The therapist should intervene when a client threatens to act out by firmly orienting the client regarding what behavior is acceptable and what is unacceptable. Option 1: This is premature. Option 2: The client should be advised of limits before this action is taken. Option 3: This is premature.

Cognitive level: Application

Nursing process: Implementation

NCLEX: Safe and Effective Care Environment

See text pages: 722, 723

5. A young male client in a therapy group relates to an older female client as one might to a mother. The younger client asks the mother figure's permission to attend activities, to socialize with others, and so forth. This phenomenon is known as
   1. a hidden agenda.
   2. corrective recapitulation.
   3. imitative behavior.
   4. resistance.

Answer: 2

Rationale: The younger client is demonstrating an emotional attachment to the older client that is similar to a relationship within a nuclear family. This phenomenon is called corrective recapitulation of the primary family group. Group feedback provides learning about the behavior. Option 1: A hidden agenda refers to having goals that are at cross purposes to the group's goals. Option 3: Imitative behavior refers to copying behavior from the leader or peers. Option 4: Resistance refers to the inability to accept change.

Cognitive level: Application

Nursing process: Assessment

NCLEX: Psychosocial Integrity

See text pages: 721, 722

6. In which stage of a group's development would the following interaction most likely occur?
   Leader: "Shall we begin?"
   Client 1: "Why do you ask us if we want to begin?"
   Client 2: "You ought to just tell us what you want us to do."
   Leader: "You seem irritated."
   Client 3: "We thought someone in this group would give us help with our problems, but you do not give us any answers."
   1. preorientation
   2. Initial phase
   3. Working phase
   4. Termination

Answer: 3

Rationale: In the working phase issues of power and control surface. Members of the group may challenge the leader and display anger with the leader for not providing autocratic leadership. In its own way this behavior helps the group move toward reliance on one another. Option 1: Preorientation refers to the time during which the leaders select members and make plans for the group. Option 2: The initial phase refers to the time during which the members get to know one another, observe each other, and begin to take steps toward the working phase. Option 4: Termination prepares members for separation.

Cognitive level: Application

Nursing process: Assessment

NCLEX: NA

See text page: 719

7. During group therapy, a client states "When I first started in this group, B wasn't able to make a decision. Now she can. She has made a lot of progress. I am beginning to think that maybe I can conquer my fears, too." According to Yalom, this statement reflects
   1. Hope
   2. Altruism
   3. Catharsis
   4. Cohesiveness

Answer: 1

Rationale: The client's profession that he may be able to learn to cope more effectively reflects hope. Groups can instill hope in individuals who are demoralized or pessimistic. Option 2: Altruism refers to unselfish regard for others. Option 3: Catharsis refers to expression of strong emotion. Option 4: Cohesion refers to coming together and togetherness.

Cognitive level: Application

Nursing process: Assessment

NCLEX: Psychosocial Integrity

See text page: 722

8. During a group therapy session a client addresses the group, saying "I have been thinking about the way I feel about my husband. I am angry with him. He has no right to hit me or call me names. I feel hurt, too. I wonder what I have done to deserve this abuse." The client begins to sob. This can be assessed as
   1. Transference
   2. Cohesiveness
   3. Ventilation
   4. Altruism

Answer: 3

Rationale: Ventilation is the expression of one's feelings. Option 1: Transference is an emotional attachment to the therapist based on experience in the primary family. Option 2: Cohesiveness refers to the "togetherness" of the group. Option 4: Altruism refers to learning that one can be useful to others.

Cognitive level: Application
Nursing process: Assessment
NCLEX: Psychosocial Integrity
See text page: NA

9. During a group therapy session, a newly admitted client suddenly says to the nurse "How old are you? You do not act old enough to be helpful to any of us." The most appropriate response the nurse might make is
   1. "I wonder why you ask."
   2. "I am old enough to be a nurse."
   3. "My age should not really concern you."
   4. "You are wondering whether I have enough experience to lead this group."

Answer: 4
Rationale: A question such as this is common in the initial phase of group development when the members are getting to know one another and testing the leader. Option 4 permits the leader to explore the underlying issue with the client. Option 1 does not get at the underlying issue. Options 2 and 3 are defensive.

Cognitive level: Application
Nursing process: Implementation
NCLEX: Psychosocial Integrity
See text page: 719

10. A client in a group therapy session listens for a time and then remarks "I used to think I was the only one who felt afraid. It is nice to know that I am not alone." This is an example of
    1. ventilation.
    2. altruism.
    3. universality.
    4. group cohesiveness.

Answer: 3
Rationale: Realizing that one is not alone and that others share one's problems and feelings is called universality. Option 1: Ventilation refers to expressing emotions. Option 2: Altruism refers to learning that one can be of help to others. Option 4: Group cohesiveness refers to the degree of esprit de corps of the group.

Cognitive level: Application
Nursing process: Assessment
NCLEX: Psychosocial Integrity
See text pages: 721, 722

11. A nurse assigned to the well-child clinic in a low-cost housing development realizes that a number of mothers have misconceptions about the most effective ways of disciplining their children. The nurse decides that forming a group to resolve this problem would be an effective strategy. The focus of the group should be
    1. support.
    2. socialization.
    3. education.
    4. feelings.

Answer: 3
Rationale: The nurse has diagnosed a knowledge deficiency. The focus of the group should be education. The other options will be of lesser importance within the group meetings.

Cognitive level: Application
Nursing process: Planning
NCLEX: Health Promotion and Maintenance
See text page: 724

12. An appropriate outcome for a psychoeducation group composed of clients with chronic schizophrenia would be that group members would
    1. uncover dynamic material related to their illnesses.
    2. adopt roles used in their families to reduce anxiety.
    3. develop plans for relapse prevention.
    4. increase feelings of social isolation.

Answer: 3
Rationale: An appropriate psychoeducational focus for clients with schizophrenia is relapse prevention. During the group clients would identify behaviors and symptoms that signal relapse and develop plans for preventing their occurrence. Option 1: A more concrete outcome is called for. Option 2: This would not necessarily be appropriate. Option 4: This is undesirable.

Cognitive level: Analysis
Nursing process: Planning (Outcome Identification)
NCLEX: Psychosocial Integrity
See text page: 724

13. A client has talked constantly throughout the group therapy session. She has repeated the same material several times. Other members were initially attentive, then became bored, inattentive, and finally angry. Which intervention would be most effective for the nurse psychotherapist to take?
    1. Asking the group why they have permitted the client to take up their time with her repetitions
    2. Asking the group members how they felt when the client repeated herself throughout the session
    3. Mentioning that the group seems withdrawn and uninterested
    4. Telling the client she must allow others to have an opportunity to speak

Chapter 35   Therapeutic Groups

Answer: 1

Rationale: The most effective action the nurse psychotherapist can take will be the one that encourages the group to solve its own problem. Option 1 validates the other members' anger and helps them realize that they are responsible adults with the right to say what they feel. Option 2 is less direct. Option 3 skirts the issue. Option 4 does not allow the group to resolve the issue.

Cognitive level: Application
Nursing process: Implementation
NCLEX: Psychosocial Integrity
See text page: 726

14. A client with a dual diagnosis of bipolar disorder and alcoholism is referred to Alcoholics Anonymous (AA). He asks what good "meeting with a bunch of ex-drunks" is going to do him. The answer that will give the client relevant information about AA is
   1. "The group will work to help you create new defenses."
   2. "People with a common problem provide mutual support."
   3. "The group leader sets tasks for members to promote behavioral change."
   4. "You will have a sponsor who will watch you to prevent a return to drinking."

Answer: 2

Rationale: The basis for AA (and other self-help groups) is that members who have experienced a common problem can effectively provide support and encourage positive coping behaviors. Option 1 is undesirable. Option 3 is untrue. Option 4 is partially untrue.

Cognitive level: Application
Nursing process: Implementation
NCLEX: Psychosocial Integrity
See text page: 727

15. The nurse is cotherapist of a group. The guidelines followed by the therapists include focusing on changing dysfunctional behavior and thinking patterns, selecting from the unit population the clients who can profit from the group, intervening promptly, and being directive. This type of group therapy can be identified as
   1. behavioral therapy.
   2. self-help.
   3. psychoeducational.
   4. cognitive-behavioral.

Answer: 4

Rationale: The characteristics described are those of cognitive-behavioral therapy in which clients learn to reframe dysfunctional thoughts to provide more re-

alistic appraisals. Option 1: Behavioral therapy focuses on changing behavior rather than thoughts or feelings. Option 2: A self-help group is composed of clients with similar problems and has no leaders. Option 3: A description of psychoeducational therapy would describe something being taught.

Cognitive level: Application
Nursing process: Implementation
NCLEX: Psychosocial Integrity
See text page: 726

16. The nurse is to lead a sexuality group. The best setting would be
   1. the unit day room.
   2. the hospital's theater-style auditorium.
   3. the unit conference room.
   4. a corner of the music therapy room.

Answer: 3

Rationale: The conference room would provide a quiet, private area for teaching and learning. The day room and the music therapy room are too busy. The auditorium is too large and has inappropriate seating.

Cognitive level: Application
Nursing process: Planning
NCLEX: Safe and Effective Care Environment
See text page: 724

17. Which remark would the nurse expect to hear during the mature stage of group therapy?
   1. "How do I know you people will not tell others what I say?"
   2. "I am uncomfortable because two people seem to have more power in this group than the rest of us."
   3. "If we are all going to benefit, we have to make sure that everyone gets a chance to share feelings."
   4. "Telling you about that problem has made me feel better. I appreciate the support and suggestions."

Answer: 4

Rationale: In the mature stage members actively participate to help each individual to accomplish goals. Option 1, an issue of confidentiality, would be heard during the initial stage. Option 2, an issue of power, would be heard during the working stage. Option 3 is an issue of norming and would be seen in the initial stage.

Cognitive level: Application
Nursing process: Assessment
NCLEX: Psychosocial Integrity
See text page: 719

18. Three members of the therapy group share covert glances as other members of the group bring up

problems. One of them often makes a statement that subtly puts down another speaker or takes exception to a comment by the group leader. The others then nod in agreement. The group leader should suspect the occurrence of
1. cohesiveness.
2. confrontation.
3. subgrouping.
4. countertransference.

Answer: 3

Rationale: Subgrouping occurs when a small group is isolated within a larger group and functions separately, having more loyalty to the subgroup than to the larger group. Option 1: Cohesiveness refers to the "togetherness" of the group. In this case the group lacks cohesion. Option 2: Confrontation refers to questioning a member in a challenging, yet supportive, way. Option 4: Countertransference refers to the therapist's reaction to a group member.

Cognitive level: Application
Nursing process: Assessment
NCLEX: Safe and Effective Care Environment
See text page: 719

19. The nurse therapist is planning to begin a therapy group to which new clients will be added as the present clients are discharged. This qualifies the group as
1. open.
2. closed.
3. time-limited.
4. milieu therapy.

Answer: 1

Rationale: An open group is a group that adds members throughout the life of the group. Option 2: A closed group does not add new members. Option 3: Time-limited refers to a group that meets for a specific number of sessions, then terminates. Option 4: Milieu therapy refers to groups such as recreational, physical activity, creative arts, and story-telling groups.

Cognitive level: Application
Nursing process: Assessment
NCLEX: Psychosocial Integrity
See text page: 719

20. The next to last meeting of an interpersonal therapy group is taking place. The group leader's task is to
1. keep the group focused on the goals of individual members.
2. solidify progress of members in building relationships.
3. help members prepare for separation.
4. foster clear, congruent communication.

Answer: 3

Rationale: The goal for the termination phase of groups is to prepare the group for separation and prepare each member for the future. Contributions of members and the experience as a group are acknowledged as part of termination. Option 1: Individual goals should have been achieved before termination. Option 2: Relationship-building will have been completed before termination. Option 3: This is a goal for all stages and is not exclusive to termination.

Cognitive level: Application
Nursing process: Implementation
NCLEX: Psychosocial Integrity
See text page: 719

21. During an inpatient therapy group that uses existential/Gestalt theory, feelings experienced by clients at the time of their admission to the unit are discussed. As a silence falls, one member mentions "We have heard from several people who describe feeling angry. I would like to hear from some people who experienced other feelings." The nurse identifies this communication as exemplifying the group role of
1. Energizer
2. Compromiser
3. Encourager
4. Self-confessor

Answer: 3

Rationale: The member is filling the role of encourager by acknowledging those who have contributed and seeking input from others. Option 1: An energizer encourages the group to make decisions or take an action. Option 2: The compromiser yields during a conflict to preserve harmony. Option 4: A self-confessor verbalized feelings or observations unrelated to the group.

Cognitive level: Application
Nursing process: Assessment
NCLEX: Psychosocial Integrity
See text page: 720

22. The nurse conducting a support group for clients undergoing cancer treatment will use interventions that (more than one option may be correct)
1. confront ingrained behaviors and defenses.
2. foster controlled expression of feelings.
3. teach stress management techniques.
4. show acceptance and empathy.
5. provide psychoeducation.
6. encourage mutual support.

Answers: 3, 4, 5, 6

Rationale: The leader of a support group models acceptance and empathy in interactions with members as

Chapter 35   Therapeutic Groups

they express feelings, encourages mutual support, provides psychoeducation and direction as needed, and teaches stress management techniques as necessary. Additional interventions might be directed toward reducing member feelings of isolation and strengthening existing defenses of members. Option 1: Existing defenses are strengthened rather than attacked. Option 2: Open expression of feelings is fostered and support is given by the leader and group members.

Cognitive level: Application
Nursing process: Implementation
NCLEX: Psychosocial Integrity
See text page: 727

23. A nurse on the inpatient unit leads a self-care group for clients having many negative symptoms of schizophrenia. An appropriate outcome would be that clients will
   1. be able to describe the effect of medication on sexuality.
   2. exercise increased self-control over hallucinations.
   3. appear clean and neatly groomed each day.
   4. ask questions about unit routines.

Answer: 3
Rationale: This outcome relates directly to the focus of the group, self-care. The other options are desirable outcomes but are unrelated to the group's purpose.

Cognitive level: Analysis
Nursing process: Planning (Outcome Identification)
NCLEX: Psychosocial Integrity
See text page: 725

24. The nurse working with members of a support group for rape trauma victims focuses the discussion by saying "What ways have members handled the problem of fear of being alone with men?" This communication technique can be correctly identified as
   1. feedback.
   2. reflecting.
   3. questioning.
   4. clarification.

Answer: 3
Rationale: Questioning asks for information and encourages members to discuss the subject extensively. Option 1: Feedback gives members information about behaviors. Option 2: Reflecting highlights information to emphasize it or check it for accuracy. Option 4: Clarification checks the meaning of an interaction or statement and serves to decrease misunderstandings.

Cognitive level: Application
Nursing process: Implementation
NCLEX: Psychosocial Integrity
See text page: 721

25. Which client would benefit most from a symptom management group focusing on relapse prevention?
   1. A middle-aged woman with chronic schizophrenia
   2. An elderly man with early symptoms of dementia
   3. A teenage boy with obsessive-compulsive disorder
   4. A woman experiencing rape trauma syndrome

Answer: 1
Rationale: The goal for a symptom management group is that members will learn coping skills from each other, such as relapse prevention for clients with chronic schizophrenia by developing a plan for action at the first sign of losing control. Option 2: Relapse prevention is not possible. Options 3 and 4: Relapse prevention may not be the best focus for these clients. A more meaningful focus might be increased control over symptomatic behaviors.

Cognitive level: Analysis
Nursing process: Assessment
NCLEX: Psychosocial Integrity
See text page: 724

CHAPTER 36

1. The nurse can identify scapegoating as occurring within a family when
   1. the family members project the inadequacies of the family onto one particular family member.
   2. messages of hostility are sent by the identified patient to family members.
   3. the identified patient threatens separation to induce feelings of isolation and despair.
   4. family members use nonverbal techniques to disguise or qualify the meaning of verbal messages.

Answer: 1
Rationale: Scapegoating is defined as blaming family problems on a member of the family who is not very powerful. The purpose of the blaming is to keep the focus off the painful issues and problems of the blamers. The behaviors described in options 2 and 3 are dysfunctional behaviors that have no specific name. Option 4 refers to a double bind.

Cognitive level: Application
Nursing process: Assessment
NCLEX: Psychosocial Integrity
See text page: 739

2. The nurse therapist assessing a family system perceives the family to be enmeshed and determines that family members have little sense of individuality. A desirable outcome is that members will
   1. form groups of three to reduce anxiety.
   2. become more differentiated regarding values and beliefs.

456

3. become comfortable adhering to family norms and rules.
4. form two subgroups: the most capable and least capable members.

Answer: 2

Rationale: Enmeshment results from high anxiety that keeps members emotionally bound to each other and unable to define individual values and beliefs. To define individual values and beliefs would mark progress in differentiation. Triangulation (option 1) and subgrouping (option 4) are not desirable. Option 3: The members already adhere to the family norms and rules.

Cognitive level: Analysis
Nursing process: Planning (Outcome Identification)
NCLEX: Psychosocial Integrity
See text page: 746

3. A student, aged 15 years, is a school truant. His family, a second-generation Asian American family, comes to see the school nurse, who discovers that the student's parents have been having marital conflict for approximately 6 months since the paternal grandmother moved into their home. The student's parents say their son is behaving disrespectfully. The nurse determines several factors of concern in assessing the family, including (more than one option may be correct)
1. stage of family life cycle.
2. multigenerational issues.
3. sociocultural context.
4. sexual dysfunction.

Answers: 1, 2, 3

Rationale: Options 1, 2, and 3 are relevant. Sexual dysfunction is not a factor in this scenario; therefore this topic need not receive emphasis in the family assessment.

Cognitive level: Analysis
Nursing process: Assessment
NCLEX: Psychosocial Integrity
See text pages: 735, 739, 740

4. Bowen's approach to family therapy focuses on differentiation of members. A therapist using this approach would negotiate with the family to arrive at the outcome criteria. The family will
1. restructure dysfunctional triangles.
2. use straight messages without manipulation.
3. achieve greater individuation of members.
4. assess itself in terms of life cycle stage and multicultural issues.

Answer: 3

Rationale: The identification of poor differentiation of family members calls for a goal of greater differentiation, that is, members developing a greater sense of individual selves. Differentiation does not relate directly to triangulating, improving the clarity of communication, or looking at family life cycles.

Cognitive level: Application
Nursing process: Planning (Outcome Identification)
NCLEX: Psychosocial Integrity
See text pages: 735, 736

5. A client remarks to the nurse "The family therapist mentioned that our family is enmeshed. Can you tell me what that means?" The best reply from the nurse would be
1. "It means that your family members do not have a strong sense of their own individual selves."
2. "It means that your communication patterns often give double messages. Your body language does not match the meaning of what you say."
3. "Enmeshment refers to the tendency of your family to try to maintain balance. When the balance tips, you take measures to restore the balance."
4. "Enmeshment refers to blaming the weakest family member for all the troubles of the family."

Answer: 1

Rationale: Enmeshed families have unclear distinctions among family members. Option 2 refers to double-bind communication. Option 3, the seeking of balance, refers to family homeostasis. Option 4 refers to scapegoating.

Cognitive level: Application
Nursing process: Implementation
NCLEX: Health Promotion and Maintenance
See text pages: 731, 732

6. A family has revealed to the nurse that the father has begun to be verbally abusive to his wife and physically abusive to his oldest son since he lost his job 3 months ago. The son is threatening to run away and the wife has developed increased anxiety. An appropriate nursing diagnosis for the family would be
1. ineffective coping related to job loss.
2. impaired parenting related to father beating son.
3. caregiver role strain related to increased tension between parents.
4. disabled family coping related to use of verbal and physical abuse.

Answer: 4

Rationale: Disabled family coping refers to the behavior of a significant family member that disables his or her own capacity as well as another's capacity to perform tasks essential to adaptation. Option 1: Ineffective coping is inaccurate because more than one individual's coping is affected. Option 2: Impaired parenting deals with only a part of the problem. Option 3: Caregiver role strain refers to the caregiver's difficulty in performing family caregiver roles.

Cognitive level: Analysis
Nursing process: Diagnosis
NCLEX: Psychosocial Integrity
See text page: 742

7. An appropriate outcome for family therapy for a family of three in which the father became verbally abusive to his wife and physically abusive to his oldest son, resulting in the son threatening to run away and the wife developing increased anxiety, is the
   1. dysfunctional behavior of individual family members will be lessened within 3 months.
   2. family will begin to consider parental divorce within 6 weeks.
   3. sensitivity to other members' emotional needs will decrease.
   4. family system will be fully integrated into societal system within 1 year.

Answer: 1
Rationale: Assessment has shown that family members are behaving dysfunctionally. Option 2 may not be necessary. Option 3 is undesirable. Option 4 refers to a concern that has not been identified.

Cognitive level: Analysis
Nursing process: Planning (Outcome Identification)
NCLEX: Psychosocial Integrity
See text pages: 742, 743

8. When a single parent of three communicates with her children, she often refuses the requests they make but manages to give subtle nonverbal messages that indicate the child may do the opposite of what she says. The nurse who observes this should assess the behavior as
   1. permissive.
   2. dysfunctional.
   3. defensive.
   4. supportive.

Answer: 2
Rationale: Giving unclear or contradictory messages is a dysfunctional pattern of communication. Messages should be clear and unequivocal. Permissive parenting would allow the children to do as they pleased. Defensiveness would be suggested by trying to protect self from perceived attack. Supportive parenting would provide clear communication.

Cognitive level: Application

Nursing process: Assessment
NCLEX: Psychosocial Integrity
See text pages: 732, 733

9. Which of the following, if living in one household, would be identified as a nuclear family?
   1. A married couple, their son, and their daughter
   2. A grandmother, her divorced son, and his girlfriend
   3. A gay couple and a sister
   4. An engaged couple and some cousins

Answer: 1
Rationale: A nuclear family consists of a parent or parents and the child or children under the care of the parent(s).

Cognitive level: Application
Nursing process: Assessment
NCLEX: Psychosocial Integrity
See text page: 739

10. Family R is described by a neighbor: "The parents are not rich, but all the kids have what they need. They love to see their kids behave assertively. Everybody in that family knows where they stand. The kids have great people skills like their parents. When the mother was in the hospital, their daughter cooked the meals and their son cleaned. Sure, they have their disagreements, but they settle them without grudges." The family can be assessed as
    1. enmeshed.
    2. fragile.
    3. healthy.
    4. schizophrenogenic.

Answer: 3
Rationale: The family demonstrates adequate management and flexibility, allowing for differences and providing freedom to grow, emotional support, and good communication. All are characteristics of a healthy family. Option 1 refers to blending together of roles, thoughts, and feelings of family members. Option 2 refers to the lack of hardiness and resilience. Option 4 refers to an outmoded concept that maternal coldness and double-bind communication produced schizophrenic offspring.

Cognitive level: Application
Nursing process: Assessment
NCLEX: Psychosocial Integrity
See text page: 731

11. Which situation is least likely to place severe, disabling stress on a family? The
    1. need for long-term care for a man with a wife and two teenage sons who sustains severe brain injury.

458

2. divorce of the parents of three children, aged 10, 8, and 2 years.
3. death of a mother who leaves a husband and three sons younger than 12 years.
4. family in which the son leaves for college and the father retires.

Answer: 4

Rationale: Family stress is greatest when an interruption or dislocation occurs in the unfolding of the family life cycle. Options 1, 2, and 3 are such dislocations. The situation described in option 4 may be fraught with stress but the changes are not interruptions; they are to be expected.

Cognitive level: Analysis
Nursing process: Assessment
NCLEX: Psychosocial Integrity
See text page: 735

12. A woman tells the BSN-prepared community health nurse that she and her son fight all the time since the son started using drugs. The son tells his mother when she counsels against drug use that his drug use is none of her business. The most effective nursing intervention would be to
1. arrange drug detoxification and rehabilitation for the son.
2. provide family therapy for both son and mother.
3. turn the son in to the police.
4. arrange a referral to a family counselor.

Answer: 4

Rationale: A BSN-prepared nurse is not able to conduct family therapy but can determine the need for referral to counseling. Option 1 is premature. Option 3 is not a nursing intervention.

Cognitive level: Application
Nursing process: Implementation
NCLEX: Psychosocial Integrity
See text pages: 743, 744

13. The advanced practice nurse is assigned to be case manager for a client with newly diagnosed bipolar disorder who is participating in a multiple family therapy group led by the nurse. Discharge planning for the client included return to independent living with the family, attendance at a day hospital program, and maintenance medication. The responsibilities appropriate for the nurse to assume would be (more than one option may be correct)
1. providing medication psychoeducation.
2. providing ongoing assessment of family strengths.
3. coordinating services the client will receive.
4. referring the family to the National Alliance for the Mentally Ill for support.

5. planning family mobilization if relapse occurs.
6. supporting client and family as they deal with loss.

Answers: 1, 2, 3, 4, 5, 6

Rationale: The nurse will be filling roles of case manager as well as family therapist; thus all the tasks listed in the options would be appropriate for the nurse to undertake.

Cognitive level: Application
Nursing process: Implementation
NCLEX: Psychosocial Integrity
See text pages: 745, 746

14. Which option describes a healthy family?
1. Mrs. S is highly involved with their daughter; Mr. S is only peripherally involved with the child.
2. The C family has rigid family boundaries that permit their adolescent children to move in and out.
3. Mr. and Mrs. D are renegotiating their marital system as a couple now that their children have moved out.
4. The younger generation of the K family (in their 30s) is taking over completely for the older generation (in their 60s).

Answer: 3

Rationale: Option 3 is correct. Reforming as a couple is necessary when children move out of the family of origin. Option 1 refers to triangulation. Option 2: To allow adolescents to move in and out, family boundaries must be more relaxed rather than rigid. Option 4: The healthy family would allow the older generation the freedom to do as much as they can rather than push them aside.

Cognitive level: Application
Nursing process: Assessment
NCLEX: Psychosocial Integrity
See text pages: 731-734, 737, 740, 741

15. The nurse performing a family assessment determines that the parents jointly make decisions regarding family rules and apportion the family resources in ways that serve the interests of all members. Plans for the future exist but are flexible and allow for changing circumstances. The three teenage children participate in discussions but do not have responsibility for decisions. The assessment the nurse should document is
1. family management function is appropriate and adequate.
2. boundary function makes a distinction between individuals.
3. communication function of the family is healthy.
4. emotional-supportive function is dominated by conflict.

Chapter 36   Family Therapy

Answer: 1

Rationale: Family management function refers to decisions regarding issues of power, rule making, provision of financial support, goods allocation, and future planning.

The management functions described in the scenario should be assessed as healthy and appropriate. The scenario does not refer to other family functions such as boundary, communication, or emotional-supportive functions.

Cognitive level: Analysis
Nursing process: Assessment
NCLEX: Psychosocial Integrity
See text page: 731

16. The daughter in a family consisting of a father, mother, and two sons describes the family to the nurse, saying "We are like most families. Dad is always angry and expects us to know why without having to tell us his problem. Mom is always trying to smooth things over. Tom is always messing up but never takes any blame. Jim stays in his room and hides from the rest of us. And I play the part of the sweet little girl to get my own way." Assuming this is an accurate description, the nurse should make the assessment that
   1. family communication is clear and direct.
   2. family communication relies on dysfunctional patterns.
   3. family members are seeking more functional communication patterns.
   4. the socialization function of the family will permit role change with minimal stress.

Answer: 2

Rationale: A number of dysfunctional patterns are described in the scenario: Dad, Mom, Tom, and the daughter each rely on a dysfunctional strategy. Option 1: Communication is neither clear nor direct. Option 3: The scenario does not suggest that members are seeking more functional communication patterns. Option 4: The scenario describes the communication function of the family rather than the family's socialization function.

Cognitive level: Analysis
Nursing process: Assessment
NCLEX: Psychosocial Integrity
See text page: 733

17. The daughter in a family consisting of a father, mother, and two sons describes the family to the nurse, saying "We are like most families. Dad is always angry and expects us to know why without having to tell us his problem. Mom is always trying to smooth things over. Tom is always messing up but never takes any blame. Jim stays in his room and hides from the rest of us. And I play the part of the sweet little girl to get my own way." The daughter's description gives evidence of her use of
   1. projection.
   2. rationalization.
   3. generalizing.
   4. identification.

Answer: 3

Rationale: The daughter uses many global statements including "always" and "never," which defines generalization. A better alternative would be to describe specific problems or areas of conflict. Generalization is an example of a dysfunctional communication pattern. Option 1: Projection refers to attributing one's unwanted attributes onto another. Option 2: Rationalization refers to offering a socially acceptable explanation in lieu of the actual explanation. Option 3: Identification refers to adopting the attributes of another.

Cognitive level: Application
Nursing process: Assessment
NCLEX: Psychosocial Integrity
See text page: 733

18. When the daughter of a family describes herself as playing the part of the sweet little girl to get her own way, the nurse can make the assessment that the daughter is using a dysfunctional strategy called
   1. placation.
   2. distraction.
   3. blaming.
   4. manipulation.

Answer: 4

Rationale: Manipulation is an example of dysfunctional communication. Manipulation refers to controlling by being artful rather than honest. Playing the part of the sweet little girl to gain one's goal is dysfunctional. Openly and clearly asking for what is wanted is a more functional communication pattern. Option 1: Placating is a way of keeping peace. Option 2: Distraction refers to the introduction of irrelevant details into problematic issues. Option 3: Blaming serves the purpose of keeping the focus away from the self.

Cognitive level: Application
Nursing process: Assessment
NCLEX: Psychosocial Integrity
See text page: 733

19. Which example of behavior within a family system would be assessed as double-bind communication?

1. A mother tells her daughter "I do not want you to go to the mall with Sandra today."
2. A daughter tells her father "I feel as though you are treating me like a baby when you tell me I must be home by 10 PM on a school night."
3. A son tells his mother "You worry too much about what might happen."
4. A wife tells her husband "You go ahead and go bowling. If it is necessary, I will try to manage getting up and going to the bathroom with my crutches."

Answer: 4

Rationale: Option 4 suggests the wife may not be entirely comfortable getting up and using the crutches to get to the bathroom and would actually prefer that the husband stayed home to help her. This remark places the husband in a double bind, a situation in which no acceptable response exists. The husband is "damned if he does" and "damned if he doesn't." Options 1, 2, and 3 are clear, direct communications.

Cognitive level: Application
Nursing process: Assessment
NCLEX: Psychosocial Integrity
See text pages: 735, 736

20. To make the most relevant assessment of a client within the context of the family the nurse must think in terms of
   1. cause and effect.
   2. circular causality.
   3. insight orientation.
   4. emotional reactivity.

Answer: 2

Rationale: In circular causality, the presenting problem of the identified patient must be viewed from many different perspectives: stressors, strengths, family's current life cycle stage, sociocultural context, mutigenerational issues, and so forth rather than from a single cause and effect. Option 1: Cause and effect is too simplistic a framework. Option 3 is terminology without meaning to family theory. Option 4: Emotional reactivity is a term that is too narrow to be correct.

Cognitive level: Comprehension
Nursing process: Assessment
NCLEX: Psychosocial Integrity
See text page: 737

21. The nurse is to meet a family for the first family therapy session. The husband/father is an accountant who admits to being skeptical of the idea that talking can help the family strengthen its ability to cope with life stressors. The wife/mother is a teacher who states she is not skillful in conflict resolution. The son, aged 15 years, defies parents and teachers and is in academic trouble. The daughter, aged 17 years, is trying to decide whether to attend a local college and live at home or attend an out-of-state university. The family member listed on the referral as the identified patient is most likely to be the
   1. husband/father.
   2. wife/mother.
   3. son.
   4. daughter.

Answer: 3

The identified patient is the family member who is regarded as the problem. The identified patient usually bears most of the family system's anxiety and may have come to the attention of parents, teachers, or law enforcement as a result of poor coping skills. The identified patient, however, may not actually be the one who initially seeks help. The other members of the family are not likely to be considered problem members based on the information provided in the scenario.

Cognitive level: Analysis
Nursing process: Assessment
NCLEX: Psychosocial Integrity
See text page: 737

22. The nurse is to meet a family for the first family therapy session. The husband/father is an accountant who admits to being skeptical of the idea that talking can help the family strengthen its ability to cope with life stressors. The wife/mother is a teacher who states she is not skillful in conflict resolution. The son, aged 15 years, defies parents and teachers and is in academic trouble. The daughter, aged 17 years, is trying to decide whether to attend a local college and live at home or attend an out-of-state university. During the first meeting the nurse should plan to
   1. elicit the perspective of each family member.
   2. maintain the focus of all members on the here and now.
   3. provide psychoeducation regarding oppositional defiant disorder.
   4. state the expectation that members will promote and support family coping.

Answer: 1

Rationale: The perspective of each family member must be elicited and heard. Not only does the nurse gain information with this technique, but family members may be hearing the information for the first time and will come to better understand the position and feelings of other members. Option 2: This may not be appropriate because a certain amount of history may be relevant at the first meeting. Option 3: This may be premature.

Option 4: Outcomes should be negotiated by the entire family, not imposed by the nurse.

Cognitive level: Application
Nursing process: Planning
NCLEX: Psychosocial Integrity
See text page: 743, 744

23. During a multifamily psychoeducational family therapy session, a client who has persistent schizophrenia mentions "Sometimes I feel very sad that I will never have a high-level job like my brother, who is an executive. Then I dwell on it, and maybe I should not." The nurse leader can best facilitate discussion of this issue by saying
    1. "Grieving for what is lost is a normal part of having a mental disorder."
    2. "How have others in the group handled painful feelings like these?"
    3. "It is often better to focus on our successes rather than our failures."
    4. "I wonder if you might also experience feelings of anger and helplessness."

Answer: 2
Rationale: Asking for others to share their experiences will facilitate discussion of an issue. Option 1 gives information and may serve to close off discussion of the issue because it sounds final. Option 3 implies a discussion of the issue is not appropriate. Option 4 is inappropriate at this point considering the client has identified feelings of sadness and seems to have a readiness to explore this feeling.
Cognitive level: Analysis
Nursing process: Implementation
NCLEX: Psychosocial Integrity
See text page: 745

24. The nurse caring for a 40-year-old building contractor with rheumatoid arthritis realizes from what he says that his wife and 13-year-old son have taken on many new roles since he became severely debilitated. They have become caregivers, helping him dress, lifting him into his truck so he can go to building sites, and picking him up when he falls. His wife has taken over ordering building supplies and assigning work teams in addition to running her own home cleaning business. When the nurse asks the wife "How are you holding up these days?" her response is "Sometimes I wonder how long we are going to be able to provide the care he needs. He seems to be weaker every month. I feel like I am going to collapse under the strain, but I know I have to keep going. It is hard on our son, too, to see his dad so

helpless." The nursing diagnosis the nurse should consider completing is
    1. ineffective denial.
    2. defensive coping.
    3. spiritual distress.
    4. caregiver role strain.

Answer: 4
Rationale: The definition of this diagnosis is difficulty in performing family caregiver role. The information in the scenario is clearly related to this diagnosis but not directly related to any of the other options.
Cognitive level: Analysis
Nursing process: Diagnosis
NCLEX: Psychosocial Integrity
See text page: 742

25. A husband/father who is disabled with chronic back pain has progressed with rehabilitation to being able to do light household chores and care for his 5-year-old son. The wife/mother decides to attend a 2-year nursing program to provide income for the family. The husband tells everyone he is delighted with the decision, but shortly after his wife begins classes the husband finds his pain is so severe that he must return to being on bed rest and give up his household responsibilities. This scenario is an example of
    1. scapegoating.
    2. triangulation.
    3. placating.
    4. double-bind communication.

Answer: 4
Rationale: In this situation the husband's verbal response to his wife returning to school is positive, but his behavioral response is negative. The wife is placed in a no-win situation. Option 1: Scapegoating refers to blaming one family member for the family's problems. Option 2: Triangulation refers to drawing in a third person to stabilize an unstable relationship between two persons. Option 3: Placating refers to a way of keeping peace within the family by taking the blame for another's behavior.
Cognitive level: Application
Nursing process: Assessment
NCLEX: Psychosocial Integrity
See text page: 733

CHAPTER 37

1. A client tells the nurse "I always buy St. John's wort manufactured by Company X so I know what I am getting." The best response for the nurse would be
    1. "That is fine. This will ensure continuity of therapy."

2. "That is not really necessary because industry standards exist."
3. "No manufacturing standards exist, so you may get variations even from Company X."
4. "You should really use a drug rather than an herbal preparation to treat your depression."

Answer: 3

Rationale: No standards for preparation of herbal remedies exist, so dosages may vary widely even in preparations made by one company. Option 1: Continuity is not guaranteed. Option 4 is not advisable because it does not recognize the importance of the alternative treatment to the client.

Cognitive level: Application
Nursing process: Implementation
NCLEX: Physiological Integrity
See text pages: 749, 750

2. A client shows a nurse the following advertisement for a product: "Product X is a miraculous cure for a wide range of ailments, including depression, anxiety, and sleeplessness. Made from an ancient formula and containing a secret ingredient, Product X will cure you or you will receive your money back. Only $45 for a 1-month supply. Order now and receive a free month's supply." The nurse should assess this as most likely being
1. a bargain.
2. worth a try.
3. dangerous.
4. worthless.

Answer: 4

Rationale: Advertisements promising miracles are usually for products that are useless and being fraudulently marketed. Some may even be harmful. Caution clients that things that sound "too good to be true" probably are.

Cognitive level: Analysis
Nursing process: Assessment
NCLEX: Physiological Integrity
See text page: 764

3. When a client wishes to learn more about alternative or complementary treatments the nurse should refer the client to
1. The American Medical Association.
2. The American Nurses Association.
3. The National League for Nursing.
4. The National Center of Complementary and Alternative Medicine.

Answer: 4

Rationale: The National Center of Complementary and Alternative Medicine has a clearinghouse from which individuals may request information. The organizations named in the other options do not provide extensive information about this topic.

Cognitive level: Application
Nursing process: Implementation
NCLEX: Health Promotion and Maintenance
See text page: 750

4. A client informs a nurse that he is sold on the idea that aromatherapy is a viable cure for his agoraphobia and that he plans to order several hundred dollars' worth of oils from an Internet site that promises swift results when their products are used. The client mentions that the Internet provides up-to-date, reliable information. The nurse should
1. offer praise for seeking information from an independent source.
2. tell the client that aromatherapy is little more than a fraudulent money-making scam.
3. advise the client that aromatherapy has not been proven to be helpful in the treatment of phobias.
4. suggest that the client report the offer to the local police and have them investigate the Internet site.

Answer: 3

Rationale: The nurse should view alternative treatments with an open mind and try to recognize the importance of the treatment to the client while trying to give the client accurate information about the treatment.

Cognitive level: Application
Nursing process: Implementation
NCLEX: Health Promotion and Maintenance
See text page: 761

5. A client states she has taken megadoses of vitamin E for 3 months to improve her circulation but thinks she feels somewhat worse. The priority action for the nurse should be to
1. assess the client for symptoms and signs of hypervitaminosis E: headaches, fatigue, blurred vision, and thrombophlebitis.
2. remind the client that the Food and Drug Administration has not evaluated vitamin E as preventive or curative of any disease.
3. formulate the outcome that the client will use a reliable resource to investigate megadosing before her next visit.
4. evaluate the effectiveness of the vitamin by performing ultrasound examination of the legs and a mental status examination.

Answer: 1

Rationale: Megadoses of any vitamin taken over long periods may produce untoward side effects. The priority for the nurse is to assess for problems associated with megadosage and urge caution in continuing the practice. Option 2 and 3 are not as viable alternatives as option 1. Option 4: Ordering an ultrasound examination is not within the limits of the nurse's license.

Cognitive level: Analysis
Nursing process: Implementation
NCLEX: Physiological Integrity
See text page: 757

6. A client plans to go to the acupuncturist for complementary treatment of alcoholism. He asks the nurse to explain how acupuncture works. The most accurate response would be "Acupuncture is a traditional Chinese medical treatment. The Chinese believe
   1. the insertion of needles modulates the flow of energy along body meridians."
   2. taking small doses of noxious substances will alleviate illness symptoms."
   3. manipulation of the spinal column will correct energy flow problems."
   4. herbal remedies, which are natural substances, are better than synthetics."

Answer: 1
Rationale: Acupuncture involves the insertion of needles to modulate the flow of body energy (chi) along specific body pathways called meridians. Option 2 refers to homeopathy. Option 3 refers to chiropractic. Option 4: Traditional Chinese medicine is more concerned with balance than with natural versus synthetic treatments.

Cognitive level: Application
Nursing process: Implementation
NCLEX: Health Promotion and Maintenance
See text page: 760

7. A client is receiving acupuncture as a complementary treatment for alcoholism. An expected outcome would be that the client will
   1. state he has decreased desire for alcohol.
   2. experience fewer symptoms of anxiety.
   3. practice skills that promote well-being.
   4. verbalize knowledge of how to cope with relapse.

Answer: 1
Rationale: This would be an appropriate outcome for a complementary treatment for alcoholism. The other outcomes are not directly related to the client's problem.

Cognitive level: Application
Nursing process: Planning (Outcome Identification)
NCLEX: Psychosocial Integrity
See text page: 760

8. A client tells the nurse she is supplementing her selective serotonin reuptake inhibitor with St. John's wort. The priority action the nurse should take is to
   1. inquire as to what degree the depression has lifted.
   2. advise the client of the danger of selective serotonin syndrome.
   3. suggest that adding valerian to the treatment regimen may produce even better results.
   4. remind the client of the possibility of insomnia if the drugs are taken late in the day.

Answer: 2
Rationale: Research has suggested that St. John's wort inhibits serotonin reuptake by elevating extracellular sodium; thus it may interact with medication, particularly selective serotonin reuptake inhibitors, to produce selective serotonin syndrome.

Cognitive level: Application
Nursing process: Implementation
NCLEX: Health Promotion and Maintenance
See text pages: 761-763

9. A client describes herself as a social drinker, but the nurse realizes that the client's intake is excessive. The client tells the nurse that her memory has gotten a bit "spotty" so she is taking gingko biloba. The nurse will make the assessment that the combination of gingko and alcohol may produce
   1. delirium.
   2. gastrointestinal symptoms.
   3. spontaneous bleeding.
   4. thromboembolic phenomena.

Answer: 3
Rationale: Gingko interacts with anticoagulants and antiplatelet agents and may cause spontaneous bleeding. It should be used with caution by individuals who consume alcohol or who have other risk factors for hemorrhagic stroke.

Cognitive level: Application
Nursing process: Assessment
NCLEX: Health Promotion and Maintenance
See text pages: 761-763

10. A nurse tells a peer "I think all that stuff about the effectiveness of herbal remedies is bunk." The second nurse replies "Some herbs can live up to their reputations." The first nurse replies "Name one." The best response would be "Research has shown that
    1. chamomile binds with γ-aminobutyric acid receptors to produce a calming effect."
    2. St. John's wort produces side effects similar to those of selective serotonin reuptake inhibitors."

3. kava kava acts synergistically with central nervous system stimulants to elevate mood."
4. gingko produces sedation equivalent to the benzodiazepines."

Answer: 1

Rationale: Option 1 is a true statement and accounts for chamomile's calming effects. Option 2 is true but does not address the ongoing debates over the therapeutic action of St. John's wort. Options 3 and 4 are not true statements.

Cognitive level: Application
Nursing process: Implementation
NCLEX: Health Promotion and Maintenance
See text pages: 761-763

11. A client asks the nurse "What is the major difference between allopathic therapies and complementary and alternative therapies (CAM)?" The best reply for the nurse to make is "Allopathic medicine
   1. is curative, and CAM is preventive."
   2. is symptom specific, and CAM is holistic."
   3. is preventive, and CAM treats actual health problems."
   4. has been tested by research, and CAM is scientifically untested."

Answer: 4

Rationale: Allopathic medicine is also known as conventional, mainstream, regular medicine, and biomedicine. Most allopathic therapies have the benefit of having a body of scientific research that supports their use, whereas CAM remedies are not evidence based. Option 1: This difference is not the major difference. Option 2: This difference is not entirely true. Option 3 This difference is not entirely true.

Cognitive level: Application
Nursing process: Implementation
NCLEX: Health Maintenance and Promotion
See text pages: 749-751

12. The nurse asks a client to describe what it was like going to a CAM practitioner. The client is most likely to recount "The CAM practitioner
   1. prescribed a high-cost remedy."
   2. spent a long time talking with me."
   3. was more interested in my symptoms than in me as a person."
   4. told me no standards for herbal remedies exist, so safety is in question."

Answer: 2

Rationale: CAM practitioners often spend considerable time assessing the person in a holistic way. Visits often involve lengthy discussions, in contrast to visits to traditional physicians, whose visits are short. Option 1: CAM remedies are usually low cost. Option 3: CAM practitioners are holistic in their orientation. Option 4: Although this is true, it would be unlikely for the CAM practitioner to mention this.

Cognitive level: Analysis
Nursing process: Assessment
NCLEX: Psychosocial Integrity
See text pages: 749-751

13. The nurse plans to assess a client's use of nutritional supplements. The rationale for this is to
   1. permit the nurse to review related food, drug, and supplement interactions as necessary.
   2. determine whether nutritional supplements would be advisable to supplement the diet.
   3. assist the client to develop positive lifestyle habits.
   4. assess cost effectiveness of the therapy.

Answer: 1

Rationale: Whenever the nurse obtains data that the client is using supplements, the nurse should review the use of the supplement and any related food, drug, or supplement interactions to help reduce the risk of untoward reactions. The other options are not specific rationales for the assessment.

Cognitive level: Analysis
Nursing process: Assessment
NCLEX: Health Promotion and Maintenance
See text pages: 756, 757

14. A client tells the nurse that she has had problems with kidney stones three times in the past year. As assessment data related to diet and nutritional supplements is gathered, the nurse should pose questions about use of megadoses of
   1. vitamin A.
   2. vitamin C.
   3. vitamin E.
   4. SAMe.

Answer: 2

Rationale: Large doses of vitamin C are known to cause kidney stones in some individuals. Option 1: Vitamin A megadoses produces nausea, vomiting, blurred vision, and lack of muscle coordination. Option 3: Megadoses of vitamin E may lead to hemorrhage because of its anticoagulant properties. Option 4: SAMe therapy may be helpful in relieving depression.

Cognitive level: Application
Nursing process: Assessment
NCLEX: Physiological Integrity
See text pages: 756, 757

15. A client tells the nurse "Take a look at the bruises on my arms and legs. I take a multivitamin tablet daily and no other medicine. The bruises started about a week after I began taking some nutritional supplements from the health food store." The nurse should focus assessment questions on the client's use of supplements containing
1. vitamin A.
2. vitamin B.
3. vitamin C.
4. vitamin E.

Answer: 4

Rationale: Vitamin E has anticoagulant properties. Generally, a multiple vitamin tablet contains the minimum daily requirement of each vitamin. Taking nutritional supplements containing additional vitamin E would qualify as megadosing. Megadosing has the potential for causing bruising and hemorrhage. Option 1: Vitamin A megadoses produces nausea, vomiting, blurred vision, and lack of muscle coordination. Option 2: Vitamin B megadoses do not produce anticoagulant effects. Option 3: Vitamin C megadoses may produce kidney stones.

Cognitive level: Application
Nursing process: Assessment
NCLEX: Physiological Integrity
See text pages: 756, 757

16. A client relates to the nurse "I have been trying to lose weight. I am not hungry at breakfast, so I wait until lunch to eat. I have a small lunch and then use most of my calorie allotment for dinner. Lately, I have noticed that I do not have a lot of energy. I seem to be more anxious and my mood is lower." The counsel the nurse should provide is
1. "You seem to be doing what is usually effective."
2. "Perhaps you should divide your calories evenly between lunch and dinner."
3. "Eating breakfast is important. It improves mood, energy, and feelings of calm."
4. "You might want to talk with your doctor about the use of SAMe for depression."

Answer: 3

Rationale: A 2004 research study indicates regularly eating breakfast improves energy, mood, memory, and feelings of calmness. Option 1 is inappropriate because option 3 should be tried. Option 2: No evidence exists that this would be of help. Option 4: No evidence exists that this suggestion would help the client.

Cognitive level: Application
Nursing process: Implementation
NCLEX: Physiological Integrity
See text pages: 756, 757

17. A client tells the nurse "I prefer to try to treat my physical problems with CAM remedies. After all, they are natural substances and natural products are safe." The best response for the nurse to make is
1. "Natural substances do tend to be safer than conventional medical remedies."
2. "Natural and harmless are not synonyms. Natural substances can be harmful."
3. "Most natural substances have more side effects than conventional remedies."
4. "Natural remedies give you the idea that you are controlling your treatment."

Answer: 2

Rationale: CAM remedies are natural substances, but it is a fallacy that products purchased at a health food store are safer to use than conventional medicines. Natural products contain powerful ingredients that can cause illness and damage to the body if taken inappropriately. This is the most important message for the nurse to convey to the client. Option 1 is an untrue statement. Option 3: This is not uniformly true. Option 4: Although this may be the case for some clients, the issue of controlling treatment may not be true for all clients.

Cognitive level: Analysis
Nursing process: Implementation
NCLEX: Health Promotion and Maintenance
See text pages: 756, 757

18. When a client who has immigrated from India tells the nurse that his entire family uses Ayurvedic medicine, the nurse should understand that conventional medical treatment most acceptable to the client will be that which
1. is holistic.
2. focuses on cure rather than prevention.
3. offers synthetic medication rather than natural remedies.
4. stresses group responsibility for health rather than individual responsibility.

Answer: 1

Rationale: Ayurvedic medicine, which originated in India, stresses individual responsibility for health, is holistic, promotes prevention, recognizes the uniqueness of the individual, and offers natural methods of treatment.

Cognitive level: Application
Nursing process: Planning
NCLEX: Psychosocial Integrity
See text pages: 752, 753

19. The outcome proposed by the treatment team of conventional Western medical practitioners that would have greatest meaning to a client who is to

have surgery for colon cancer who has previously been treated by traditional Chinese medicine (TCM) is: Forty-eight hours after surgery the client will
1. state that his yin and yang reflect transformation toward healing.
2. develop awakening to the need for dietary change in his life.
3. express feelings of empowerment to use Western medical remedies.
4. return to baseline functioning.

Answer: 1

Rationale: Individuals treated with TCM usually believe that the goal of healing is to be in harmony with one's environment and all of creation in mind, body, and spirit and that all healing is manifested as a simultaneous yin and yang reflection of the whole being in a state of transition. Transformation is recognized as a stage of healing occurring when mutual creative active participation occurs between healers and the client toward changes in the mind, body, and spirit. For this client, this statement would suggest a desirable outcome. Option 2 may or may not be necessary for the client. Option 3 may not be an outcome desired by the client. Option 4 is an outcome easily understood by Western practitioners but is one that may not be easily understood by the user of TCM.

Cognitive level: Analysis
Nursing process: Planning (Outcome Identification)
NCLEX: Psychosocial Integrity
See text pages: 752, 753

20. Allergy shots, which are injections with an allergen solution, makes use of the theory of
   1. naturopathy.
   2. homeopathy.
   3. chiropractic.
   4. shiatsu.

Answer: 2

Rationale: Homeopathy uses small doses of a substance to stimulate the body's defenses and healing mechanisms to treat illness. Option 1: Naturopathy emphasizes health restoration rather than disease. Option 3: Chiropractic uses manipulation of the body to restore health. Option 4: Shiatsu is a type of massage.

Cognitive level: Application
Nursing process: NA
NCLEX: Physiological Integrity
See text pages: 752, 753

21. A client tells the nurse "I want to have the type of massage that makes use of acupressure points. What sort of practitioner should I try to find?" The nurse should advise the client to seek a practitioner of

1. Swedish massage.
2. shiatsu massage.
3. rolfing.
4. reflexology.

Answer: 2

Rationale: Shiatsu massage applies pressure by massaging various parts of the body identified as acupressure points. Option 1: Swedish massage provides relaxation and increases circulation but does not focus on acupressure points. Option 3: Rolfing focuses on connective tissue fascia. Option 4: Reflexology focuses on the foot.

Cognitive level: Application
Nursing process: Implementation
NCLEX: Physiological Integrity
See text page: 754

22. A client tells the nurse she plans to apply an aromatic oil to the skin over both knees to reduce knee pain. The nurse should counsel the client to (more than one option may be correct)
   1. perform a 24-hour patch test to determine if sensitivity or allergy exist.
   2. read directions carefully to avoid damage from underuse.
   3. exercise caution to avoid inhaling fumes if she is asthmatic.
   4. avoid use of the oil near an open flame.

Answers: 1, 3, 4

Rationale: Apply a small amount of diluted oil to a patch on the forearm, keep the patch in place for 24 hours, then inspect for redness or rash. If sensitivity exists the oil should not be applied to the skin in another area of the body. Option 3: Aromatic oils can trigger respiratory problems in those with asthma, bronchitis or emphysema. Option 4: Aromatic oils are flammable. Option 2: Overuse is a greater problem.

Cognitive level: Application
Nursing process: Implementation
NCLEX: Health Promotion and Maintenance
See text page: 761

23. A nurse who is to provide health education for a client who will be receiving warfarin (Coumadin) for several weeks after knee replacement surgery should include caution to avoid the CAM remedy of
   1. black cohosh.
   2. kava kava.
   3. valerian.
   4. gingko biloba.

Answer: 4

Rationale: Gingko biloba has anticoagulant effects and can cause bleeding in individuals using anticoagulants and antiplatelet agents. Option 1: Black cohosh is a popular treatment for hot flashes. Option 2: Kava kava is considered to have analgesic properties and may potentiate the effects of alcohol and benzodiazepines. Option 3: Valerian has calming, sleep-inducing effects.

Cognitive effects: Application
Nursing process: Implementation
NCLEX: Physiological Integrity
See text pages: 761-763

24. A client reports to the nurse that last night she had difficulty falling sleep. She states she returned home from a social evening with friends, during which she consumed several alcoholic drinks. When unable to fall sleep after half an hour in bed, she brewed herself two cups of herbal tea containing valerian. In the morning she awakened with a severe headache and blurred vision. The nurse should explain that
   1. valerian should be taken before use of alcohol to avoid unpleasant side effects.
   2. the side effects are those of "hangover" from excessive alcohol use.
   3. valerian may potentiate the effects of other central nervous system depressants.
   4. herbal teas contain several active ingredients that may produce unpleasant effects.

Answer: 3
Rationale: Valerian has sedative properties. In high doses side effects include blurred vision and headache. Valerian is known to potentiate the central nervous system depressant effects of other drugs with this action. The nurse should advise caution in ingesting alcohol and valerian for these reasons. Option 1 is untrue. Option 2 is not entirely correct. Option 4 is not relevant to this situation.

Cognitive level: Analysis
Nursing process: Implementation
NCLEX: Health Maintenance and Promotion
See text pages: 761-763